Medical Management of Chronic Myelogenous Leukemia

BASIC AND CLINICAL ONCOLOGY

Editor

Bruce D. Cheson, M.D.

*National Cancer Institute
National Institutes of Health
Bethesda, Maryland*

1. Chronic Lymphocytic Leukemia: Scientific Advances and Clinical Developments, *edited by Bruce D. Cheson*
2. Therapeutic Applications of Interleukin-2, *edited by Michael B. Atkins and James W. Mier*
3. Cancer of the Prostate, *edited by Sakti Das and E. David Crawford*
4. Retinoids in Oncology, *edited by Waun Ki Hong and Reuben Lotan*
5. Filgrastim (r-metHuG-CSF) in Clinical Practice, *edited by George Morstyn and T. Michael Dexter*
6. Cancer Prevention and Control, *edited by Peter Greenwald, Barnett S. Kramer, and Douglas L. Weed*
7. Handbook of Supportive Care in Cancer, *edited by Jean Klastersky, Stephen C. Schimpff, and Hans-Jörg Senn*
8. Paclitaxel in Cancer Treatment, *edited by William P. McGuire and Eric K. Rowinsky*
9. Principles of Antineoplastic Drug Development and Pharmacology, *edited by Richard L. Schilsky, Gérard A. Milano, and Mark J. Ratain*
10. Gene Therapy in Cancer, *edited by Malcolm K. Brenner and Robert C. Moen*
11. Expert Consultations in Gynecological Cancers, *edited by Maurie Markman and Jerome L. Belinson*
12. Nucleoside Analogs in Cancer Therapy, *edited by Bruce D. Cheson, Michael J. Keating, and William Plunkett*
13. Drug Resistance in Oncology, *edited by Samuel D. Bernal*
14. Medical Management of Hematological Malignant Diseases, *edited by Emil J Freireich and Hagop M. Kantarjian*
15. Monoclonal Antibody-Based Therapy of Cancer, *edited by Michael L. Grossbard*
16. Medical Management of Chronic Myelogenous Leukemia, *edited by Moshe Talpaz and Hagop M. Kantarjian*

ADDITIONAL VOLUMES IN PREPARATION

Cancer Screening: Theory and Practice, *edited by Barnett S. Kramer, John K. Gohagan, and Philip C. Prorok*

Expert Consultations in Breast Cancer: Critical Pathways and Clinical Decision Making, *edited by William N. Hait, David A. August, and Bruce Haffty*

Medical Management of Chronic Myelogenous Leukemia

edited by

Moshe Talpaz
Hagop M. Kantarjian

*University of Texas M.D. Anderson Cancer Center
Houston, Texas*

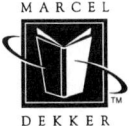

MARCEL DEKKER, INC.   NEW YORK · BASEL · HONG KONG

Library of Congress Cataloging-in-Publication Data

Medical management of chronic myelogenous leukemia / edited by Moshe Talpaz, Hagop M. Kantarjian.
p. cm. — (Basic and clinical oncology; 16)
Includes bibliographical references and index.
ISBN 0-8247-9901-1 (alk. paper).
1. Myelocytic leukemia—treatment. I. Talpaz, Moshe. II. Kantarjian, Hagop. III. Series.
[DNLM: 1. Leukemia, Myeloid, Chronic—therapy. W1BA813W v. 16 1998]
RC643.M434 1998
616.99'419—dc21
DNLM/DLC
for Library of Congress 98-38123
CIP

This book is printed on acid-free paper.

Headquarters
Marcel Dekker, Inc.
270 Madison Avenue, New York, NY 10016
tel: 212-696-9000; fax: 212-685-4540

Eastern Hemisphere Distribution
Marcel Dekker AG
Hutgasse 4, Postfach 812, CH-4001 Basel, Switzerland
tel: 44-61-261-8482; fax: 44-61-261-8896

World Wide Web
http://www.dekker.com

The publisher offers discounts on this book when ordered in bulk quantities. For more information, write to Special Sales/Professional Marketing at the headquarters address above.

Copyright © 1999 by Marcel Dekker, Inc. All Rights Reserved.

Neither this book nor any part may be reproduced or transmitted in any form or by any means, electronic or mechanical, including photocopying, microfilming, and recording, or by any information storage and retrieval system, without permission in writing from the publisher.

Current printing (last digit)
10 9 8 7 6 5 4 3 2 1

PRINTED IN THE UNITED STATES OF AMERICA

Preface

Historically, the therapeutic objective in CML was the normalization of blood counts with the basic understanding that this action will have little impact on the predictable fatal outcome of the disease. With the development of allogeneic bone marrow transplant came the notion that the disease is a potential target for curative therapy. This effect was, however, confined to only a fraction of the patients. Interferon alpha (IFN-α) was initially given to CML patients in the early 1980s and gradually became the foundation for nontransplant treatment of the disease. This is based on its ability to obtain survival prolongation in most of the patients and a complete sustained remission in a fraction of the patients. Our current therapeutic issues include the formation of therapeutic algorithms that will enable adequate incorporation of the two aforementioned therapeutic modalities and improvement of the existing therapies by developing combination therapies (IFN-α combined with Ara-C) or new allo-transplantation strategies, such as matched unrelated donor (MUD) transplantation.

This book summarizes new developments in the therapy of CML. Because the major therapies (IFN and bone marrow transplantation) are discussed in more than one chapter, the reader will be subjected to different points of view as to the significance of each therapy and its priority in the global therapeutic schema of CML.

CML has also been the subject of an intense effort to decipher its underlying molecular defect. The knowledge accumulated has provided the basis for the current approaches in investigational therapies. These rational approaches toward the treatment of CML, which include antisense oligonucleotides to bcr-abl and C-Myb transcripts, bcr-abl kinase inhibitors, and bcr-abl–based immunotherapy, are discussed in this book and provide the link to future therapies of this disease.

In addition to the extensive coverage of therapies for CML, this book also provides information on the rapidly evolving disease-monitoring molecular techniques such as fluorescent in situ hybridization (FISH), polymerase chain reaction (PCR) amplification of the bcr-abl gene product, and the bcr Southern blot assay. The value of these methods for disease monitoring and their possible advantages over the commonly used cytogenetic assays are discussed as well.

Special attention is given to two uncommon leukemias [e.g., chronic myelomonocytic leukemia (CMML) and Philadelphia-negative CML (CML Ph–)]. There is insufficient information on the course and therapy of both of these conditions. In this book we made an attempt to address this deficiency.

This book is directed to hematologists, clinical investigators, and oncologists who treat myeloproliferative disorders, and we hope that they will find it a timely and useful addition to the available literature on CML.

Moshe Talpaz
Hagop M. Kantarjian

Contents

Preface	*iii*
Contributors	*ix*

CML Introduction

1. Chronic Myelogenous Leukemia—A Brief Review   1
   Hagop M. Kantarjian and Moshe Talpaz

2. Chronic Myelomonocytic Leukemia   43
   John F. Seymour and Jorge E. Cortes

3. Animal Models of Chronic Myelogenous Leukemia   77
   Richard A. Van Etten

4. Natural History and Prognostic Factors in Chronic Myelogenous Leukemia: Past, Present, and Future   103
   Sergio Giralt

Chemotherapy and Interferons

5. Changing Nature of Conventional Therapy in Chronic Myelogenous Leukemia   113
   Rüdiger Hehlmann and Andreas Hochhaus

6. Interferon Therapy: Is It the Standard of Care?   141
   Sante Tura and Michele Baccarani

7. Practical Management of Interferon Therapy and Side Effects 161
   Susan O'Brien, Hagop M. Kantarjian, and Moshe Talpaz

8. Treatment of Chronic Myelogenous Leukemia by Interferon
   and Cytarabine 173
   François Guilhot

9. Chronic Myeloid Leukemia: Australian Experience with Interferon
   Combinations and High-Dose Interferon 185
   Christopher K. Arthur

Bone Marrow Transplantation

10. Allografting for Chronic Myelogenous Leukemia 215
    David G. Savage and John Michael Goldman

11. Treatment Algorithm in CML: Bone Marrow Transplantation as
    Frontline Therapy 259
    Reginald A. Clift

12. Autologous Stem Cell Transplantation for Chronic Myeloid
    Leukemia 273
    *Josy Reiffers, F. X. Mahon, J. M. Boiron, H. Chahine, C. Faberes,
    T. Cousin, P. Cony-Makhoul, A. Pigneux, A. Agape, A. Broustet,
    and G. Marit*

13. Philadelphia Chromosome-Negative Chronic Myelogenous
    Leukemia 285
    Jorge E. Cortes and John F. Seymour

Monitoring Therapy and Minimal Residual Disease

14. Monitoring Changes in the Breakpoint Cluster Region During
    Therapy for CML: The M.D. Anderson Cancer Center Experience 303
    Claire F. Verschraegen

15. Monitoring the Course of Chronic Myelogenous Leukemia by
    Fluorescence In Situ Hybridization 317
    *Chu-Myong Seong, Hagop M. Kantarjian, Moshe Talpaz, Richard
    Champlin, and Michael Siciliano*

Contents

16. Molecular Monitoring of CML During Interferon Treatment: Insights from the Cancer and Leukemia Group B Experience   327
    Wendy Stock

Developmental Therapies

17. Oligonucleotide Therapeutics for Chronic Myelogenous Leukemia   341
    Alan M. Gewirtz

18. Role of Cytokines and Adhesion Molecules in Chronic Myelogenous Leukemia   363
    Luis Fayad and Zeev Estrov

19. ABL Protein Tyrosine Kinase Inhibitors: Potential Clinical Role in CML   395
    Brian J. Druker

20. Immunotherapy of Chronic Myelogenous Leukemia   413
    David A. Scheinberg, Monica Bocchia, and Richard O'Reilly

Index   *429*

Contributors

A. Agape Université Victor Segalen, Bordeaux 2, Bordeaux, France

Christopher K. Arthur, M.B., B.S., F.R.A.C.P., F.R.C.P.A. Haematology and Transfusion Medicine Department, Royal North Shore Hospital, Sydney, Australia

Michele Baccarani, M.D. Professor, Department of Hematology and Bone Marrow Transplantation, Udine University, Udine, Italy

Monica Bocchia, M.D. Memorial Sloan-Kettering Cancer Center, New York, New York

J. M. Boiron Université Victor Segalen, Bordeaux 2, Bordeaux, France

A. Broustet Université Victor Segalen, Bordeaux 2, Bordeaux, France

H. Chahine Université Victor Segalen, Bordeaux 2, Bordeaux, France

Richard Champlin Professor and Chairman (ad interim), Department of Bone Marrow Transplantation, Department of Hematology, M. D. Anderson Cancer Center, Houston, Texas

Reginald A. Clift Senior Staff Scientist, Clinical Research Division, Fred Hutchinson Cancer Research Center, Seattle, Washington

P. Cony-Makhoul Université Victor Segalen, Bordeaux 2, Bordeaux, France

Jorge E. Cortes, M.D. Assistant Professor, Leukemia Department, M.D. Anderson Cancer Center, Houston, Texas

T. Cousin Université Victor Segalen, Bordeaux 2, Bordeaux, France

Brian J. Druker, M.D. Associate Professor, Division of Hematology and Medical Oncology, Oregon Health Sciences University, Portland, Oregon

Zeev Estrov, M.D. Associate Professor, Department of Bioimmunotherapy, M.D. Anderson Cancer Center, Houston, Texas

C. Faberes Université Victor Segalen, Bordeaux 2, Bordeaux, France

Luis Fayad, M.D. Department of Bioimmunotherapy, M.D. Anderson Cancer Center, Houston, Texas

Alan M. Gewirtz, M.D. Professor, Department of Pathology and Laboratory Medicine and Internal Medicine, University of Pennsylvania, Philadelphia, Pennsylvania

Sergio Giralt, M.D. Assistant Professor, Section of Blood and Bone Marrow Transplantation, M.D. Anderson Cancer Center, Houston, Texas

John Michael Goldman, D.M., F.R.C.P., F.R.C.Path. Professor, Department of Haematology, Imperial College School of Medicine, Hammersmith Hospital, London, England

François Guilhot, M.D. Department of Hematology and Medical Oncology, Centre Hospitalier Universitaire de Poitiers, Poitiers, France

Rüdiger Hehlmann, M.D. Professor, Medizinische Klinik, Klinikum Mannheim, University of Heidelberg, Mannheim, Germany

Andreas Hochhaus, M.D. III. Medizinische Klinik, Klinikum Mannheim, University of Heidelberg, Mannheim, Germany

Hagop M. Kantarjian, M.D. Professor and Chairman (ad interim), Leukemia Department, M.D. Anderson Cancer Center, Houston, Texas

G. Marit Université Victor Segalen, Bordeaux 2, Bordeaux, France

F. X. Mahon Université Victor Segalen, Bordeaux 2, Bordeaux, France

Susan O'Brien, M.D. Associate Professor of Medicine, Associate Director of Hematology Center, Leukemia Department, M.D. Anderson Cancer Center, Houston, Texas

Contributors

Richard O'Reilly, M.D. Memorial Sloan-Kettering Cancer Center, New York, New York

A. Pigneux Université Victor Segalen, Bordeaux 2, Bordeaux, France

Josy Reiffers, M.D. Professor, Department of Hematology, Université Victor Segalen, Bordeaux 2, Bordeaux, France

David G. Savage, M.D. Associate Professor, Hematology/Oncology Division, College of Physicians & Surgeons, Columbia University, New York, New York

David A. Scheinberg, M.D., Ph.D. Chief, Leukemia Service, Department of Medicine, Memorial Sloan-Kettering Cancer Center, New York, New York

Chu-Myong Seong Ewha Woman's University, Seoul, Korea, and Section of Pheresis, Department of Hematology, M.D. Anderson Cancer Center, Houston, Texas

John F. Seymour, M.B., B.S., F.R.A.C.P. Medical Oncologist, Department of Clinical Hematology and Medical Oncology, Royal Melbourne Hospital, Parkville, Australia

Michael Siciliano Professor, Department of Molecular Genetics, M.D. Anderson Cancer Center, Houston, Texas

Wendy Stock Loyola University Medical Center, Maywood, Illinois

Moshe Talpaz, M.D. Professor and Chairman (ad interim), Department of Bioimmunotherapy and Professor of Medicine, M.D. Anderson Cancer Center, Houston, Texas

Sante Tura, M.D. Professor of Hematology, Institute of Hematology and Medical Oncology, University of Bologna, Bologna, Italy

Richard A. Van Etten, M.D., Ph.D. Associate Professor, Center for Blood Research, Department of Genetics, Harvard Medical School, Boston, Massachusetts

Claire F. Verschraegen, M.D. Assistant Professor, Department of Clinical Investigation, M.D. Anderson Cancer Center, Houston, Texas

Medical Management of Chronic Myelogenous Leukemia

1
Chronic Myelogenous Leukemia— A Brief Review

Hagop M. Kantarjian and Moshe Talpaz
M.D. Anderson Cancer Center, Houston, Texas

INTRODUCTION

The prognosis of patients with chronic myelogenous leukemia (CML) has changed markedly since 1856, when the use of arsenical (Fowlers solution) was first advocated. In the early 1900s, systemic or splenic irradiation therapy was shown to be effective in controlling CML and became the standard of care for the next 50 years (1). In the 1950s, oral alkylating agents were found to be more effective than radiation therapy, and busulfan became the mainstay of treatment (2). In the 1970s, hydroxyurea became more favored because of its manageable marrow suppression and lack of pulmonary and other organ toxicities (3). In the 1980s, interferon-alpha (IFN-α) was studied in CML (4), and IFN-α-containing regimens have recently become first-line therapy for the majority of CML patients. Younger patients with matched sibling donors benefit from allogeneic stem cell transplantation (SCT) as first-line therapy instead of IFN-α-containing regimens (5). Over the past few years, several important studied related to the biology and the treatment of Philadelphia chromosome (Ph)-positive CML have matured. These include single- and multi-institutional programs with allogeneic SCT, IFN-α, autologous SCT, and other investigational agents or modalities (5). These investigations have answered some questions, but raised new ones. In this review, we will discuss (1) CML biology, natural history, and prognostic features; (2) standard therapy with IFN-α regimens and allogeneic SCT; (3) the value of additional investigational agents and modalities; and (4) specific treatment and ancillary parameters in CML management.

NATURAL HISTORY AND PROGNOSTIC FEATURES

CML accounts for 7% to 15% of adult leukemias. The median age at presentation is 50 to 60 years. In earlier reports, 50% to 65% of patients were 60 years or older, but this incidence had decreased in recent reports to below 20%, a consequence of earlier detection, referral of young patients to large centers, or the exclusion of patients with CML-like disorders prevalent in older populations such as myeloproliferative disorders, Ph-negative CML, and chronic myelomonocytic leukemia (CMML) (6,7).

The etiology of CML is unknown. There is little evidence for genetic factors linked to CML, and no correlation in monozygotic twins, suggesting that CML is acquired. There may be some correlation with HLA antigens CW3 and CW4 (8), and with exposure to irradiation, either accidental (9) or therapeutic (10). Chemicals have not been associated with increased risk of CML. A recent intriguing study reported the detection of the Ph-related molecular abnormality by polymerase chain reaction (PCR for BCR-ABL) using a modified technology to detect one abnormal cell in 10^8 cells: 22 of 73 (30%) samples from normal adults were PCR-positive compared to only 1 of 44 (2%) samples from infant or cord blood. This suggested that abnormal clones may occur in adults at very low levels, but become clinically important in only 1 of 20,000 such occurrences in susceptible individuals (11).

Definitions of CML Phases

Precise definitions of CML phases and of prognostic groups is important in the analysis of therapeutic results (12). CML has a biphasic or triphasic course: it usually presents in an indolent or chronic phase and evolves into an accelerated phase that may last for <1 to 1.5 years, and then a blastic phase which results in the patient's death within 3 to 6 months. Twenty percent to 25% of patients die in accelerated phase while another 20% to 25% progress directly from chronic to blastic phase without a discernible intermediate accelerated phase. Standard definitions of the accelerated and blastic phases of CML have been proposed (Table 1) (12–14).

Prognostic Factors and Risk Groups

Prognostic systems have allowed the categorization of patients with CML into good-, intermediate-, and poor-risk groups (Table 2) with respective median survivals of 6, 3–4, and 2 years in patients receiving conventional therapy (15–18). Some models have been applied to IFN-α-treated populations (19–22). Recent studies in CML show an increase in the percentage of good-prognosis patients (Table 2) but also an improved prognosis in each risk group. The median

Table 1 Definitions of Accelerated and Blastic Phases of CML

A. Blastic phase CML
   30% or more blasts in the marrow or peripheral blood
   Extramedullary disease with localized immature blasts
B. Accelerated phase CML
   1. Multivariate analysis-derived criteria
      Peripheral blasts 15% or more
      Peripheral blasts plus promyelocytes 30% or more
      Peripheral basophils 20% or more
      Thrombocytopenia <100 × 10^9/L unrelated to therapy
      Cytogenetic clonal evolution
   2. Other commonly used criteria
      Increasing drug dosage requirement
      Splenomegaly unresponsive to therapy
      Marrow reticulin or collagen fibrosis
      Marrow or peripheral blasts ≥10%
      Marrow or peripheral basophils ± eosinophils 10% or greater
      Triad of WBC >50 × 10^9/L, hematocrit <25% and platelets <100 × 10^9/L not controlled with therapy
      Persistent unexplained fever or bone pains

survivals in the good-, intermediate-, and poor-risk groups are 9, 7.5, and 4–5 years, respectively (Table 3). Good-risk patients now account for 45% to 50% of CML cohorts, reflecting earlier diagnosis and screening tests. Improved survival in modern CML studies should be analyzed in the context of the change of risk group distribution, and within risk groups. IFN-α therapy has not been associated with a change in the significance of prognostic factors derived from conventional chemotherapy studies (Table 2) (20). In multivariate analyses, the percent of blasts and thrombocytoses have correlated with response to IFN-α therapy; splenomegaly, marrow basophilia, anemia, and percent of blasts have been associated with survival (20–24). Patients with good-risk CML treated with IFN-α have an expected major cytogenetic response rate of about 50% and an expected median survival of >8 years, while patients with poor-risk CML have an expected major cytogenetic response rate of 14% to 26%, and an expected median survival of 4–5 years (20).

The in vivo response to IFN-α is the dominant treatment-associated prognostic factor. Achieving a complete hematologic remission (CHR) at 3 to 8 months, a cytogenetic response at 12 months, or a major cytogenetic response at 24 months is associated with a significant survival prolongation (23–26). Combining pretreatment features with response to IFN-α may allow early risk-oriented treatment modification (27). Patients who do not achieve a CHR after 6–8 months, or a cytogenetic response after 12 months of IFN-α therapy, may

Table 2 Poor Prognostic Factors in Ph-Positive CML

A. Individual poor prognostic factors

Clinical	Hematologic	Marrow
older age	anemia	increased blasts or basophils
symptoms at diagnosis	thrombocytopenia/cytosis	megakaryocytopenia
splenomegaly	leukocytosis	cytogenetic clonal evolution
hepatomegaly	increased blasts or basophils	collagen or reticulin fibrosis grade 3–4
significant weight loss		
poor performance		
black race		

Other
  hypoalbuminemia
  extramedullary disease

B. Synthesis staging model

CML phase	Clinical characteristics	Stage	Definition
chronic	age ≥60 years	1	0 or 1 characteristics
	spleen ≥10 cm below costal margin		
	blasts ≥3% in blood or ≥5% in marrow	2	2 characteristics
	basophils >7% in blood or ≥3% in marrow		
	platelets ≥700 × 10^9/L	3	≥3 characteristics
accelerated	cytogenetic clonal evolution	4	≥1 characteristic defines accelerated phase (regardless of characteristics for chronic phase)
	blasts ≥15% in blood		
	blasts + promyelocytes ≥30% in blood		
	basophils ≥20% in blood		
	platelets <100 × 10^9/L		

Table 3 Median Survival (in Months) in CML by Modality and Risk Group

Risk group	Before IFN-α therapy	IFN-α programs
Good	53	102–104
Intermediate	39	82–95
Poor	25	47–62

Source: Refs. 5, 20.

be taken off IFN-α and offered allogeneic SCT or other options if the aim of IFN-α therapy is the achievement of durable cytogenetic response. The Medical Research Council (MRC) trial suggested that continued IFN-α therapy may still be appropriate for patients who do not have an allogeneic SCT option, even if cytogenetic remission is not achieved (26). However, in most trials, achieving a minimal disease burden (CHR, cytogenetic response) has been associated with survival prolongation independently (discussed later).

CML BIOLOGY AND PATHOPHYSIOLOGY
Philadelphia (Ph) Chromosome

The presence of a chromosomal marker, the Ph abnormality, is found in >90% of patients with a morphologic diagnosis of CML (28). Quantitative analysis of Ph or Ph-related molecular abnormalities have become a major surrogate marker for therapeutic success in CML (28–37). The Ph chromosome is a shortened chromosome 22 (22q-) from a reciprocal translocation t(9;22),(q34;q11), which transposes the *c-sis* proto-oncogene from chromosome 22 to chromosome 9 and the cellular Abelson (*c-abl*) proto-oncogene from chromosome 9 to chromosome 22, close to the breakpoint cluster region gene (*bcr*) (38–40). The latter hybrid *bcr-abl* oncogene produces an abnormal 8.5 kb RNA (41) which encodes for a 210 kD (P210) fusion protein. This protein exhibits tyrosine kinase activity and shows considerable homology to the catalytic subunit of 3′,5′-cAMP (42).

Ph-positive CML patients and 20% to 25% of Ph-positive acute lymphoblastic leukemia (ALL) and acute myelogenous leukemia (AML) have breakpoints on chromosome 22 which cluster in a 5.8-kb region, termed the major BCR (M-bcr). The breakpoints within M-bcr have been assigned to 3′ or 5′ locations. Depending on whether the hybrid oncogene involves exon 3 or exon 2 of the M-bcr and exon 2 of *abl*, two distinct RNA messages are produced: b3a2 or b2a2. While the 3′ *bcr* breakpoints often result in b3a2 and 5′ breakpoints in b2a2 messages, some patients with 5′ breakpoints produce b3a2 message. The hybrid b3a2 mRNA and the protein for which it codes differ in size by 75 bases and 25 amino acids, respectively, from b2a2 and its product. This spectrum of abnormalities at the DNA and RNA levels have been variably associated with different disease features (e.g., thrombocytosis), but not with conclusive evidence of different prognoses (43,44). In Ph-negative patients with a clinical diagnosis of CML, Southern blot analysis for *bcr* rearrangement will identify Ph-negative, BCR-positive CML in 30% to 50% of patients. They have similar response to IFN-α therapy and similar prognosis as Ph-positive CML; the remaining ones with Ph-negative, BCR-negative CML have a worse prognosis (6,7,45).

Pathophysiology

The mechanisms conferring the growth advantage of CML over normal hematopoietic cells are unknown. A reduced stroma-CML hematopoietic cell interaction, attributed to abnormalities in the patterns of adherence of CML cells to the stromal matrix (46,47), may abrogate normal maturation of cell surface moieties (cytoadhesion molecules HLA-DR), required for a normal proliferation-maturation sequence. IFN-α in vitro reverses adhesion abnormalities (48,49). Discordant nuclear : cytoplasmic maturation in CML may also confer a CML growth advantage (50). A causal association between the Ph chromosome and the initiation and perpetuation of CML has been established in a number of models (51,52). In one study, c-DNA encoding for P210 was introduced into mouse marrow cells, which were reinfused into lethally irradiated mice (51). After 2 to 8 weeks, some mice developed CML-like disorders, including leukocytosis, splenomegaly, monocyte/macrophage extramedullary tumors, and ALL. This spectrum of disorders, recapitulating the pathogenesis of human CML-like disease, suggests that BCR-ABL may be sufficient not only for development of chronic phase CML, but also for its transformation into blastic phase disease, and lends support to strategies aimed at suppressing the Ph-positive clones, as a means to improve prognosis in CML. Additional mechanisms proposed for CML growth advantage and evolution have involved failure of programmed cell death, as well as RAS-mutation pathways involving CRKL, GRB-2, MYB, and other abnormalities (53–56).

Ph-Positive Disorders

About 20% of adults and 5% of children with ALL have Ph-positive blasts with Ph-positive blasts. Children with Ph-positive ALL are older than Ph-negative ALL patients (median 8 years), and have a higher median white cell count (WBC), more frequent L2 blast morphology, and pre-B CALLA-positive disease. Their prognosis is poor. Fifty percent to 80% of patients have a breakpoint within the m-bcr region, proximal to the M-bcr region, which results in a 7.5-kb mRNA encoding for a 190-kD (P190) protein. In contrast to P190 acute leukemia, a second chronic-phase disease may follow induction therapy in some patients with P210 Ph-positive acute leukemia. However, the clinical features and prognoses are similar in P210 and P190 acute leukemias (57).

About 10% of "CML" patients lack the Ph abnormality by cytogenetic studies. These patients are usually older, have less frequent leukocytosis basophilia and thrombocytosis, and have more frequent monocytosis and thrombocytopenia. They respond poorly to therapy, and have a shorter survival time than Ph-positive CML. In 35% of Ph-negative CML patients, the BCR-ABL rearrangement is detectable: these Ph-negative, BCR-ABL-positive patients have a clinical course and prognosis similar Ph-positive CML. G6PD isozyme studies indicate that Ph-negative, BCR-ABL-negative "CML" cells are clonal, originating in a neoplastic multipotential stem cell. These patients usually have myeloproliferative disorders other than CML, often clonal myelodysplastic syndromes, most commonly CMML or refractory anemia with excess blasts.

True Ph-negative, BCR-ABL-negative CML patients may have a lower propensity for blastic transformation than BCR-ABL positive patients and an intermediate prognosis between CMML and BCR-ABL-positive CML (6,7). Some patients with "neutrophilic" or "thrombocythemia" CML have been found to have a c3a2 BCR-ABL junction. Too few patients have been described to have a precise picture of its incidence and implications (58).

CML in children may either be a Ph-positive disorder like adult Ph-positive CML or occur as juvenile form of Ph-negative CML (59). The peak age incidence in juvenile is at 1–2 years. No consistent associated cytogenetic abnormalities occur. Juvenile CML patients respond poorly to cytotoxic therapy. Prognosis is poor, with a median survival from time of diagnosis <1 year. Some patients with juvenile CML respond to retinoids. Occasionally, Ph-positive CML may present only with thrombocytosis; hence cytogenetic and molecular studies in patients with thrombocytosis (or essential thrombocytosis) are required to diagnose and treat appropriately the occasional patient with "masked" Ph-positive CML disease.

ESSENTIAL CLINICAL AND LABORATORY FEATURES

Chronic phase CML is often asymptomatic. Asymptomatic presentation has increased over the last decade from 15% to 45% (12). Symptoms usually include fatigue, anorexia, weight loss, sweating, left upper quadrant discomfort, and early satiety because of splenomegaly. Splenomegaly was documented in 70% of patients in older reports but has decreased to 50% in recent studies (Table 4). Hepatomegaly is less common (10% to 40% of patients). Lymphadenopathy is uncommon in chronic phase CML, and its appearance suggests accelerated or blastic phase disease (13,14). Rare manifestations of severe leukocytosis and thrombocytosis may include hyperviscosity, priapism, headaches, dizziness, mental changes, neuropathies, digital gangrene, organ failures (respiratory, cardiac, renal), tinnitus, stupor, visual changes, retinal hemorrhages, cerebrovascular accidents, marrow necrosis, and diabetes insipidus (60). Some patients have wide cyclic variations in the WBC count of up to an order of magnitude in 50- to 70-days cycles (61). This can be mistaken as disease resistant to IFN-α therapy; it may require continuation or resumption of hydroxyurea in the first 3-6 months of IFN-α therapy. Extremes of thrombocytosis ($>10^6/\mu L$), basophilia ($\geq 20\%$), or thrombocytopenia ($<10^5/\mu L$), and cytogenetic clonal evolution are

Table 4 Presenting Features and Risk Groups in Early Chronic Phase Ph-Positive CML by Year of Referral

Characteristic	Category	Percentage	
		Before 1983	Since 1983
Age (years)	≥60	16	13
Asymptomatic*	Yes	18	37
Hepatomegaly*	Yes	45	13
Splenomegaly*	Yes	74	50
Hemoglobin (g/dL)*	<12	58	45
WBC count (10^9/L)*	≥100	68	53
Platelet ($\times 10^9$/L)**	>700	24	18
Peripheral blasts*	Yes	63	52
Peripheral basophils (%)	≥7	14	13
Marrow blasts (%)*	≥5	12	7
Marrow basophils (%)**	≥3	35	29
Prognostic risk group*	Good	35	41
	Intermediate	44	47
	Poor	21	12

*$p < 0.01$.
**$0.05 < p < 0.01$.

unusual in chronic phase and may indicate disease resistance to IFN-α therapy or acceleration. Fibrosis may be evident at diagnosis and increases with disease progression. About 30% of CML patients have focal or diffuse increases in marrow reticulin fibers (reticulin fibrosis) at presentation, which may suggest worse prognosis (62). Fibroblasts are not derived from the leukemia clone but represent a secondary reaction to leukemic infiltration. About 20% of patients in older series developed extensive marrow collagen fibrosis and died of complications of marrow fibrosis or failure. This is now a rare occurrence of CML evolution in recent series, and may be due to lesser use of busulfan or the effect of IFN-α in preventing the progressive fibrosis (63).

The accelerated phase is based on peripheral blood and/or bone marrow findings (Table 1). Blastic phase is often symptomatic with weight loss, fever, night sweats, and bone pains. Anemia, infectious complications, and bleeding are common. Subcutaneous nodules, hemorrhagic tender skin lesions, and lymphadenopathy are more common in blastic phase, and central nervous system (CNS) leukemia may occur particularly with lymphoid blastic transformation (30% cumulative incidence of CNS leukemia). Tissue infiltration can occur in blastic phase, often in lymph nodes, skin, subcutaneous tissues, and bone (13). Disseminated intravascular coagulation may be seen in blastic phase.

Blastic phase CML resembles acute leukemia (13). Its diagnosis requires the presence of at least 30% of blasts in the bone marrow or peripheral blood, or extramedullary deposits of leukemia. Patients in blastic phase usually die within 3 to 6 months. Approximately 50% of patients have a myeloid blastic phase, 25% lymphoid, and 25% undifferentiated. Patients with lymphoid blastic phase often have CALLA-positive, myeloid marker-positive disease and respond to ALL therapy (CR rate 50% to 60%); their median survival is better than myeloid or undifferentiated cases (9 months versus 3 months) (64).

A cytogenetic clonal evolution has been considered a criterion for acceleration. A recent analysis suggests that its prognostic effect depends on the specific abnormality, its predominance in marrow metaphases, and the time of appearance (65). Patients with chromosome 17 abnormalities, ≥25% abnormal metaphases, clonal evolution >25 months after diagnosis, and no prior therapy with IFN-α have the worst outcome. The median survival for patients with none of these features is 51 months, compared to 24, 14, and 7 months when one, two, three, or four features are present. Clonal evolution may be suppressed with IFN-α therapy (66).

THERAPY OF CML

Previously Accepted Conventional and Other Chemotherapies

Busulfan allows long periods of hematologic control and is inexpensive. A Medical Research Council (MRC) randomized controlled trial established the superiority of busulfan therapy over irradiation. Subsequent comparisons with dibromomannitol, chlorambucil, 6-mercaptopurine, 6-thioguanine, cyclophosphamide, and melphalan documented the superiority or equivalence of busulfan to these agents. Busulfan can cause unpredictable severe myelosuppression, which may be fatal, and delayed as well as severe idiosyncratic pulmonary reaction, interstitial fibrosis (busulfan lung), marrow fibrosis, endocardial fibrosis, skin pigmentation, disorders of menstruation and infertility, Addison's-like disease, cataract, sicca syndrome, and myasthenia gravis. The dose of busulfan is usually 0.1 mg/kg daily until the WBC is reduced by 50% for each halving of the WBC count, discontinued when the WBC is 20×10^9/L, and restarted when it is $>50 \times 10^9$/L.

Hydroxyurea, a cycle-specific inhibitor of DNA synthesis, has a better toxicity profile than busulfan. It produces rapid but more transient control of hematologic manifestations, and requires more frequent follow-ups. It is usually given at a dose of 40 mg/kg daily, and reduced by 50% with each halving of the WBC count. Recent studies have followed the leads of IFN-α therapy and adjusted the individual hydroxyurea dose to keep the WBC at $2-5 \times 10^9$/L with the platelets $>60 \times 10^9$/L. One study used higher doses of hydroxyurea, 2 g/m^2/day, until the absolute neutrophil count reached $<1 \times 10^9$/L (67). Patients achieving a cytogenetic response were given additional cycles until maximal response. Fourteen of 25 cycles administered to 14 patients in chronic phase resulted in ≥25% Ph-negative cells, and one complete cytogenetic response was achieved, but responses were transient. Hydroxyurea is well tolerated and has few side effect, including nausea, anorexia, skin rashes, and occasionally ulcers in the mucous membranes and skin. Hydroxyurea may cause marked red cell macrocytosis and megaloblastic changes in the marrow.

Both agents can control the hematologic manifestations of CML in more than 80% of patients. In a recent randomized study (67), 458 patients were received hydroxyurea or busulfan therapy in early chronic phase. The 232 patients randomized to hydroxyurea therapy had a significantly longer median survival (56 versus 44 months, $p = 0.01$) than the 226 patients who received busulfan, and the survival advantage was evident in all prognostic subgroups. The median duration of chronic phase in the hydroxyurea cohort was significantly longer (47 versus 37 months; $p = 0.04$). There were no serious hydroxyurea-related adverse events, in contrast to serious adverse events including prolonged marrow aplasia or pulmonary toxicity in 6% of patients receiving busulfan. Neither agent as routinely used produces significant or durable cytogenetic remissions. Exposure to busulfan prior to allogeneic SCT affects patient outcome adversely (69). Based on these studies, hydroxyurea is now preferred over busulfan, except in patients who are not candidates for SCT and who do not wish to have frequent follow-ups, or who have hydroxyurea related toxicities.

In two reports, low-dose ara-C as single-agent therapy induced cytogenetic responses in seven of nine patients treated in chronic phase (70,71). Agents like 6-mercaptopurine, melphalan, 6-thioguanine, dibromomannitol, and thioTEPA have been used infrequently, either alone or in combination. None have obvious advantages over hydroxyurea but could be used as alternatives in hydroxyurea-intolerant patients. ThioTEPA may effectively control thrombocytosis resistant to other modalities, as do IFN-α and anagrelide.

Allogeneic Stem Cell Transplantation

Summary of Allogeneic SCT Results

The International and European Bone Marrow Transplantation Registries (IB-MTR and EBMT) have reported event free survival (EFS) rates of 40% to 45% (72,73). These rates are less encouraging than the initial reports, but several points should be considered.

1. Registries include smaller transplant programs, in which patient outcome may be worse than in larger institutions with extensive transplant experi-

Table 5 Allogeneic SCT in Chronic-Phase CML

Study (reference)	No. of patients	EFS % (at x year)
IBMTR (72)	1426	45% (5)
EBMT (73)	1082	39% (5)
Goldman; IBMTR (69)	450	No busulfan, 61% (3)
		Prior busulfan, 45% (3)
Biggs (79)	62	58% (3)
Clift (85)	69	CY-TBI, 66% (3)
	73	BU-CY, 70% (3)
Synder (78)	94	64% (5)

ence (74); on the other hand, possible selective favorable data registration may also occur.

2. When the IBMTR analyzed only patients transplanted with non-T-cell-depleted marrow in chronic-phase CML, the 5-year EFS was about 50% (69).

3. EFS and survival after allogeneic SCT are not similar. Many patients who relapse in chronic-phase postallogeneic SCT have a favorable survival, and can be reinduced into a cytogenetic remission with immunomodulatory approaches including IFN-α or donor lymphocyte infusions. The 6-year probability of survival after relapse in chronic-phase postallogeneic SCT was 36% (75). Of among 189 patients transplanted in early chronic phase (i.e., within 12 months from diagnosis), the 4-year EFS rate was 60%, but the survival rate was about 80% (76).

4. Recent studies from single institutions show 2- to 5-year EFS rates of 60% or more (77–79). Improvement in allogeneic SCT outcome has also been reported in the EBMT. This may be due to (a) improved allogeneic SCT management, (b) different patient selection, (c) short follow-up with early censoring, (d) greater graft-versus-host disease (GVHD) prophylaxis and therapy (cyclosporin plus methotrexate, FK506), (e) the use of ganciclovir with or without Ig therapy and prophylaxis against cytomegalovirus, and (f) improved supportive care (antibiotics and colony-stimulating factors) (80–83). Different preparative regimens have not contributed to improved outcome: reductions in relapse rates with more intensive regimens have been counterbalanced by higher treatment-related mortality, with consequent similar EFS rates (84–86).

As studies of allogeneic SCT continue to mature, its indications and timing in relation to other modalities will be continuously reevaluated. Results are summarized in Table 5.

Salvage Therapy Postallogeneic SCT Relapse

Patients who relapse postallogeneic SCT can be reinduced into cytogenetic remission with several modalities.

The most exciting salvage approach is immunomodulation by donor lymphocyte reinfusion (87,88). In an update of 84 CML patients treated post-SCT relapse, 54 (72%) of 75 evaluable patients achieved cytogenetic complete response: 82% among patients treated in cytogenetic relapse, 78% among patients treated in hematologic relapse in chronic phase, and 12% among patients treated in CML transformed phases. Forty-two of 44 patients tested in cytogenetic remission were also negative for the BCR-ABL RNA transcripts by polymerase chain reaction (PCR) analysis. The 3-year survival after lymphocyte reinfusions was 67%. The hypothesis behind this treatment is that donor T lymphocyte induce a graft-versus-leukemia (GVL) effect that suppresses the Ph-positive clones and allows the normal donor cells to reexpand (89). Marrow suppression (50% of patients treated for hematologic relapse) and acute GVHD (59% to 80%) have been significant problems; the 1-year mortality rate was 18%. These complications may be reduced by earlier use of donor lymphocyte reinfusions at the time of cytogenetic relapse (myelosuppression rate, 13%) or as prophylaxis among high-risk patients for relapse (accelerated or blastic phase). Modulation of the dose and subsets of T lymphocytes reinfused may also reduce GVHD and improve GVL (90,91).

Other immunomodulatory approaches include interleukin-2, granulocyte colony-stimulating factor, linomide, or IFN-α (92–95). IFN-α induces cytogenetic remission in 20% to 40% patients with cytogenetic relapse in chronic phase. A second allogeneic SCT may be effective among patients who are beyond 12 months from their first SCT, but is associated with a high incidence of transplant-related complications and mortality.

Allogeneic SCT in Transformation

Treatment results in blastic-phase CML have been poor. The long-term EFS rates from the IBMTR and EBMT are 10% or less, because of a high relapse rate of 60% to 80%.

Patient outcome in accelerated phase has been variable with EFS rate to 15% to 40%. Some studies have attributed their better results to improved preparative regimens (e.g. busulfan-cyclophosphamide (96). However, this may be due to a less strict definition of accelerated-phase CML, which shifted a proportion of chronic-phase patients into the accelerated-phase category. This may falsely improve the EFS curves of both chronic and accelerated-phase patients; the only change is the ratio of chronic- to accelerated-phase patients. Thus, when analyzing the results of allogeneic BMT in CML, the selection criteria for accelerated-phase CML, and the ratio of chronic- to accelerated-phase patients should be considered. In the EBMTR study, the ratio was 4.3:1 (72); in two other studies, they were about 2.4:1 (7) and 1:2 (97). Defining strict objective and reproducible accelerated-phase criteria may help in the comparative analyses of such studies.

Chronic Myelogenous Leukemia

Clonal evolution as the only criterion of accelerated-phase CML has been associated with an EFS rate of 60% (98). Clonal evolution does not bear a uniformly poor outcome with standard therapy, and prognosis may depend on the specific cytogenetic abnormality (65).

Allogeneic SCT in Older Patients

A recent study from Seattle (77) reported on 33 patients (23 aged 50 to 55 years and 10 aged 56 to 60 years) undergoing matched related allogeneic SCT. The estimated 2-year survival rate was 80%, which suggests significant selection of patients treated, but indicates the feasibility and success of the procedure among such selected patients (77). In the IBMTR studies, patients >50 years of age had a 5-year EFS rate of 30% (72). In the EBMT studies, 71 patients >45 years old has a 47% transplant-related mortality and a 25% 5-year EFS rate (73).

Timing of Allogeneic SCT in Chronic Phase

Although every patient with a matched (or 1 antigen mismatch) related donor should be offered allogeneic SCT before disease transformation, the timing of allogeneic SCT in chronic phase is controversial. Most groups advocate allogeneic SCT as early as possible based on the original Seattle and later IBMTR studies showing a significantly worse EFS with later transplant (1 year from diagnosis). This was because of a higher transplant-associated mortality and may be due to confounding variables increasing transplant mortality (prior busulfan therapy, older age, and others). In the EBMTR studies, patients transplanted within the first year, in the second year, or subsequently had similar 5-year EFS rates of about 35% to 40% (73). An update of the Seattle data indicates that patients transplanted within the first year or in the second year do equally well (76). A recent IBMTR analysis of the outcome of allogeneic SCT by Horowitz et al. shows no adverse effect by prior IFN-α exposure, but also a similar outcome whether patients were transplanted within or beyond 12 months from diagnosis (99).

The timing of allogeneic SCT chronic phase has to be considered in relation to (1) expected outcome, patient age, and institutional experience; (2) the projected survival optimal non-SCT approaches; and (3) the anticipated worsening from delaying the procedure. As discussed later, about half of the patients in recent CML series have good-risk disease, and their median survival with IFN-α regimens is about 102 months (20). Patients achieving major cytogenetic responses have excellent long-term survival rates (>80% at 5 to 7 years, mostly with major durable cytogenetic responses (20).

When allogeneic SCT is delayed, several considerations are brought up: (1) the worse outcome with delayed BMT (discussed above); (2) the unpredictable course of CML and sudden blastic transformation; and (3) the possible worse outcome of allogeneic BMT with IFN-α exposure (presumably from marrow fibrosis).

With IFN-α therapy, the incidence of blastic transformation is <5% yearly in the first 2 years and is often preceded by disease resistance in chronic phase. Among 274 patients evaluated on IFN-α studies, 11 (4%) had a blastic transformation in the first year; six had lymphoid blastic transformation, and all responded (five CR and one partial response) to anti-ALL therapy. Thus, the loss rate from unpredictable transformation is low.

Among 41 patients evaluated on IFN-α therapy over a period of 2 to 3 years, marrow reticulin fibrosis remained the same in 22 (54%), increased in 8 (20%), and decreased in 12 (26%) (63). The inaspirability of marrow samples on IFN-α therapy is not due to marrow fibrosis, but perhaps to its antiproliferative or cytoadhesion-induced effect (63).

In comparing the outcome after allogeneic BMT, Giralt et al. (100) found no significant differences in the incidences of graft failure and GVHD, time to engraftment, and long-term prognosis by prior IFN-α exposure. This has also been confirmed in several other studies including the larger recent IBMT analysis (99–102). Only one study, by Beelen et al., reported different results. Exposure to IFN-α for >12 months before allogeneic SCT was associated with a significantly worse outcome (5-year survival rate of 22% vs. 55%; $p < 0.01$), primarily due to graft failure in 7 of 17 patients receiving related mismatched or unrelated SCT (49% in incidence), which has not been seen in other studies. Factors contributing to this (preparative regimen, stem cell infusion, CML phase, and marrow fibrosis) should be analyzed.

Role of Matched Unrelated Donor (MUD) Transplant

Follow-up results of MUD SCT in CML show high incidences of graft failure (15%), severe acute (54%) and extensive chronic (52%) GVHD, and 2-year mortality (>50%). Still, MUD is curative in selected patient subsets (104,105). The estimated 2-year EFS rates among patients <30 years old were 43% with matched donor and 31% with a 1 antigen mismatched donor. For older patients, the estimated 2-year EFS rates were 27% and 14%, respectively. Thus, optimal candidates for MUD SCT are younger (<30 years) patients in chronic phase who have a matched donor and have exhibited resistance to IFN-α therapy. Older patients and those with ≥1 antigen mismatch donor may be offered the procedure if disease acceleration develops, because the outcome of MUD SCT in chronic or accelerated phase is not much different. Many groups still advocate MUD SCT in chronic phase to a broader selection of patients (older, 1 antigen mismatch) based on the potential curability and continued improvement of MUD SCT results.

Alpha Interferon Therapy

Single-Arm Studies

In 1983, IFN-α was identified as the first agent capable of inducing significant and durable cytogenetic responses in CML without causing marrow ablation (106,107). In comparing the results of IFN-α studies in CML, uniform criteria for hematologic and cytogenetic responses, as proposed originally, will be used (20). A CHR refers to a complete normalization of the peripheral counts (WBC $<10 \times 10^9$/L), platelets $<450 \times 10^9$/L, absence of immature cells and all signs and symptoms of disease including palpable organomegaly. CHR is further classified by the degree of Ph suppression (cytogenetic response): Complete cytogenetic response (Ph = 0%), partial cytogenetic response (Ph 1% to 34%), and minor cytogenetic response (Ph 35% to 90%). A major cytogenetic response includes complete and partial cytogenetic responses (Ph <35%).

Long-term follow-up of IFN-α studies at our institution were positive. Among 274 patients treated from 1982 through 1990 with IFN-α programs using IFN-α at 5 MU/m^2 daily or the maximally tolerated lower dose schedule, 80% achieved CHR and 58% had a cytogenetic response (complete 26%, major 38%). The median survival was 89 months (confidence interval 66 to 102 months). A cytogenetic response after 12 months of therapy resulted in significantly longer survival by landmark analysis: the 5-year survival dated from 12 months into therapy was 90% for complete cytogenetic response, 88% for partial cytogenetic response, 76% for minor cytogenetic response, and 38% for other response categories. A multivariate analysis including major cytogenetic response as a time-dependent variable showed it to be an independent prognostic factor for survival: patients achieving a major cytogenetic response had a 0.21 risk of death per unit time compared with the total study group (20). Thus, cytogenetic response did not merely identify "an intrinsically more favorable group" since cytogenetic response had an independent positive effect after accounting for the prognostic effect of pretreatment variables by multivariate analysis. This is also confirmed by the favorable effect of cytogenetic response within prognostic risk groups by landmark analysis (Table 6).

Studies from many single institutions and cooperative groups have confirmed the efficacy of CML (Table 7). Alimena et al. reported that IFN-α therapy in early chronic-phase CML produced a CHR rate of 46% and a cytogenetic response rate of 55% (major 12%) (108). Patients randomized to IFN-α 5 MU/m^2 had better results than those treated with 2 MU/m^2 three times weekly, (CHR 57% versus 38%), which led to subsequent use of IFN-α 5 MU/m^2 daily. The Cancer and Leukemia Group B (CALGB) increased the intended dose of IFN-α from 2 MU/m^2 five times weekly to 5 MU/m^2 daily after observing poor responses among the first 16 patients on study (excluded from subsequent analy-

Table 6 Cytogenetic Response Status at 12 Months and Survival Within Prognostic Groups (Synthesis Model)

Prognostic group	Cytogenetic response	Estimate 4-year[a] survival %	p value
Good	Yes	79	<0.01
	No	62	
Intermediate	Yes	82	<0.01
	No	35	
Poor	Yes	83	<0.01
	No	39	

[a]Survival rate from 1 year after start of interferon-α therapy; i.e., estimated percentage of patients surviving 5 years after starting interferon-α therapy.

sis). The hematologic response rate was 59% (CHR 22%, partial 36%), the cytogenetic response rate was 29% (complete 18% among 78 evaluable patients; 13% among the total 107 study patients), and the median survival was 66 months (109). The median dose schedule of IFN-α delivered was 3.2 MU/m² daily. There was no relationship between achieving a cytogenetic response and survival, but the number of patients with major (and complete) cytogenetic response was low. Mahon et al. treated 101 patients with IFN-α 5 MU/m² daily (24). The CHR rate was 79%, the major cytogenetic response rate 42% (complete 32%), and the estimated 5-year survival rate 72%. Survival was signifi-

Table 7 Results of IFN-α Therapy in Early Chronic-Phase CML

Study (Ref.)	No. pts.	Median daily dose IFN-α (MU/m²) delivered	CHR (%)	Cytogenetic response (%)			Median survival (mo)
				Any	Major	Complete	
Alimena (108)	65	—	46	55	12	—	—
Ohnishi (111)	80	4.0	39	44	7.5	9	65+
Mahon (24)	101	5	78	—	42	32	60+
Ozer (109)	107	3.2	59	—	29	13	66
Hehlmann (110)	133	3	31	18	10	7	66
ICSG-CML (25)	218	4.3	62	55	19	8	72
MDACC (20)	274	5	80	56	38	26	89
Allan (26)	293	2 (3.2)	68	22	11	6	61
Guilhot (112,113)	324	5	54	—	22	7	60+

cantly influenced by the achievement of CHR 3 months ($p = 0.01$) and of major ($p < .0003$) or complete cytogenetic response ($p = 0.0001$). Significant predictors for achievement of a major cytogenetic remission were the achievement of CHR within 3 months ($p < 0.0001$), and of a minor cytogenetic response at 3 months ($p = 0.0014$).

Randomized Studies

Four randomized studies of IFN-α versus conventional chemotherapy in CML have been reported (25,26,110,111). In three studies IFN-α therapy prolonged survival and delayed progression to the blastic phase when compared with conventional therapy with hydroxyurea or busulfan (26,26,111). In the fourth study, by Hehlmann et al. (110), IFN-α was superior to busulfan but not to hydroxyurea (110). In all four randomized trials, IFN-α therapy produced a higher rate of major and complete cytogenetic response than conventional chemotherapy.

Italian Cooperative Study Group on CML (ICSG-CML). Patients were randomized IFN-α 5 MU/m^2 daily or conventional therapy with hydroxyurea or busulfan (15). The 218 patients randomized to IFN-α therapy had a higher major cytogenetic response rate (19% versus 1%; $p < 0.01$), which was complete in 8%. They also had significantly longer survival (median survival 72 versus 52 months; $p = 0.002$), and time to progression to accelerated or blastic phase (median time >72 versus 45 months; $p < 0.001$). Six-year survival rate was 50% with IFN-α versus 29% with chemotherapy ($p = 0.002$). The median dose of IFN-α delivered was 4.3 MU/m^2 daily. IFN-α treatment was discontinued in 31%, in 16% for IFN-α-related adverse events (predominantly influenza-like, gastrointestinal, neurologic); 18% had IFN-α dose reductions of >50%. By landmark analysis, achieving CHR after 8 months of therapy was associated with better survival (5-year survival rate 78% versus 48%; $p < 0.001$), as was achieving a cytogenetic response after 24 months of therapy (5-year survival rate 88% versus 65%; $p < 0.001$).

German/Swiss Studies. Patients were randomized to IFN-α, hydroxyurea, or busulfan therapy (110). Patients treated with either IFN-α or hydroxyurea had significantly better survivals than those receiving busulfan (median survivals of 66, 56, and 45 months, respectively; $p < 0.01$). There was no survival difference with IFN-α versus hydroxyurea therapy ($p = 0.44$). The median IFN-α dose delivered after the first 4 weeks was 3 MU/m^2 daily. Twenty-five percent of patients had IFN-α therapy discontinued. Karyotypic analysis was carried out in only 63% of patients receiving IFN-α therapy; only 15 patients (7%) had complete cytogenetic response. The estimated 3-year survival rates were 100% for cytogenetic responders versus 72% for nonresponders ($p = 0.20$).

Possible reasons for the lack of a demonstrable survival advantage in the IFN-α cohort may be (1) the lower dose of IFN-α therapy actually delivered; (2) different entry criteria allowing treatment of only symptomatic disease (more advanced patients); (3) a higher percentage of poor-risk patients on study (25%) as well as of patients with advanced/accelerated disease (15%); and (4) early IFN-α requirement for monotherapy, possibly causing early discontinuation in about 20% of patients, half of whom later received busulfan, an inferior therapy (22).

MRC Study. The MRC study randomized patients to maintenance therapy with IFN-α or cytotoxic therapy, usually hydroxyurea (26). The 293 patients randomized to IFN-α had longer survival than the 294 patients who received hydroxyurea or busulfan (median survivals 61 and 41 months, respectively; $p = 0.0009$). Only 59 patients (22%) had any cytogenetic response (complete 5%; partial 6%). The 5-year survival rates were 100% with a complete cytogenetic response, 92% with a partial cytogenetic response, 59% with a minor cytogenetic response, and 47% with no cytogenetic response. Five-year survival rates were 52% in the IFN-α cohort and 34% in the chemotherapy cohort ($p = 0.004$). The median daily dose of IFN-α actually received was 3.2 MU, or about 1.9 MU/m^2. Patients achieving CHR did significantly better than those who had lesser degrees of hematologic response ($p = 0.01$). Patients treated with IFN-α survived longer than those treated with conventional therapy even if they had not demonstrably achieved a cytogenetic response. An update of the results (114) showed the superiority of IFN-α versus hydroxyurea ($p = 0.05$) and similar survivals with hydroxyurea or busulfan, this contrasting with the results of Hehlmann et al. (110).

Japanese Study. Patients were randomized to IFN-α 5 MU/m^2 daily (80 patients) or busulfan (79 patients) (111). IFN-α therapy resulted in a higher major cytogenetic response rate (16% versus 5%; $p = 0.046$), and better projected 5-year survival rate (54% versus 32%; $p = 0.03$). Patients achieving any cytogenetic response with either IFN-α or busulfan therapy survived significantly longer than patients who did not.

In most studies, achieving minimal hematologic (CHR) or cytogenetic tumor burden correlated with survival prolongation (Table 8). In two studies that failed to show this prognostic association, a low rate of major cytogenetic response rate was noted, possibly because of low doses of IFN-α administered (Table 7). Two studies showing a correlation between cytogenetic response and survival also reported that patients on IFN-α therapy who did not achieve a cytogenetic response resulted in equivalent survival as conventional chemotherapy (20,25). In contrast, the MRC study showed a survival advantage for IFN-α even without achieving a cytogenetic response, although patients achieving a cytogenetic response also had a better survival than those who did not (26).

Table 8 Minimal Disease Burden and Survival with IFN-α Therapy

Study (Ref.)	Survival advantage with achievement of	
	CHR	Cytogenetic response
MDACC (20)	+	+
Ozer (109)	ND	—
Mahon (24)	+	+
ICSG-CML (25)	+	+
Hehlmann (110)	+	trend
Allan (26)	+	+
Ohnishi (111)	ND	trend
Guilhot (112,113)	+	+

NA = not applicable; ND = not done.

Dose Intensity of IFN-α and Response in Lower Versus Higher Dose Schedules

CHR rates in similar study populations of early chronic phase CML have ranged from 31% to 80%. Variability in CHR rates may be due to different population characteristics, response criteria, or protocol treatment designs. IFN-α monotherapy in the German/Swiss and CALGB studies (as opposed to allowing the addition of initial chemotherapy in others) may have produced lower CHR rates. This, however, may not explain the large differences in cytogenetic (18% to 58%), major cytogenetic (10% to 38%), and complete cytogenetic (6% to 26%) response rates. These may be due to: (1) different risk group distributions, (2) patient and physician motivation, (3) actual IFN-α dose delivered, (4) frequency of cytogenetic studies, (5) inclusion of advanced or accelerated phase patients, or (6) IFN-α monotherapy as induction with consequent higher early dropout rates. When IFN-α effect was analyzed for response and survival within risk group, IFN-α showed better results in each risk group and higher cytogenetic response rates even in the poor-risk group in our studies, compared with cooperative groups (5). This suggested the value of IFN-α dose intensity to increase the quality of cytogenetic response and to prolong survival. As with any new anticancer therapy, a "learning curve" exists, which improves the results as experience is gained. The complete cytogenetic response rate in our first IFN-α CML study was 14%, similar to some current multicenter results, and may be in part due to unfamiliarity with IFN-α-related toxicities and management.

Comparing the median dose of IFN-α delivered among responders versus nonresponders is misleading since many studies have built-in dose reductions after achieving a response, and dose escalations with resistant disease (25,26,110), thus precluding meaningful analyses of the relationship of IFN-α dose-intensity with response. Comparison of the actual median dose of IFN-α delivered versus response rate among different studies may help demonstrating the dose-response phenomenon (Table 7).

A study by Schofield et al. indicated that lower dose schedules of IFN-α (2 MU/m^2 three times weekly) were as effective as the higher dose schedules (5 MU/m^2 daily) recommended for CML (weekly dose 6 MU/m^2 versus 35 MU/m^2) (115). The lower dose schedule would be less toxic and less expensive. Comparison of the M.D. Anderson Cancer Center (Houston) cohort of 274 patients equivalent to those in the Denver cohort (early chronic phase) indicated similar hematologic response rates, but higher incidences of overall and major cytogenetic responses with the higher IFN-α dose schedules (Table 9). This is supported by the initial CALGB experience with the lower IFN-α dose schedule, the comparative study of Alimena et al. with the two IFN-α dose schedules, and other studies of low-dose IFN-α schedules (108,116,117). Another issue is the relationship between IFN-α response and risk groups (5). The 27 patients reported by the Denver group belonged predominantly to a good-risk subgroup, in whom the expected major cytogenetic response rate would be 46% to 52% (rather than 22%) and the projected median survival 8 to 9 years (5,115). Randomized studies of lower versus higher-dose IFN-α schedules are ongoing to clarify the role of IFN-α dose intensity in the management of CML. This question may, however, become less relevant with combination studies (e.g., IFN-α plus ara-C or homoharringtonine).

Importance of Achieving Minimal Tumor Burden in CML

In human malignancies, achieving a minimal burden (complete remission) is a prerequisite for improving prognosis and cures. The causal association between

Table 9 IFN-α Dose Schedules and Response in CML

Study (Ref.)	IFN-α schedule	No. patients	CHR (%)	Cytogenetic responses (%)		
				Any	Major	Complete
MDACC (20)	5 MU/m^2 daily	274	80	58	38	26
Schofield et al. (115)	2 MU/m^2 TIW	27	70	33	22	7
Alimena et al. (108)	5 MU/m^2 TIW	30	63	NS	NS	NS
	2 MU/m^2 TIW	30	24	NS	NS	NS
Freund et al. (116)	5 MU/m^2 TIW	10	33	0	0	0
Anger et al. (117)	3 MU/m^2 TIW	9	22	20	0	0

TIW = three times a week; NS = not stated.

Chronic Myelogenous Leukemia

Ph-related molecular events and the development of CML encourages the acceptance of Ph suppression as a surrogate marker for tumor burden and subsequent long-term prognosis. Reduction in hematologic tumor burden, reflected by CHR, has been associated with significant survival prolongation in all studies in which it has been examined (5,24–26,110,111,113).

Achieving a minimal cytogenetic burden was also associated with a survival prolongation by landmark and/or multivariate analysis in five of eight studies, (20,24–26,113), with a positive trend in two others (110,111). In the Japanese study mentioned above, achieving a cytogenetic response was associated with a significantly better duration of chronic phase CML (5-year rates 79% versus 22%; $p = 0.0017$) but only a trend for better survival ($p = 0.10$) (111). Thus, most current data suggest that achieving a minimal CML tumor burden (hematologic, cytogenetic) will impact outcome favorably, and should be pursued as a therapeutic objective in future investigations.

Management of IFN-α-Related Problems

Tachyphylaxis to the early adverse effects of IFN-α (fever, chills, postnasal drip, and anorexia) develops within 1 to 2 weeks; these are usually not dose-limiting. Their severity is increased with high WBC counts (levels of leukotriene C4 which may induce an inflammatory response). These are reduced by tumor debulking with hydroxyurea (until the leukocyte count is $<20 \times 10^9$/L) before institution IFN-α therapy, premedication with acetaminophen, nighttime injections, and by starting therapy at 25% to 50% of the recommended dose for the first week, and increasing dosage as tachyphylaxis occurs. Delayed adverse effects are dose-limiting in 10% to 30% of patients, and include persistent fatigue, weight loss, neurotoxicity, depression, insomnia, alopecia, marrow hypoplasia, and infrequent immune-mediated complications, (hemolysis or thrombocytopenia, collage vascular disorders such as rheumatoid arthritis and systemic lupus erythematosus, nephrotic syndrome, and hypothyroidism) (118,119). Rare cardiac dysfunction (arrhythmias, congestive heart failure) has been reported.

A triad of depression, fatigue, and insomnia is common and can be improved with amitriptyline 25–50 mg at bedtime. Some patients respond better to other antidepressants (e.g., fluoxetine, sertraline) if one component of the symptom triad is more prominent; in such cases a neuropsychiatric consult is helpful. Practical guidelines to IFN-α therapy are summarized in Table 10 (120).

Duration of IFN-α Therapy and Monitoring of Response

Though major cytogenetic remissions induced by IFN-α therapy are durable, it is uncertain how long they can last after IFN-α is stopped. One approach is to

Table 10 Practical Guidelines on IFN-α Therapy

Therapy initiation
    Hydroxyurea to obtain initial cytoreduction (WBC: 10–20 × 10^9/L)
    Slow dose escalation: 3 MU daily for a week; then 5 MU daily for a week; then 5 MU/m^2 daily or maximally tolerated individual dose
    Cyclic WBC phenomenon may be noted in first 3 months; does not indicate resistance; requires reinstitution of hydroxyurea intermittently if WBC >10 × 10^9/L
Improve tolerance
    Premedicate with acetaminophen
    Evening self-injection
    Tricyclic antidepressants for neurologic side effects (insomnia, depression, fatigue)
Therapeutic monitoring
    Complete blood counts weekly until counts stable, then every 2–4 weeks
    Maintain WBC between 2–4 × 10^9/L and platelets >50 × 10^9/L
    Cytogenetic evaluation on bone marrow aspirate every 3–4 months in the first year then every 4–6 months
    Recent introduction of BCR quantification, and interphase FISH (iFISH) monitoring in peripheral blood; acceptable until PH <20% (false positive with iFISH), then shift to hypermetaphase FISH analysis on bone marrow. Regular cytogenetic studies at least every 12 months to look for cytogenetic clonal evolution
Dose modifications
    Interrupt IFN-α for grade 3 to 4 toxicities then resume at 50%
    Reduce IFN-α dose by 25% for grade 2 persistent toxicities
    Do not reduce IFN-α dose schedule for "low counts" unless WBC is <2 × 10^9/L or platelets <50 × 10^9/L; 25% dose reduction is then appropriate
    Hold IFN-α for moderate acute intercurrent disease
Efficacy assessment
    Hematologic remission at 6–8 months
    Cytogenetic response by 12 months
    Major cytogenetic response by 18–24 months

continue IFN-α therapy until continuous complete response is documented for 3 years.

Fluorescent in situ hybridization (FISH) techniques has allowed a more precise evaluation of patient response and status on therapy (121). More sensitive techniques such as PCR for BCR-ABL detect rare cells with a BCR rearrangement in most patients with CML in remission after IFN-α therapy (35). However, these patients may remain in remission (sometimes even after discontinuing therapy), do not develop blastic phase CML, and have prolonged survival. The PCR technique may be detecting nonclonogeneic cells, or patient's immune system may be able to control such minimal residual disease and prevent relapse. Kurzrock et al. recently showed that about half of the patients in continued complete cytogenetic response may become PCR-negative for BCR-ABL: the median duration of complete cytogenetic response was 42 months in PCR-negative patients, and 12 months in PCR-positive patients, suggesting the need for longer therapy duration to achieve better-quality remissions, and perhaps the potential curability of CML with IFN-α therapy (122).

Combined Modality Therapies with IFN-α

IFN-α plus chemotherapy agent combinations were investigated as to whether they would produce higher CHR or cytogenetic response rates than IFN-α alone. IFN-α combinations with hydroxyurea and ara-C were initially investigated in patients with late chronic-phase disease (123,124). Results of IFN-α plus hydroxyurea seemed to prolong late chronic phase duration in contrast to patients treated with IFN-α or cytotoxics alone (123). Ara-C selectively suppressed the growth of CML cells over that of normal hematopoietic cells in vitro, and induced in vivo cytogenetic responses in seven of nine patients treated (70,71). Our initial study of IFN-α and ara-C used a regimen of IFN-α 5 MU/m^2 daily plus ara-C 15 mg/m^2 daily for 7 days, repeated every 28 days (124). Forty patients in late chronic phase and 20 patients in accelerated phase were treated. The combination regimen produced higher CHR (55% versus 28%; $p = 0.02$) and 3-year survival rates (75% versus 48%; $p < 0.01$) than IFN-α alone. Guilhot et al. reported in 1993 on a pilot study of 24 patients, 12 previously untreated, who received IFN-α and hydroxyurea induction followed by IFN-α and ara-C maintenance (112). Ara-C was given at 10–20 mg/m^2 daily for 10–15 days, repeated every 28 days, to 10 patients who did not achieve CHR or a durable cytogenetic response, with IFN-α; the combination was not highly effective in these resistant patients.

Anger et al. documented the efficacy of IFN-α and hydroxyurea in a small cohort of newly diagnosed CML patients (117). Arthur et al. reported on 30 patients treated in early chronic phase CML with IFN-α and low dose ara-C (125), 20 mg/m^2 daily for 21 days, repeated every 42 days. Repeated cycles of ara-C were given for 12 months, after which IFN-α alone was continued. The CHR rate was 93%, and the cytogenetic response rate 67% (major 53%, complete 33%). In a recent update, at a median follow-up of 6 years, the projected survival was 76%, and the median survival not reached (Arthur, personal communication): nine patients are dead—six from allogeneic SCT-related complications, and three from CML progression. Only one patient discontinued the regimen because of adverse events.

Two studies of IFN-α and ara-C were conducted by our group (126) in a cohort of 148 patients in early chronic phase. Patients received IFN-α 5 MU/m^2 daily plus ara-C 15 mg/m^2 daily for 7 days, repeated every 28 days (47 patients treated between 1989 and 1992) or plus ara-C 10 mg daily (101 patients

Table 11 Result of IFN-α Plus Low-Dose ara-C in Ph-Positive Early Chronic Phase CML

Parameter	IFN + LD ara-C 7 d/mo	IFN + LD ara-C daily
% CHR	84	95
% CG response		
overall	64	78 $p = 0.08$
major	38	54 $p = 0.10$
complete	20	30
% 4 yr survival	78	84

treated from 1993 to 1997). Fifty-two percent had good-risk CML; 15% had poor-risk CML. Results are shown in Table 11. The daily ara-C schedule may be superior to the 7 days every month ara-C, and to IFN-α alone.

In a CALGB study (127), IFN-α plus ara-C (IFN-α 5 MU/m² daily and ara-C 15 mg/m² twice daily) were given until a WBC <2 × 10⁹/L; therapy was then discontinued and resumed when the WBC was >5 × 10⁹/L. In the first 35 patients, six exhibited grade 3 gastrointestinal toxicity; subsequently the dose of ara-C was reduced to 10 mg/m² twice daily. Among 88 evaluable patients, 63 (72%) had CHR, 9 of 63 (15%) achieved cytogenetic response, and 15% had a major cytogenetic response. The estimated 5-year survival rate was 58%.

Thaler et al. reported on 10 patients resistant to IFN-α, four of whom responded when ara-C was added (128). They later treated additional patients with IFN-α plus ara-C regimen (IFN-α 3.5 MU daily, and ara-C 10 mg/m² daily for 10 days every 28 days) (129). Initially all patients received hydroxyurea until they had a WBC <20 × 10⁹/L, at which time IFN-α/ara-C maintenance therapy began. Among 84 evaluable patients, 45 (54%) achieved CHR, and 21 (25%) achieved a major cytogenetic response (complete in 18%). The estimated overall survival at 4 years was 65%. Sixteen patients (19%) discontinued therapy due to adverse events.

In a recent study by Guilhot et al. (113), patients with early chronic-phase CML were randomized to receive IFN-α 5 MU/m² daily either alone or combined with monthly courses of ara-C 20 mg/m²/day for 10 days. All patients underwent a cytoreductive induction phase with hydroxyurea and IFN-α. Of 745 patients randomized, 646 were evaluable. The 324 patients randomized to IFN-α plus ara-C had significantly higher incidences of CHR at 6 months (67% versus 54%; $p = 0.002$), of major cytogenetic response at 12 months (39% versus 22%; $p < 0.001$), and of complete cytogenetic response (15% versus 7%; $p < 0.001$). The IFN-α plus ara-C combination was associated with a significantly longer survival and time to development of accelerated or blastic phase dura-

Chronic Myelogenous Leukemia

tions (3-year survival rates 84% versus 76%; $p = 0.006$). The resistance, the Ph-negative collection rate was 27%, and 43% of patients had Ph-positive cells <35%. Peripheral stem cell collections were "cleaner" than marrow collections in 23% of patients (134). Similar findings were reported by others (135). The treatment-related mortality in chronic phase was 7% (134,135). Intensive chemotherapy may be beneficial as part of combined-modality therapy in poor-risk patients and those with advanced-transformed disease.

Homoharringtonine

Homoharringtonine (HHT), a synthetic derivative of a Chinese plant alkaloid, had demonstrated activity in CML in "lower-dose, longer-exposure" schedule which almost eliminated the cardiovascular side effects. Homoharringtonine was first investigated in late chronic phase CML at 2.5 mg/m^2 by continuous infusion for 14 days for remission induction, then for 7 days every month as maintenance. Among 72 patients treated, 72% achieved CHR, and 31% had a cytogenetic response (major in 15%) (136). These figures compared favorably with the results of IFN-α alone or with ara-C in late chronic phase CML, albeit in different study groups as defined by prior IFN-α exposure and resistance.

This encouraged us to combine HHT and ara-C and administer the regimen to patients in late chronic phase CML who had exhibited IFN-α resistance; many had been exposed to HHT (30%) or ara-C (28%) (i.e., more extensively treated group than in the HHT alone regimen). Patients received HHT 2.5 mg/m^2 daily by continuous infusion for 5 days and ara-C 15 mg/m^2/day for 5 days divided into two daily subcutaneous doses. The combination was given at 28-day intervals. Sixty-six percent of patients achieved a CHR, and 17% had a major cytogenetic response (137). Similar results were reported by Ernst et al. (138).

HHT for six cycles followed by IFN-α maintenance was also investigated in early chronic median dose of IFN-α delivered was 5 MU/m^2 daily in both cohorts, and 22% of patients in both arms discontinued therapy because of adverse events. The results of the IFN-α plus ara-C regimens are summarized in Table 12.

INVESTIGATIONAL MODALITIES

Some investigational approaches have focused on suppression of the Ph-positive clones. These include: (1) intensive chemotherapy, alone or followed by autologous SCT; (2) new chemotherapy agents such as homoharringtonine (HHT) and decitabine; (3) immunomodulation (e.g., linomide); (4) addition of various

Table 12 Results with IFN-α Plus Ara-C Therapy in Early Chronic Phase CML

Study	No. pts	IFN/day	Ara-C/28days	CHR	Major cytogenetic	Complete cytogenetic	% Survival (at x year)
MDACC (126)	45	5 MU/m^2	105 mg/m^2	84	38	20	78 (5)
MDACC (126)	93	5 MU/m^2	180 mg/m^2	95	53	30	84 (5)
Guilhot et al. (113)	322	5 MU/m^2	200 mg/m^2	67	39	15	88 (3)
Arthur et al. (125)	30	5 MU/m^2	280 mg/m^2	93	53	33	76 (6)
Thaler et al. (129)	84	3.5 MU	100 mg/m^2	54	25	18	74 (3)
CALGB (127)	88	5 MU/m^2	180 mg/m^2 BID as required	72	51	15	72 (4)

agents to IFN-α (e.g., HHT, azidothymidine, GM-CSF); and (5) genetic-targeted therapy.

Intensive Chemotherapy

Intensive AML-like chemotherapy induced remission in 60% to 70% of patients, and complete cytogenetic responses in 35% to 50% (130). Initial intensive chemotherapy for three cycles followed by IFN-α maintenance did not increase the rate of long-term cytogenetic response compared with IFN-α alone (131). Simonsson et al. treated 120 patients with CML with IFN-α for 6 months, followed by three different intensive chemotherapy regimens and autologous SCT using Ph-negative collected cells. The projected 5-year survival rate was 68%, and 11 of 26 autografted patients remain Ph-negative up to 48 months post-BMT (132).

Intensive chemotherapy has been used recently for in vivo purging to collect marrow or peripheral diploid-rich stem cells during early hematopoietic recovery. Carella et al. reported 50% of patients collected in chronic phase CML to be 100% diploid in the peripheral stem cell collections (133). In our study, in patients with longer chronic phase duration and with IFN-α phase CML (139). Among 90 patients treated, the CHR rate after six cycles of HHT was 92%, and the cytogenetic response rate 68% (major 27%). The long-term follow-up results were favorable with trends for higher hematologic and cytogenetic response rates at 3 years with the combination compared with IFN-α alone. Results of HHT studies are shown in Table 13.

Autologous Stem Cell Transplantation (SCT)

In chronic-phase CML, unpurged autologous SCT was associated with recovery with some Ph-negative cells in 30% to 77% of patients (140), but only occa-

Table 13 Results of Single-Agent Homoharringtonine Therapy in Chronic-Phase CML

Parameter	Early chronic phase[a]	Late chronic phase[b]
No. treated	90	72
% CHR	92	72
% CG response		
overall	68	31
major (CR + partial)	27	15
complete	4	7

[a]Results after six cycles of HHT with best response coded.
[b]CHR rate is based on 58 patients with active CML; cytogenetic response rates were based on the 58 patients with active CML and 13 in CHR treated to assess cytogenetic response. The cytogenetic response rates were 28% versus 46%, respectively.

sional patients maintained Ph negativity with long-term follow-up. Some studies suggested a survival advantage with autologous SCT with 4- to 5-year survival rates of 56% to 70% posttransplant (141–143). Our analysis of 22 patients undergoing SCT and compared to matched historical controls showed median survivals of 34 versus 49 months, respectively (p value not significant) (144). However, these patients had late chronic phase CML (median time to transplant 43 months) and proven resistance to IFN-α therapy, while patients in other studies were transplanted in earlier chronic phase and had little or no IFN-α exposure. The value of unpurged autologous SCT for survival prolongation in CML remains controversial and is under investigation (145).

Since infused tumor cells contribute partly to relapse postautologous SCT (146), purged autologous SCT is an exciting investigational approach. In vitro methods for purging have included long-term liquid (Dexter) cultures, in vitro incubation with chemotherapy or biological agents (interferon), negative selection of Ph-positive (CD 34+, HLA Dr+) cells, positive selection for normal (CD34+, HLA DR−) stem cells, and purging with antisense oligonucleotides against different oncogenic products (e.g., BCR-ABL, c-MYB) (147–155). In vivo purging methods have included stem cell collections following IFN-α or intensive chemotherapy, as discussed earlier (132,156).

The Vancouver group investigated long-term culture in vitro purging for autologous SCT. Of 87 patients, 36 (40%) exhibited normal cell growth advantage, and 22 underwent purged autologous BMT. Marrows with 100% diploid cells were observed in 13 of 16 patients who recovered, this lasting for a median of 12 months. Five patients maintained Ph-negative status, two with IFN-α maintenance and three without maintenance. The 3-year survival rate was 75% (147). In the study by Simonsson et al., 26 of the 120 patients with CML treated with the sequence of IFN-α, intensive chemotherapy, and autologous SCT, have undergone SCT. Eleven (46%; 9% of total) maintain a Ph-negative status. The 6-year actuarial survival rate of the study group was 68% (132).

In the study of Carella et al., 16 patients (11 chronic, five accelerated) have undergone autologous SCT using diploid stem cells collected during early hematopoietic recovery: five remain in cytogenetic CR on IFN-α maintenance at 5+ to 29+ months (133).

In our studies, 22 patients with CML (10 chronic, nine accelerated, three blastic) underwent autologous SCT using stem cells collected during hematopoietic recovery from intensive chemotherapy. There was a correlation between the percent of Ph-positive cells infused and recovered. The median time to loss of cytogenetic response was 12 months for patients infused with <35% Ph-positive cells, and 5 months for those infused with >35% Ph-positive cells (156).

Improved results with autologous SCT may result from improvements in preparative regimens (157), purging methods (158), or immunomodulation strategies (159). Alpha interferon, or interleukin-2, and linomide are candidate approaches (159,160). Rowe et al. treated 12 patients who underwent unpurged autologous BMT with linomide up to 0.2 mg/kg orally twice weekly; three patients have maintained a Ph-negative status for 12+, 13+, and 16+ months (159).

Other Investigations

Decitabine

Hypermethylation of DNA, an indicator of tumor progression and aggressiveness, is found in 50% of patients in chronic-phase CML, and in 100% in blastic phase. Decitabine, a potent hypomethylating agent, was investigated in 37 patients in accelerated (17 patients) or blastic phases (20 patients) (161). Decitabine was given at 100 mg/m^2 IV over 6 hours at 12-hour intervals for 10 doses (1000 mg/m^2 per course) in 13 patients, and at 75 g/m^2 IV over 6 hours at 12-hour intervals for 10 doses (750 mg/m^2 per course) in 24 patients. CHR was achieved in 29% of patients in accelerated phase and in 10% in blastic phase. Two patients achieved a cytogenetic response. Prolonged myelosuppression was the most significant side effect; the median time to platelet recovery >30 × 10^9/L was 31 days, and to granulocyte recovery >0.5 × 10^9/L was 48 days. Studies of lower doses (e.g., 500 mg/m^2/course) of decitabine plus IFN-α in CML should be considered.

Retinoids

These have shown activity in hematologic and solid tumors (acute promyelocytic leukemia, juvenile CML, T cell lymphoid, head and neck and cervical

Chronic Myelogenous Leukemia

cancer). Retinoids synergize with IFN-α and induce differentiation and apoptosis, events considered favorable in reversing CML pathophysiology (162). In a study by Meyskens et al., the addition of vitamin A to busulfan improved survival significantly compared with busulfan therapy alone (163).

In a pilot study, 13 patients with CML (seven late chronic phase, five accelerated phase, one blastic phase; all extensively pretreated, 12 had failed IFN-α therapy) received ATRA 175 mg^2 orally in two divided doses daily. Four of five accelerated phase patients, and one of seven late chronic phase patients showed a transient decrease in blast, promyelocyte, and/or basophil percentage (164). While ATRA may not be effective in these advanced IFN-α refractory patients, its addition to IFN-α in early chronic phase may of value.

Growth Factors

In patients who show hematologic or minor cytogenetic response to IFN-α, the normal stem cell population suppressed to a point that they cannot regrow after leukemic clones have been partially controlled by IFN-α. We investigated adding GM-CSF 30–60 μL/m^2 daily to the therapy of 10 patients with CML who had a hematologic response but failed to achieve or lost a major cytogenetic response on IFN-α therapy (165). Three patients (30%) achieved a major cytogenetic response with the combination; a fourth had a partial cytogenetic response which evolved to a complete cytogenetic response after stopping therapy, and persisted for over 4 years. Thus, the addition of GM-CSF may be beneficial in some patients with IFN-α-sensitive disease but unsatisfactory cytogenetic response. Combination of cytokines and IFN-α may be worth further investigations.

TREATMENT OPTIONS

Most patients with CML (75% to 80%) do not have the option for related (match, 1 antigen mismatch) allogeneic SCT. Following an initial trial of IFN-α-based therapy, patients who achieve CHR by 6 to 8 months, and a cytogenetic response by 12 months, may continue on therapy as long as the cytogenetic response persists, or for at least 3 years in cytogenetic complete response. Patients who do not have a cytogenetic response after 12 months may either continue on IFN-α (based on MRC studies) or be offered investigations aimed to suppress Ph-positive disease (HHT, purged autologous SCT, new agents), or MUD SCT in chronic or transformed phase depending on patient age and degree of donor-host matching. Since the median interval between the initiation of a preliminary search for a donor and MUD transplant may be long (~8 months), a preliminary MUD search soon after diagnosis among eligible patients is preferred.

Patients who have a related donor may be offered allogeneic SCT initially or after a trial of IFN-α therapy based on patient age, patient and physician preferences, and experience with allogeneic SCT and IFN-α. In general, patients may undergo allogeneic SCT as initial therapy if the expected related mortality is low (<20% at 2 years) of if the experience with IFN-α in terms of achieving a cytogenetic response is poor. Patients who have an expected mortality of >20% with SCT may undergo initial IFN-α therapy, and would be offered related allogeneic SCT later if no cytogenetic response is observed after 12 months or is lost later on.

FUTURE DIRECTIONS

Investigations will incorporate known active regimens and agents in the most effective and least toxic combinations and sequences. Interferon-alpha, ara-C, retinoids, HHT, and decitabine are candidate agents for such regimens.

Immunomodulatory approaches with linomide, interleukin-2, newer agents, SCT with allogeneic incremental donor lymphocyte infusions, and modified expanded autologous lymphocytes are under consideration. An extension to this concept is the development of CML vaccines using modifications that would render CML cells more recognizable as "foreign" to the host autologous T lymphocytes (166).

CML-targeted therapies aimed at the BCR-ABL molecular abnormalities or at molecular events associated with disease progression should be investigated. These include BCR-ABL antisense molecules (possibly liposomally encapsulated), ribozymes directed at the BCR-ABL mRNA, tyrosine kinase inhibitors, and agents directed against the RAS oncogene pathways (RAS antisense, farnesyl transferase inhibitors), GRB-2, IL-1 (e.g., IL-1 receptor antagonists), and MYB (167,168). Some of these approaches have already been investigated with promising results. Others, such as inhibitors of BCR-ABL protein kinase, will soon undergo clinical trials.

In all these therapeutic strategies, appropriate biologic correlates should be conducted to understand the reasons behind the success (or failure) of various strategies, identify specific patient subsets that have a selected benefit from particular modalities, and modulate future regimens based on these results.

REFERENCES

1. Pusey W. Report of cases treated with roentgen rays. JAMA 38; 911:1902.
2. Report of the MRC Working Party. Comparison of radiotherapy and busulfan therapy in chronic granulocytic leukemia. Br Med J 1968; 1:201.

3. Kennedy B, Yarbro K. Metabolic and therapeutic effects of hydroxyurea in chronic myeloid leukemia. JAMA 1966; 195:1038.
4. Talpaz M, Kantarjian H, McCredie K, et al. Clinical investigation of human alpha interferon in chronic myelogenous leukemia. Blood 1987; 69:1280.
5. Kantarjian H, O'Brien S, Anderlini P, et al. Treatment of chronic myelogenous leukemia: current status and investigational options. Blood 1996; 87:3069.
6. Cortes J, Talpaz M, O'Brien S, et al. Philadelphia-chromosome negative chronic myelogenous leukemia with rearrangement of the breakpoint cluster region: long-term follow-up results. Cancer 1995; 75:464.
7. Kantarjian H, Kurzrock R, Talpaz M. Philadelphia chromosome-negative chronic myelogenous leukemia and chronic myelomonocytic leukemia. Hematol Oncol Clin North Am 1990; 4:389.
8. Bortin M, D'Amaro J, Bach F, et al. HLA associations with leukemia. Blood 1987; 70:227.
9. Lange R, Moloney W, Yamawaki T. Leukemia in atomic bomb survivors. 1. General observations. Blood 1954; 9:514.
10. Boice J, Day N, Andersen A, et al. Second cancer following radiation treatment for cervical cancer. An international collaboration among cancer registries. J Natl Cancer Inst 1985; 74:955.
11. Biernaux C, Loos M, Sels A, Huez G, Stryckmans P. Detection of major bcr-abl gene expression at a very low level in blood cells of some healthy individuals. Blood 1995; 86:3118.
12. Kantarjian H, Deisseroth A, Kurzrock R, et al. Chronic myelogenous leukemia: a concise update. Blood 1993; 82:691.
13. Kantarjian H, Keating M, Talpaz M, et al. Chronic myelogenous leukemia in blast crisis. Analysis of 242 patients. Am J Med 1987; 83:445.
14. Kantarjian H, Dixon D, Keating M, et al. Characteristics of accelerated disease in chronic myelogenous leukemia. Cancer 1988; 61:1441.
15. Kantarjian H, Smith T, McCredie K, et al. Chronic myelogenous leukemia: a multivariate analysis of the association of patient characteristics and therapy with survival. Blood 1985; 66:1326.
16. Sokal J, Cox E, Baccarani M, et al. Prognostic discrimination in "good risk" chronic granulocytic leukemia. Blood 1984; 63:789.
17. Tura S, Baccarani M, Corbelli G, et al. Staging of chronic myeloid leukaemia. Br J Haematol 1981; 47:105.
18. Kantarjian H, Keating M, Smith T, et al. Proposal for a simple synthesis prognostic staging system in chronic myelogenous leukemia. Am J Med 1990; 88:1.
19. Italian Cooperative Study Group on Myeloid Leukaemia. Prospective confirmation of a prognostic classification for Ph-positive chronic myeloid leukaemia. Br J Haematol 1988; 69:463.
20. Kantarjian H, Smith T, O'Brien S, et al. Prolonged survival following achievement of cytogenetic response with alpha interferon therapy in chronic myelogenous leukemia. Ann Intern Med 1995; 122:254.
21. Hehlmann R. Chronic myelogenous leukemia: does interferon alpha prolong life? Leukemia 1996; 10:193–196.
22. Tura S, Zuffa E. Interferon-α and hydroxyurea in early chronic myeloid leukemia:

a comparative analysis of the Italian and German chronic myeloid leukemia trials with interferon-α. Blood 1996; 87:5384–5391.
23. Mahon F, Montastruc M, Faberes C, et al. Predicting complete cytogenetic response in chronic myelogenous leukemia patients treated with recombinant interferon. Blood 1994; 84:3592.
24. Mahon F, Fabères C, Boiron J, et al. High response rate using recombinant alpha interferon in patients with newly diagnosed chronic myeloid leukemia—analysis of predictive factors. Blood 1996; 88(suppl 1):638a. Abstract.
25. Tura S, Baccarani M, Zuffa E. Interferon alfa-2a as compared with conventional chemotherapy for the treatment of chronic myeloid leukemia. N Engl J Med 1994; 330:820.
26. Allan N, Richards S, Shepherd P, et al. UK Medical Research Council randomized multicenter trial of interferon-αn1 for chronic myeloid leukemia: improved survival irrespective of cytogenetic response. Lancet 1995; 345:1392.
27. Sacchi S, Kantarjian HM, Smith TL, et al. Early treatment decisions with interferon alpha therapy in early chronic phase chronic myelogenous leukemia. In preparation.
28. Rowley JD. A new consistent chromosomal abnormality in chronic myelogenous leukaemia identified by quinacrine fluorescence and Giemsa banding. Nature 1973; 243:290.
29. Bilhou-Nabera C, Viard F, Marit G, et al. Complete cytogenetic conversion in chronic myelocytic leukemia patients undergoing interferon α therapy: follow-up with reverse polymerase chain reaction. Leukemia 1992; 6:595.
30. Bilhou-Nabera C, Bernard P, Marit G, et al. Serial cytogenetic studies in allografted patients with chronic myeloid leukemia. Bone Marrow Transplant 1992; 9:263.
31. Cross N, Hughes T, Mackinnon S, et al. Minimal residual after allogeneic bone marrow transplantation for chronic myeloid leukaemia in chronic phase: correlations with probability of relapse. Br J Haematol 1993; 84:67.
32. DeLage R, Soiffer R, Dear K, et al. Clinical significance of bcr-abl rearrangement detected by polymerase chain reaction after allogeneic bone marrow transplantation in chronic myelogenous leukemia. Blood 1991; 78:2759.
33. Guerrasio A, Martinelli G, Saglio G, et al. Minimal residual disease status in transplanted chronic myelogenous leukemia patients: low incidence of polymerase chain reaction positive cases among 48 long disease-free subjects who received unmanipulated allogeneic bone marrow transplants. Leukemia 1992; 6:507.
34. Hughes T, Morgan G, Martiat P, et al. Detection of residual leukemia after bone marrow transplant for chronic myeloid leukemia: role of polymerase chain reaction in predicting relapse. Blood 1991; 77:874.
35. Lee M, Kantarjian H, Talpaz M, et al. Detection of minimal residual disease by polymerase chain reaction in Philadelphia chromosome-positive chronic myelogenous leukemia following interferon therapy. Blood 1992; 79:1920.
36. Lion T, Henn T, Gaiger A, et al. Early detection of relapse after bone marrow transplantation in patients with chronic myelogenous leukaemia. Lancet 1993; 341:275.
37. Seong D, Giralt S, Fischer H, et al. Usefulness of detection of minimal residual

disease by "hypermetaphase" fluorescent in situ hybridization after allogeneic BMT for chronic myelogenous leukemia. Bone Marrow Transplant 1997; 19:565–570.
38. Bartram C, de Klein A, Hagemeijer A, et al. Translocation of c-abl oncogene correlates with the presence of a Philadelphia chromosome in chronic myelocytic leukemia. Nature 1983; 306:277.
39. De Klein A, Geurts van Kessel A, Grosfeld G, et al. A cellular oncogene is translocated to the Philadelphia chromosome in chronic myelocytic leukaemia. Nature 1982; 300:765.
40. Kurzrock R, Gutterman J, Talpaz M. The molecular genetics of Philadelphia chromosome-positive leukemias. N Engl J Med 1988; 319:990.
41. Gale R, Canaani E. An 8-kilobase *abl* RNA transcript in chronic myelogenous leukemia. Proc Natl Acad Sci USA 1984; 81:5648.
42. Ben-Neriah Y, Daley GQ, Mes-Masson AM, et al. The chronic myelogenous leukemia specific p210 protein is the product of the bcr/abl hybrid gene. Science 1986; 223:212.
43. Mills K, Benn P, Birnie G. Does the breakpoint within the major cluster region influence the duration of the chronic phase in chronic myeloid leukemia? An analytical comparison of current literature. Blood 1991; 78:1155.
44. Verschraegen CF, Kantarjian HM, Hirsch-Ginberg C, et al. The breakpoint cluster region site in patients with Philadelphia chromosome-positive chronic myelogenous leukemia. Cancer 1995; 76:992–997.
45. Kurzrock R, Kantarjian H, Shtalrid M, et al. Philadelphia chromosome-negative chronic myelogenous leukemia without breakpoint cluster region rearrangement: a chronic myeloid leukemia with a distinct clinical course. Blood 1990; 75:445.
46. Dowding C, Guo AP, Osterholz J, et al. Interferon-α overrides the deficient adhesion of chronic myeloid leukemia primitive progenitor cells to bone marrow stromal cells. Blood 1991; 78:499.
47. Gordon M, Dowding C, Riley G, et al. Altered adhesive interactions with marrow stroma of hematopoietic progenitor cells in chronic myeloid leukemia. Nature 1987; 328:342.
48. Upadhyaya G, Guba S, Sih S, et al. Interferon-alpha restores the deficient expression of the cytoadhesion molecule lymphocyte function antigen-3 by chronic myelogenous leukemia progenitor cells. J Clin Invest 1991; 88:2131.
49. Bhatia R, Wayner E, McGlave P, et al. Interferon-α restores normal adhesion of chronic myelogenous leukemia hematopoietic progenitors to bone marrow stroma by correcting impaired β1 integrin receptor function. J Clin Invest 1994; 94:384.
50. Clarkson B, Strife A. Linkage of proliferative and maturational abnormalities in chronic myelogenous leukemia and relevance to treatment. Leukemia 1993; 7:1683.
51. Daley G, Van Etten R, Baltimore D. Induction of chronic myelogenous leukemia in mice by the $P210^{bcr/abl}$ gene of the Philadelphia chromosome. Science 1990; 247:824.
52. Elefanty AG, Hariharan IK, Cory S. *bcr-abl*, the hallmark of chronic myeloid leukaemia in man, induces multiple haemopoietic neoplasms in mice. EMBO J 1990; 9:1069.

53. Tauci T, Boswell HS, Leibowitz D, Broxmeyer HE. Coupling between p210 bcr/abl and She and Grb2 adaptor proteins in hematopoietic cells permits growth factor-independent link to Ras activation pathway. J Exp Med 1994; 179:167.
54. Puil L, Liu J, Gish G, et al. Bcr-Abl oncoproteins bind directly to activators of the Ras signalling pathway. EMBO J 1994; 13:764.
55. ten Hoeve J, Arlinghaus RB, Guo JQ, Heisterkamp N, Groffen J. Tyrosine phosphorylation of CRKL in Philadelphia$^+$ leukemia. Blood 1994; 84:1731–1736.
56. Druker B, Okuda K, Matulonis U, Salgia R, Roberts T, Griffin JD. Tyrosine phosphorylation of rasGAP and associated proteins in chronic myelogenous leukemia cell lines. Blood 1992; 79:2215.
57. Kantarjian HM, Talpaz M, Dhingra K, et al. Significance of the p210 versus p1990 molecular abnormalities in adults with Philadelphia chromosome-positive acute leukemia. Blood 1991; 78:2411–2418.
58. Mittre H, Leymarie P, Macro M, Leporrier M. A new case of chronic myeloid leukemia with c3/a2 BCR/ABL junction. Is it really a distinct disease? Blood 1997; 89:4239.
59. Gamis A, Haake R, McGlave P, et al. Unrelated-donor bone marrow transplantation for Philadelphia chromosome-positive myelogenous leukemia in children. J Clin Oncol 1993; 11:834.
60. Suri R, Goldman J, Catovsky D, et al. Priapism complicating chronic granulocytic leukemia. Am J Hematol 1980; 9:295.
61. Inbal A, Akstein E, Barak I, et al. Cyclic leukocytosis and long survival in chronic myeloid leukemia. Acta Haematol 1983; 69:353.
62. Dekmezian R, Kantarjian H, Keating M, et al. The relevance of reticulin stain-measured fibrosis at diagnosis in chronic myelogenous leukemia. Cancer 1987; 59:1739.
63. Wilhelm M, Ramos C, O'Brien S, et al. Effect of interferon-alpha therapy on bone marrow fibrosis in chronic myelogenous leukemia. Blood 1996; 88(suppl 1):202b. Abstract.
64. Walters R, Kantarjian H, Keating M, et al. Therapy of lymphoid and undifferentiated chronic myelogenous leukemia in blast crisis with continuous vincristine and adriamycin infusions plus high dose decadron. Cancer 1987; 60:1708.
65. Majlis A, Smith T, Talpaz M, O'Brien S, Rios MB, Kantarjian H. Significance of cytogenetic clonal evolution in chronic myelogenous leukemia. J Clin Oncol 1996; 14:196–203.
66. Cortes J, Kantarjian H, O'Brien S, et al. Suppression of clonal evolution in patients with Philadelphia chromosome-positive chronic myelogenous leukemia on interferon-alpha therapy. Blood 88(suppl 1):232a. Abstract 918.
67. Kolitz J, Kempin S, Schluger A, et al. A phase II pilot trial of high-dose hydroxyurea in chronic myelogenous leukemia. Semin Oncol 1992; 19(suppl 9):27.
68. Hehlmann R, Heimpel H, Hasford J, et al. Randomized comparison of busulfan and hydroxyurea in chronic myelogenous leukemia: prolongation of survival by hydroxyurea. Blood 1993; 82:398.
69. Goldman J, Szydlo R, Horowitz M, et al. Choice of pretransplant treatment and timing of transplants for chronic myelogenous leukemia in chronic phase. Blood 1993; 82:2235.

70. Sokal J, Leong S, Gomez G. Preferential inhibition by cytarabine of CFU-GM from patients with chronic granulocytic leukemia. Cancer 1987; 59:197.
71. Robertson M, Tantravahi R, Griffin J, et al. Hematologic remission and cytogenetic improvement after treatment of stable-phase chronic myelogenous leukemia with continuous infusion of low-dose cytarabine. Am J Hematol 1993; 43:95.
72. Bortin M, Horowitz M, Rowlings P, et al. Report from the International Bone Marrow Transplant Registry. Bone Marrow Transplant 1993; 12:97.
73. Gratwohl A, Hermans J, Niederwieser D, et al. Bone marrow transplantation for chronic myeloid leukemia: long-term results. Bone Marrow Transplant 1993; 12:509.
74. Horowitz MM, Przepiorka D, Champlin RE, et al. Should HLA-identical sibling bone marrow transplants for leukemia be restricted to large centers? Blood 1992; 74:2771.
75. Arcese W, Goldman JM, D'Arcangelo E, et al. Outcome for patients who relapse after allogeneic bone marrow transplantation for chronic myeloid leukemia. Blood 1993; 82:3211.
76. Clift R, Appelbaum F, Thomas E. Bone marrow transplantation for chronic myelogenous leukemia. Blood 1994; 83:2752.
77. Clift RA, Appelbaum FR, Thomas ED. Treatment of chronic myeloid leukemia by marrow transplantation. Blood 1993; 82:1954.
78. Snyder D, Negrin R, O'Donnell M, et al. Fractionated total-body irradiation and high dose etoposide as a preparatory regimen for bone marrow transplantation for 94 patients with chronic myelogenous leukemia in chronic phase. Blood 1994; 84:1672.
79. Biggs J, Szer J, Crilley P, et al. Treatment of chronic myeloid leukemia with allogeneic bone marrow transplantation after preparation with BUCy2. Blood 1992; 82:1352.
80. Storb R, Deeg HJ, Pepe M, et al. Methotrexate and cyclosporine versus cyclosporine alone for prophylaxis of graft-versus-host disease in patients given HLA-identical marrow grafts for leukemia: long-term follow-up of a controlled trial. Blood 1989; 73:1729.
81. Nash RA, McSweeney PA, Storb R, et al. FK506 in combination with methotrexate for the prevention of graft-versus-host disease after marrow transplantation from phenotypically HLA-identical unrelated donors. Blood 1994; 84:394a. Abstract.
82. Goodrich JM, Bowden RA, Fisher L, et al. Ganciclovir prophylaxis to prevent cytomegalovirus disease after allogeneic marrow transplant. Ann Intern Med 1993; 118:173.
83. Goodrich JM, Mori M, Gleaves CA, et al. Early treatment with ganciclovir to prevent cytomegalovirus disease after allogeneic bone marrow transplantation. N Engl J Med 1991; 325:1601.
84. Clift RA, Buckner CD, Appelbaum FR, et al. Allogeneic marrow transplantation in patients with chronic myeloid leukemia in the chronic phase. A randomized trial of two irradiation regimens. Blood 1991; 77:1660.
85. Clift RA, Buckner CD, Thomas ED, et al. Marrow transplantation for chronic myeloid leukemia: a randomized study comparing cyclophosphamide and total body irradiation with busulfan and cyclophosphamide. Blood 1994; 84:2036.

86. Anderson JE, Appelbaum FR, Storb R. Anasetti C. Busulfan and cyclophosphamide with or without total body irradiation as preparative regimens for patients undergoing allogeneic bone marrow transplantation for myelodysplastic syndrome. Blood 1993; 82:377a. Abstract.
87. Kolb HJ, Mittermuller J, Clemm CH, et al. Donor leukocyte transfusions for treatment of recurrent chronic myelogenous leukemia in marrow transplant patients. Blood 1990; 76:2462.
88. Kolb HJ, Schattenberg A, Goldman J, et al. Graft-versus-leukemia effect of donor lymphocyte transfusions in marrow grafted patients. Blood 1995; 86:2041.
89. Antin JH. Graft-versus-leukemia: no longer an epiphenomenon. Blood 1993; 82: 2273.
90. MacKinnon S, Papadopoulos EB, Carabasi MH, et al. Adoptive immunotherapy evaluating escalating doses of donor leukocytes for relapsed chronic myeloid leukemia after allogeneic bone marrow transplantation-separation of graft-versus-host leukemia responses from graft-versus-host disease. Blood 1995; 86:1261.
91. Giralt S, Hester J, Huh Y, et al. CD8+ depleted donor lymphocyte infusion as treatment for relapsed chronic myelogenous leukemia after allogeneic bone marrow transplantation: graft vs leukemia without graft vs host disease. Blood 1994; 84(suppl 1):538a.
92. Giralt S, Champlin R. Leukemia relapse after allogeneic bone marrow transplant: a review. Blood 1994; 83:3603.
93. Mrsic M, Horowitz MM, Atkinson K, et al. Second HLA-identical sibling transplants for leukemia recurrence. Bone Marrow Transplant 1992; 9:269.
94. Higano CS, Raskind WH, Singer JW. Use of α interferon for the treatment of relapse of chronic myelogenous leukemia in chronic phase after allogeneic bone marrow transplantation. Blood 1992; 80:1437.
95. Giralt S, Escudier S, Kantarjian H, et al. Preliminary results of treatment with filgrastim for relapse of leukemia and myelodysplasia after allogeneic bone marrow transplantation. N Engl J Med 1993; 329:757.
96. Tutschka PJ, Copelan EA, Klein JP. Bone marrow transplantation for leukemia following a new busulfan and cyclophosphamide regimen. Blood 1987; 70: 1382.
97. McGlave P, Arthur D, Haake R, et al. Therapy of chronic myelogenous leukemia with allogeneic bone marrow transplantation. J Clin Oncol 1987; 5:1033.
98. Clift R, Buckner C, Thomas E, et al. Marrow transplantation for patients in accelerated phase of chronic myeloid leukemia. Blood 1994; 84:4368.
99. Horowitz MM, Giralt S, Szydlo R, et al. Effect of prior interferon therapy on outcome of HLA-identical sibling bone marrow transplants for chronic myelogenous leukemia in first chronic phase. Blood 1996; 88(suppl 1):682a. Abstract.
100. Giralt S, Kantarjian H, Talpaz M, et al. Effect of prior interferon alpha therapy on the outcome of allogeneic bone marrow transplantation for chronic myelogenous leukemia. J Clin Oncol 1993; 11:1055.
101. Zuffa E, Bandini G, Bonini A, et al. Outcome of allogeneic transplant in CML patients previously treated with alpha-interferon. Analysis in a single institution. Bone Marrow Transplant 1995; 15(S2):S18.
102. Shepherd P, Richards S, Allan N. Survival after allogeneic bone marrow trans-

plantation (BMT) in patients randomized into a trial of IFN-α versus chemotherapy: no significant adverse effect of prolonged IFN-α administration. Blood 1995; 86:94a, Abstract, Suppl 1.
103. Beelen DW, Graeven U, Elmaagacli AH, et al. Prolonged administration of interferon-α in patients with chronic-phase Philadelphia chromosome-positive chronic myelogenous leukemia before allogeneic bone marrow transplantation may adversely affect transplant outcome. Blood 1995; 85:2981.
104. McGlave P, Bartsch G, Anasetti C, et al. Unrelated donor marrow transplantation for chronic myelogenous leukemia: initial experience of the National Marrow Donor Program. Blood 1993; 81:543.
105. Beatty P, Anasetti C, Hansen J, et al. Marrow transplantation from unrelated donors for treatment of hematologic malignancies: effect of mismatching for one HLA locus. Blood 1993; 81:249.
106. Talpaz M, Mavligit G, Keating M, et al. Human leukocyte interferon to control thrombocytosis in chronic myelogenous leukemia. Ann Intern Med 1983; 99:789.
107. Talpaz M, Kantarjian H, McCredie K, et al. Hematologic remission and cytogenetic improvement induced by recombinant human interferon alpha A in chronic myelogenous leukemia. N Engl J Med 1986; 314:1065.
108. Alimena G, Morra E, Lazzarino M, et al. Interferon alpha-2b as therapy for Ph-positive chronic myelogenous leukemia: a study of 82 patients treated with intermittent or daily administration. Blood 1988; 72:642.
109. Ozer H, George S, Schiffer C, et al. Prolonged subcutaneous administration of recombinant alfa-2b interferon in patients with previously untreated Philadelphia chromosome-positive chronic-phase chronic myelogenous leukemia: effect on remission duration and survival. Cancer and Leukemia Group B Study 8583. Blood 1993; 82:2975.
110. Hehlmann R, Heimpel H, Hasford J, et al. Randomized comparison of interferon-α with busulfan and hydroxyurea in chronic myelogenous leukemia. Blood 1994; 84:4064.
111. Ohnishi K, Ohno R, Tomonaga M, et al. A randomized trial comparing interferon-α with busulfan for newly diagnosed chronic myelogenous leukemia in chronic phase. Blood 1995; 86:906.
112. Guilhot F, Abgrall J, Harousseau, J, et al. A multicenter randomized study of alfa 2b interferon and hydroxyurea with or without cytosine-arabinoside in previously untreated patients with Ph+ chronic myelocytic leukemia: preliminary cytogenetic results. Leuk Lymph 1993; 11(suppl 1):181.
113. Guilhot F, Chastang C, Guerci A, et al. Interferon-alpha 2b and cytarabine increase survival and cytogenetic response in chronic myeloid leukemia: results of a randomized trial. Blood 1996; 88(suppl 1):141a. Abstract.
114. Allan NC, Richards SM, Shepherd PCA. Interferon-α therapy with busulphan (BU) or hydroxyurea (HU) compared with either BU or HU alone in treatment of chronic phase CML. Results from MRC CML III Trial. Int J Hematol 1996; 64(suppl 1):S68. Abstract.
115. Schofield J, Robinson W, Murphy J, et al. Low doses of interferon a are as effective as higher doses in inducing remissions and prolonging survival in chronic myeloid leukemia. Ann Intern Med 1994; 121:736.

116. Freund M, von Wussow P, Diedrich H, et al. Recombinant human interferon alpha-2b in chronic myelogenous leukaemia: dose dependency of response and frequency of neutralizing anti-interferon antibodies. Br J Haematol 1989; 72:350.
117. Anger B, Porzsolt F, Leichtle R, et al. A phase I/II study of recombinant interferon alpha 2a and hydroxyurea for chronic myelocytic leukemia. Blut 1989; 58:275.
118. Sacchi S, Kantarjian H, O'Brien S, Cohen PR, Pierce S, Talpaz M. Immune-mediated and unusual complications during interferon alfa therapy in chronic myelogenous leukemia. J Clin Oncol 1995; 13:2401–2407.
119. Talpaz M, Kantarjian H, Kurzrock R, et al. Bone marrow hypoplasia and aplasia complicating interferon therapy for chronic myelogenous leukemia. Cancer 1992; 69:410.
120. O'Brien S. Guidelines for chronic myelogenous leukemia treatment with alpha interferon. Leuk Lymph 1996; 23:247.
121. Seong D, Kantarjian H, Ro J, et al. Hypermetaphase fluorescence in situ hybridization for quantitative monitoring of Philadelphia chromosome-positive cells in patients with chronic myelogenous leukemia during treatment. Blood 1995; 86: 2343.
122. Kurzrock R, Estrov Z, Kantarjian H, Talpaz M. Conversion of interferon-induced, long-term cytogenetic remissions in chronic myelogenous leukemia to PCR negativity. Submitted.
123. Giles F, Aitchison R, Syndercombe-Court D, et al. Recombinant alpha 2B interferon in combination with oral chemotherapy in late chronic phase chronic myeloid leukaemia. Leuk Lymph 1992; 7:99.
124. Kantarjian H, Keating M, Estey E, et al. Treatment of advanced stages of Philadelphia chromosome-positive chronic myelogenous leukemia with interferon-α and low-dose cytarabine. J Clin Oncol 1992; 10:772.
125. Arthur C, Ma D. Combined interferon alfa-2a and cytosine arabinoside as first-line treatment for chronic myeloid leukemia. Acta Haematol 1993; 89(suppl 1): 15.
126. Kantarjian H, O'Brien S, Keating M, et al. Interferon alpha and low-dose cytosine arabinoside therapy in Philadelphia chromosome (Ph) positive chronic myelogenous leukemia. Proc Am Soc Clin Oncol 1997; 16:13a. Abstract.
127. Silver R, Szatrowski T, Peterson B, et al. Combined a-interferon and low dose cytosine arabinoside for Ph+ chronic phase chronic myeloid leukemia. Blood 1996; 88(suppl 1):638a. Abstract.
128. Thaler J, Fluckinger T, Huber H, et al. Treatment of 11 patients with chronic myelogenous leukemia with interferon-alpha-2c and low dose ara-c. Leuk Res 1993; 17:711.
129. Thaler J, Hilbe W, Apfelbeck U, et al. Interferon-alpha-2c and low dose ara-C for the treatment of patients with CML: results of the Austrian multi-center phase II study. Leuk Res 1997; 21:75.
130. Kantarjian HM, Vellekoop L, McCredie KB, et al. Intensive combination chemotherapy (ROAP 10) and splenectomy in the management of chronic myelogenous leukemia. J Clin Oncol 1985; 3:192.
131. Kantarjian HM, Talpaz M, Keating MJ, et al. Intensive chemotherapy induction

followed by interferon-alpha maintenance in patients with Philadelphia chromosome-positive chronic myelogenous leukemia. Cancer 1991; 68:1201.
132. Simonsson B, Oberg G, Kollander A, et al. Intensive treatment in order to minimize the Ph-positive clone in chronic myelogenic leukemia (CML). Bone Marrow Transplant 1994; 14:(suppl 3)S55.
133. Carella AM, Frassoni F, Negrin RS. Autografting in chronic myelogenous leukemia—new questions. Leukemia 1995; 9:365.
134. Kantarjian HM, Talpaz M, Hester J, et al. Collection of peripheral blood diploid cells from chronic myelogenous leukemia patients early in the recovery phase from myelosuppression induced by intensive-dose chemotherapy. J Clin Oncol 1995; 13:553.
135. Chalmers EA, Franklin IM, Kelsey S, et al. Mobilization of Ph-negative peripheral blood stem cells in CML with idarubicin and cytaragine. Bone Marrow Transplant 1994; 14(suppl 3):34.
136. O'Brien S, Kantarjian H, Keating M, et al. Homoharringtonine therapy induces long-term responses in patients with chronic myelogenous leukemia in late chronic phase. Blood 1995; 86:3322.
137. Kantarjian H, O'Brien S, Keating M, et al. Homoharringtonine and low-dose cytosine arabinoside combination therapy has significant activity in patients with late phase Philadelphia chromosome positive chronic myelogenous leukemia. Blood 1996; 88(suppl 1):578a.
138. Ernst T, Shuman L, Grossbard M. Treatment of the chronic phase of CML with a combined continuous infusion of homoharringtonine and cytarabine. Blood 1995; 86(suppl 1):529a. Abstract.
139. O'Brien S, Kantarjian H, Feldman E, et al. Sequential homoharringtonine and interferon produce high hematologic and cytogenetic response rates in Philadelphia chromosome positive chronic myelogenous leukemia. Proc ASCO 1995; 14:336 Abstract.
140. Brito-Babapulle F, Bowcock SJ, Marcus RE, et al. Autografting for patients with chronic myeloid leukaemia in chronic phase: peripheral blood stem cells may have a finite capacity for maintaining haemopoiesis. Br J Haematol 1989; 73:76.
141. McGlave PB, De Fabritis P, Deisseroth A, et al. Autologous transplants for chronic myelogenous leukaemia: results from eight transplant groups. Lancet 1994; 343:1486.
142. Reiffers J, Goldman JM, Meloni JM, et al. Autologous stem cell transplantation in chronic myelogenous leukemia. A retrospective analysis of the European Group for Bone Marrow Transplantation. Bone Marrow Transplant 1994; 14:407.
143. Hoyle C, Gray R, Goldman J. Autografting for patients with CML in chronic phase: an update. Br J Haematol 1994; 86:76.
144. Khouri IF, Kantarjian HM, Talpaz M. High-dose chemotherapy and unpurged autologous stem cell transplantation for chronic myelogenous leukemia: the M.D. Anderson experience. Blood 1994; 84:537a. Abstract.
145. O'Brien SG, Goldman J. Current approaches to hemopoietic stem-cell purging in chronic myeloid leukemia. J Clin Oncol 1995; 13:541.
146. Deisseroth AB, Zu Z, Claxton D, et al. Genetic marking shows that Ph+ cells

present in autologous transplants of chronic myelogenous leukemia (CML) contribute to relapse after autologous bone marrow in CML. Blood 1994; 83:3068.
147. Barnett MJ, Eaves CJ, Phillips GL, et al. Autografting with cultured marrow in chronic myeloid leukemia. Results of a pilot study. Blood 1994; 84:724.
148. Carlo Stella C, Mangoni L, Piovani G, et al. In vitro marrow purging in chronic myelogenous leukemia. Effect of mafosfamide and recombinant granulocyte-macrophage colony-stimulating factor. Bone Marrow Transplant 1991; 8:265.
149. McGlave PB, Arthur D, Miller WJ, et al. Autologous transplantation for CML using marrow treated ex vivo with recombinant human interferon gamma. Bone Marrow Transplant 1990; 6:115.
150. Verfaillie CM, Miller WJ, Boylan K, et al. Selection of benign primitive hematopoietic progenitors in chronic myelogenous leukemia on the basis of HLA-DR antigen expression. Blood 1992; 79:1003.
151. van Denderen J, ten Hacken P, Berendes P, et al. Antibody recognition of the tumor-specific b3-a2 junction of bcr-abl chimeric proteins in Philadelphia-chromosome-positive leukemias. Leukemia 1992; 6:1107.
152. Kirkland MA, O'Brien SG, McDonald C, et al. BCR-ABL antisense purging in chronic myeloid leukaemia. Lancet 1993; 342:614. Letter.
153. Ratajczak MZ, Hijiya N, Catani L, et al. Acute- and chronic-phase chronic myelogenous leukemia colony-forming units are highly sensitive to the growth inhibitory effects of c-myb antisense oligodeoxynucleotides. Blood 1992; 79: 1956.
154. Luger SM, Ratajczak MZ, Stadtmauer EA, et al. Autografting for chronic myeloid leukemia (CML) with C-MYB antisense oligodeoxynucleotide purged bone marrow. A preliminary report. Blood 1994; 84(suppl 1):151a. Abstract.
155. De Fabritiis P, Lisci E, Montefusco M, et al. Autograft after in vitro purging with BCR-ABL antisense oligonucleotides for patients with CML in advanced phase. Bone Marrow Transplant 1994; 14(suppl 3):S80.
156. Talpaz M, Kantarjian H, Liang J, et al. Percentage of Philadelphia chromosome Ph-negative and Ph-positive cells found after autologous transplantation for chronic myelogenous leukemia depends on percentage of diploid cells induced by conventional-dose chemotherapy before collection of autologous cells. Blood 1995; 85:3257–3263.
157. Giralt S, Davis M, O'Brien S, et al. Studies of decitabine with allogeneic progenitor cell transplantation. Leukemia (suppl) 1997. In press.
158. Gewirtz A. Treatment of chronic myelogenous leukemia (CML) with c-myb antisense oligodeoxynucleotides. Bone Marrow Transplant 1994; 14(suppl 3):S57.
159. Rowe J, Ryau H, Nilsson BL, et al. Chronic myelogenous leukemia treated with autologous bone marrow transplantation followed by Roquiminex. Blood 1994; 84:204a. Abstract.
160. Vey N, Baume D, Lafage M, et al. Recombinant interleukin-2 induces cytogenetic responses in patients with chronic myelogenous leukemia in chronic phase. Blood 1996; 88(suppl 1):202b. Abstract.
161. Kantarjian HM, O'Brien SM, Keating M, et al. Results of decitabine therapy in the accelerated and blastic phases of chronic myelogenous leukemia. Leukemia 1997. In press.

162. McGahon A, Bissonnette R, Schmitt M, Cotter KM, Green DR, Cotter TG. BCR-ABL maintains resistance of chronic myelogenous leukemia cells to apoptotic cell death. Blood 1994; 83:1179–1187.
163. Meyskens FK, Kopecky KJ, Appelbaum FR, Balcerzak SP, Samlowski W, Hynes H. Effects of vitamin A on survival in patients with chronic myelogenous leukemia: a SWOG randomized trial. Leuk Res 1995; 19:605–612.
164. Cortes J, Kantarjian H, O'Brien S, Beran M, Keating M, Talpaz M. A pilot study of all-trans retinoic acid in patients with Philadelphia chromosome-positive chronic myelogenous leukemia. Leukemia 1997. In press.
165. Cortes J, Kantarjian H, O'Brien S, et al. GM-CSF can improve the cytogenetic response obtained with interferon-alpha therapy in patients with chronic myelogenous leukemia. Blood 1996; 88(suppl 1):232a. Abstract.
166. Choundhury A, Gajewski J, Liang J, et al. Use of leukemic dendritic cells for the generation of antileukemic cellular cytotoxicity against Philadelphia chromosome-positive chronic myelogenous leukemia. Blood 1997; 89:1133.
167. Martiat P, Lewalle P, Taj A, et al. Retrovirally transduced antisense sequences stably suppress $P210^{BCR/ABL}$ and inhibit the proliferation of bcr/abl-containing cell lines. Blood 1993; 81:502.
168. Estrov Z, Kurzrock R, Wetzler M, et al. Suppression of chronic myelogenous leukemia colony growth by IL-1 receptor antagonist and soluble IL-1 receptors: a novel application for inhibitors of IL-1 activity. Blood 1991; 78:1476.

2
Chronic Myelomonocytic Leukemia

John F. Seymour
Royal Melbourne Hospital, Parkville, Australia

Jorge E. Cortes
M. D. Anderson Cancer Center, Houston, Texas

INTRODUCTION

Chronic myelomonocytic leukemia (CMML) is an uncommon but distinct morphological, molecular, and clinical disorder. At times it can be difficult to clearly distinguish from instances of Philadelphia chromosome-negative chronic myeloid leukemia (CML), underlining the need for specific diagnostic criteria. For many years our understanding of the clinical features, natural history, and optimal therapy of CMML has been hampered by the practice of grouping patients with CMML together with other disease entities in most descriptive and therapeutic studies. Fortunately, with the increasing recognition of the unique aspects of this disease, this practice is becoming less common, thus facilitating the timely evaluation of the emerging therapeutic options for patients and increasing the rate of acquisition of knowledge of the natural history of this disorder.

HISTORY

The first report of a malignancy involving the monocytic lineage was a case of acute monocytic leukemia described by Reschad and Schilling-Torgau in 1913 (1). The existence of a distinct "chronic" counterpart of acute monocytic leukemia was not recognized during this era, although in retrospect a number of reports from the 1930s included cases with a clear smoldering nature (2–4). The 1934 report of Doan and Wiseman (4) made specific note of the concomitant involvement of the myeloid lineage but did not speculate further on the pathogenetic implications of this observation, for at this time it was not considered possible for a leukemic clone to involve the "separate and distinct" myeloid and monocytic lineages.

In his 1937 review Osgood (5) considered 11% of the 133 reported cases of monocytic leukemia from the literature to have displayed a "chronic" course but did not recognize any distinct clinical or morphological features in these "chronic" cases. The first suggestions that the "chronic" form of monocytic leukemia may have distinguishing clinicopathological features came from the reports of Beattie et al. (6) and Sinn and Dick (7) in the 1950s. These authors clearly recognized the predilection for chronic monocytic leukemia to afflict the elderly, preferentially men, and to present with symptomatic anemia and constitutional symptoms. Sinn and Dick (7) specifically noted the common prodrome of refractory anemia, the frequent findings of hepatosplenomegaly and a hypercellular marrow despite peripheral cytopenias, the development of skin involvement late in the natural history of the disorder, and, in distinction from acute monocytic leukemia, the rarity of gum infiltration.

This increasing recognition of "chronic monocytic leukemia" as a distinct disease process was popularized in the early 1970s by Linman (8,9), who additionally noted the frequent occurrence of morphological dysplasia in both the monocyte and myeloid lineages, leading to the promulgation of the term "myelomonocytic." It should be noted, however, that similar cases had been reported a few years earlier without drawing widespread comment (10). The term "myelomonocytic" is now accepted without dispute as a morphologically useful and pathophysiologically accurate descriptor of CMML, but it was not always the case. Indeed the term was first used by Osgood in 1969 (11) in an editorial in the journal Blood in which he ironically argued *against* the dual lineage involvement by the malignant cells of chronic monocytic leukemia, suggesting the myeloid component to be "reactive" in nature.

The 1972 report by Zittoun and colleagues in Paris further popularized the concept of CMML as a discrete and separate clinicopathological entity, although they used the designation "subacute" (12). By 1975, three other European groups reported confirmatory clinical series (13–15), leading to the formal recognition of CMML in the historic 1976 report by the French-American-British Cooperative Group (FAB) (16). They noted the now widely accepted features of a peripheral blood monocytosis ($>1.0 \times 10^9$/L), morphologically atypical monocytes, and variable neutrophilia together with marrow hypercellularity. The current understanding of the morphological features of CMML has not changed significantly since; indeed, Zittoun's 1976 review of the clinical and laboratory features remains an accurate description of this disease despite the passage of two decades (17). A few investigators have suggested that there may be a separate entity of true chronic monocytic leukemia distinct from CMML (18), al-

Table 1 Diagnostic Criteria for CMML According to FAB Classification

Morphological evidence of dysplastic hematopoiesis
Absolute peripheral blood monocytosis ($>1.0 \times 10^9$/L)
Peripheral blood blasts <5%
Bone marrow blasts ≤20%
Auer rods not present

Source: Ref. 19.

though if it indeed does exist, such an entity is exceedingly rare and awaits thorough characterization.

CLASSIFICATION (Myelodysplastic Syndrome Versus Myeloproliferative Disorder)

According to the accepted FAB diagnostic criteria, the defining features of CMML are the presence of an absolute peripheral blood monocytosis of $>1 \times 10^9$/L together with morphological evidence of dysplasia and the absence of Auer rods (Table 1) (19). It is the shared presence of morphological evidence of dysplastic hematopoiesis that persuaded the FAB to include CMML as one of the myelodysplastic syndromes (MDS). Conversely, CMML has a number of distinct manifestations of a proliferative disorder which clearly sets it apart from the other MDS, where bone marrow failure is the dominant manifestation (20). The difficulty in reconciling this duality of features has led to much of the controversy over the optimal classification of this disorder.

A careful recent study by the members of the FAB (21) has demonstrated the feasibility of reproducibly distinguishing CMML from typical or atypical CML and related disorders. In the peripheral blood the major features identified which were able to distinguish CMML were the absence of basophilia, a low percentage of immature granulocytic forms, minimal granulocytic dysplasia, a high percentage of monocytes, and within the marrow an increased proportion of erythroid precursors. Recent excellent reviews have more fully discussed many of these morphological issues (22,23).

INCIDENCE AND ETIOLOGY

There are very few studies which accurately define the incidence of CMML. Earlier studies reported the frequency of CMML relative to other diseases; for example, Zittoun (24) reported that CMML comprised 2.8% of the 1345 adult leukemias seen over a 10-year period in a referral center. A number of studies have reported the frequency of CMML as a percentage of all cases of MDS seen, with most larger series describing incidence figures of between 12% and 22% (25–30) but with one large population-based study reporting 31.2% of all MDS cases to be CMML (31).

There have only been three population-based incidence studies of CMML reported. The most recent of these described an overall incidence of 0.67 cases per 100,000 population per year (1.03 in men and 0.30 in women), with a mean age of 78 years at diagnosis and a steep increase in incidence over the age of 65 years (32). These figures were based on cases diagnosed between 1980 and 1990 in the Cote d'Or region of France and did not show any significant variation in the rate with time over the study period. An earlier study in the Dusseldorf region from 1976 to 1990 described an age-dependent rise in the overall incidence of MDS, peaking in the 70- to 80-year-old age group, with a rising incidence over time, most likely due to changes in diagnostic procedures (33). Over the most recent period of this Dusseldorf study, the annual incidence of CMML was 0.03 per 100,000 population aged <50 years, 0.73 in the 50- to 70-year-old age group, and rising to 3.95 in the population ≥70 years of age, again with a male predominance in all age strata. A third population-based study from the Bournemouth district of the United Kingdom confirmed this age-related increase in incidence, without evidence of a plateau (31). Assuming a constant distribution of MDS subtypes across age strata, the annual incidence of CMML from the Bournemouth study would be 0.16 per 100,000 population aged <50, 4.7 in the 50- to 69-year-old group, and 15.3 in the 70- to 79-year-old age group.

In contrast to the other MDS categories where exposure to environmental or therapeutic mutagens are significant etiological factors, such exposures are apparently very uncommon in patients with CMML. In a review of seven series carefully examining 233 patients with CMML, only 3.4% of patients were found to have an identifiable prior exposure to a potentially mutagenic agent (24). Similarly, the population-based Dusseldorf study (33) did not find a higher-than-expected rate of occupational exposures among CMML cases.

A recent study by Sandler et al. (34) has clearly established a link between cigarette smoking and the development of acute myeloid leukemia in the elderly, particularly those associated with adverse chromosomal abnormalities. Perhaps unexpectedly, this group did not find a significantly increased risk of MDS among smokers, although the total number of cases encountered was small and the wide confidence intervals could not exclude a moderately increased risk (adjusted odds ratio 1.64; 95% confidence interval 0.53–5.07).

There are no data to support any familial risk for the development of CMML, and the only reported predisposing genetic condition is Noonan syn-

Chronic Myelomonocytic Leukemia

drome, a rare autosomal-dominant disorder characterized by facial and skeletal anomalies together with a specific congenital heart disorder (35).

MOLECULAR BIOLOGY AND CYTOGENETICS

Approximately one-third of the patients with CMML have identifiable cytogenetic abnormalities at diagnosis. However, no unique cytogenetic abnormality has been identified in these patients. Among the most frequent cytogenetic abnormalities encountered are monosomy 7, trisomy 8, and abnormalities of the short arm of chromosome 12 (12p) (35a). New chromosomal abnormalities, including isochromosome (17q), may appear as the disease progresses. A translocation involving chromosomes 5 and 12, t(5;12)(q31;p12), has been reported in a small subgroup of patients with CMML who present also with eosinophilia (35b).

Although no disease-specific molecular abnormalities have been identified in patients with CMML, Ras mutations can be found in 57–69% of cases (35c,35d). This incidence is similar to that seen in patients with Philadelphia chromosome-negative, bcr rearrangement-negative CML, and contrasts with the very infrequent occurrence of these mutations in patients with Philadelphia chromosome-positive CML. In patients with the t(5;12), the translocation juxtaposes the PDGF receptor β to a novel ets-like gene, suggesting that a PDGFRβ may participate in the oncogenesis of at least some cases of CMML (35e).

PRESENTING FEATURES

Clinical

In between 15% and 20% of cases, the diagnosis of CMML is established incidentally while the patient is asymptomatic (15,16,36–38). Among patients who are symptomatic, the onset of the disease is usually insidious. The mean duration of symptoms prior to diagnosis described in the literature has ranged from 2.5 to 12 months (15,24,39,40). The median age of patients in published series ranges between 64 and 80 years, corresponding to the reported age distribution of other subtypes of MDS, with more than 90% of patients being over the age of 50 at diagnosis. Cases in childhood are extraordinarily uncommon and are likely to represent misclassified instances of juvenile CML. In his 1992 literature review, Zittoun noted a male predominance (male : female = 1.83) (24), and analysis of seven subsequent series describing more than 430 patients confirms this clear male predominance with a nearly identical ratio of 1.82 : 1.0 (32,41–45).

From the very thorough review of 326 patients in 11 published series by Zittoun (24), the most common symptoms present at diagnosis were fatigue and weight loss (in 25% of patients), symptomatic anemia (31%), infections, often recurrent (19%), and hemorrhagic manifestations (21%).

The spleen is clinically enlarged in 25–40% of patients at diagnosis, although symptomatic splenomegaly is present in <5%, whereas hepatomegaly is found in approximately 30% (24). Although often considered a characteristic feature of CMML, serous effusions are distinctly uncommon at presentation, occurring in only 1–2% of patients. However, they do occur with increasing frequency late in the disease process, and are related to the degree of peripheral blood monocytosis (38,46). Other manifestations of tissue infiltration at diagnosis include lymphadenopathy (in 11% of patients) and leukemic skin infiltrate (2.5%) which usually take the form of widespread erythematous maculopapular lesions. Anecdotal evidence suggests that the appearance of skin infiltration portends an aggressive disease course with a survival of 1 to 3 months from onset in the small series of Duguid et al. (47) but a less adverse outlook in another report (48). Although very common in acute monocytic leukemia, gum infiltration is rare in CMML; in fact, it was not described at presentation in any of 198 patients from five series where this was specifically sought (13,36,37,40,49).

Although the actual incidence is uncertain, some investigators have reported an increased risk of autoimmune phenomena (including polymyalgia rheumatica, inflammatory bowel disease, and cutaneous vasculitis) in patients with CMML (50,51,51a).

Hematological

Except for the monocytosis, most peripheral blood manifestations of CMML are nonspecific. From a review of 220 patients from nine series, anemia was present in 83% of patients, although this was usually mild to moderate (24). Thrombocytopenia was present in 56% of patients, although a platelet count of $<75 \times 10^9$/L was seen in only 20% of cases. By definition, all patients must have a peripheral blood monocyte count of $>10 \times 10^9$/L. This is usually in the range of $2–5 \times 10^9$/L, but in approximately 25% of patients is minimal ($1–2 \times 10^9$/L). Monocyte counts of as high as $10–30 \times 10^9$/L are reported, but extremely uncommon at diagnosis. Most patients will also have a moderate degree of neutrophilia contributing to the reported median leukocyte count at presentation of $10–50 \times 10^9$/L (13–16,37,40,49,52,53). In contrast to patients with CML, the degree of left shift in the myeloid series in the peripheral blood is usually minimal, although very occasional blasts may be present, and eosinophilia or basophilia are not characteristically seen.

As with the other MDS, the bone marrow is usually hypercellular; in patients with CMML this is due to both granulocytic and monocytic hyperplasia. Blasts may be increased, but are usually <5% (by definition, according to the FAB, those with >20% blasts are classified as having refractory anemia with excess blasts in transformation—RAEBt). The diagnosis of CMML requires the presence of morphologic dysplasia, although the degree is usually less than that seen in other types of MDS. Dysplastic monocytes (hyperlobulation, cytoplasmic granules, increased basophilia) are usually prominent, with promonocytes being more frequently seen in the marrow than the peripheral blood (54). Some degree of marrow fibrosis is recognized in up to 15% of cases (13,37, 40,49).

Although the FAB's definition of CMML specifically excludes those patients with recognizable Auer rods, it is not clear that this is biologically or prognostically justified (55). The few patients who present with the features of CMML but are classified according to the FAB definition as having RAEBt solely on the basis of the presence of Auer rods, have clinical features and a survival expectation indistinguishable from other patients with CMML and probably should be considered to have an identical disease process and be treated equivalently (56).

Laboratory

A characteristic feature of the disease is a greatly increased serum or urinary lysozyme level in 70–95% of cases, reflecting an increased monocyte pool (57,58). The serum lysozyme level is directly proportional to the monocyte count (59). As observed in the spectrum of myeloproliferative disorders, serum levels of vitamin B_{12} and the transcobalamins may be elevated in up to 80% of patients with CMML, although these are of a much lesser degree than seen in CML.

Although not recognized in many of the early series, the serum level of LDH is very commonly elevated in patients with CMML. In the four published studies with LDH data, between 50% and 73% of patients have levels above the upper limit of normal (39,43,45,60). In the authors' experience, serial measurements of the serum level of LDH are also a useful surrogate indicator of disease activity. As with other myeloproliferative disorders, the serum level of uric acid has been reported to be elevated in 35% of patients with CMML at diagnosis (43).

Additionally, the presence of polyconal hypergammaglobulinemia has been reported in up to 30% of patients, monoclonal immunoglobulin bands in as many as 12%; Coombs' positivity has also been described infrequently in patients with CMML.

Table 2 Survival of Patients with CMML from Selected Reported Series

Author	No. patients	Median survival	Risk of transformation
Alessandrino 1985 (36)	30	18 months	No data
Mufti 1985 (25)	31	22 months	13%
Group Français 1986 (61)	120	27.4 months	No data
Kerkhofs 1987 (27)	35	>60 months	18% @ 5 years
Fenaux 1987 (37)	60	28 months	22%
Ribera 1987 (39)	29	8.2 months	24%
Stark 1987 (59)	97	18 months	4%
Worsley 1988 (38)	53	17 months	13%
Fenaux 1988 (41)	107	30 months	17%
Sanz 1989 (29)	70	12 months	15% @ 5 years
Tefferi 1989 (42)	41	36 months	24%
del Cañizo 1989 (43)	70	12 months	14% @ 3 years
Storniolo 1990 (62)	30	41 months	53%
Aul 1992 (30)	25	19 months	0%
Morel 1993 (63)	125	21 months	16% @ 2 years
Aul 1994 (45)	43	16 months	9%
Catalano 1996 (64)	77	17 months	14% (@ median 8 mo.)

NATURAL HISTORY (Distinguishing Features from CML)
Survival

The major feature in the natural history of CMML distinguishing it from typical CML is the absence of the classical triphasic pattern of disease evolution. In patients with CMML, the disease pattern is most commonly one of gradual progression without a distinct "blastic" phase. The frequency of transformation to acute leukemia, conventionally defined as the attainment of ≥30% bone marrow blasts, has ranged from 0% to 53% (Table 2). However, most series report transformation rates of 10–25% at 3–5 years (Table 2) (65). Given the median survival of 12–30 months reported from most series, this indicates that the majority of patients with CMML succumb to their leukemia while still in a "chronic" phase. This distinct pattern of evolution is shared by patients given the diagnosis of Philadelphia chromosome-negative, BCR-negative CML, supporting the contention that this disease is indistinguishable from CMML (66). Also distinct from the findings in CML, patients with advanced CMML usually manifest increasing degrees of visceral infiltration, serous effusions, and leukemia cutis, in addition to worsening cytopenias and progressive peripheral blood monocytosis.

Prognostic Factors

Following the recognition of CMML as a distinct clinical entity, investigators were struck by the extremely variable disease course, and much early work focused on attempts to identify patients whose outlook justified intervention with the relatively ineffective therapies available. Despite the widespread acceptance of the diagnostic criteria proposed by the FAB, many of these early studies are difficult to accurately interpret due to the use of what are now considered to be nonstandard diagnostic criteria allowing the inclusion of patients with a lesser degree of peripheral blood monocytosis (27,37,62) or with 20–30% bone marrow blasts (37,40,41). Whether such rigid distinctions are biologically justified, however, is a separate and unresolved issue.

Largely due to the rarity of CMML, many analyses of prognostic factors reported used only univariate analysis, or had inadequate patient numbers for informative multivariate analysis. The factors predictive of an inferior survival in these univariate analyses are given in Table 3. Based on studies in other categories of MDS, many of these studies emphasized the influence of peripheral blood cytopenias on outcome. However, it should be noted that numerous

Table 3 Adverse Prognostic Factors in CMML—Univariate Analyses

Adverse prognostic factors	References
WBC >10.0	36,41,43
Marrow blasts >5%	30,36,41–43,62,67
Blasts present in the peripheral blood	36,41,43,67
Anemia (<13 g/dL male, <11.5 g/dL female)	27,41–43,67
Neutropenia (<1.8)	27
Thrombocytopenia (<50 or <140 × 10^9/L)	27
(continuous variable)	39,41
Pseudo-Pelger-Huet anomaly	27
Monoclonal protein	27
Splenomegaly	39,41
Peripheral blood monocyte count	
(continuous variable)	39
(≥5.0 × 10^9/L)	59
(>2.6 × 10^9/L)	38,41
Raised serum lysozyme	41,59
Neutrophilia	
(>16 × 10^9/L)	38
(continuous variable)	41
Elevated serum LDH	30
Erythroblasts in the peripheral blood	43
Bone marrow cellularity >80%	43

studies also reported the adverse influence of various indicators of the "proliferative" component of CMML: increased bone marrow blasts, the presence of circulating blasts, splenomegaly, the peripheral blood monocyte count, the degree of neutrophilia, and an elevated serum LDH level (Table 3).

The development of the "Bournemouth score" was the first attempt to synthesize these prognostic factors into a predictive index (25). In this model based on a cohort of 141 patients with various MDS, including 31 with CMML, a score of 1 point is allocated for the presence of any of the following: bone marrow blasts $\geq 5\%$; platelets $\leq 100 \times 10^9$/L; hemoglobin ≤ 10.0 g/dL; and neutrophils $\leq 2.5 \times 10^9$/L (Table 4). When the whole cohort of 141 patients where then grouped according to the derived score (0 or 1, 2 or 3, and 4), survival was significantly different, ranging from a median of 62 months (score of 0 or 1) to 8.5 months (score of 4).

Although very useful in the other categories of myelodysplasia, the Bournemouth score was unfortunately not able to stratify patients with CMML (Table 4). This failure was attributed to the rarity of neutropenia in patients with CMML. To address this deficiency, Worsley et al. (38) subsequently proposed a "modified Bournemouth score" specifically for patients with CMML which allocated 1 point for the presence of any of the following: bone marrow blasts $>5\%$; platelets $<100 \times 10^9$/L; hemoglobin <10.0 g/dL; and neutrophils <2.5 or $>16 \times 10^9$/L. When the resulting scores were grouped as 0 or 1, versus ≥ 2, survival was significant different ($p < 0.001$) (Table 5). Although able to identify patients with a differing prognosis, these indices are relatively crude and did not fully utilize the discriminatory capacity of the features associated with the "proliferative" component of the disease process.

After the publication of the modified Bournemouth score, larger clinical studies were published which included multivariate analyses of factors associated with survival specifically in CMML (Table 6). The factors consistently found to be associated with a shorter survival are bone marrow blasts $>5\%$,

Table 4 Criteria for the Bournemouth Score in CMML

Score 1 point for the presence of any of:
- bone marrow blasts $\geq 5\%$
- platelets $\leq 100 \times 10^9$/L
- hemoglobin ≤ 10.0 g/dL
- neutrophils $\leq 2.5 \times 10^9$/L

Median survival of patients with CMML according to the Bournemouth score:
- Score of 0 or 1 (84% of patients) 23 months
- Score of 2 or 3 (16% of patients) 11 months
- Score of 4 (no patients included)

Source: Ref. 25.

Table 5 Criteria for the "Modified" Bournemouth Score in CMML

Score 1 point for the presence of any of:
- bone marrow blasts >5%
- platelets <100 × 10^9/L
- hemoglobin <10.0 g/dl
- neutrophils <2.5, or >16.0 × 10^9/L

Median survival:
- Score of 0 or 1: 32 months
- Score of 2, 3, or 4: 8.9 months

Source: Ref. 38.

anemia, thrombocytopenia, higher blood monocyte counts, and an elevated serum LDH level. In 1992 Aul et al. (30), based in Dusseldorf, proposed another modification of a prognostic scoring system for patients with MDS. One of the aims of the group was to develop a system which was equally applicable to patients with CMML as with other categories of MDS. The major innovation was the incorporation of the serum LDH level (Table 7). Unlike the Bournemouth score, the "Dusseldorf score," as it soon became known, was able to discriminate effectively among patients with CMML. This was confirmed in the analysis of a second independent cohort of patients by the same group (45).

There are few studies available that specifically address the possible prognostic significance of cytogenetic abnormalities in patients with CMML. The study of Kerkhofs et al. (27) arbitrarily grouped patients into those with "single" or "complex" abnormalities. With a total of only nine of the 26 analyzed patients with CMML having cytogenetic abnormalities of either category, not surprisingly they were unable to demonstrate any prognostic impact of cytogenetics. The larger study of Morel et al. (63) included 125 patients with CMML among a total of 408 patients with MDS. In the whole cohort by multivariate analysis they found a markedly inferior outcome for those patients with complex cytogenetic abnormalities (those involving at least three chromosomes). Unfortunately, no separate analysis of the CMML patients was performed. However, the recent study of Wattel et al. (68) demonstrates the applicability of these findings specifically to patients with CMML. Within the randomized therapeutic study of hydroxyurea versus VP-16, these investigators analyzed the prognostic significance of karyotype. By multivariate analysis within each treatment arm, the presence of either complex cytogenetic abnormalities or isolated monosomy 7 were associated with inferior survival (both $p \leq 0.001$) (Fig. 1).

Currently, both the modified Bournemouth score (38) and the Dusseldorf score (30,45) are similarly able to segregate patients with CMML into two groups of comparable size with median survivals of approximately 1 year and 2.5–3 years, respectively. Although the poor-prognosis group derived by either

Table 6 Adverse Prognostic Factors in CMML—Multivariate Analyses

Reference	No. patients	Adverse prognostic factors
Solal-Celigny 1984 (40)	35	No factors identified
Fenaux 1987 (37)	60	Elevated bone marrow blasts
		Lower hemoglobin
		Higher blood monocyte count
Ribera 1987 (39)	29	Splenomegaly
		Blood monocyte count (continuous)
Stark 1987 (59)	97	Elevated serum lysozyme level
Worsley 1988 (38)	53	Modified Bournemouth score
Fenaux 1988 (41)	107	Bone marrow blasts (continuous)
		Anemia (continuous)
Tefferi 1989 (42)	41	Bone marrow blasts >5%
del Cañizo 1989 (43)	70	WBC >10.0 × 10^9/L
		bone marrow blasts >5%
Aul 1992 (30)	25	Bone marrow blasts >5%
		Elevated serum LDH
		Hemoglobin ≤9 g/dL
		Platelets ≤100 × 10^9/L
Aul 1994 (45)	43	Bone marrow blasts >5%
		Anemia ≤9 g/dL
		Platelets ≤100 × 10^9/L
		Elevated serum LDH
		Increasing age
Catalano 1996 (64)	77	Thrombocytopenia
		Anemia
		Leukocytosis
Wattel 1996 (68)	105	Anemia (not further specified)
		Complex karyotype[a]/monosomy 7

[a]See text for details.

index is relatively homogeneous, with a 2-year survival expectation of approximately 20%, neither index is able to identify the 30% of "good-prognosis" patients who are destined to die in the first year following diagnosis, nor the 20–30% of patients with a genuinely "chronic" leukemia who will remain alive with stable disease beyond 5 years. Further studies are needed in this area to allow accurate identification of these patients.

None of the currently applied prognostic indices utilize any cytogenetic or molecular data. With the increasing realization of the cytogenetic and molecular heterogeneity of patients with CMML, these features are likely to provide the capacity to identify more homogeneous prognostic categories.

Table 7   Criteria for the Düsseldorf Score in CMML

Score 1 point for the presence of any of:
- bone marrow blasts ≥5%
- elevated serum LDH
- hemoglobin ≤9.0 g/dL
- platelets ≤100 × 10^9/L

Median survival:
- Score of 0: No patients included
- Score of 1 or 2 (58% of patients): 32 months
- Score of 3 or 4 (42% of patients): 11 months

Source: Ref. 30.

THERAPY

There are two major difficulties in evaluating the published literature on the treatment of patients with CMML: there are no uniformly accepted response criteria, and most reports have included patients with CMML in studies with other categories of MDS without describing outcomes separately. In comparative studies, the lack of accepted response criteria can be overcome through the use of survival as the primary endpoint. This is not applicable to single-arm Phase II studies. In this setting responses have traditionally been assessed through the description of degree of reduction in organomegaly, amelioration of cytopenias, or reduction in monocytosis. Unfortunately, the details of such criteria vary among studies, making literature comparisons impossible. Further, it is unclear whether the attainment of any of these response criteria has any favorable impact on the natural history of the disease or result in improved survival or quality of life for patients.

More recently, the more rigid and reproducible criteria for complete remission developed for acute myeloid leukemia have been applied to therapeutic studies in CMML. The designation of complete remission (CR) usually requires normalization of peripheral blood counts and white cell differential, absence of morphological dysplasia, a normocellular bone marrow without increased blasts or monocytes, and, where initially abnormal, reversion to a diploid karyotype. In the following discussion, this definition of CR is used as the major measure of efficacy of therapy.

VP-16

There are four small single-institution reports documenting the activity of VP-16 in CMML (69–72). Of the total of 25 patients reported, 17 were claimed by the authors to have obtained some degree of hematological or clinical benefit, although only one patient attained a CR as defined above. The doses of VP-16 used varied from 50 mg orally twice weekly to 50 mg/day for 10–20 days repeated at monthly intervals. Although the majority of responses were claimed for the higher-dose schedule (72), response criteria and patient characteristics are too variable to conclude that a definite dose-response relationship exists. These encouraging early results provided the basis for the randomized comparison of VP-16 with hydroxyurea discussed below.

Hydroxyurea

Hydroxyurea is considered by most clinicians to be standard treatment for patients with CMML who manifest proliferative disease features. This conclusion appears to be based more on clinical experience than on published prospective studies, as there are very few Phase II data thoroughly evaluating the efficacy of hydroxyurea, or indeed any other agents, in patients with CMML. In retrospective series where treatment details are provided, the proportion of patients with CMML treated with hydroxyurea has ranged from 8% (39) to 71% (40), reflecting physician preference.

The recently published results of a prospective randomized study of hydroxyurea versus oral VP-16 in patients with poor-prognosis CMML has provided objective data to support the role of hydroxyurea as the standard treatment of patients not participating in clinical trials (68). In this European collaborative project, previously untreated patients fulfilling the FAB definition of CMML (but with up to 30% bone marrow blasts allowed) without molecular evidence of the Philadelphia chromosome were eligible if they had poor prognostic features, as defined by either:

1. Presence of two or more of (a) neutrophils $>16 \times 10^9$/L, (b) hemoglobin <10 g/dL, (c) platelets $<100 \times 10^9$/L, (d) bone marrow blasts >5%, or (e) splenomegaly >5 cm
2. Visceral involvement (other than spleen, liver, or lymph nodes)

Both treatment arms specified a dose escalation schema for initially nonresponsive patients, and the definition of CR was as discussed above, but the investigators additionally defined "good" and "minor" responses on the basis of control of myeloproliferative features and diminished organomegaly. Between October 1991 and October 1994, 105 patients were randomized. The baseline features were balanced between the treatment arms and were typical of patients with CMML in that the median age was 71 years, 70% were male, and a very small percentage of patients had skin infiltrate (8.6%) or serous effusions (2.9%). The objective response rates (sum of complete, good, and minor responses) were relatively low in both treatment arms, but significantly favored hydroxyurea; 60% (2% CR) vs. 36% (0% CR) ($p = 0.02$). Other indices of therapeutic efficacy

Chronic Myelomonocytic Leukemia

also favored hydroxyurea over VP-16; median time to response (2.1 versus 3.5 months; $p = 0.003$), median response duration (24 vs. 9 months; $p = 0.0004$). Overall survival was the primary endpoint of the study, and this also revealed a major advantage for hydroxyurea-treated patients—median survival 20 months vs. 9 months ($p < 10^{-4}$) (Fig. 2).

This study is noteworthy for a number of reasons. This is the first report of a prospectively randomized study specifically and exclusively designed to address a therapeutic question in patients with CMML. The results discussed above clearly establish the superiority of hydroxyurea over VP-16 in this patient group, but also suggest that the application of effective cytoreductive treatment actually prolongs survival. The extremely low CR rate of 2% with hydroxyurea is in striking contrast to the demonstrated survival benefit. This suggests that the attainment of CR (as defined) is an unduly restrictive surrogate endpoint for therapeutic efficacy in CMML. However, there are currently no alternative objective and reproducible measures of biologic activity. Thus, while establishing hydroxyurea as an interim "gold standard," the demonstrated survival benefit also provides a great impetus for the development of more effective therapies, utilizing both more active single agents, and rationally designed combination therapies, with the recognition of the great need for prognostically meaningful and objectively verifiable surrogate endpoints for drug activity.

Low-Dose ara-C

In the early 1980s there was much enthusiasm for the use of low-dose ara-C in an attempt to induce leukemic cell differentiation, rather than cytotoxicity. The experimental basis for this mode of action of ara-C is tenuous, and the capacity of the drug to induce such terminal differentiation in vivo remains to be proven. Regardless, a number of small studies have specifically reported the results of this therapy in patients with CMML (Table 8), although it should be noted that five of the reports described five or fewer patients, making both selection and reporting biases likely. Nevertheless, the overall confirmed CR rate was 13.8% (95% confidence intervals 7.1–23%), with very few data on response duration reported. Despite the low dose of ara-C, the majority of patients developed significant cytopenias on therapy consistent with a predominantly cytotoxic action, and two studies described therapy-related deaths.

This apparently modest efficacy should be seen in perspective, however. As discussed above, hydroxyurea, the gold standard treatment of CMML, induced a CR in only 2% patients in a randomized study. If the claimed degree of activity of ara-C in CMML is confirmed in larger prospective studies, it would certainly be an active agent with the potential for either combination or sequential use with other cytotoxics. The potential for GM-CSF to enhance leukemic cell survival and proliferation discussed below suggests that the addition

Table 8 Low-Dose ara-C in CMML

Author	No. pts.	No. CR (%)	Comments
Solal-Celigny 1984 (40)*	6	4 (67)	10 mg/m^2 SC bd for 21–25 days
Cheson 1986 (73)	11	2 (18)	Literature review, cases from Solal-Celigny 1984 (40) excluded
Fenaux 1986 (37)	2	0 (0)	Patients may be also be included in subsequent report (74)
Fenaux 1987 (74)	17	1 (6)	2 fatal toxicities, median survival 2.5 months
Powell 1988 (75)	4	1 (25)	No toxic deaths
Aul 1989 (76)*	12	1 (8)	2 deaths on therapy, CR duration = 4 months
Höffken 1990 (77)	2	0 (0)	With concurrent GM-CSF
Hellström-Lindberg 1992 (78)	5	0 (0)	2 partial responses (5-month duration)
Miller 1992 (79)	8	0 (0)	Randomized study vs supportive care; no advantage in ara-C
Aul 1992 (80)	9	2 (22)	Literature review; cases marked "*" have been excluded
Gerhartz 1994 (81)	4	0 (0)	With concurrent GM-CSF
Total	**80**	**11 (13.8)**	**95% confidence intervals for CR rate 7.1–23.0%**

of this growth factor to treatments such as low-dose ara-C with a very low likelihood of eradication of the malignant clone is of questionable benefit, and may indeed be detrimental.

A study by Hellström-Lindberg et al. (78) attempted to identify patients with MDS likely to obtain a hematologic response from treatment with low-dose ara-C. This study included only five patients with CMML. They identified a platelet count of $>150 \times 10^9$/L as the major predictor of response (overall objective response rate of 55%). Among patients with a platelet count below this level, the following factors were associated with a greater likelihood of response: bone marrow cellularity <70%; absence of ringed sideroblasts; and fewer than two chromosomal aberrations. By applying a derived scoring system, they identified patient groups with low (3%), intermediate (24%), and high (53%) response rates to low-dose ara-C. It is unclear, however, whether this scoring system is applicable specifically to patients with CMML.

6-Mercaptopurine

Although 6-mercaptopurine has been reported as the primary treatment of patients with CMML in as many as 77% of patients in some series (39), there are no published response data on which to base such use.

Busulfan

As with many of the other agents discussed, retrospective series have anecdotally described the effective use of this agent in patients with CMML (39,42), although no estimate of the objective response rate is possible.

Anthracyclines

There are few data available on the efficacy of single-agent anthracyclines in CMML. Small series have described the used of oral idarubicin, with either intermittent dosing (82) or a low-dose chronic administration schedule (83). None of the seven patients with CMML included in these reports obtained an objective response. Further, two patients with CMML were included in a Phase II study of low-dose intravenous aclarubicin, again without evidence of biological activity (84).

Intensive Chemotherapy

Standard induction therapy for patients with acute myeloid leukemia usually consists of 7 days of ara-C together with an anthracycline. A number of studies have prospectively applied such intensive treatment strategies to younger patients with CMML. The available data are summarized in Table 9. Overall, 29.7% of the 37 patients reported attained a CR (95% confidence intervals 15.9–47.0%). Where reported, the duration of these remissions was relatively brief. Although the number of patients reported is small, those regimens lacking an anthracycline (85,89,91) appear to have a similar response rate to those incorporating such drugs. The lack of any evidence for the activity of single-agent anthracyclines in patients with CMML discussed above raises some doubts as to the therapeutic value of the anthracycline component of these therapies. Certainly additional studies of novel anthracyclines are warranted. However, in the interim, it is possible that dose-intensive single-agent ara-C may be as effective as, and certainly less toxic than, anthracycline-containing combinations. Although patient selection on the basis of age and other factors is likely to influence the reported outcome for various therapeutic strategies, it does appear that intensive chemotherapy regimens incorporating ara-C are more likely to attain

Table 9 Results of Intensive Chemotherapy in CMML

Author	Regimen	No. patients	Median age (range)	No. CR (%)	Comments
Mertelsmann 1980 (85)	Ara-C & 6-TG (& daunorubicin in 1)	10	51.5	5 (50)	4 pts. with Auer rods excluded from original report, median remission duration 6.2 mo.
Armitage 1981 (86)	Variable	7	70 (44–79)	0 (0)	Median survival 1 mo., anthracycline and/or Ara-C applied in only 3 pts.
Fenaux 1988 (87)	Ara-C & rubidazone	2	39 (21–56)	0 (0)	1 toxic death
Fenaux 1991 (88)	Ara-C & zorubicine	7	54 (18–68)	2 (29)	1 toxic death, median survival 10 mo.
Estey 1994 (89)	Fludarabine & Ara-C (& G-CSF in 5)	7	Not given	2 (29)	All patients had cytogenetic abnormality and/or platelets $<50 \times 10^9/L$
de Witte 1995 (90)	Ara-C & idarubicin	4	46	2 (50)	8% toxic death rate among whole cohort of 50 pts., median age is for entire cohort.
Total		37	—	11 (29.7%)	95% confidence intervals 15.9–47.0%

a complete remission than "low-dose" ara-C regimens. Whether this higher CR rate would translate into an overall survival benefit for patients remains unproven, but probable.

Vitamin D Derivatives and Retinoids

There is a large body of preclinical data demonstrating the capacity of vitamin D derivatives to stimulate the terminal differentiation of leukemic cell lines and primary cultures of leukemic blasts (92). The initial attempts to apply such "differentiation induction" therapy clinically in patients with MDS were limited by a high frequency of the development of hypercalcemia (93). However, a few patients with CMML have been so treated, and the report of a single patient who attained a prolonged complete morphological remission following treatment with oral 25-OH-vitamin D (94) demonstrates that this approach to treatment has significant potential and merits further investigation once noncalcemic analogs of vitamin D reach clinical trials.

Based on a similar principle of differentiation-induction, a number of retinoid derivatives have been applied in patients with various forms of MDS, including a small number of patients with CMML (95–97), with seven of 22 assessable patients manifesting some degree of hematological improvement with 13-*cis*-retinoic acid, but none of three attaining a major response to all-*trans*-retinoic acid alone (98). Many patients are intolerant of long-term retinoid therapy, and although not impacting on the moderate efficacy, the addition of alpha-tocopherol has been reported to reduce the toxicity of 13-*cis*-retinoic acid compared with historical controls (99). Similarly, a more recent study reported the use of all- trans-retinoic acid in combination with low-dose oral hydroxyurea in 10 patients with CMML (100); there were no complete hematological responses seen. However, this study did note interesting biological activity, with two patients developing manifestations suggestive of the "ATRA syndrome" as first described in patients with acute promyelocytic leukemia receiving all-*trans*-retinoic acid (101). These patients had a rapid rise in white cell count, unexplained fever, fluid retention, and pulmonary infiltrates. It was not clear whether the rise in white cell count was due to proliferation, or differentiation of the malignant clone. A number of patients treated with the combination of all-*trans*-retinoic acid and hydroxyurea had a significant improvement in cytopenias, reduction in transfusion requirements, or disappearance of organomegaly, although the relative contribution of the all-*trans*-retinoic acid versus the hydroxyurea is uncertain.

Hexamethylene Bisacetamide (HMBA)

Together with DMSO, HMBA is a member of the class of polar-planar solvents which have significant capacity to induce the terminal differentiation of transformed cell lines in vitro (102). This property leads to the evaluation of HMBA in patients with MDS in two studies, including six patients with CMML (103,104). Based on in vitro data, the agent has been administered by prolonged continuous intravenous infusion at 20–24 g/m^2/day. The 5-day administration schedule studied of Rowinsky et al. did not induce any meaningful hematologic improvements in four patients, despite achieving the targeted plasma HMBA levels of 1–2 nM (103). Conversely, one of the two CMML patients treated with 10 days of HMBA by Andreeff et al. achieved a 4-month partial remission and resolution of leukemia skin infiltrates (104). The majority of patients treated in both studies developed significant and at times prolonged posttreatment cytopenias, suggesting that the few beneficial responses may not be solely attributable to any putative differentiative actions of HMBA. Transient adverse neurological and metabolic effects were seen less frequently.

Although some promising biologic activity was seen with HMBA, the low rate of responses together with the prominent cytopenias suggest that as currently applied, this agent may be acting as a cytotoxic, rather than differentiating, agent. Further preclinical evaluation of the emerging novel polar-planar compounds may lead to more effective application in patients with CMML.

Bone Marrow Transplantation

As with the other MDS, allogeneic bone marrow transplantation is often touted as a potentially curative therapy for patients with CMML (105). As with the other categories of MDS, the upper age limit for eligibility of 50–60 years and the low frequency of HLA-matched siblings or alternative donors, render this therapy even hypothetically applicable to a small minority of patients with CMML. Further, the few published cases of the use of allogeneic bone marrow transplantation do not yet allow us to conclude that the potential for cure has been proven, although this is likely to be the case. There are reports from five groups describing series of allogeneic transplants in MDS which include a total of 15 adult patients with CMML (106–113). The high degree of selection is evidenced by the median age of patients from these series ranging from 23 to 41 years. The preparative regimens used were variable: busulfan and cyclophosphamide; cyclophosphamide and TBI; busulfan, cyclophosphamide and TBI; or busulfan and VP-16. As with most other therapeutic studies in MDS, it is often difficult to specifically determine the outcome of the patients with CMML. The first reported cases were from the City of Hope hospital (111,112) and described two patients with CMML. One died from procedure-related complications, and the other remained alive in ongoing CR 3 years posttransplant. Nevill et al. (109) also describe a single patient with CMML alive in ongoing CR beyond 2 years. Overall, these series have described nonrelapse mortality rates of 32–68% and very consistent relapse rates of 19–28%, resulting in overall disease-free survival rates of 23–45% at 3–6 years posttransplant. The Seattle group has attempted to identify factors predictive of outcome for patients with MDS who undergo an allogeneic bone marrow transplant and have reported age <40 years, the use of combination GVHD prophylaxis including methotrexate, and a normal karyotype as the major determinants of overall survival in multivariate analysis (106,107). Again, the applicability of these factors specifically to patients with CMML remains speculative. Overall, there are certainly data to support the further investigation of allogeneic bone marrow transplantation in patients with CMML; however, the consistent relapse rate suggests that novel disease-directed preparative regimens are required. Given the high procedure-related mortality rates, the development of effective preparative regimens without unacceptable toxicity will be a difficult task. The observation that the use of a donor other than a matched sibling may diminish the incidence of disease relapse suggests that immunotherapeutic strategies may be worth pursuing, even in the absence of total myeloablative therapy (113a).

Topotecan

The recently reported studies from the M.D. Anderson identify topotecan, a topoisomerase-I inhibitor, as one of the most active agents in CMML (114,115). A total of 60 patients with MDS, including 30 with CMML, were treated with 2 mg/m^2 of topotecan by continuous intravenous infusion over 24 hours daily for 5 days, with courses repeated every 4–8 weeks according to toxicity. Full data have been presented for the first 25 CMML patients treated (114), who did not appear to be highly selected, with 84% aged 60 years or older and the majority manifesting both anemia and thrombocytopenia prior to treatment. A true CR, including disappearance of cytogenetic abnormalities where initially present, was obtained in six of 16 previously untreated patients (38%) and one of nine (11%) previously treated patients (overall CR rate 28%), and lasted a median of 7.5 months. However, 17% of patients died from myelosuppression-related complications during treatment, and the period of pancytopenia was relatively prolonged. For responders, the median time to recovery of granulocytes above 0.5×10^9/L was 24 days and platelets above 30×10^9/L was 25 days. This period of pancytopenia was complicated by documented infection in 47% of patients, and grade 3 or 4 mucositis in 19% of patients.

This study has clearly demonstrated the potent activity of topotecan against CMML, however, with substantial associated morbidity and mortality using this schedule in an elderly patient group. It is unknown whether lower doses or alternative schedules may improve the therapeutic index of topotecan. Given that this agent has obtained the highest CR rate of any of the single agents investigated to date in CMML, it is a high priority to optimize its delivery and to explore combination regimens.

Interferons

Given the striking efficacy of interferon-α (IFN-α) in CML and the similarities between this disease and CMML, there was significant enthusiasm regarding the application of IFN-α in CMML. Most early series included a small number of CMML patients together with other MDS categories (116–121), and only one study specifically in patients with CMML has been reported (122). The doses applied have been in the lower range, usually between 3×10^6 units 3 days per week and 3×10^6 units/m^2/day, with all reported studies describing the use of single-agent IFN-α. Overall, 31 patients have been reported, with just one complete response of 9.5 months described (118). Evidence of biological activity with reduced monocytosis, improved neutrophil or platelet counts, or diminished transfusion requirements were documented in a total of 16 patients (52%). Although the studies have been generally small, it does appear that IFN-α has greater efficacy in patients with CMML than in other MDS, consistent with its "myeloproliferative" character. There are no data available on the potential effectiveness of IFN-α maintenance following chemotherapeutic cytoreduction. Given the moderate activity displayed in these studies, this application of IFN-α merits further investigation, particularly given the availability of new agents with a greater capacity to induce true complete remissions in this disease.

Conversely, the few available data do not suggest that IFN-γ is an agent worth pursuing in patients with CMML. The one patient treated progressed to frank AML on therapy (123).

Nucleoside Analogs

2-Chlorodeoxyadenosine (2-CdA) a purine nucleoside analog with proven efficacy in indolent lymphoproliferative disorders, particularly hairy cell leukemia (124), has been studied in patients with CMML. Krieger et al. (125) treated seven elderly patients with CMML using 0.2 mg/kg/day of 2-CdA for 5 days every 4 weeks for a planned three cycles. All patients demonstrated a rapid reduction in peripheral blood monocyte counts with the first cycle of therapy, and overall, one patient attained a CR of 4 months' duration, and four patients attained partial responses of 3- to 6-month durations. The major complications were those associated with myelosuppression and subsequent infectious complications. This degree of activity confirms the initial observation of Tallman et al. (126) in four patients with CMML treated with 2-CdA 0.1 mg/kg/day for 5–7 days. Although no patients achieved a sustained response in this study, the mean monocyte count was reduced from 14.0 before treatment to 0.62 after just one cycle of 2-CdA therapy. Based on the initial experience in this small group of patients, 2-CdA has major biological activity and certainly merits further investigation in CMML.

Chronic Myelomonocytic Leukemia

The other class of nucleoside analogs under active investigation in CMML and other myelodysplastic syndromes are 5-azacytidine and 5-aza-2'-deoxycytidine, analogues of 2'-deoxycytidine (127). In early studies in heterogeneous groups of patients with MDS (including CMML), both of these agents demonstrated the capacity to induce trilineage hematological improvements (128–132), although patients with CMML were not analyzed separately. Where specific data have been provided for CMML patients (133), 5-aza-2'-deoxycytidine was able to produce complete remissions in two of six patients without unacceptable toxicity, establishing this as another active agent in this disease. Given the in vitro data demonstrating synergistic cytotoxicity with 2'-deoxy-5-azacytidine and topotecan (134), another active single agent in CMML, such combination studies merit further investigation.

Colony-Stimulating Factors

In the early years of the clinical application of the hematopoietic colony-stimulating factors, patients with CMML were occasionally included in studies primarily designed to investigate the capacity of either G-CSF or GM-CSF to ameliorate the neutropenia associated with bone marrow failure states and MDS (135). The reported studies contain an aggregate of seven patients with CMML who were treated with GM-CSF (136–139). All four of the patients described who received "standard" doses of 100–500 $\mu g/m^2$/day had clear evidence of acceleration of their disease with increases in both peripheral blood and marrow blasts (136–137). Thus the use of standard-dose GM-CSF treatment in patients with CMML appears detrimental. Of interest, one of two patients treated with significantly lower doses of 5–10 $\mu g/m^2$/day manifested improved neutrophil counts in the absence of signs of disease acceleration (138), raising the prospect that in some cases there may be a potentially safe dose range for this factor.

This evidence of disease acceleration by GM-CSF is consistent with the observation that a proportion of cases of CMML, like juvenile CML (140), display hypersensitivity to exogenous GM-CSF (141). GM-CSF has been proposed to have an autocrine role in the proliferation of CMML cells, based on the observations that conditioned media from the growth of fresh CMML cells contain biologically active GM-CSF (142) and that neutralizing antibodies to GM-CSF inhibit spontaneous colony formation (143).

There are no clinical data available relating to the safety or efficacy of G-CSF in this setting (144), although the published in vitro data suggest that CMML cells do not proliferate in response to G-CSF.

An area of recent active investigation in the treatment of patients with CMML is the possible therapeutic role of growth-inhibitory cytokines. Initial studies focused on interleukin-4 following a report documenting potent suppression of spontaneous colony formation by fresh CMML cells in vitro (143). This inhibitory effect was suggested to be mediated via inhibition of autocrine production of both GM-CSF and IL-6, two potent stimulatory factors for CMML cells (142). However more recent studies suggest that this inhibitory capacity is frequently lost during disease progression, with many patients with advanced CMML having enhanced proliferation in response to IL-4 (145). This is consistent with the preliminary results from clinical studies of IL-4 in patients with advanced CMML where profound disease stimulation was seen.

Interleukin-10 has a number of negative-regulatory activities within the immune and hematopoietic systems (146,147). Preliminary reports of in vitro colony formation studies with fresh patient leukemic cells have demonstrated a profound, specific, dose-dependent inhibition of spontaneous colony formation by IL-10 in 10 of 11 cases studied (148). This inhibitory effect could be overcome by the addition of exogenous GM-CSF, and abolished by the addition of exogenous GM-CSF (148). These observations, together with the demonstration of reduced GM-CSF mRNA expression in leukemic cells following treatment with IL-10, demonstrate that one mode of action of IL-10 is through the inhibition of autocrine GM-CSF secretion by CMML cells (148,149). There are no clinical studies of IL-10 in patients with CMML yet reported, but the above laboratory studies provide a compelling rationale for such trials.

If indeed IL-10 does act solely through inhibition of autocrine GM-CSF production, similar beneficial effects may be achieved by direct antagonism of GM-CSF. An inhibitory peptide analog of GM-CSF, known as E21R, has been developed which selectively binds to the GM-CSF receptor α-chain while preventing subsequent interaction of the resulting complex with the GM-CSF receptor β-chain, which is essential for signal transduction (150). In vitro E21R is completely devoid of any agonist activity and is able to completely, and specifically, antagonize the proliferative actions of GM-CSF on cells lines and primary human cultures of human AML cells, resulting in apoptotic cell death (151). As yet, there are no data available on the effects of E21R on the spontaneous colony growth of CMML cells in vitro. However, this analog has shown potent inhibitory action against primary cultures of juvenile CML cells (152), which are similarly hypersensitive to exogenous GM-CSF.

Other growth factors that have been reported to enhance the proliferation or colony formation by CMML cells include IL-6 (142) and IL-3 (140), making interruption of these pathways in vivo also a potential therapeutic target in this disease. The observation of greatly enhanced, but reversible, monocytosis in one of three patients with CMML included in a Phase I study of IL-3 is consistent with its potential role as a proliferative stimulus in this disorder (153).

Other Agents

Small retrospective series have suggested a benefit from danazol, 200 mg orally three times daily, in improving the platelet count in patients with MDS, including CMML (154). A newly developed therapeutic agent, bryostatin, which may act through the protein kinase C pathway, has demonstrated the capacity to inhibit the spontaneous colony formation by CMML cells in vitro (155), making it an appealing agent to explore in future studies in this disease.

REFERENCES

1. Reschad H, Schilling-Torgau V. Ueber eine neue leukämie durch echte uebergangsformen (splenozytenleukämie) und ihre bedeutung für die selbstständigkeit dieser zellen. München Med Wchnschr 1913; 60:1981–1984.
2. Böhne C, Huismans L. Beiträge zur kenntnis der chronischen leukämischen reticuloendotheloisen. Virch Arch Path Physiol Klin Med 1932; 283:575–592.
3. Orr JW, Belf MD. Monocytic leukæmia: two cases. Lancet 1933; 1:403–407.
4. Doan CA, Wiseman BK. The monocyte, monocytosis, and monocytic leukosis: a clinical and pathological study. Ann Intern Med 1934; 8:383–416.
5. Osgood EE. Monocytic leukemia: report of six cases and review of the one hundred and twenty-seven cases. Arch Intern Med 1937; 59:931–951.
6. Beattie JW, Seal RME, Crowther KV. Chronic monocytic leukaemia. Q J Med 1951; 20:131–139.
7. Sinn CM, Dick FW. Monocytic leukemia. Am J Med 1956; 20:588–602.
8. Linman JW. Myelomonocytic leukemia and its preleukemic phase. J Chron Dis 1970; 22:713–716.
9. Saarni MI, Linman JW. Myelomonocytic leukemia: disorderly proliferation of all marrow cells. Cancer 1971; 27:1221–1230.
10. Seligsohn U, Ramot B. Chronic monocytic leukemia: a case with an eight year survival. Isr J Med Sci 1967; 3:868–874.
11. Osgood EE. Acute monocytic leukemia as an explanation for "hiatus leukemicus" and "myelo-monocytic leukemia." Blood 1969; 3:268–273.
12. Zittoun R, Bernadou A, Bilski-Pasquier G, Bousser J. Les leucémies myélo-monocytaires subaiguës. Étude de 27 cas et revue de la littérature. Semin Hop Paris 1972; 48:1943–1956.
13. Miescher PA, Farquet JJ. Chronic myelomonocytic leukemia in adults. Semin Hematol 1974; 11:129–139.
14. Sexauer J, Kass L, Schnitzer B. Subacute myelomonocytic leukemia: clinical, morphological and ultrastructural studies of 10 cases. Am J Med 1974; 57:853–861.
15. Geary CG, Catovsky D, Wiltshaw E, et al. Chronic myelomonocytic leukaemia. Br J Haematol 1975; 30:289–302.
16. Bennett JM, Catovsky D, Daniel M-T, et al. Proposals for the classification of the acute leukaemias. French-American-British (FAB) Co-operative Group. Br J Haematol 1976; 33:451–458.
17. Zittoun R. Subacute and chronic myelomonocytic leukaemia: a distinct haematologic entity. Br J Haematol 1976; 32:1–7.
18. Bearman RM, Kjeldsberg CR, Pangalis GA, Rappaport H. Chronic monocytic leukemia in adults. Cancer 1981; 48:2239–2255.

19. Bennett JM, Catovsky D, Daniel MT, et al. Proposals for the classification of the myelodysplastic syndromes. Br J Haematol 1982; 51:189–199.
20. Michaux J-L, Martiat P. Chronic myelomonocytic leukaemia (CMML)—a myelodysplastic or myeloproliferative syndrome? Leuk Lymph 1993; 9:35–41.
21. Bennett JM, Catovsky D, Daniel MT, et al. The chronic myeloid leukaemias: guidelines for distinguishing chronic granulocytic, atypical chronic myeloid, and chronic myelomonocytic leukaemia. proposals by the French-American-British Cooperative Leukaemia Group. Br J Haematol 1994; 87:746–754.
22. Kouides P, Bennett JM. Morphology and classification of the myelodysplastic syndromes and their pathologic variants. Semin Hematol 1996; 33:95–110.
23. Rosati S, Anastasi J, Vardiman J. Recurring diagnostic problems in the pathology of the myelodysplastic syndromes. Semin Hematol 1996; 33:111–126.
24. Zittoun R. Chronic myelomonocytic leukemia. In: Mufti GJ, Galton DAG, eds. The Myelodysplastic Syndromes. Edinburgh: Churchill Livingstone, 1992:65–88.
25. Mufti GJ, Stevens JR, Oscier DG, Hamblin TJ, Machin D. Myelodysplastic syndromes: a scoring system with prognostic significance. Br J Haematol 1985; 59:425–433.
26. Vallespì T, Torrabadella M, Julia A, et al. Myelodysplastic syndromes: a study of 101 cases according to the FAB classification. Br J Haematol 1985; 61:83–92.
27. Kerkhofs H, Hermans J, Haak HL, Leeksma CHW. Utility of the FAB classification for myelodysplastic syndromes: investigation of prognostic factors in 237 cases. Br J Haematol 1987; 65:73–81.
28. Group Francais de Morphologie Hematologique. French registry of acute leukemia and myelodysplastic syndromes: age distribution and hemogram analysis of the 4496 cases recorded during 1982–1983 and classified according to FAB criteria. Cancer 1987; 60:1385–1394.
29. Sanz GF, Sanz MA, Vallespí T, et al. Two regression models and a scoring system for predicting survival and planning treatment in myelodysplastic syndromes: a multivariate analysis of prognostic factors in 370 patients. Blood 1989; 74:395–408.
30. Aul C, Gattermann N, Heyll A, Germing U, Derigs G, Schneider W. Primary myelodysplastic syndromes: analysis of prognostic factors in 235 patients and proposals for an improved scoring system. Leukemia 1992; 6:52–59.
31. Williamson PJ, Kruger AR, Reynolds PJ, Hamblin TJ, Oscier DG. Establishing the incidence of myelodysplastic syndrome. Br J Haematol 1994; 87:743–745.
32. Maynadié M, Verret C, Moskovtchenko P, et al. Epidemiological characteristics of myelodysplastic syndrome in a well-defined French population. Br J Cancer 1996; 74:288–290.
33. Aul C, Gattermann N, Schneider W. Age-related incidence and other epidemiological aspects of myelodysplastic syndromes. Br J Haematol 1992; 82:358–367.
34. Sandler DP, Shore DL, Anderson JR, et al. Cigarette smoking and risk of acute leukemia: associations with morphology and cytogenetic abnormalities in bone marrow. J Natl Cancer Inst 1993; 85:1994–2002.
35. Bader-Meunier B, Tchernia G, Thomas C, Dommergues JP. Occurrence of chronic myelomonocytic leukemia (CMML) in patients with the Noonan syndrome. Br J Haematol 1996; 93(suppl 2):68. Abstract 265.

35a. Groupe Francais de Cytogenetique Hematologique. Cytogenetics of chronic myelomonocytic leukemia. Cancer Genet Cytogenet 1986; 21:11–30.
35b. Wessels JW, Fibbe WE, van der Keur D, et al. t(5;12)(q31;p12): a clinical entity with features of both myeloid leukemia and chronic myelomonocytic leukemia. Cancer Genet Cytogenet 1993; 65:7–11.
35c. Padua RA, Carter G, Hughes D, et al. RAS mutations in myelodysplasia detected by amplification, oligonucleotide hybridization, and transformation. Leukemia 1988; 2:503–510.
35d. Hirsch-Ginsberg C, LeMaistre AC, Kantarjian H, et al. RAS mutations are rare events in Philadelphia chromosome-negative/bcr gene rearrangement-negative chronic myelogenous leukemia, but are prevalent in chronic myelomonocytic leukemia. Blood 1990; 76:1214–1219.
35e. Golub TR, Barker GF, Lovett M, Gilliland DG. Fusion of PDGF receptor β to a novel ets-like gene, tel, in chronic myelomonocytic leukemia with t(5;12) chromosomal translocation. Cell 1994; 77:307–316.
36. Alessandrino EP, Orlandini E, Brusamolino E, et al. Chronic myelomonocytic leukemia: clinical features, cytogenetics, and prognosis in 30 consecutive cases. Hematol Oncol 1985; 3:147–155.
37. Fenaux P, Jouet JP, Zandecki M, et al. Chronic and subacute myelomonocytic leukaemia in the adult: a report of 60 cases with special reference to prognostic factors. Br J Haematol 1987; 65:101–106.
38. Worsley A, Oscier DG, Stevens J, et al. Prognostic features of chronic myelomonocytic leukaemia: a modified Bournemouth score gives the best prediction of survival. Br J Haematol 1988; 68:17–21.
39. Ribera JM, Cervantes F, Rozman C. A multivariate analysis of prognostic factors in chronic myelomonocytic leukaemia according to the FAB criteria. Br J Haematol 1987; 65:307–311.
40. Solal-Celigny P, Desaint B, Herrera A, et al. Chronic myelomonocytic leukemia according to FAB classification: analysis of 35 cases. Blood 1984; 63:634–638.
41. Fenaux P, Beuscart R, Lai JL, Jouet JP, Bauters F. Prognostic factors in adult chronic myelomonocytic leukemia: an analysis of 107 cases. J Clin Oncol 1988; 6:1417–1424.
42. Tefferi A, Hoagland HC, Therneau TM, Pierre RV. Chronic myelomonocytic leukemia: natural history and prognostic determinants. Mayo Clin Proc 1989; 64:1246–1254.
43. del Cañizo MC, Sanz G, San Miguel JF, et al. Chronic myelomonocytic leukemia—clinicobiological characteristics: a multivariate analysis in a series of 70 cases. Eur J Haematol 1989; 42:466–473.
44. Goasguen J-E, Garand R, Bizet M, et al. Prognostic factors of myelodysplastic syndromes—a simplified 3-D scoring system. Leuk Res 1990; 14:255–262.
45. Aul C, Gattermann N, Germing U, Runde V, Heyll A, Schneider W. Risk assessment in primary myelodysplastic syndromes: validation of the Düsseldorf score. Leukemia 1994; 8:1906–1913.
46. Mufti GJ, Oscier DG, Hamblin TJ, Nightingale A, Darlow S. Serous effusions in monocytic leukaemias. Br J Haematol 1984; 58:547–552.

47. Duguid JKM, Mackie MJ, McVerry BA. Skin infiltration associated with chronic myelomonocytic leukaemia. Br J Haematol 1983; 53:257–264.
48. Copplestone JA, Oscier DG, Mufti GJ, Hamblin TJ. Monocytic skin infiltration in chronic myelomonocytic leukemia. Clin Lab Haematol 1986; 8:115–119.
49. Briére J, Dresch C, Briére JF, Faille A. Leucémies myélomonocytaires subaiguës ou chroniques de l'adulte. Étude clinique et données cinétiques à propos de 46 observations. Actualités Hématol 1977; 10:53–80.
50. Kouides P, Bennett J. Myelodysplastic syndromes. In: Abeloff M, Armitage J, Lichter A, et al., eds. Clinical Oncology. New York: Churchill Livingstone, 1995: 1977–1995.
51. Poullin P, Saddier P, Nicolino-Brunet C, et al. Evidence of immunologic abnormalities in myelodysplastic syndromes. A matched case-control study. Br J Haematol 1996; 93(suppl 2):66. Abstract 257.
51a. Hebbar M, Kozlowski D, Wattel E, et al. Association between myelodysplastic syndromes and inflammatory bowel diseases. Report of seven new cases and review of the literature. Leukemia 1997; 11:2188–2191.
52. Hurdle ADF, Garson OM, Buist DGP. Clinical and cytogenetic studies in chronic myelomonocytic leukaemia. Br J Haematol 1972; 22:773–782.
53. Ohyashiki K, Ohyashiki J, Oshimura M, et al. Cytogenetic and in vitro culture studies on chronic myelomonocytic leukemia. Cancer 1984; 54:2468–2474.
54. Ho PJ, Gibson J, Vincent P, Joshua D. The myelodysplastic syndromes: diagnostic criteria and laboratory evaluation. Pathology 1993; 25:297–304.
55. Seymour JF, Estey EH. The contribution of Auer rods to the classification and prognosis of myelodysplastic syndromes. Leuk Lymph 1995; 17:79–85.
56. Seymour JF, Estey EH. The prognostic significance of auer rods in myelodysplasia. Br J Haematol 1993; 85:67–76.
57. Perillie PE, Kaplan SS, Lefkowitz E, Rogarvay W, Finch S. Studies of muramidase (lysozyme) in leukemia. JAMA 1968; 203:317–322.
58. Perillie PE, Finch SC. Muramidase studies with Philadephia chromosome-positive and chromosome-negative chronic granulocytic leukemia. N Engl J Med 1970; 283:456–459.
59. Stark AN, Thorgood J, Head C, Roberts BE, Scott CS. Prognostic factors and survival in chronic myelomonocytic leukaemia (CMML). Br J Cancer 1987; 56: 59–63.
60. Garcia S, Sanz MA, Amigo V, et al. Prognostic factors in chronic myelodysplastic syndromes: a multivariate analysis in 107 cases. Am J Hematol 1988; 27:163–168.
61. Group Français de Cytogénétique Hématologique. Cytogenetics of chronic myelomonocytic leukemia. Cancer Genet Cytogenet 1986; 21:11–30.
62. Storniolo AM, Moloney WC, Rosenthal DS, Cox C, Bennett JM. Chronic myelomonocytic leukemia. Leukemia 1990; 4:766–770.
63. Morel P, Hebbar M, Lai J-L, et al. Cytogenetic analysis has strong independent prognostic value in de novo myelodysplastic syndromes and can be incorporated in a new scoring system: a report on 408 cases. Leukemia 1993; 7:1315–1323.
64. Catalano L, Improta S, de Laurentiis M, et al. Prognosis of chronic myelomonocytic leukemia. Haematologica 1996; 81:324–329.
65. Hornsten P, Wahhlin A, Rudolphi O, Nordenson I. Myelodysplastic syndromes—a

population based study on transformation and survival. Acta Oncol 1995; 34:473–478.
66. Kurzrock R, Kantarjian HM, Shtalrid M, Gutterman JU, Talpaz M. Philadelphia chromosome-negative chronic myelogenous leukemia without breakpoint cluster region rearrangement: a chronic myeloid leukemia with a distinct clinical course. Blood 1990; 75:445–452.
67. Zittoun R, Cardiou M, Kouzan S. Les éléments du prognostic des leucémies myélo-monocytaires subaiguës et chroniques. Ann Med Interne 1982; 133:80–83.
68. Wattel E, Guerci A, Hecquet B, et al. A randomized trial of hydroxyurea versus VP-16 in adult chronic myelomonocytic leukemia. Blood 1996; 88:2480–2487.
69. Labedzki L, Illiger HJ. Erfolgreiche behandlung der chronischen myelomonozytären leukämie mit VP 16-213. Blut 1979; 38:421–424.
70. Oscier DG, Worsley A, Hamblin TJ, Mufti GJ. Treatment of chronic myelomonocytic leukaemia with low dose etoposide. Br J Haematol 1989; 72:468–471.
71. Sato K, Ushijima T, Ohbayashi Y, Sato H, Urabe A. Low-dose etoposide in the treatment of chronic myelomonocytic leukemia. Rinsho Ketsueki 1990; 31:521–522.
72. Doll DC, Kasper LM, Sanchez-Deeter R, Taetle R, List AF. Low dose oral etoposide is effective treatment for chronic myelomonocytic leukemia (CMML). Blood 1994; 84(suppl 1):518a. Abstract 2059.
73. Cheson BD, Jasperse DM, Simon R, Friedman MA. A critical appraisal of low-dose cytosine arabinoside in patients with acute non-lymphocytic leukemia and myelodysplastic syndromes. J Clin Oncol 1986; 4:1857–1864.
74. Fenaux P, Jouet JP, Bauters F. Low-dose cytosine arabinoside in adult chronic myelomonocytic leukemia. J Clin Oncol 1987; 5:1129–1130. Letter.
75. Powell BL, Capizzi RL, Jackson DV, et al. Low dose ara-C for patients with myelodysplastic syndromes. Leukemia 1988; 3:153–156.
76. Aul C, Schneider W. The role of low-dose cytosine arabinoside and aggressive chemotherapy in advanced myelodysplastic syndromes. Cancer 1989; 64:1812–1818.
77. Höffken K, Overkam F, Stirbu J, et al. Recombinant human granulocyte-macrophage colony-stimulating factor and low-dose cytosine arabinoside in the treatment of patients with myelodysplastic syndromes. A Phase II study. Onkologie 1990; 13:33–37.
78. Hellström-Lindberg E, Robèrt K-H, Gahrton G, et al. A predictive model for the clinical response to low dose ara-C: a study of 102 patients with myelodysplastic syndromes or acute leukemia. Br J Haematol 1992; 81:503–511.
79. Miller KB, Kyungmann, K, Morrison FS, et al. The evaluation of low-dose cytarabine in the treatment of myelodysplastic syndromes: a Phase-III intergroup study. Ann Hematol 1992; 65:162–168.
80. Aul C, Gatterman N. The role of low-dose chemotherapy in myelodysplastic syndromes. Leuk Res 1992; 16:207–215.
81. Gerhartz HH, Marcus R, Delmer A, et al. A randomized phase II study of low-dose cytosine arabinoside (LD-AraC) plus granulocyte-macrophage colony-stimulating factor (rhGM-CSF) in myelodysplastic syndromes (MDS) with a high risk of developing leukemia. Leukemia 1994; 8:16–23.

82. Lowenthal RM, Lambertenghi-Deliliers G. Oral idarubicin as treatment for advanced myelodysplastic syndrome. Haematologica 1991; 76:398–401.
83. Greenberg BR, Reynolds RD, Charron CB, et al. Treatment of myelodysplastic syndromes with daily oral idarubicin. A phase I–II study. Cancer 1993; 71:1989–1992.
84. Shibuya T, Teshima T, Harada M, Taniguchi S, Okamura S-I, Niho Y. Treatment of myelodysplastic syndrome and atypical leukemia with low-dose aclarubicin. Leuk Res 1990; 14:1611–1617.
85. Mertelsmann R, Thaler HT, To L, et al. Morphological classification, response to therapy, and survival in 263 patients with acute nonlymphoblastic leukemia. Blood 1980; 56:773–781.
86. Armitage JO, Dick FR, Needleman SW, Burns CP. Effect of chemotherapy for the dysmyelopoietic syndrome. Cancer Treat Rep 1981; 65:601–605.
87. Fenaux P, Lai JL, Jouet JP, Pollet JP, Bauters F. Aggressive chemotherapy in adult primary myelodysplastic syndromes. A report on 29 cases. Blut 1988; 57:297–302.
88. Fenaux P, Morel P, Rose C, Lai JL, Jouet JP, Bauters F. Prognostic factors in adult de novo myelodysplastic syndromes treated by intensive chemotherapy. Br J Haematol 1991; 77:497–501.
89. Estey E, Thall P, Andreeff M, et al. Use of granulocyte colony-stimulating factor before, during, and after fludarabine plus cytarabine induction therapy of newly diagnosed acute myelogenous leukemia or myelodysplastic syndromes: comparison with fludarabine plus cytarabine without granulocyte colony-stimulating factor. J Clin Oncol 1994; 12:671–678.
90. de Witte T, Suciu S, Peetermans M, et al. Intensive chemotherapy for poor prognosis myelodysplasia (MDS) and secondary acute myeloid leukemia (sAML) following MDS of more than 6 months duration. A pilot study by the Leukemia Cooperative Group of the European Organisation for Research and Treatment of Cancer (EORTC-LCG). Leukemia 1995; 9:1805–1811.
91. Estey E, Pierce S, Kantarjian H, et al. Treatment of myelodysplastic syndromes with AML-type chemotherapy. Leuk Lymph 1993; 11(suppl 2):59–63.
92. Paquette RL, Koeffler HP. Differentiation therapy. Hematol/Oncol Clin North Am 1992; 6:687–706.
93. Mehta AB, Kumaran TO, Marsh GW, McCarthy DM. Treatment of advanced myelodysplastic syndrome with alfacalcidiol. Lancet 1984; 2:761.
94. Mellibovsky L, Díez A, Nogues X, Pérez-Vila E, Serrano S, Recker RR. Longstanding remission after 25-OH D3 treatment in a case of chronic myelomonocytic leukaemia. Br J Haematol 1993; 85:811–812.
95. Gold EJ, Mertelsmann RH, Itri LM, et al. Phase I clinical trial of 13-*cis*-retinoic acid in myelodysplastic syndromes. Cancer Treat Rep 1983; 67:981–986.
96. Greenberg BR, Durie BGM, Barnett TC, Meyskens FL Jr. Phase I–II study of 13-*cis*-retinoic acid in myelodysplastic syndrome. Cancer Treat Rep 1985; 69:1369–1374.
97. Koeffler HP, Heitjan D, Mertelsmann R, et al. Randomized study of 13-*cis*-retinoic acid versus placebo in the myelodysplastic disorders. Blood 1987; 71:703–708.

98. Kurzrock R, Estey E, Talpaz M. All-*trans*-retionoic acid: tolerance and biologic effects in myelodysplastic syndrome. J Clin Oncol 1993; 11:1489–1495.
99. Besa EC, Abrahm JL, Bartholomew MJ, Hyzinski M, Nowell PC. Treatment with 13-*cis*-retinoic acid in transfusion-dependent patients with myelodysplastic syndrome and decreased toxicity with addition of alpha-tocopherol. Am J Med 1990; 89:739–747.
100. Cambier N, Wattel E, Menot ML, Guerci A, Chomienne C, Fenaux P. All-*trans*-retinoic acid in adult chronic myelomonocytic leukemia: results of a pilot study. Leukemia 1996; 10:1164–1167.
101. Frankel SR, Eardley A, Lauwers G, Weiss M, Warrell R. The "retinoic acid syndrome" in acute promyelocytic leukemia. Ann Intern Med 1992; 117:292–301.
102. Spremulli EN, Dexter DL. Polar solvents: a novel class of antineoplastic agents. J Clin Oncol 1984; 2:227–241.
103. Rowinsky EK, Conley BA, Jones RJ, Spivak JL, Auerbach M, Donehower RC. Hexamethylene bisacetamide in myelodysplastic syndrome: effect of five-day exposure to maximal therapeutic concentrations. Leukemia 1992; 6:526–534.
104. Andreeff M, Stone R, Michaeli J, et al. Hexamethylene bisacetamide in myelodysplastic syndrome and acute myelogenous leukemia: a phase II clinical trial with a differentiation-inducing agent. Blood 1992; 80:2604–2609.
105. de Witte T, Gratwhol A. Bone marrow transplantation for myelodysplastic syndrome and secondary leukaemias. Br J Haematol 1993; 84:361–364.
106. Anderson JE, Applebaum FR, Fisher LD, et al. Allogeneic bone marrow transplantation for 93 patients with myelodysplastic syndrome. Blood 1993; 82:677–681.
107. Anderson JE, Applebaum FR, Storb R. An update on allogeneic marrow transplantation for myelodysplastic syndrome. Leuk Lymph 1995; 17:95–99.
108. Anderson JE, Appelbaum FR, Schoch G, et al. Allogeneic marrow transplantation for myelodysplastic syndrome with advanced disease morphology: a phase II study of busulfan, cyclophosphamide, and total-body irradiation and analysis of prognostic factors. J Clin Oncol 1996; 14:220–226.
109. Nevill TJ, Shepherd JD, Reece DE, et al. Treatment of myelodysplastic syndrome with busulfan-cyclophosphamide conditioning followed by allogeneic BMT. Bone Marrow Transplant 1992; 10:445–450.
110. de Witte T, Zwaan F, Hermans J, et al. Allogeneic bone marrow transplantation for secondary leukaemia and myelodysplastic syndrome: a survey by the Leukaemia Working Party of the European Bone Marrow Transplantation Group (EB-MTG). Br J Haematol 1990; 74:151–157.
111. O'Donnell MR, Nademanee AP, Snyder DS, et al. Bone marrow transplantation for myelodysplastic and myeloproliferative syndromes. J Clin Oncol 1987; 5:1822–1826.
112. Forman SJ, O'Donnell MR, Blume KG, Feinstein DI. Allogeneic bone marrow transplantation as primary therapy for chronic myelomonocytic leukemia. Blut 1987; 54:189–192.
113. Demuynck H, Verhoef GEG, Zachee P, et al. Treatment of patients with myelodysplastic syndromes with allogeneic bone marrow transplantation from genotypically HLA-identical siblings and alternative donors. Bone Marrow Transplant 1996; 17:745–751.

113a. Grigg A, Bardy P, Seymour JF, Szer J. Fludarabine-based non-myeloablative chemotherapy followed by infusion of HLA-identical stem cells for relapsed leukemia and lymphoma. Bone Marrow Transpl 1998, in press.
114. Beran M, Kantarjian H, O'Brien S, et al. Topotecan, a topoisomerase I inhibitor, is active in the treatment of myelodysplastic syndrome and chronic myelomonocytic leukemia. Blood 1996; 88:2473–2479.
115. Beran M, O'Brien S, Estey E, Keating M, Kantarjian H. Topotecan, a topoisomerase I inhibitor, induces complete remissions in myelodysplastic syndrome (MDS) and chronic myelomonocytic leukemia (CMML). Blood 1996; 88(suppl 1):580a. Abstract 2308.
116. Elias L, Hoffman R, Boswell S, Tensen L, Bonnem EM. A trial of recombinant α-interferon in the myelodysplastic syndromes. I. Clinical results. Leukemia 1987; 1:105–111.
117. Gisslinger H, Chott A, Linkesch W, Fritz E, Ludwig H. Long-term α-interferon therapy in myelodysplastic syndromes. Leukemia 1990; 4:91–94.
118. Nand S, Ellis T, Messmore H, Fisher SG, Gaynor E, Fisher RI. A phase II study of interferon alpha 2a in myelodysplastic syndromes. Blood 1990; 76(suppl):303a. Abstract 1203.
119. Aul C, Gattermann N, Schneider W. Treatment of advanced myelodysplastic syndromes with recombinant interferon-alpha2b. Eur J Haematol 1991; 46:11–16.
120. Yataganas X, Eliopoulos G, Koulcheri S, et al. The effect of recombinant α-inteferon on natural killer cell activity and clinical course in patients with myelodysplastic syndrome. Ann Hematol 1991; 62:225–229.
121. Petti MC, Latagliata R, Avvisati G, et al. Treatment of high-risk myelodysplastic syndromes with lymphoblastoid alpha interferon. Br J Haematol 1996; 95:364–367.
122. Catalano L, Majolino I, Musto P, et al. Alpha inteferon in the treatment of chronic myelomonocytic leukemia. Haematologica 1989; 74:577–581.
123. Schwarzinger I, Stain C, Bettelheim P, Hinterberger W, Lechner K. Gamma-interferon in myelodysplastic syndromes: a pilot study. Oncology 1990; 47:322–326.
124. Seymour JF, Kurzrock R, Freireich EJ, Estey EH. 2-Chlorodeoxyadenosine induces durable remissions and prolonged suppression of CD4+ lymphocyte counts in patients with hairy cell leukemia. Blood 1994;83:2906–2911.
125. Krieger O, Kasparu H, Girschkofsky M, et al. 2-Chlorodeoxyadenosine (2-CDA) in the therapy of high risk CMML. Br J Haematol 1996; 93(suppl 2):231. Abstract 867.
126. Tallman M, Saven A, Hakimian D, et al. 2-Chlorodeoxyadenosine (2-CdA) in the treatment of myelomonocytic leukemias. Proc Am Soc Clin Oncol 1995; 14:340. Abstract 1022.
127. Pinto A, Zagonel V. 5-aza-2′-deoxycytidine and 5-azacytidine in the treatment of acute myeloid leukemia and myelodysplastic syndromes: past, present, and future trends. Leukemia 1993; 7(suppl 1):51–60.
128. Silverman LR, Holand JF, Nelson D, et al. Trilineage (TLR) response of myelodysplastic syndromes (MDS) to subcutaneous (SQ) azacytidine (Aza C). Proc Am Soc Clin Oncol 1991; 10:222. Abstract 747.

129. Silverman LR, Holand JF, Demakos EP, et al. Subcutaneous 5-azacytidine in myelodysplastic syndromes (MDS): the experience at Mount Sinai hospital. Proc Am Soc Clin Oncol 1995; 14:340. Abstract 1021.
130. Zagonel V, Lo Re G, Marotta G, et al. 5-aza-2′-deoxycytidine (decitabine) is an effective agent for the treatment of advanced myelodysplastic syndromes (MDS). Proc Am Soc Clin Oncol 1992; 11:262. Abstract 858.
131. Rugo HH, Damon L, Ries C, Linker C. Treatment of myelodysplastic syndromes (MDS) with subcutaneous 5-azacytidine (Aza C). Blood 1994; 84(suppl 1):317a. Abstract 1254.
132. Chitambar CR, Libnoch JA, Matthaeus WG, Ash RC, Ritch PS, Anderson T. Evaluation of continuous infusion low-dose 5-azacytidine in the treatment of myelodysplastic syndromes. Am J Hematol 1991; 37:100–104.
133. Zagonel V, Lo Re G, Marotta G, et al. 5-aza-2′-deoxycytidine (decitabine) induces trilineage response in unfavourable myelodysplastic syndromes. Leukemia 1993; 7(suppl 1):30–35.
134. Anzai H, Frost P, Abbruzzese JL. Synergistic cytotoxicity with 2′-deoxy-5-azacytidine and topotecan in vitro and in vivo. Cancer Res 1992; 52:2180–2185.
135. Ganser A, Hoelzer D. Treatment of myelodysplastic syndromes with hematopoietic growth factors. Hematol/Oncol Clin North Am 1992; 6:633–653.
136. Herrmann F, Lindemann A, Klein H, Lübbert M, Schulz G, Mertelsmann R. Effect of recombinant human granulocyte-marcophage colony-stimulating factor in patients with myelodysplastic syndrome with excess blasts. Leukemia 1989; 3: 335–338.
137. Ganser A, Völkers B, Greher J, et al. Recombinant human granulocyte-macrophage colony-stimulating factor in patients with myelodysplastic syndromes—a phase I/II trial. Blood 1989; 73:31–37.
138. Rosenfeld CS, Suulecki M, Evans C, Shadduck RK. Comparison of intravenous versus subcutaneous recombinant human granulocyte-macrophage colony-stimulating factor in patients with primary myelodysplasia. Exp Hematol 1991; 19: 273–277.
139. Estey EH, Kurzrock R, Talpaz M, et al. Effects of low doses of recombinant human granulocyte-macrophage colony stimulating factor (GM-CSF) in patients with myelodysplastic syndromes. Br J Haematol 1991; 77:291–295.
140. Emanuel PD, Bates LJ, Castleberry RP, Gualtieri RJ, Zuckerman KS. Selective hypersensitivity to granulocyte-macrophage colony-stimulating factor by juvenille chronic myeloid leukemia hematopoietic progenitors. Blood 1991; 77:925–929.
141. Emanual PD, Zhu S-W, Bates LJ, Zuckerman KS. Hypersensitivity to hemopoietic growth factors in chronic myelomonocytic leukemia (CMML). Blood 1991; 78(suppl 1):156a. Abstract 613.
142. Everson MP, Brown CB, Lily MB. Interleukin-6 and granulocyte-macrophage colony-stimulating factor are candidate growth factors for chronic myelomonocytic leukemia cells. Blood 1989; 74:1472–1476.
143. Akashi K, Shibuya T, Harada M, et al. Interleukin 4 suppresses the spontaneous growth of chronic myelomonocytic leukemia cells. J Clin Invest 1991; 88:223–230.
144. Negrin RS, Greenberg PL. Filgrastim (r-metHuG-CSF) for the treatment of my-

elodysplastic syndromes. In: Morstyn G, Dexter TM, eds. Filgrastim (r-metHuG-CSF) in Clinical Practice. New York: Marcel Dekker, 1994:211–229.

145. Yanagisawa K, Hatta N, Watanable I, Hoiuchi T, Hasegawa H, Fujita S. IL-4 stimulates the growth of chronic myelomonocytic leukemia cells (CMMoL) once leukemic transformation has occurred. Leukemia 1995; 9:1056–1059.

146. Cortes JE, Talpaz M, Cabanillas F, Seymour JF, Kurzrock R. Serum levels of interleukin-10 in patients with diffuse large cell lymphoma: lack of correlation with prognosis. Blood 1995; 85:2516–2520.

147. Chernoff AE, Granowitz EV, Shapiro L, et al. A randomized, controlled trial of IL-10 in humans. Inhibition of inflammatory cytokine production and immune responses. J Immunol 1995; 154:5492–5499.

148. Geissler K, Öhler L, Födinger M, et al. Interleukin-10 inhibits growth and granulocyte/macrophage colony-stimulating factor production in chronic myelomonocytic leukemia cells. J Exp Med 1996; 184:1377–1384.

149. Oehler L, Foedinger M, Koeller M, et al. Interleukin-10 inhibits spontaneous colony-forming unit-granulocyte-macrophage growth from human peripheral blood mononuclear cells by suppression of endogenous granulocyte-macrophage colony-stimulating factor release. Blood 1997; 89:1147–1153.

150. Hercus TR, Bagley CJ, Cambareri B, et al. Specific human granulocyte-macrophage colony-stimulating factor antagonists. Proc Natl Acad Sci USA 1994; 91: 5838–5842.

151. Iverson PO, To LB, Lopz AF. Apoptosis of hemopoietic cells by the human granulocyte-macrophage colony-stimulating factor mutant E21R. Proc Natl Acad Sci USA 1996; 93:2785–2789.

152. Iverson PO, Rodwell RL, Pitcher L, Taylor KM, Lopez AF. Inhibition of proliferation and induction of apoptosis in juvenile myelomonocytic leukemic cells by the granulocyte-macrophage colony-stimulating factor analogue E21R. Blood 1996; 88:2634–2639.

153. Kurzrock R, Talpaz M, Estrov Z, Rosenblum MG, Gutterman JU. Phase-I study of recombinant human interleukin-3 in patients with bone marrow failure. J Clin Oncol 1991; 9:1241–1250.

154. Marini B, Bassan R, Barbui T. Therapeutic efficacy of danazol in myelodysplastic syndromes. Eur J Cancer Clin Oncol 1988; 24:1481–1489.

155. Lilly M, Brown C, Pettit G, Kraft A. Bryostatin 1: a potential anti-leukemic agent for chronic myelomonocytic leukemia. Leukemia 1991; 5:283–287.

3
Animal Models of Chronic Myelogenous Leukemia

Richard A. Van Etten
Harvard Medical School, Boston, Massachusetts

INTRODUCTION

Chronic myelogenous leukemia (CML) is one of the most intensively studied and best understood human malignancies. In part, this is due to a large effort in the development of animal model systems of the disease. A great deal has been learned about the molecular mechanisms of transformation by the product of the Philadelphia chromosome, *BCR/ABL*, from expression of this oncogene in tissue culture cells. However, a complete understanding of leukemogenesis requires that the oncogenic process be studied within the context of the hematopoietic system, a level of complexity which cannot be attained by any available cell culture system. In this regard, animal models of CML have proven invaluable for establishing the central role of *BCR/ABL* in the pathogenesis of the disease, and for furthering our understanding of the molecular pathophysiology of CML and related diseases (1,2). This chapter will summarize the current state of knowledge in this area with particular emphasis on what we have learned from specific models, the usefulness and limitations of animal models, and prospects for the future.

PROPAGATION OF HUMAN CML CELLS IN MICE

One approach to modeling human CML in animals is to grow primary cells or cell lines from CML patients in immunodeficient mice, such as *bg/nu/xid* mice (3) or mice with severe combined immunodeficiency (SCID) (4). To date, most of the published work has utilized SCID mice as the host. Due to a defect in V(D)J recombination, SCID mice lack functional B and T cells and will accept human xenografts. Both normal (5,6) and leukemic (7–12) human hematopoietic cells have been propagated in SCID mice and in a derivative of SCID mice (SCID-hu mice) which has been engrafted with human fetal lymphoid and bone tissue (13–16). In general, engraftment of SCID mice with myeloid cells, either normal or malignant, appears to be more difficult than lymphoid engraftment, and is facilitated by coadministration of exogenous human cytokines (5).

Although there have been no cell lines isolated from chronic phase CML patients, there are several well-characterized lines established from CML patients in blast crisis, including the prototypic myeloid leukemia cell line K562 (17). Like most leukemic cell lines, CML blast crisis cell lines grow in liquid medium supplemented with serum but without requiring additional growth factors. Not surprisingly, such blast crisis lines are readily propagated in SCID mice after intravenous injection, without requiring exogenous growth factors (18,19). Cells are detectable first in peripheral blood and marrow, and later in metastatic tumor sites such as the central nervous system and peritoneal cavity, ultimately causing death. This system has been utilized for testing the in vivo effectiveness of antisense oligonucleotide therapy (19). As a model of human CML or blast crisis, however, the use of cell lines is complicated by the likelihood that the malignant cells may have acquired additional abnormalities during establishment or passage and therefore may no longer accurately reflect the human disease.

Efforts have also been made to propagate primary cells from CML patients in the SCID mouse system. Initial efforts yielded some success with cells from CML patients in blast crisis (9,15,18,20), with cells injected either intraperitoneally, beneath the kidney capsule, or subcutaneously. However, engraftment of primary chronic phase CML cells was not possible (18,20). In one study, focal growth of mature human myeloid cells at the site of implantation of chronic phase CML cells was occasionally seen, but no sustained growth after 20 weeks was observed and there was no dissemination (18).

Recently, these difficulties have been overcome by using a very high cell inoculum, allowing engraftment of SCID mice with human hematopoietic cells from CML patients in chronic phase (21). SCID mice were inoculated intravenously with either peripheral blood or bone marrow from newly diagnosed CML patients, with subsequent detection of between 1% and 10% human cells in the recipient bone marrow at 30–60 days postinoculation, as judged by flow cytometric analysis of the human-specific CD45 cell surface antigen or analysis of genomic DNA with a human-specific DNA probe. Human myeloid (CD13$^+$), B lymphoid (CD19$^+$), and progenitor (CD34$^+$) cells as well as multilineage colony-forming cells (CFC) were detected in recipient mice. Efficient engraftment required a high cell inoculum ($\geq 8 \times 10^7$ cells), with very low engraftment observed at the lower doses ($2–4 \times 10^7$ cells) traditionally used for SCID mouse repopulation. Peripheral blood and bone marrow appeared equally efficacious as sources of repopulating cells.

Surprisingly, treatment of the mice with exogenous cytokines was not required for efficient engraftment, in contrast to mice transplanted with normal marrow (5). Genotyping of CFC by reverse transcriptase polymerase chain reaction (RT-PCR) for *BCR/ABL* transcripts showed that, on average, only a third of colonies were derived from Ph$^+$ progenitors. In agreement with earlier studies, primary cells from patients with CML myeloid or lymphoid blast crisis engrafted SCID mice very efficiently at low cell doses without cytokines, with the engrafted cells maintaining a morphological and cell surface phenotype similar to that of the original transplanted population (21).

This system and related transplant models utilizing immunodeficient mice hold great promise as tools for studying CML. To list a few potential applications, the system could be useful for functionally defining the nature of the clonogenic leukemic cell in CML (11), for investigating the nature of the prominent graft versus leukemia effect in CML (22) or for testing new therapies for CML such as antisense oligonucleotide and gene therapy approaches. Given the striking difference in transplantability of chronic phase and blast crisis cells, it is also possible that the SCID mouse transplant model might yield useful prognostic information when serially performed with peripheral blood samples from the same patient. As it currently stands, however, the model has several limitations, and a number of issues must be clarified. The degree of engraftment of individual mice inoculated with cells from the same patient varies considerably, making it difficult to make the SCID repopulation assay quantitative. Although the fate of mice followed posttransplant for long periods is not known, the growth of the transplanted CML cells appears restricted to the marrow, with no dissemination to the peripheral blood, spleen, or liver, and no evidence of evolution to blast crisis. Thus, the SCID model may lack important pathological features of human CML. Finally, the preferential engraftment of SCID mice with Ph$^-$ progenitors may simply reflect the tendency of Ph$^-$ hematopoiesis to predominate over Ph$^+$ under some circumstances, such as long-term in vitro culture (23). However, in conjunction with the very large cell dose required for engraftment, the possibility also arises that cytokine production from the Ph$^+$ CML cells (24,25) mediates the engraftment that is observed. Despite these problems, there is certain to be renewed interest in these CML model systems, and we can expect that many of these issues will be resolved in the near future.

PROPAGATION OF *BCR/ABL*-TRANSFORMED CELL LINES IN MICE

Although there are important advantages to animal models employing primary cells directly isolated from CML patients, there are drawbacks to these systems as well. Chief among these is the difficulty in manipulating the system experimentally, such as expressing different forms of the bcr/abl protein or introducing other modulatory genes and proteins. In addition, because humans are genetically heterogeneous, it is difficult to infer that properties of primary CML isolates are a consequence of expression of the *BCR/ABL* gene, and appropriate negative controls are often lacking. These problems can be circumvented by use of murine factor-dependent hematopoietic cell lines.

Hematopoietic factor-dependent lines are derived from long-term in vitro culture of murine bone marrow, can be of either myeloid or lymphoid phenotype, and typically are absolutely dependent on a given hematopoietic growth factor or cytokine for survival and proliferation. Examples of myeloid factor-dependent cell lines include 32D (26), an IL-3-dependent line, and FDCP-1 (27), which requires either IL-3 or GM-CSF, while Ba/F3 is a commonly used B-lymphoid IL-3-dependent line (28). In the absence of the required growth factor, these cells undergo rapid death by apoptosis. When introduced subcutaneously into nude mice or intravenously into syngeneic immunocompetent mice, the parental factor-dependent cells are unable to form tumors or induce leukemia.

Interestingly, these cell lines can be transformed by a number of tyrosine kinase oncogenes, including v-*abl* and *BCR/ABL*, to become independent of exogenous growth factors for survival and proliferation (24,29–32). Although in some cases production of low levels of cytokines by the transformed cells is detectable (24), the mechanism of transformation of such cells to factor-independence by *BCR/ABL* does not involve autocrine stimulation. Importantly, transformation to growth factor independence correlates with acquisition of the ability of the cells to form tumors in nude mice (24,31). More recently, it has been shown that introduction of *BCR/ABL*-transformed factor-independent cells intravenously into syngeneic mice results in in vivo proliferation and a rapidly fatal leukemia (33,34). This system thus constitutes a model system for *BCR/ABL*-induced leukemia in vivo. It had the advantage that the cells employed are permanent lines which can be genetically manipulated and extensively characterized in culture, then assayed for leukemia induction in vivo. Because the parental factor-dependent cells and their *BCR/ABL*-transformed derivatives are identical except for the presence or absence of the *BCR/ABL* gene, it is possible to ascribe differences in leukemogenicity directly to the action of *BCR/ABL*.

These systems have been utilized for a number of different purposes. One line of investigation has determined which of the many functional domains of the bcr/abl protein are required for transformation of hematopoietic factor-dependent cells and leukemogenesis by these cells in vivo. Although the structural requirements for bcr/abl transformation of fibroblasts have been extensively studied (35–38), it has become apparent that there are significant differences in the requirements for transformation of hematopoietic cells. For example, while myristoylation greatly facilitates transformation of NIH 3T3 fibroblasts by bcr/abl and v-Abl (39), it is not required for these proteins to transform Ba/F3 cells (40). Similarly, the phosphotyrosine-binding function of the Abl SH2 domain is absolutely required for bcr/abl and activated c-abl to transform fibroblasts (41–43), but the SH2 domain is dispensable for transformation of factor-dependent myeloid and lymphoid cell lines and for leukemogenesis in syngeneic hosts (34). Interestingly, in the latter studies there was a significant difference between the leukemogenicity of cells transformed with *BCR/ABL* constructs containing either a point mutation or a complete deletion of the SH2 domain (34). These results emphasize that there are important differences between transformation of fibroblasts and hematopoietic cells by *BCR/ABL*, and that in vivo leukemogenicity is a complex process whose outcome cannot necessarily be inferred from cell culture studies.

Factor-dependent hematopoietic cells transformed by *BCR/ABL* also comprise an attractive system for screening for new drugs which might be useful in the treatment of human Ph$^+$ leukemia. A derivative of the Ba/F3 cell line in which the bcr/abl protein is expressed from the *BCR* promoter has been used as a cell-based assay in a high-throughput screen of chemical and natural product libraries for compounds that decrease transcription from the *BCR* promoter or decrease intracellular phosphotyrosine levels (44). A similar cell line is currently used by the National Cancer Institute as part of a panel for screening potential antitumor agents. When a promising lead compound is identified, its in vivo activity can be quickly assessed by testing whether the compound can prolong the survival of syngeneic mice inoculated with the same cells. In this manner, a potent and selective inhibitor of the Abl tyrosine kinase has recently been shown to specifically inhibit tumor formation by *BCR/ABL*-transformed 32Dcl3 cells in syngeneic C3H/HEJ mice (45).

Another exciting application of *BCR/ABL*-transformed factor-dependent hematopoietic cell lines is the investigation of antitumor immunity in vivo. *BCR/ABL*-transformed 32Dc13 myeloid cells induce a rapidly fatal leukemia after intravenous inoculation of syngeneic C3H/HEJ mice, but when the same cells are modified to express the T-cell costimulatory cell surface protein B7-1 (46), animals that receive an intermediate cell dose eradicate the leukemia by an mechanism which requires CD8$^+$ cells (33). Such animals are protected from further rechallenges with the fully leukemogenic parental *BCR/ABL*-32D line. Further studies have shown that B7-1 is superior to the related B7 family member B7-2 in generating an antileukemic effect (47). The identity of the tumor-specific antigen(s) responsible for the induction of this antitumor response is not known, but it is possible that the bcr/abl protein itself plays such a role, because others have shown that peptides representing the junction between the bcr and abl sequences can elicit T-cell responses in mice (48) and humans (49) (see Chap. 19). The relationship of the antileukemia response observed in this mouse model system to the prominent graft-versus-leukemia effect observed in human CML remains to be defined. Nevertheless, this system will provide an important tool for future investigation into methods to induce or improve the immune response against human cancers, and particularly against Ph$^+$ leukemias.

BCR/ABL TRANSGENIC MICE

Despite their advantages, the usefulness of factor-dependent hematopoietic cell lines as a model of human CML is limited by several problems. Although the parental factor-dependent cells are nonleukemogenic, they are still immortalized cell lines which are aneuploid and doubtless have many abnormalities relative to primary hematopoietic cells. In addition, the disease phenotype induced by *BCR/ABL*-transformed cells is one of an acute leukemia and does not accurately reflect the pathophysiology of chronic phase CML, where myeloid differentiation is effectively preserved. In fact, introduction of *BCR/ABL* into 32D cells has the paradoxical effect of blocking G-CSF-induced differentiation into neutrophils (32). Because of these problems, much effort has gone into developing methods to express *BCR/ABL* directly in the hematopoietic system of mice. One such approach is the generation of transgenic strains of mice carrying a *BCR/ABL* gene.

Initial attempts to generate *BCR/ABL* transgenic mice were carried out before a *BCR/ABL* cDNA clone was widely available, and instead utilized a facsimile of the human *BCR* gene fused to the mouse v-*abl* gene (50). The resulting transgene differed from the bona fide P210$^{BCR/ABL}$ gene by lacking some *BCR* and *ABL* sequences in the region of the junction between the two genes, and by having murine *abl* sequences instead of the closely related human *ABL* gene. In spite of these differences, the results were instructive and the lessons learned have proven relevant to subsequent efforts.

Two different promoter/enhancer constructs were used to direct the expression of the transgene: a murine immunoglobulin heavy-chain enhancer and V$_H$ promoter (EµV$_H$), which functions mainly in pre-B and pre-T lymphocytes, and the promoter/enhancer of the long terminal repeat (LTR) of the mouse myeloproliferative sarcoma virus (MPSV), which was known to express at high levels in many differentiated hematopoietic cell types and in undifferentiated embryonal carcinoma cells. Compared to the customary efficiency of generating transgenic offspring from microinjected eggs, there was a decreased yield of transgenic pups after injection of the *BCR*/v-*abl* transgene, particularly the MPSV-*BCR*/v-*abl* construct, suggesting that expression of the transgene during early embryonic development was deleterious. Lymphoid tumors developed in a minority of primary transgenic mice and in some breeding lines; no myeloid leukemias were observed. The tumors were predominantly T-lymphomas with a small number of B-lymphomas, were clonal by analysis of T-cell receptor or immunoglobulin genes, and expressed the *BCR*/v-*abl* transgene at high levels. Significantly, healthy *BCR*/v-*abl* transgenic mice exhibited no hematologic abnormalities and did not express the transgene, even in pre-T and pre-B cells. This sharply contrasts with Eµ-*myc* transgenic mice, which uniformly express c-*myc* constitutively in early B cells, leading to a premalignant expansion of this population and subsequently clonal B-lymphomas (51). These observations implied that the *BCR*/v-*abl* transgene was silenced during development, perhaps because of toxicity, and induced sporadic lymphoid tumors only after chance somatic activation in these cells. Therefore, while confirming the leukemogenic potential of *BCR/ABL*, these studies did not provide a suitable transgenic model of human CML.

Concurrent efforts by others to generate *BCR/ABL* transgenic mice provided support for the notion that expression of the *BCR/ABL* gene during early development is toxic to the embryo. With a construct utilizing the native *BCR* promoter, which is widely expressed in somatic cells (52) and during fetal development (53), to drive expression of the P210$^{BCR/ABL}$ gene, there was a greatly decreased yield of pups from injected eggs (6% versus 20–40% with other constructs), and no live transgenic progeny were obtained despite multiple attempts (54). To investigate the nature of the failure of injected eggs to develop to term, reimplanted foster mothers were sacrificed at different stages of pregnancy. Analysis of early pregnancies (embryonic day 9.5–13.5) showed an abnormally increased number of decidual swellings, over 40% of which were positive for the *BCR/ABL* transgene by PCR and therefore likely represented degenerating transgenic embryos; in addition there were some visibly normal embryos, about 20% of which were transgenic by Southern blot. Analysis of later (ed 17.5–18.5) pregnancies showed that about 10% of embryos surviving to this stage were transgenic, some of which were clearly abnormal and lacked any apparent vascular system. There was no morphological evidence of leukemia in these embryos. RT-PCR and Northern blot analyses showed that the transgene was expressed in most of these embryos. These observations suggest that a *BCR/ABL* transgene can indeed have pleiotropic deleterious effects on embryonic development. The precise mechanism of toxicity was not identified, but the lack of identifiable leukemia in the transgenic embryos makes it plausible that the fetal demise was a consequence of expression of the *BCR/ABL* transgene outside the hematopoietic system.

However, the same group of investigators were successful in generating transgenic mice carrying the P190 form of *BCR/ABL* (55). The transgene was expressed from a mouse metallothionein-1 (MT-1) promoter which is inducible by heavy metals (56) but in vivo is constitutively and widely expressed in transgenic mice (57). In the initial set of experiments, 10 transgenic progeny were obtained (a frequency of 17%), eight of which rapidly developed fatal leukemias within 58 days of birth; three of the animals died within 13 days of birth, suggesting that the leukemogenic process had likely initiated in utero. The two other animals were chimeric and failed to express the transgene or develop disease. Two diseased animals were thought to have myeloid leukemias with some degree of differentiation toward mature neutrophils, but definitive analysis was not possible because both animals were found dead. The lack of myeloid leukemias in subsequent experiments with the MT-P190 transgene (58) suggests that these animals may have been misdiagnosed.

The phenotype of the leukemias in all the other animals was consistent with that of a early B-cell lymphoma, with the tumor cells positive for the B-cell-specific murine cell surface antigen B220 and leukemic involvement of peripheral blood, spleen, bone marrow, and occasionally lymph nodes. The status of the immunoglobulin heavy-chain genes of the tumors were found to be germline, consistent with an early or pro-B-cell malignancy, making it difficult to assess the clonality of the tumors. Surprisingly, the transgene was expressed in several nonhematopoietic organs in these mice, including brain and skeletal muscle, yet this widespread expression did not lead to malignancies in these tissues (at least during the period of observation) or, apparently, to any embryonic toxicity of the sort seen with the *BCR* promoter construct. Subsequent studies further clarified the nature of leukemogenesis in this transgenic model. Generation of additional founders and some transgenic breeding lines indicated that the animals developed exclusively B-cell lymphoma. The lymphoma cells express P190 protein at high levels and produce disease after adoptive transfer into syngeneic mice (58). Expression of the transgene is detected at significant levels in nonhematopoietic organs, particularly brain and kidney, yet tumors of these tissues were not observed, again suggesting that the oncogenic action of *BCR/ABL* is restricted to the hematopoietic system. Although the overall penetrance of the disease phenotype in transgenic animals was only 67%, several transgenic lines were established where 100% of offspring developed leukemia by 6 months of age.

An important issue is whether the leukemias that develop in these mice are polyclonal, as would be expected if the presence of $P190^{BCR/ABL}$ alone were sufficient for leukemogenesis, or whether they are oligo- or monoclonal, which would imply that additional, relatively rare events are required to develop full-blown leukemia. Detailed studies of the karyotype and IgH gene rearrangement status of primary cells and cell lines established from these mice have not yielded a clear answer to this question. Karyotype analysis of advanced primary leukemias and secondary transplants (59) and in cell lines established from these mice (60) indicated that multiple nonrandom cytogenetic abnormalities developed in the leukemic cells from individual mice, with a preference for trisomy involving chromosomes 10, 12, 14, and 17.

Analysis of IgH gene rearrangements confirmed that multiple individual

Animal Models

IgH rearrangements can be detected in primary animals and secondary recipients, suggesting that clonal evolution and progression are prominent features of the advanced stages of this leukemic process. However, it appears that the earliest leukemic cells have a normal karyotype, because the majority of metaphases in several mice with greatly elevated (>$100 \times 10^3/\mu L$) peripheral blood white blood counts were normal (59). While the early leukemic cells lack clonal karyotypic abnormalities, this does not necessarily imply that they are not clonal. While several mice with advanced leukemia were found to have only germline bands on analysis of IgH gene rearrangements, it was difficult to distinguish whether the population of leukemic cells had polyclonal rearrangements of a single IgH allele or both IgH genes were germline (60). In theory, this could be determined utilizing a PCR assay for IgH gene rearrangement (61) on this population. If both IgH alleles were found to be germline, then an additional test for clonality looking for nonrandom X-chromosome inactivation could be employed (62). Without these data, it is difficult to draw definitive conclusions about whether P190$^{BCR/ABL}$ alone is sufficient to induce B-cell leukemia in these mice. In other experiments where *BCR/ABL* genes are transferred ex vivo into bone marrow-derived B-lymphoid progenitors (63) (see next section), expression of P190 alone appeared to be insufficient for development of a fully tumorigenic phenotype.

Another puzzling feature of these mice is the lack of myeloid leukemias. One possibility is that the P190 form of *BCR/ABL*, which is almost exclusively associated with acute B-lymphoblastic leukemia in humans, is incapable of inducing leukemia in myeloid cells. The ability of P190 to transform myeloid cells in vitro and the detection of P190 in some cases of human acute myelogenous leukemia (64) make this unlikely. Alternatively, the MT-P190 transgene may not be expressed at high levels in myeloid cells. Although expression of the transgene in bone marrow is detected by RT-PCR in utero and throughout postnatal life in a disease-prone transgenic line (58), it is not known whether any of this expression is in myeloid cells. Interestingly, transgene expression is not found in peripheral blood of newborn mice from this line, but becomes detectable by about 30 days after birth. This may reflect the sequestration of leukemic cells in the marrow until physical crowding, loss of adhesive interactions, or acquisition of stromal independence allows migration into the blood. On the other hand, because around half of murine peripheral blood cells are mature myeloid cells, this also implies that the transgene is not expressed in these cells. Further study is required to understand the lack of myeloid disease in these mice.

Recently, several groups have reported the first success in generating transgenic mice with the P210$^{BCR/ABL}$ gene (65,66). These studies used versions of the same MT-1 promoter employed to express P190. In the first study, six primary transgenic animals were born, and two developed T-cell leukemia/lymphoma, with one of these founders generating a transgenic line which developed similar disease with a penetrance of about 30% (65). The leukemic cells expressed high levels of P210 protein, were positive for Thy-1.2 antigen, and exhibited rearrangements of TCR-β and -γ gene loci, although it is not entirely clear whether the rearrangements were clonal. Analysis of expression of the transgene in different tissues by RT-PCR showed sporadic expression in kidney in two transgenic lines that did not develop disease, and widespread expression in kidney, liver, heart, brain, spleen, and particularly thymus (but not bone marrow) in mice from the disease-prone line. The tendency of these P210 transgenic mice to develop T-lymphoma is reminiscent of the *BCR/v-abl* transgenic mice and suggests that P210 and P190 transgenes may induce different diseases in transgenic mice. The lack of myeloid disease is again puzzling, but might be explained by lack of transgene expression in bone marrow myeloid cells. The high level of premalignant thymic transgene expression raises the possibility that a somatic event in the thymus, such as TCR rearrangement, might activate expression of the transgene specifically in T cells, but no rearrangements of the transgene were apparent by Southern blot analysis of the tumors.

In the second study, a distinct difference in the leukemogenic action of P210 and P190$^{BCR/ABL}$ was definitively confirmed, because one of the MT-P210 constructs utilized an MT promoter identical to that used for P190, allowing a direct comparison of the two strains (66). Several transgenic founders and transgenic lines were generated, and these animals developed both B- and T-cell leukemia/lymphoma with penetrance of around 50% by 44 weeks of age. This is considerably slower than leukemogenesis in MT-P190 mice, which typically had >90% disease incidence by 24 weeks and were never observed to develop T-cell disease. The clonality of the lymphoid tumors was not assessed. Again there was a striking absence of myeloid leukemias, with only one animal having a myeloblastic leukemia positive for the myeloid cell-surface antigen GR-1$^+$. By RT-PCR analysis, the transgene was expressed at low levels both in nonhematopoietic tissues (testes and brain) and in bone marrow and spleen of nondiseased animals in utero and after birth, but not in the peripheral blood. Interestingly, peripheral blood expression of the MT-P210 transgene seemed to be a prerequisite for developing disease, as is the case with the MT-P190 transgene, but development of leukemia did not necessarily immediately follow, as some animals that developed transgene expression in circulating leukocytes remained disease-free for months. These observations suggest that unlike P190, expression of P210 in primary hematopoietic cells is insufficient to induce the dysregulation of growth and differentiation that we phenotypically recognize as leukemia. These inferences are supported by studies of expression of P210 in primary bone marrow-derived B cells (67,68) (see next section).

What conclusions can we draw from these extensive efforts to generate *BCR/ABL* transgenic mice? First, *BCR/ABL* is indeed an oncogene, and furthermore would appear to be a leukemia-specific oncogene, because malignancies of nonhematopoietic tissues were not observed in these mice despite widespread expression of *BCR/ABL*. This is in stark contrast to some other oncogenes such as v-*ras* or SV40 large T antigen, which will induce malignant transformation in practically any organ where they are expressed (69,70). The reasons for this striking specificity are unknown, but one might speculate that hematopoietic cells are permissive for *BCR/ABL*-induced transformation because they contain unique effector molecules necessary for the oncogenic action of bcr/abl. Second, there are distinct differences in the in vivo leukemogenicity of the two forms of *BCR/ABL*. P190$^{BCR/ABL}$ efficiently and preferentially transforms B-lymphoid cells and may be sufficient for leukemic transformation of primary hematopoietic cells, while P210$^{BCR/ABL}$ can induce both T- and B-lymphoid leukemias but does so quite inefficiently, suggesting that other events are necessary for progression to overt leukemia. Third, the existing *BCR/ABL* transgenic mice do not develop myeloid leukemia at a significant frequency, and certainly do not exhibit a myeloproliferative syndrome characteristic of CML. The lack of myeloid disease might simply be due to a failure of the MT-1 promoter to express well in myeloid progenitor cells, although other explanations are possible. Finally, it is clear that some *BCR/ABL* transgenes are toxic to embryonic development. The mechanism of the embryonic toxicity is not known, but may be related to the potent growth suppressive activity observed with c-abl and some activated forms of abl in vitro (71).

Why this toxicity is seen with some transgene constructs and not with others is not clear, although it may be related to the relative levels and tissue distribution of transgene expression within the developing embryo. Currently, there does not seem to be any reliable way to predict whether a given *BCR/ABL* transgene might be toxic, although it is plausible to expect that promoter/enhancers that are widely and highly expressed in the embryo might be more problematic. Recognizing transgene toxicity with a new *BCR/ABL* construct should not be difficult, as one might expect difficulty in generating transgenic pups, and those transgenic animals that are born may have decreased or absent transgene expression in the tissues where the transgene is expected to be active.

Even though they do not accurately model CML, these *BCR/ABL* transgenic mice will have many uses. They may be valuable for testing potential therapies or for examining the interaction of *BCR/ABL* activity with other oncogenes and tumor suppressor genes, and they provide an important reagent for biochemical investigation of the physiological consequences of expression of *BCR/ABL* in primary hematopoietic cells. However, it is clear that efforts to develop a transgenic model of CML must continue.

There are several plausible strategies available. One approach is to utilize promoters that are specific for hematopoietic stem cells or myeloid cells in order to avoid potential toxicity and ensure transgene expression in progenitor or myeloid cells. Currently, there are no stem cell-specific promoters that have been demonstrated to function in transgenic mice, but there are a number of promoters that have been shown to direct expression of reporter genes in early and more differentiated myeloid cells in transgenic mice, including the CD11b (72), c-*fms* (73), and cathepsin G (74) promoters. Transgenic mice with either the P210 or P190$^{BCR/ABL}$ genes under the control of the CD11b promoter have been generated (75). Similar to the *BCR*/v-*abl* transgenic mice, these mice developed sporadic B- and T-lymphomas but not myeloid leukemias, and had low to absent transgene expression in monocytes and macrophages, which is suggestive of toxicity. Because of the unpredictability of this phenomenon, other myeloid-specific promoters should certainly be tried.

Another worthwhile strategy is the use of binary transgene systems, where the product of one transgene controls the expression of a second target transgene. Several types of binary systems are in use, employing either transcription factors [such as yeast Gal4p (76)] or DNA recombinases [such as the Cre protein of bacteriophage P1 (77)] to modulate target transgene expression, with the goals of improving the tissue-specific expression of a transgene and allowing easier propagation of mice bearing cancer-inducing oncogenes.

A third approach involves expression of *BCR/ABL* in embryonic stem (ES) cells, followed by generation of chimeric mice through blastocyst injection. This method could allow the analysis of leukemic phenotypes without requiring germline transmission of the oncogene (78), and could be combined with homologous recombination (79) or Cre/loxP expression (80) to produce a rearrangement of the endogenous murine *bcr* and *abl* genes and generate an analog of the Philadelphia chromosome in mice.

Finally, the use of inducible transcription systems, such as the tetracycline-responsive transactivator/operator (81), deserves consideration as a means of avoiding embryonic toxicity by preventing expression of *BCR/ABL* in transgenic mice until after birth. Clearly, there is no shortage of potential experimental strategies, and enthusiasm is tempered only by the appreciation that these approaches are very labor-intensive. Given the paucity of knowledge of what might work and the importance of the problem, further effort in these areas appears warranted.

EX VIVO TRANSFER OF *BCR/ABL* INTO MURINE BONE MARROW

Perhaps the most faithful and informative animal model of CML involves transfer of the *BCR/ABL* gene into primary mouse hematopoietic cells ex vivo. In almost all cases, defective murine retroviral vectors have been used for the gene transfer step because of their unparalleled efficiency at introducing new genetic material into hematopoietic progenitor and stem cells, and because the retroviral provirus, after integration into the recipient cell chromosomal DNA, serves as a unique clonal marker of that cell and its descendants. Following gene transfer, the genetically modified cells can be analyzed in various in vitro culture systems, or introduced into irradiated syngeneic recipient mice to assess the in vivo consequences of *BCR/ABL* expression.

The earliest experiments in this area involved infection of mouse bone marrow with a *BCR/ABL* retrovirus followed by long-term liquid culture of infected cells under conditions which favor expansion of B-lymphoid cells [Whitlock-Witte cultures (82)]. Uninfected marrow will undergo expansion to densities of $2-4 \times 10^5$ cells/mL over a 6-week period, and the resulting cell population, a mixture of immature and more differentiated B-lymphoid cells, is nontumorigenic and able to reconstitute B-cell immune functions in SCID mice. In contrast, marrow infected with a retrovirus carrying the $P210^{BCR/ABL}$ gene proliferates to higher densities ($4-10 \times 10^5$ cells/mL) over the same time period, due to oligoclonal outgrowth of P210-expressing pre-B cells (67).

Unlike cultures infected with Abelson murine leukemia virus, which become independent of the stromal layer by 4–8 weeks and are highly malignant in vivo (83), the P210-infected lines remained stromal-dependent for up to 15 weeks and were only weakly leukemogenic after intraperitoneal inoculation of syngeneic mice. Substitution of a cloned stromal cell line for the bone marrow-derived adherent layer in these cultures allowed isolation of clonal P210-expressing B-progenitor lines which underwent Ig gene rearrangements in vitro and in vivo and were nonleukemogenic, confirming the ability of P210 to stimulate growth without arresting differentiation (68).

Other studies established that $P190^{BCR/ABL}$ appeared more potent than P210 at stimulating oligoclonal outgrowth in this system, but P190 also appeared insufficient to induce full leukemic transformation (63). Initial efforts to alter the culture conditions (84) to favor myeloid transformation by *BCR/ABL* were unsuccessful (85). Subsequently, $P210^{BCR/ABL}$ infection was shown to decrease the requirement for IL-3 or stem cell factor for the growth of multipotential CFC in soft agar, allowing the isolation of clonal mast cell, macrophage, granulocyte-macrophage, and B-lymphoid cell lines which eventually became growth-factor-independent but remained nontumorigenic (86,87). Together, these experiments provide strong support for the concept that the primary consequence of *BCR/ABL* expression in hematopoietic cells is a very subtle stimulation of growth without an appreciable effect on differentiation.

To assess the in vivo leukemogenic potential of *BCR/ABL*-infected marrow, it can be transplanted into a syngeneic recipient mouse whose marrow has been ablated by ionizing radiation. These experiments were modeled on the original transfer of the v-*fms* oncogene into mice, which results in multilineage hematopoietic disorders including some myeloproliferative-like syndromes (88).

After considerable effort, a breakthrough was finally achieved when several groups were able to induce a CML-like myeloproliferative syndrome and several other hematologic malignancies in mice reconstituted with marrow infected with a $P210^{BCR/ABL}$ retrovirus (89–92).

The CML-like syndrome was a rapidly progressive and fatal illness characterized by striking elevations in the peripheral blood white cell count, composed largely of mature neutrophils but with an excess of early myeloid cells such as metamyelocytes and myelocytes, and hepatosplenomegaly with extensive neutrophil infiltration. Myeloid cells carry the $P210^{BCR/ABL}$ provirus and express active P210 protein, confirming that the disease is directly induced by BCR/ABL. In addition, the provirus was present in the majority of day 12 spleen colonies (CFU-S_{12}) (93) generated in a secondary transplant experiment, suggesting that the target cell which is infected by the $P210^{BCR/ABL}$ retrovirus to induce the CML-like syndrome is an early multipotential progenitor which can give rise to CFU-S_{12}.

This was a striking finding, because it suggested that the target cells for retroviral infection of mouse bone marrow in this system and for the Philadelphia chromosome translocation in human CML were similar or identical. Further support for a progenitor/stem cell origin of the CML-like syndrome came from secondary transplant studies. Marrow and/or splenocytes from primary animals with the CML-like syndrome were able to induce an identical syndrome in secondary recipients, confirming that this disorder represents a true malignancy (92,94). Surprisingly, other secondary transplant recipients developed clonally related acute leukemias of myeloid, B-lymphoid, or T-lymphoid origin, strongly implicating the stem cell nature of the murine CML-like syndrome, and mimicking the blast crisis phase of human CML. Also reminiscent of human CML, no cell lines could be isolated from cultures of marrow and spleen from mice with the CML-like syndrome. Overall, these experiments demonstrate that $P210^{BCR/ABL}$ induces a disease in mice that is a remarkably close pathophysiological match to human CML.

In addition to the CML-like syndrome, which was observed in up to 25% of transplanted mice, other recipients developed a number of distinct hematological malignancies, including B-lymphoblastic leukemia, tumors of monocytic/macrophage lineage, and occasionally erythroleukemia and T-cell leukemia (89–91). The B-lymphoblastic leukemia involved marrow and spleen, with less prominent involvement of peripheral blood and lymph nodes, and generally appeared 10–30 weeks posttransplant. The malignant cells expressed P210 protein and had a pre-B-cell phenotype. The tumor cells were $B220^+$ with clonal rearrangement of one or both IgH genes, but germline configurations of κ and λ light chain Ig genes, were easily transplanted to secondary recipients, and readily established permanent lines in cultures supplemented with 2-mercaptoethanol but no other growth factors. This disease therefore appears to be a reasonable facsimile of human Ph$^+$ acute B-lymphoblastic leukemia, and is also similar to the disease induced in adult Balb/c mice by Abelson murine leukemia virus (95).

The macrophage disease was characterized by discrete tumors in the liver, spleen, bone marrow, and mesentery, with occasional malignant ascites or lung involvement, which appeared at lengthy intervals (up to 50 weeks) after transplant and pathologically resembled a reticulum cell sarcoma or malignant histiocytosis, neither of which is associated with a Philadelphia chromosome translocation in humans. These cells expressed P210, had large vacuolated cytoplasm, and were esterase-positive, as is typical for cells of monocytic origin. They grew poorly in culture but could transfer the disease to secondary recipients. Interestingly, some of the animals with extensive macrophage tumors were observed to have modest expansion of neutrophils in peripheral blood, marrow, and spleen, suggestive of a myeloproliferative syndrome, but when it was possible to isolate pure populations of neutrophils, these cells were found to lack the P210 provirus and therefore were not part of the malignant clone (89,90). It is likely that increased neutrophils in these mice were secondary to cytokine production by the macrophage tumors, as significant levels of GM-CSF and G-CSF were detected by bioassay of serum from several of the mice (90). These results emphasize the complexity of the leukemic process in vivo and show that demonstration of the *BCR/ABL* provirus within the granulocyte lineage is a necessary part of the clinicopathological definition of the CML-like syndrome in mice.

Why do different recipients of the same infected marrow develop distinctly different hematological diseases? A likely explanation is that these diseases are the consequence of infection of different target cells in the bone marrow. Several animals were afflicted with multiple leukemias—for example, macrophage tumors in conjunction with either the CML-like syndrome or pre-B ALL. When pure populations of the two tumors are analyzed by Southern blot, they are generally found to have two distinct proviral integrations, consistent with the existence of distinct targets (89). Other studies showed that a variation in the retrovirus infection conditions such as changing the length of infection period or including different cytokines during infection could alter the spectrum of disease which develops, as would be expected if different conditions favored the infection or survival of different target cells (96). In vitro soft agar culture of *BCR/ABL*-infected marrow cells also showed that the target cells for B-lymphoid and myeloid colony formation were distinct (97). Importantly, analysis of animals with ALL or macrophage disease has shown that the retroviral provirus is restricted to the tumor cells in these mice, is not found in other myeloid and lymphoid lineages, and is absent from the CFU-S$_{12}$ population (98). These results suggest that the target cells for these diseases represent lineage-restricted committed lymphoid or myeloid progenitors. However, other studies have indicated that clonal cell lines isolated from *BCR/ABL*-infected mice can alternatively exhibit erythroid, mast cell, and monocyte/macrophage characteristics during in vitro culture (99), implying that some myeloid *BCR/ABL* target cells are multipotential. Further studies are necessary to definitively define the target cells responsible for induction of different diseases by *BCR/ABL*.

Several features of the *BCR/ABL* bone marrow infection/transplantation model deserve further comment. First, some of the experiments have been conducted with *BCR/ABL* retroviral stocks that were free of replication-competent Moloney murine leukemia virus ("helper" virus) (89,90,92), while others included helper virus in order to boost infection efficiency (91). Although similar results have been obtained with both systems, the helper-free system is probably superior because of the high frequency of multilineage disease in animals transplanted with marrow infected with helper-containing stocks, and the tendency of the Moloney MuLV to induce thymic lymphoma in animals followed for longer than several months (100). An additional concern is spread of the *BCR/ABL* virus within the animal after transplantation, compromising the use of proviral integration as a clonal marker, although in practice this has apparently not been prevalent.

Second, the question of polyclonal disease versus monoclonal disease, raised earlier in the discussion of *BCR/ABL* transgenic mice, is also relevant to this system, as studies in humans have suggested that the Ph chromosome translocation may not be the initiating event in CML (101). In the bone marrow infection/transplant model, only monoclonal cases of the CML-like syndrome have been observed (89,92), but because the target cell for the CML-like syndrome might be rare and poorly infectable, it cannot be concluded that P210 alone is insufficient to induce CML in mice.

Third, one report found a difference in efficiency of transplantation of the CML-like syndrome into secondary recipients depending on whether the disease appeared early (4–20 weeks) after transplant or later (after 20 weeks), suggesting that only late-onset disease represented a true malignancy involving hematopoietic stem cells (92). However, data from different research groups demonstrates that there is a wide variability in the onset of the CML-like myeloproliferative syndrome after transplant (89,92,96), and subsequent secondary transplant experiments from donors with early-onset CML-like disease have yielded efficient transfer of the syndrome into secondary recipients (102). The difference in disease latency is therefore more likely to be a variable induced by differences in the infection and transplant protocols between different groups, rather than a fundamental difference in target cell or disease characteristics. Because retrovirus-infected hematopoietic stem cells can remain quiescent for lengthy periods of time after transplant (103), it is possible that some transplant conditions favor immediate proliferation of *BCR/ABL*-infected stem cells while other induce quiescence. Even with efficient transfer of the CML-like syndrome, many recipient animals do not develop disease yet engraft with provirus-negative hematopoiesis of donor origin. This suggests that normal stem cells exist in the marrow of animals with the CML-like syndrome. Similar observations have been made in human CML patients treated with high-dose chemotherapy or α-interferon, and provide a rationale for consideration of autologous bone marrow transplantation in CML (104,105) (see Chap. 12).

Fourth, in agreement with results obtained with transgenic mice, different forms of *BCR/ABL* appear to have distinctly different activities in the bone marrow infection/transplantation model system. A direct comparison of the leukemogenic activity of P210 and P190$^{BCR/ABL}$ in a bone marrow infection experiment utilizing helper virus showed that the phenotypes of leukemia induced by the two forms of *BCR/ABL* were similar, but the disease latency with P190 was significantly shorter, with 50% of P190-infected animals dying by 50 days posttransplant compared with 70 days for P210 animals (106). In addition to acceleration of disease onset, different oncogenic forms of *ABL* may also induce a different spectrum of leukemia, as the v-*abl* gene failed to induce a CML-like syndrome in this system (107). An earlier report suggested v-*abl* could also induce the CML-like syndrome (91), but presence of the provirus in the neutrophil lineage was not confirmed. Further studies will be necessary to resolve this important issue.

Finally, it is apparent that the strain of inbred mice utilized for the transplant experiment greatly influences the disease phenotypes that are obtained, as does the nature of the retroviral LTR sequence used to express the *BCR/ABL* gene. For unknown reasons, the CML-like myeloproliferative syndrome has only been observed in a Balb/c background, but not in DBA/2 or C57B1/6 mice (96). Similarly, while *BCR/ABL* retroviruses derived from Moloney MuLV are capable of inducing B-cell leukemia after bone marrow infection (67), only viruses with LTR sequences derived from the closely related Moloney sarcoma virus (92) and myeloproliferative sarcoma virus (89,96) have been successful in inducing the CML-like syndrome. Specific mutations in the LTR enhancer of these viruses may allow them to avoid inactivation and promote expression in undifferentiated stem cells (108). However, the reasons for these peculiarities of host strain and vector are not known, but understanding these phenomena may reveal important clues to the complex pathophysiology of CML.

In summary, the bone marrow infection/transplantation model system has been very successful at recapitulating the complex physiology of CML in mice and has established beyond any reasonable doubt that *BCR/ABL* is the cause of human CML. The model has also been useful in defining differences between the leukemogenic activity of different *BCR/ABL* genes and in emphasizing that the leukemogenic consequence of *BCR/ABL* expression can vary greatly depending on the cell context, both of which have significant implications for the diagnosis and therapy of human Ph$^+$ leukemia (2). In theory, this model system could have many additional applications ranging from investigation of the molecular mechanisms of disease progression or graft-versus-leukemia effects to testing potential therapies. However, most of these uses will require that the generation of animals with the CML-like syndrome be made more efficient and reproducible. Fortunately, recent efforts appear to have made considerable progress toward this goal. The development of transient retroviral packaging systems (109,110) has led to improvements in titers of *BCR/ABL* retroviral stocks and allows the rapid generation of different high-titer viruses. In addition, the use of retroviral vectors capable of expressing two cooperating genes, such as *BCR/ABL* and *SHC* (111) or *GRB-2* (102), through the use of dual promoters or an internal ribosome entry site, has the potential to boost the efficiency of induction of the CML-like syndrome. Through systematic application of these improvements, we can anticipate that the bone marrow infection/transplantation model system, already a valuable tool, will become even better.

SUMMARY AND FUTURE PROSPECTS

It is apparent that we have learned an enormous amount about chronic myelogenous leukemia in the past several decades, and few clinicians and scientists would argue with the proposition that it is perhaps the best understood of all human cancers. However, the central biological mystery of CML remains: how does the bcr/abl protein, acting in a hematopoietic stem cell, perturb the delicate regulatory balance and lead to uncontrolled production of maturing myeloid cells? Is it through changes in sensitivity to negative growth signals in the marrow microenvironment? Is it mediated by loss of adhesive interactions with the stroma? What are the key domains of the Bcr/Abl kinase, and with which critical signaling molecules do they interact? The answers to such questions are of course unknown, but are likely to be revealed not through studies of human patients or cultured cells, but rather by careful and creative application of the animal model systems we have considered here.

ACKNOWLEDGMENTS

I thank Dr. George Q. Daley for helpful comments and for reading the manuscript. This work was supported in part from a grant from the Lucille P. Markey Charitable Trust, and by NIH grant CA57593. The author is a Lucille P. Markey Scholar in Biomedical Science and The Carl and Margaret Walter Scholar in Blood Research at Harvard Medical School.

REFERENCES

1. Daley GQ, Ben-Neriah Y. Implicating the *bcr/abl* gene in the pathogenesis of Philadelphia chromosome-positive human leukemia. In: Van de Woude GF,

Klein G, eds. Advances in Cancer Research. Vol. 57. San Diego: Academic Press, 1991:151–184.
2. Van Etten RA. The molecular pathogenesis of the Philadelphia-positive leukemias: implications for diagnosis and therapy. In: Freireich EJ, Kantarjian H, eds. Leukemia: Advances in Treatment and Research. Norwood, MA: Kluwer Academic Publishers, 1993:294–325.
3. Andriole GL, Mule JJ, Hansen CT, Linehan WM, Rosenberg SA. Evidence that lymphokine-activated killer cells and natural killer cells are distinct based on an analysis of congenitally immunodeficient mice. J Immunol 1985; 135:2911.
4. Bosma GC, Custer RP, Bosma MJ. A severe combined immunodeficiency mutation in the mouse. Nature 1983; 301:527–530.
5. Lapidot T, Pflumio F, Doedens M, Murdoch B, Williams DE, Dick JE. Cytokine stimulation of multilineage hematopoiesis from immature human cells engrafted in SCID mice. Science 1992; 225:1137–1141.
6. Vormoor J, Lappidot T, Pflumio F, et al. Immature human cord blood progenitors engraft and proliferate to high levels in severe combined immunodeficient mice. Blood 1994; 83:2489–2497.
7. Kamel-Reid S, Letarte M, Sirard C, et al. A model of human acute lymphoblastic leukemia in immune-deficient SCID mice. Science 1989; 246:1597–1600.
8. DeLord C, Clutterbuck R, Titley J, et al. Growth of primary human acute leukemia in severe combined immunodeficient mice. Exp Hematol 1991; 19:991.
9. Cesano A, Hoxie JA, Lange B, Nowell PC, Bishop J, Santoli D. The severe combined immunodeficient (SCID) mouse as a model for human myeloid leukemias. Oncogene 1992; 7:827.
10. Chelstrom L, Gunther R, Simon J, et al. Childhood acute myeloid leukemia in mice with severe combined immunodeficiency. Blood 1994; 84:20–26.
11. Lapidot T, Sirard C, Vormoor J, et al. A cell initiating human acute myeloid leukaemia after transplantation into SCID mice. Nature 1994; 367:645–648.
12. Uckun FM, Sather H, Reaman G, et al. Leukemic cell growth in SCID mice as a predictor of relapse in high-risk-B-lineage acute lymphoblastic leukemia. Blood 1995; 85:873–878.
13. Namikawa R, Weilbaecher KN, Kaneshima H, Yee EJ, McCune JM. Long-term human hematopoiesis in the SCID-hu mouse. J Exp Med 1990; 172:1055–1063.
14. Kyoizumi S, Baum CM, Kaneshima H, McCune JM, Yee EY, Namikawa R. Implantation and maintenance of functional human bone marrow in SCID-hu mice. Blood 1992; 79:1704–1711.
15. Namikawa R, Ueda R, Kyoizumi S. Growth of human myeloid leukemias in the human marrow environment of SCID-hu mice. Blood 1993; 82:2526–2536.
16. Chen BP, Galy A, Kyoizumi S, et al. Engraftment of human hematopoietic precursor cells with secondary transfer potential in SCID-hu mice. Blood 1994; 84: 2497.
17. Lozzio BB, Lozzio CB, Machado E. Human myelogenous (Ph^+) leukemia cell line: transplantation into athymic mice. J Natl Cancer Inst 1976; 56:627.
18. Sawyers CL, Gishizky ML, Quan S, Golde DW, Witte ON. Propagation of human blastic myeloid leukemias in the SCID mouse. Blood 1992; 79:2089–2098.
19. Ratajczak MZ, Kant JA, Luger SM, et al. In vivo treatment of human leukemia

in a *scid* mouse model with *c-myb* antisense oligodeoxynucleotides. Proc Natl Acad Sci USA 1992; 89:11823–11827.
20. Yan Y, Dennig D, Salomon O, O'Reilly RJ. Subcutaneous growth of human leukemias in immunodeficient SCID mice. Blood 1994; 84(suppl 1):48a.
21. Sirard C, Lapidot T, Vormoor J, et al. Normal and leukemic SCID-repopulating cells (SRC) coexist in the bone marrow and peripheral blood from CML patients in chronic phase, whereas leukemic SRC are detected in blast crisis. Blood 1996; 87:1539–1548.
22. Kolb HJ, Schattenberg A, Goldman JM, et al. Graft-versus-leukemia effect of donor lymphocyte transfusions in marrow grafted patients. Blood 1995; 86:2041–2050.
23. Coulombel L, Kalousek DK, Eaves CJ, Gupta CM, Eaves AC. Long-term marrow culture reveals chromosomally normal hematopoietic progenitor cells in patients with Philadelphia chromosome-positive chronic myelogenous leukemia. N Engl J Med 1983; 308:1493–1498.
24. Hariharan IK, Adams JM, Cory S. bcr-abl oncogene renders myeloid cell line factor independent: potential autocrine mechanism in chronic myeloid leukemia. Oncogene Res 1988; 3:387–399.
25. Sirard C, Laneuville P, Dick JE. Expression of *bcr-abl* abrogates factor-dependent growth of human hematopoietic M07E cells by an autocrine mechanism. Blood 1994; 83:1575.
26. Greenberger JS, Sakakeeny MA, Humphries RK, Eaves CJ, Eckner RJ. Demonstration of permanent factor-dependent multipotential (erthyroid/neutrophil/basophil) hematopoietic progenitor lines. Proc Natl Acad Sci USA 1983; 80:2931–2935.
27. Dexter TM, Garland J, Scott D, Scolnick E, Metcalf D. Growth of factor-dependent hematopoietic precursor cell lines. J Exp Med 1980; 152:1036.
28. Palacios R, Steinmetz M. IL3-dependent mouse clones that express B-220 surface antigen, contain Ig genes in germ-line configuration, and generate B lymphocytes in vivo. Cell 1985; 41:727–734.
29. Cook WD, Metcalf D, Nicola NA, Burgess AW, Walker F. Malignant transformation of a growth factor-dependent myeloid cell line by Abelson virus without evidence of an autocrine mechanism. Cell 1985; 41:677–683.
30. Mathey-Prevot B, Nabel G, Palacios R, Baltimore D. Abelson virus abrogation of interleukin-3 dependence in a lymphoid cell line. Mol Cell Biol 1986; 6:4133–4135.
31. Daley G, Baltimore D. Transformation of an interleukin 3-dependent hematopoietic cell line by the chronic myelogenous leukemia-specific P210 *bcr/abl* protein. Proc Natl Acad Sci USA 1988; 85:9312–9316.
32. Laneuville P, Heisterkamp N, Groffen J. Expression of the chronic myelogenous leukemia-associated p210 *brc/abl* oncoprotein in a murine IL-3 dependent myeloid cell line. Oncogene 1991; 6:275–282.
33. Matulonis UA, Dosiou C, Lamont C, et al. Role of B7-1 in mediating an immune response to myeloid leukemia cells. Blood 1995; 85:2507–2515.
34. Ilaria RL Jr, Van Etten RA. The SH2 domain of $P210^{BCR/ABL}$ is not required for

transformation of hematopoietic factor-dependent cells. Blood 1995; 86:3897–3904.
35. Muller AJ, Young JC, Pendergast A, et al. BCR first exon sequences specifically activate the BCR/ABL tyrosine kinase oncogene of Philadelphia chromosome-positive leukemias. Mol Cell Biol 1991; 11:1785–1792.
36. McWhirter JR, Wang JYJ. Activation of tyrosine kinase and microfilament-binding functions of c-*abl* by bcr sequences in *bcr/abl* fusion proteins. Mol Cell Biol 1991; 11:1785–1792.
37. McWhirter JR, Galasso DL, Wang JYJ. A coiled-coil oligomerization domain of Bcr is essential for the transforming function of Bcr-Abl oncoproteins. Mol Cell Biol 1993; 13:7587–7595.
38. Pendergast AM, Quilliam LA, Cripe LD, et al. BCR-ABL-induced oncogenesis is mediated by direct interaction with the SH2 domain of the GRB-2 adaptor protein. Cell 1993; 75:175–185.
39. Daley GQ, McLaughlin J, Witte ON, Baltimore D. The CML-specific P210*bcr/abl* protein, unlike v-*abl*, does not transform NIH/3T3 fibroblasts. Science 1987; 237:532–535.
40. Daley GQ, Van Etten RA, Jackson PK, Bernards A, Baltimore D. Non-myristoylated Abl proteins transform a factor-dependent hematopoietic cell line. Mol Cell Biol 1992; 12:1864–1871.
41. Mayer BJ, Jackson PK, Van Etten RA, Baltimore D. Point mutations in the *abl* SH2 domain coordinately impair phosphotyrosine binding in vitro and transforming activity in vivo. Mol Cell Biol 1992; 12:609–618.
42. Mayer BJ, Baltimore D. Mutagenic analysis of the roles of SH2 and SH3 domains in regulation of the Abl tyrosine kinase. Mol Cell Biol 1994; 14:2883–2894.
43. Afar DEH, Goga A, McLaughlin J, Witte ON, Sawyers CS. Differential complementation of Bcr-Abl point mutants with c-myc. Science 1994; 264:424.
44. Van Etten RA, Stam K, Goddard C, Foulkes JG. Unpublished observations.
45. Druker BJ, Tamura S, Buchdunger E, et al. Effects of a selective inhibitor of the Abl tyrosine kinase on the growth of Bcr-Abl positive cells. Nature Med 1996; 2:561–566.
46. Chen L, Ashe S, Brady WA, et al. Costimulation of antitumor immunity by the B7 counterreceptor for the T lymphocyte molecules CD28 and CTLA-4. Cell 1992; 71:1093.
47. Matulonis U, Dosiou C, Freeman G, et al. B7-1 is superior to B7-2 costimulation in the induction and maintenance of T cell-mediated antileukemia immunity. J Immunol 1996; 156:1126–1131.
48. Chen W, Peace DJ, Rovira DK, You S-G, Cheever MA. T-cell immunity to the joining region of p210 BCR-ABL protein. Proc Natl Acad Sci USA 1992; 89:1468.
49. Bocchia M, Korontsvit T, Xu Q, et al. Specific human cellular immunity to bcr-abl oncogene-derived peptides. Blood 1996; 87:3587–3592.
50. Hariharan IK, Harris AW, Crawford M, et al. A *bcr*-v-*abl* oncogene induces lymphomas in transgenic mice. Mol Cell Biol 1989; 9:2798–2805.
51. Langdon WY, Harris AW, Cory S, Adams JM. The c-myc oncogene perturbs B lymphocyte development in E-mu-myc transgenic mice. Cell 1986; 47:11–18.

52. Shah NP, Witte ON, Denny CT. Characterization of the *BCR* promoter in Philadelphia chromosome-positive and -negative cell lines. Mol Cell Biol 1991; 11: 1854–1860.
53. Lifshitz B, Fainstein E, Marcelle C, et al. *bcr* Genes and transcripts. Oncogene 1988; 2:113–117.
54. Heisterkamp N, Jenster G, Kioussis D, Pattengale PK, Groffen J. Human *bcr-abl* gene has a lethal effect on embryogenesis. Transgenic Res 1991; 1:45–53.
55. Heisterkamp N, Jenster G, ten Hoeve J, Zovich D, Pattengale PK, Groffen J. Acute leukemia in bcr/abl transgenic mice. Nature 1990; 344:251–253.
56. Stuart GW, Searle PF, Chen HY, Brinster RL, Palmiter RD. A 12 base-pair DNA motif that is repeated several times in metallothionein gene promoters confers metal regulation to a heterologous gene. Proc Natl Acad Sci USA 1984; 81:7318.
57. Palmiter RD, Norstedt G, Gelinas RE, Hammer RE, Brinster RL. Metallothionein-human GH fusion gene stimulates growth of mice. Science 1983; 222:809.
58. Voncken JW, Griffiths S, Greaves MF, Pattengale PK, Heisterkamp N, Groffen J. Restricted oncogenicity of BCR/ABL p190 in transgenic mice. Cancer Res 1992; 52:4534–4539.
59. Voncken JW, Morris C, Pattengale P, et al. Clonal development and karyotype evolution during leukemogenesis of *BCR/ABL* transgenic mice. Blood 1992; 79: 1029–1036.
60. Griffiths SD, Healy LE, Ford AM, et al. Clonal characteristics of acute lymphoblastic cells derived from *BCR/ABL* p190 transgenic mice. Oncogene 1992; 7: 1391–1399.
61. Schlissel M, Baltimore D. Activation of immunoglobulin kappa gene rearrangement correlates with induction of germline kappa gene transcription. Cell 1989; 58:1001–1007.
62. Gilliland DG, Blanchard KL, Bunn HF. Clonality in myeloproliferative disorders: analysis by means of the polymerase chain reaction. Proc Natl Acad Sci USA 1991; 88:6848–6852.
63. McLaughlin J, Chianese E, Witte ON. Alternative forms of the *bcr/abl* oncogene have quantitatively different potencies for stimulation of immature lymphoid cells. Mol Cell Biol 1989; 9:1866–1874.
64. Kurzrock R, Shtalrid M, Talpaz M, Kloetzer WS, Gutterman JU. Expression of *c-abl* in Philadelphia-positive acute myelogenous leukemia. Blood 1987; 70:1584–1588.
65. Honda H, Fujii T, Takatoku M, et al. Expression of p210*bcr/abl* by metallothionein promoter induced T-cell leukemia in transgenic mice. Blood 1995; 10:2853–2861.
66. Voncken JW, Kaartinen V, Pattengale PK, Germeraad WTV, Groffen J, Heisterkamp N. *BCR/ABL* P210 and P190 cause distinct leukemia in transgenic mice. Blood 1995; 86:4603–4611.
67. McLaughlin J, Chianese E, Witte ON. In vitro transformation of immature hematopoietic cells by the P210 *bcr/abl* oncogene product of the Philadelphia chromosome. Proc Natl Acad Sci USA 1987; 84:6558–6562.
68. Scherle PA, Dorshkind K, Witte ON. Clonal lymphoid progenitor cell lines ex-

pressing the *BCR/ABL* oncogene retain full differentiative function. Proc Natl Acad Sci USA 1990; 87:1908–1912.
69. Cardiff RD, Leder A, Kuo A, Pattengale PK, Leder P. Multiple tumor types appear in a transgenic mouse with the ras oncogene. Am J Pathol 1993; 142:1199–1207.
70. Suda Y, Aizawa S, Hirai S, et al. Driven by the same Ig enhancer and SV40 T promoter, ras induced lung adenomatous tumors, myc induced pre-B lymphomas, and SV40 large T antigen a variety of tumors in transgenic mice. EMBO J 1987; 6:4055–4065.
71. Wen S-T, Jackson PK, Van Etten RA. The cytostatic function of c-Abl is controlled by multiple nuclear localization signals, and requires the *p53* and *Rb* tumor suppressor gene products. EMBO J 1996; 15:1583–1595.
72. Dziennis S, Van Etten RA, Pahl HL, et al. The CD11b promoter directs high level expression of reporter genes in macrophages in transgenic mice. Blood 1995; 85:319–329.
73. Jin DI, Jameson SB, Reddy MA, Schenkman D, Ostrowski MC. Alterations in differentiation and behavior of monocytic phagocytes in transgenic mice that express dominant suppressors of ras signaling. Mol Cell Biol 1995; 15:693–703.
74. Grisolano JL, Sclar GM, Ley TJ. Early myeloid cell-specific expression of the human cathepsin G gene in transgenic mice. Proc Natl Acad Sci USA 1994; 91:8989–8993.
75. Dziennis S, Zhang P, Van Etten RA, Tenen DG. Unpublished observations.
76. Ornitz DM, Moreadith RW, Leder P. Binary system for regulating transgene expression in mice: Targeting *int*-2 gene expression with yeast *GAL4/UAS* control elements. Proc Natl Acad Sci USA 1991; 88:698–702.
77. Kühn R, Schwenk F, Aguet M, Rajewsky K. Inducible gene targeting in mice. Science 1995; 269:1427–1429.
78. Nagy A, Rossant J. Targeted mutagenesis: analysis of phenotype without germline transmission. J Clin Invest 1996; 97:1360–1365.
79. Corral J, Lavenir I, Impey H, et al. An *MLL-AF9* fusion gene made by homologous recombination causes acute leukemia in chimeric mice: a method to create fusion oncogenes. Cell 1996; 85:853–861.
80. van Deursen J, Fornerod M, van Rees B, Grosveld G. Cre-mediated site-specific translocation between nonhomologous mouse chromosome. Proc Natl Acad Sci USA 1995; 92:7376–7380.
81. Furth PA, St. Onge L, Boger H, et al. Temporal control of gene expression in transgenic mice by a tetracycline-responsive promoter. Proc Natl Acad Sci USA 1994; 91:9302–9306.
82. Whitlock CA, Witte ON. Long-term culture of B lymphocytes and their precursors from murine bone marrow. Proc Natl Acad Sci USA 1982; 79:3608–3612.
83. Whitlock CA, Ziegler SF, Witte ON. Progression of the transformed phenotype in clonal lines of Abelson virus-infected lymphocytes. Mol Cell Biol 1983; 3:596–604.
84. Dexter TM, Allen T, Lajtha L. Conditions controlling the proliferation of haematopoietic stem cells in vitro. J Cell Physiol 1977; 91:335–344.

85. Young JC, Witte ON. Selective transformation of primitive lymphoid cells by the *bcr/abl* oncogene expressed in long-term lymphoid or myeloid cultures. Mol Cell Biol 1988; 8:4079–4087.
86. Gishizky ML, Witte ON. Initiation of deregulated growth of multipotent progenitor cells by *bcr-abl* in vitro. Science 1992; 256:836–839.
87. Gishizky ML, Witte ON. *BCR/ABL* enhances growth of multipotent progenitor cells but does not block their differentiation potential in vitro. Curr Topics Micro Immunol 1992; 182:65–72.
88. Heard JM, Roussel MF, Rettenmier CW, Sherr CJ. Multilineage hematopoietic disorders induced by transplantation of bone marrow cells expressing the v-*fms* oncogene. Cell 1987; 51:663–673.
89. Daley GQ, Van Etten RA, Baltimore D. Induction of chronic myelogenous leukemia in mice by the $P210^{bcr/abl}$ gene of the Philadelphia chromosome. Science 1990; 247:824–830.
90. Elefanty AG, Hariharan IK, Cory S. *bcr-abl*, The hallmark of chronic myeloid leukemia in man, induces multiple hematopoietic neoplasms in mice. EMBO J 1990; 9:1069–1078.
91. Kelliher MA, McLaughlin J, Witte ON, Rosenberg N. Induction of a chronic myelogenous leukemia-like syndrome in mice with v-abl and bcr-abl. Proc Natl Acad Sci USA 1990; 87:6649–6653.
92. Gishizky MI, Johnson-White J, Witte ON. Efficient transplantation of *BCR/ABL*-induced chronic myelogenous leukemia-like syndrome in mice. Proc Natl Acad Sci USA 1993; 90:3755–3759.
93. Siminovitch L, McCulloch EA, Till JE. Distribution of colony-forming cells among spleen colonies. J Cell Comp Phys 1963; 62:327.
94. Daley GQ, Van Etten RA, Baltimore D. Blast crisis in a murine model of chronic myelogenous leukemia. Proc Natl Acad Sci USA 1991; 88:11335–11338.
95. Risser R, Potter M, Rowe WP. Abelson virus-induced lymphomagenesis in mice. J Exp Med 1978; 148:714–726.
96. Elefanty AG, Cory S. Hematologic disease induced in BALB/c mice by a bcr/abl retrovirus is influenced by infection conditions. Mol Cell Biol 1992; 12:1755–1763.
97. Kelliher MA, Weckstein DJ, Knott AG, Wortis HH, Rosenberg N. ABL oncogenes directly stimulate two distinct target cells in bone marrow from 5-fluorouracil-treated mice. Oncogene 1993; 8:1249–1256.
98. Van Etten RA, Ilaria RL. Unpublished observations.
99. Elefanty AG, Cory S. bcr-abl-Induced cell lines can switch from mast cell to erythroid or myeloid differentiation in vitro. Blood 1992; 79:1271–1281.
100. Davis BR, Brightman BK, Chandy KG, Fan H. Characterization of a preleukemic state induced by Moloney murine leukemia virus: evidence for two infection events during leukemogenesis. Proc Natl Acad Sci USA 1987; 84:4875–4879.
101. Fialkow PH, Martin PJ, Naifield, Penfold GK, Jacobson RJ, Hansen JA. Evidence for a multistep pathogenesis of chronic myelogenous leukemia. Blood 1981; 58:158–163.
102. Pear WS. Personal communication.

103. Lemischka IR, Raulet D, Mullligan RC. Developmental potential and dynamic behavior of hematopoietic stem cells. Cell 1986; 45:917–927.
104. Kantarjian H, Talpaz M, LeMaistre CF, et al. Intensive combination chemotherapy and autologous bone marrow transplantation leads to reappearance of Philadelphia chromosome-negative cells in chronic myelogenous leukemia. Cancer 1991; 67:2959.
105. Daley GQ, Goldman JM. Autologous transplant for CML revisited. Exp Hematol 1993; 21:734–737.
106. Kelliher M, Knott A, McLaughlin J, Witte ON, Rosenberg N. Differences in oncogenic potency but not target cell specificity distinguish the two forms of the *BCR/ABL* oncogene. Mol Cell Biol 1991; 11:4710–4716.
107. Scott ML, Van Etten RA, Daley GQ, Baltimore D. v-*abl* causes hematopoietic disease distinct from that caused by *bcr-abl*. Proc Natl Acad Sci USA 1991; 88:6506–6510.
108. Stocking C, Kollek R, Bergholz U, Ostertag W. Long terminal repeat sequences impart hematopoietic transformation properties to the myeloproliferative sarcoma virus. Proc Natl Acad Sci USA 1985; 82:5746–5750.
109. Pear WS, Nolan GP, Scott ML, Baltimore D. Production of high-titer helper-free retroviruses by transient transfection. Proc Natl Acad Sci USA 1993; 90:8392–8396.
110. Finer MH, Dull TJ, Qin L, Farson D, Roberts M. *kat*: A high-efficiency retroviral transduction system for primary human T lymphocytes. Blood 1994; 83:43–50.
111. Goga A, McLaughlin J, Afar DE, Saffran DC, Witte ON. Alternative signals to RAS for hematopoietic transformation by the BCR-ABL oncogene. Cell 1995; 82:981–988.

4
Natural History and Prognostic Factors in Chronic Myelogenous Leukemia: Past, Present, and Future

Sergio Giralt
M.D. Anderson Cancer Center, Houston, Texas

PROGNOSTIC FACTORS: DEFINITION, DISCOVERY, AND RELEVANCE

The art or science of predicting the length, behavior, and eventual outcome of any disease process has been one of the major components of medical practice. Modern physicians have predicted individual patients' disease outcome based on the presence or absence of various signs and symptoms and comparing them to their prior experience or the body of existing knowledge known as "the literature." These signs and symptoms of a disease entity that permit a practitioner to predict the behavior of a disease in an individual patient with certain degree of accuracy are known as prognostic factors.

Definition of factors that influence eventual outcomes of disease has evolved from simple observational bias to complex statistical techniques. In modern clinical medicine, prognostic variables are determined prospectively or retrospectively first through univariate statistical analysis and then through more complex, multivariate analysis to define the independent prognostic variables.

The study of prognostic factors has assisted in: (1) providing insights into the mechanism of a disease; (2) planning therapy for the individual patient; (3) designing clinical trials; (4) comparing treatment outcomes among different groups of patients; and (5) assisting in identifying and developing new therapeutic and preventive strategies (1).

Prognostic factors can be used to predict response to therapy; although usually determined at diagnosis, they can be defined at any time in the natural history of the disease. Prognostic factors can be derived from the response to a specific medical intervention. Traditionally, prognostic factors have been elements of the patient's history or data from basic clinical or conventional laboratory examination. More recent developments have now identified genetic and molecular markers of prognosis that are rapidly being incorporated into prognostic models.

In chronic myelogenous leukemia (CML), the study of prognostic factors began in the 1920s, when the progression of the disease from a stable phase to a rapidly aggressive and fatal phase was described by Minot and collaborators, as well as the potential beneficial effects of radiation therapy. In this chapter we will describe the prognostic factors for CML before and after the interferon era and the use of these prognostic factors in making therapeutic decisions for the individual patient (2).

PROGNOSTIC FACTORS IN CML PRIOR TO THE INTERFERON ERA

In 1924 Minot reported a series of 166 patients with CML and the effects of radiation therapy on survival. The average survival of untreated patients was 3.05 years, versus 3.5 years for treated patients. This report defined the progression of the disease from a stable phase to an accelerated phase with progressive resistance to radiotherapy (2). With the advent of busulfan and hydrea, multiple investigators developed models to predict disease course for patients receiving these treatment modalities (3–9).

These prognostic models incorporated clinical and laboratory parameters. Many but not all parameters were shared by the different proposed models. These models grouped patients in three or four prognostic categories with different survival probabilities. A synthesis model has been proposed grouping elements from all the proposed models that resulted in three categories of patients with expected median survivals of 2, 3.5, and >5 years, respectively (9). In these models, age, organomegaly, increased peripheral blood or bone marrow basophilia, increased peripheral blood or bone marrow blasts, and clonal evolution emerged as important adverse prognostic factors (Table 1).

Appropriate and consistent identification of prognostic groups is extremely relevant in CML if one wants to compare efficacy of different treatments such as different bone marrow transplant regimens. Loose definitions of accelerated phase or poor prognosis disease will make the results of therapy for patients in the such defined categories of chronic phase or accelerated phase spuriously better due to the phenomenon of stage migration (10).

Table 1 Prognostic Models for CML

	Univariate (p)	Multivariate (p)	Survival at 5 years
Cervantes 1982	Splenomegaly (<0.02) Hepatomegaly (<0.02) Anemia (<0.05) PB normoblasts (<0.01) BM blasts >5% (<0.005)	Splenomegaly (0.0064) Hepatomegaly (0.012) PB normoblasts (0.066) BM blasts >5% (0.022) Hb <8.5 g/dL (0.38)	Stage 1: 0–1 factor: 70% Stage 2: 2 factors: 30% Stage 3: >2 factors: 15%
Tura 1981	Spleen >15 cm (<0.02) Hepatomegaly (<0.0005) Platelets (<0.0005) WBC >100,000 (<0.005) PB blasts >1% (<0.001) WBC precursors >20% (<0.01)	Not stated	Stage 1: 0–1 factor: 60% Stage 2: 2–3 factors: 32% Stage 3: >3 factors: 12%
Sokal 1984	Spleen size (0.000001) Liver size (0.00001) PB blast (0.000001) Platelets (0.001) WBC count (0.001) Anemia (0.0004)	PB blasts (0.000001) Spleen size (0.00005) Age (0.001) Platelet count (0.004)	Solve regression equation Stage I: 55% Stage II: 35% Stage III: 15%
Synthesis 1990	Not applicable	Age ≥60 Spleen ≥10 cm PB blast ≥3% BM blast ≥5% Platelets ≥700,000 PB basophils ≥7% Accelerated phase Criteria[a]	Stage 1: 45% Stage 2: 35% Stage 3: 18% Stage 4: 18%

PB: peripheral blood, BM: bone marrow, WBC: white blood cell count, Hb: hemoglobin.
[a] Cytogenetic clonal evolution, ≥15% blasts in PB, ≥30% blasts and progranulocytes in PB, ≥20% basophils in PB, <100,000 platelets/μL.

PROGNOSTIC FACTORS IN THE INTERFERON ERA

More than 200 patients with early chronic phase Ph-positive CML have been on interferon based programs at M.D. Anderson Cancer Center. Complete hematologic remission was achieved in 80% of these patients, 38% achieved a major cytogenetic response (<35% of Ph^+ metaphases), and 26% had at least one evaluable cytogenetic analysis with no detectable Ph^+ metaphases. The median overall survival for all patients was 89 months with an estimated 5-year survival rate of 63%. Five-year survival was 90%, 85%, 70%, and 30% for patients with complete, partial, minor, or no cytogenetic remission after 12 months of therapy, respectively (11).

Four large randomized trials comparing interferon to conventional chemotherapy have been reported (Table 2) (12–15). In all studies interferon therapy produced a higher rate of major cytogenetic remission rate, delayed the progression to blast crisis, and improved survival when compared to busulfan (13–15). However, the survival benefit is not as dramatic when comparison is made with hydroxyurea therapy although the incidence of cytogenetic remissions is higher in the interferon group (12,13,15).

Analysis of the M.D. Anderson Cancer Center data revealed that interferon therapy improved survival in all risk categories of patients with chronic phase CML. The major survival benefit was seen in patients in the good risk group. However, survival benefits were seen in all disease categories, but were limited to patients achieving a cytogenetic remission. A multivariate analysis revealed that cytogenetic response was the most important independent prognostic factor for survival in patients with newly diagnosed CML (11,16). Therefore, defining factors that can predict a cytogenetic response to interferon is essential in helping physicians decide who should get this form of therapy (17).

The percentage of peripheral blood blasts was the most important predictor for a cytogenetic response in both the M.D. Anderson and Italian Cooperative Group experiences (11,12). Splenomegaly, symptomatic disease, anemia, thrombocytosis, and white blood cell count at the time of diagnosis were also important prognostic factors reported in at least one of the studies (11). Time from diagnosis and interferon dose have been also suggested as important predictors for cytogenetic response to interferon therapy in CML (18).

Patients receiving interferon therapy can still be segregated in three distinctive prognostic groups with median survivals of 102, 90, and 47 months using the same prognostic factors derived from the chemotherapy era. Therefore, existing prognostic models continue to be relevant for interferon-treated patients.

BIOLOGICAL AND MOLECULAR CORRELATES

Surrogate markers for survival and response to interferon therapy would be useful in CML. Molecular markers that could predict a high or low likelihood

Table 2 Randomized Trials of Interferon Versus Chemotherapy for CML

	Tura (IFN vs. hydrea)	Allen (IFN vs. chemo)	Hehlmann (IFN vs. busulfan)	Hehlmann (IFN vs. hydrea)	Ohnishi (IFN vs. busulfan)
% Major Cytogenetic responses IFN vs. control	24 vs. 1	11 vs. 2	2.4 vs. 1	2.4 vs. 1	7 vs. 2.5
% Complete cytogenetic response IFN vs. control	17 vs. 0	NS	7 vs. 0	7 vs. 1	9 vs. 2.5
Median survival IFN vs. control (months)	72 vs. 52	61 vs. 41	66 vs. 45	66 vs. 58	60+ vs. 40

of response to interferon could assist the physician in guiding therapy. Likewise, molecular markers predictive of transformation or disease progression could guide physicians and patients toward more aggressive and novel forms of therapy such as bone marrow transplantation or new drug combinations.

To date only cytogenetic clonal evolution has been consistently predictive of disease transformation and poor survival. The mean survival for patients with chromosome 17 abnormalities or chromosomal translocations other than t (9,22) without any other feature of disease acceleration was 6 months, as opposed to 54 months for those without these additional chromosome abnormalities (19).

The breakpoint site in the breakpoint cluster region (bcr) has been proposed as a possible prognostic factor. Patients with a 3' breakpoint have in some studies a shorter survival and more rapid onset of transformation than patients with a 5' breakpoint (20). This observation has not been confirmed by other investigators (21,22).

Other biological markers that have been reported to be associated with increasing risk of transformation and decreased survival include: interleukin-1 beta levels, DNA-image cytometry, and calcitonin gene hypermethylation. However, these and other biological markers have not been sufficiently studied to determine if they may be of practical use in guiding therapy (23–25).

NATURAL HISTORY OF CML: INTERFERON ERA

The median survival for patients with CML has improved from 32 months in 1975 to 72 months in the 10 years spanning 1983 to 1993. The improvement in survival is in large part due to earlier diagnosis. The presenting features of CML have changed due to the availability of routine hematological examination. Up to 45% of patients present without symptoms, versus 15% in the past. Likewise, the percentage of patients presenting with high-risk features has decreased from 21% before 1982 to 11% after 1982, and the incidence of good-risk patients has increased from 35% to 45% during the same time period (17).

Improved survival during this time period has also been due to improved therapy. Patients achieving any type of cytogenetic response while on interferon therapy will have an estimated survival rate of approximately 95% at 2 years and 80% at 4 years regardless of prognostic group at the time of diagnosis. Patients not achieving a cytogenetic response will, on the other hand, have an estimated survival rate at 4 years of between 62% and 39% depending on the prognostic group at the time of presentation.

Patients undergoing allogeneic bone marrow transplantation also have a major change in the natural history of their disease, with 50–60% of them achieving long-term disease control (26,27). Even the 10–20% of these patients who relapse can still obtain a second remission with interferon or donor lympho-

Table 3 Summary of Prognostic Factors in CML

Clinical	Variable	Unfavorable
	Age	>60
	Spleen	>10 cm
Laboratory		
	Blood blast %	≥3%
	Basophilia	≥7%
	Clonal evolution	
	Thrombocytosis	

cyte infusions (28,29). However, for many patients the risk of early mortality is high enough to abrogate any potential survival benefit, and actually may be deleterious (30).

PROGNOSTIC FACTORS

Prior to interferon and allogeneic bone marrow transplantation, prognostic factors had little practical utility except to advise the patient of their impending transformation and death. With the advent of two strategies that can change the natural course of the disease, with different efficacy and toxicity profiles, this has changed. The use of prognostic factors to assist the physician in deciding among therapies is becoming essential for the rational practice of CML therapy.

Most patients will fall between the extremes of an elderly patient diagnosed with CML serendipitously, and the 15-year-old presenting with a large spleen and peripheral blood blast. The relative weight that an individual physician places on the prognostic factors for disease progression versus response to interferon and transplant related toxicity will determine the treatment that physician will recommend to that particular patient. The parameters most commonly used are summarized in Table 3 and have helped us develop our current treatment algorithms summarized elsewhere (16).

SUMMARY

Allogeneic bone marrow transplantation and interferon therapy have been major therapeutic developments for CML. These therapies can induce durable complete cytogenetic remissions, which translate into improved survival. The use of existing prognostic factors and the continued study of surrogate markers are essential in providing patients with CML the optimal therapy with the best risk/

benefit ratio at any specific stage of their disease process. Future studies aimed at improving the quality of cytogenetic remissions with interferon and improving the safety of transplant may make current prognostic factors obsolete. However, until that day, therapeutic planning for CML patients should be guided by a risk-oriented approach using the known prognostic models.

REFERENCES

1. Armitage P, Gehan E. Statistical methods for the identification and use of prognostic factors. Int J Cancer 1974; 13:16–36.
2. Minot G, Buckman T, Isaacs R. Chronic myelogenous leukemia. JAMA 1924; 82: 1489–1494.
3. Galton D. Myeleran in chronic myeloid leukemia. Lancet 1953; 1:208–213.
4. Kennedy B, Yarbro K. Metabolic and therapeutic effects of hydroxyurea in chronic myeloid leukemia. JAMA 1996; 195:1038–1043.
5. Cervantes F, Rozman C. A multivariate analysis of prognostic factors in chronic myeloid leukemia. Blood 1982; 60:1298–1304.
6. Kantarjian H, Smith T, McCredie K, et al. Chronic myelogenous leukemia: a multivariate analysis of the associations of patient characteristics and therapy with survival. Blood 1985; 66:1326–1335.
7. Sokal J, Cox E, Baccarani M, et al. Prognostic discrimination "good risk" chronic granulocytic leukemia. Blood 1984; 63:789–799.
8. Tura S, Baccarani M, Corbelli G, et al. Staging of chronic myeloid leukaemia. Br J Haematol 1981; 47:105–119.
9. Kantarjian H, Keating M, Smith T, et al. Proposal for a simple synthesis prognostic staging system in chronic myelogenous leukemia. Am J Med 1990; 88:1–15.
10. Dent M. Improving cancer survival by artifact—Will Rogers and The Stage Migration Phenomenom. S Afr Med J 1996; 86:645.
11. Kantarjian H, Smith T, O'Brien S, et al. Prolonged survival in chronic myelogenous leukemia after cytogenetic response to interferon-alpha therapy. Ann Intern Med 1995; 122:254–261.
12. Tura S, Baccarani M, Zuffa E. Interferon alfa-2a as compared with conventional chemotherapy for the treatment of chronic myeloid leukemia. N Engl J Med 1994; 330;820–825.
13. Allan N, Richards S, Shepard P. UK Medical Research Council randomized trial of interferon alpha-n-1 for chronic myeloid leukemia: improved survival irrespective of cytogenetic response. Lancet 1995; 345:1392–1397.
14. Ohnishi K, Ohno R, Tomonaga M, et al. A randomized trial comparing interferon-alpha with busulfan for newly diagnosed chronic myelogenous leukemia in chronic phase. Blood 1995; 86:906–916.
15. Hehlmann R, Heimpel H, Hasford J, et al. Randomized comparison of interferon-alpha with busulfan and hydroxyurea in chronic myelogenous leukemia. Blood 1994; 84:4064–4077.

16. Kantarjian H, Deisseroth A, Kurzrock R, Estrov Z, Talpaz M. Chronic myelogenous leukemia: a concise update. Blood 1993; 82:691–703.
17. Giralt S, Kantarjian H, Talpaz M. The natural history of chronic myelogenous leukemia in the interferon era. Semin Hematol 1995; 32:152–158.
18. Giralt S, Kantarjian H, Talpaz M. Treatment of chronic myelogenous leukemia. Semin Oncol 1995; 22:396–404.
19. Majlis A, Smith T, Talpaz M, O'Brien S, Rios M, Kantarjian H. Significance of cytogenetic clonal evolution in chronic myelogenous leukemia. J Clin Oncol 1996; 14:196–203.
20. Mills K, MacKenzie E, Birnie G. The site of the breakpoint within the bcr is a prognostic factor in Philadelphia-positive CML patients. Blood 1989; 73:1745–1746.
21. Verschraegen C, Kantarjian H, Hirsch-Ginsberg C, et al. The breakpoint cluster region site in patients with Philadelphia chromosome-positive chronic myelogenous leukemia. Clinical, laboratory and prognostic correlations. Cancer 1995; 76:992–997.
22. Sheperd P, Suffolk R, Halsey J, Allan N. Analysis of molecular breakpoint and m-RNA transcripts in a prospective randomized trial of interferon in chronic myeloid leukaemia: no correlation with clinical features, cytogenetic response, duration of chronic phase, or survival. Br J Haematol 1995; 89:546–554.
23. Wetzler M, Kurzrock R, Estrov Z, et al. Altered levels of interleukin-1 beta and interleukin-1 receptor antagonist in chronic myelogenous leukemia: clinical and prognostic correlates. Blood 1994; 84:314–317.
24. Muller C, Kropff M, Biesterfeld S, et al. Detection of high risk patients in chronic myelogenous leukemia by DNA-image cytometry. Anticancer Res 1991; 11:617–623.
25. Malinen T, Palotie A, Pakkala S, Peltonen L, Ruutu T, Jansson S. Acceleration of chronic myeloid leukemia correlates with calcitonin gene hyper methylation. Blood 1991; 77:2435–2440.
26. Goldman J, Apperley J, Jones L, et al. Bone marrow transplantation for chronic myeloid leukemia. N Engl J Med 1986; 314:202–207.
27. Clift R, Appelbaum F, Thomas E. Bone marrow transplantation for chronic myelogenous leukemia. Blood 1994; 83:2752–2753.
28. Arcese W, Goldman J, D'Arcangelo E, et al. Outcome for patients who relapse after allogeneic bone marrow transplantation for chronic myeloid leukemia. Blood 1993; 82:3211–3219.
29. Kolb H, Schattenberg A, Goldman J, et al. Graft-versus-leukemia effect of donor lymphocyte transfusions in marrow grafted patients. Blood 1995; 86:2041–2050.
30. Italian Cooperative Study Group on Chronic Myeloid Leukemia. Evaluating survival after allogeneic bone marrow transplant for chronic myeloid leukemia in chronic phase: a comparison of transplant versus no-transplant in a cohort of 258 patients first seen in Italy between 1984 and 1986. Br J Haematol 1993; 85:292–299.

5
Changing Nature of Conventional Therapy in Chronic Myelogenous Leukemia

Rüdiger Hehlmann and Andreas Hochhaus
Klinikum Mannheim, University of Heidelberg, Mannheim, Germany

INTRODUCTION

Until recently the notion prevailed that natural course and survival time of chronic myelogenous leukemia (CML) were determined by intrinsic factors of the disease rather than therapy (1,2). Conventional therapy of CML was mainly palliative, differences in survival depending less on the mode of therapy than on patient selection and exclusion of high-risk patients such as Philadelphia (Ph)-negative or preblastic ones. There seems to be general agreement now that interferon-alpha (IFN-α) and, to a lesser extent, also hydroxyurea (HU) can prolong life in CML, which represents a considerable advance of CML therapy. Although drug therapy most probably still does not cure CML, it remains of particular importance, since the only curative therapy, allogenous bone marrow transplantation (allo-BMT), can be offered only to a minority of patients of sufficiently young age who have an HLA-compatible donor (3,4). It appears that the best effect can be obtained with most treatment modalities (IFN-α, intensive chemotherapy, allo-BMT, autografting), if treatment is started early in chronic phase (5–8). Once blast crisis has developed, median survival is only 2–3 months, hardly influenced by any therapy. The purpose of this chapter is to review the evolution of conventional therapy and to show where recent progress has been made, how natural course and survival time of CML are changing with the use of new drugs and procedures, and what at present the lines of research for future improvements appear to be. Figure 1 shows the historic development of CML therapies. Table 1 gives an overview of the survival times reported under the various CML therapies.

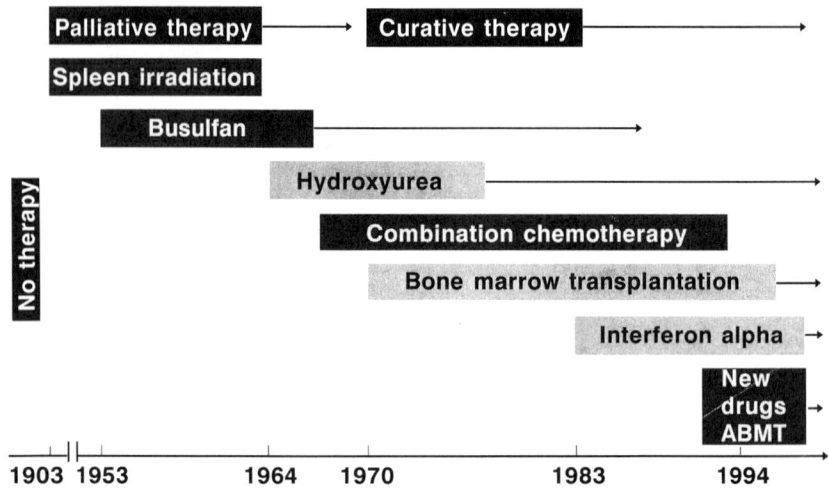

Figure 1 Historic development of CML therapies.

SPLENIC IRRADIATION

The mainstay of CML therapy during the first half of the century was splenic irradiation (9,10). Its effect was palliative, particularly for splenomegaly-related symptoms, but of limited duration, and, frequently, repeated courses of splenic irradiation had to be given. It was largely replaced by busulfan when this drug became available in the 1950s and is reserved for special indications.

BUSULFAN AND OTHER MONOTHERAPIES

Busulfan was considered the drug of choice for palliation during the chronic phase for about 30 years, since it reliably controlled CML-related signs and

Table 1 Median Survival in CML

Therapy	Months	Ref.
None	31	9
Splenic irradiation	28	10
Busulfan	35–45	11
Hydroxyurea	48–67	32, 37, 59
Intensive chemotherapy	45–55	93, 94
Interferon-α	55–89	42, 53, 54, 58, 62
Allogeneic BMT	40–80% (5-year survival rate)	95–97
Autografting	>50% (5-year survival rate)	88

symptoms in 95% of patients for at least 3 months (1). All studies had shown its efficacy and reliability since its introduction in 1953 (11). The only true alternative was hydroxyurea (HU), which was introduced 10 years later (12). Most other cytostatic drugs had been shown to be either inferior to busulfan or to lack any clear advantage.

Table 2 lists the most relevant studies comparing busulfan with other monotherapies during the chronic phase. The Southeastern Study Group compared busulfan with chlorambucil and 6-mercaptopurine (13,14). The response rate of chlorambucil was, with 12 out of 21, clearly inferior to that of busulfan, which induced remissions in all 21 patients studied (13). Similarly, the response rate of 6-mercaptopurine (5 out of 15) was much lower than that of busulfan (42 out of 47) (14). Cyclophosphamide was also clearly inferior to busulfan not only in response rates (14 out of 21 vs. 19 out of 20), but also in quality and duration of remission (15).

Several studies have compared splenic irradiation and busulfan with regard to survival. The best known of these studies is a randomized study conducted by the British Medical Research Council, which found a median survival of 28 months for irradiated patients and of 40 months for patients treated with busulfan (10). The study has been criticized because the modalities of radiotherapy were not defined well enough. Therefore, doubts remain as to whether the radiotherapy groups were really treated homogeneously and optimally. A retrospective German study concluded that the best survival is accomplished by a combination of initial splenic irradiation and busulfan maintenance therapy (16). In other retrospective studies splenic irradiation was clearly inferior to busulfan (17,18). Further studies examined thioguanine (19), dibromomannitol (20), and melphalan (21), none of which showed any clear advantage over busulfan. Dibromomannitol was shown in a randomized study to be comparable to busulfan with regard to survival (22). The median survival in both types of treatment was 44 months. Remissions were induced faster by dibromomannitol, but the duration of the remissions was shorter. Melphalan was reported to have a small advantage by controlling busulfan-resistant thrombocytosis (21). Other monotherapies such as leukapheresis or treatment with radioactive phosphorus are of limited use (23,24). Leukapheresis may be useful when the number of leukocytes has to be reduced quickly in symptomatic patients, e.g., with leukostasis syndrome. The expense of material and personnel, however, is considerable and the duration of cell reduction only brief.

CORRELATION OF TUMOR BURDEN WITH SURVIVAL

One therapeutic concept of prolonging the chronic phase of CML is based on the consideration that a reduction of clonal, genetically unstable cells should also reduce the rate of secondary genetic changes and thereby postpone blast

Table 2 Comparison of Busulfan with Other Monotherapies During the Chronic Phase

Study group	Ref.	Treatment	Patients (n)	Median survival (months)	Comparison of busulfan
Haut et al. 1961	98	Busulfan	78	41^a	—
Rundles et al. 1959	13	Chlorambucil vs. busulfan	42	—	Response rates: 12/21 vs 21/21
Southeastern Study Group 1963	14	6-Mercaptopurine vs. busulfan	49	—	Response rates: 5/15 vs. 42/47
Kaung et a. 1971	15	Cyclophosphamide vs. busulfan	41	—	Response rates 14/21, 7 relapses vs. 19/20
MRC 1968	10	Splenic irradiation vs. busulfan	102	28 vs. 40	Not superior
Musshof et al. 1969	16	Splenic irradiation vs. busulfan	308	30, 42^a	Combination superior
Gollerkerl u. Shah 1971	17	Splenic irradiation vs. busulfan	113	21	Inferior
Conrad 1973	18	Splenic irradiation vs. busulfan	99	24 vs. 41^a (30 vs. 43^a)	Inferior
Spiers et al. 1975	19	Thioguanine	7	19+–40+	Not superior
D. Coop. Study Group 1973	20	Dibromomannitol	73	43	Similar
Canellos et al. 1975	22	Dibromomannitol vs. busulfan	40	44	Shorter remissions
Hauch et al. 1978	21	Melphalan	33	29^a	Advantage for thrombocytosis
Bolin et al. 1982	35	Busulfan vs. HU	53 (30/14/11)	48 vs. 90	HU superior?
Rushing et al. 1982	36	Busulfan vs. HU	67	45 vs. 51	HU less toxic
Hehlmann et al. 1993	37	Busulfan vs. HU	371	45 vs. 58	HU superior

[a]Mean.

crisis (25). According to this concept, the degree of reduction of tumor burden directly correlates with prolongation of the chronic phase and of survival. This concept, however, would only work with drugs of sufficiently low toxicity and mutagenicity to permit the necessary reduction of tumor burden. Reduction of tumor burden in CML is usually determined by the degrees of leukocyte reduction and/or cytogenetic response.

INTENSIVE COMBINATION THERAPIES

Long survival times of CML patients with busulfan-induced mosaicisms, i.e., reduction of Ph-positive cells and the simultaneous presence of normal Ph-negative cells (26–29), led to trials to eliminate the Ph-positive cell clones by intensive combination chemotherapy. Table 3 summarizes the results of cytostatic combination therapies during the chronic phase of CML. The therapies essentially comprise combinations of arabinosylcytosine, thioguanine, 6-mercaptopurine, anthracyclines, busulfan, vincristin, methotrexate, cyclophosphamide partially combined with asparaginase and/or splenic irradiation, and splenectomy. The remarkable feature of these studies was the observation of reductions of the Ph-positive cells in up to 70% of the cases studied and, in some instances, of complete cytogenetic remissions. In at least six studies comprising about 200 patients, more than 20 complete cytogenetic remissions were observed (30).

This observation is of special interest in the context of similar observations reported after IFN therapy. The duration of cytogenetic improvement after combination chemotherapy was relatively brief, lasting only 6–8 months. Al-

Table 3 Survival and Cytogenetic Response After Intensive Combination Chemotherapies During Chronic Phase of CML

Study group	Ref.	Patients (n)	Survival (months)	Ph status
Brodsky et al.	99	23	4–133	Ph reduction
Cunningham et al. (L-5)	93	37	50 (median)	Ph reduction in 12/37, 7 CR
Sharp et al.	100	12	NI	Ph reduction in 7/12, 1 CR
Goto et al. (L-15)	101	28	NI	Ph reduction in 50%, some CR
Kantarjian et al.	94	34	52 (median)	Ph reduction in 24/34, 10 CR
Kantarjian et al.	31	97	55 (median)	
Total		197	50–55 (median)	>20 CR

NI = no information; CR = complete cytogenetic remission.

though there was no special maintenance therapy, the survival of these patients as a group was longer. These trials were uncontrolled and the patient numbers small; a significant advantage over conventional therapy (mostly busulfan or HU) was demonstrated in only one study (31). Morbidity after intensive chemotherapy was considerable, discouraging randomized studies.

HYDROXYUREA

More recently, HU, an inhibitor of ribonucleotide reductase, became increasingly popular because of its rapid action and low level of adverse effects (12,32). Initially it was given when busulfan could not be given any more because of drug resistance or intolerable side effects. Tumor burden can be reduced rapidly with little toxicity. Some early retrospective studies on small series of patients indicated survival advantages of HU-treated patients, which, however, were not significant. Kennedy (12) reported in a retrospective study on 20 patients with unknown Ph status that HU controlled all CML-related symptoms as well as busulfan, that it did not prevent progression to blastic crisis, but that it possibly prolonged the duration of the chronic phase compared to busulfan. Schwarzenberg et al. (33) found in a study of 43 patients who were treated with HU, leukapheresis, and splenectomy, a median survival that was similar to that after busulfan therapy. Schwartz and Canellos (34) treated 35 patients, mostly resistant to busulfan and/or in accelerated phase, with HU with good therapeutic results. Bolin et al. (35) reported in a retrospective study on 30 busulfan- and 14 HU-treated patients that he expected for the busulfan group, after a median observation period of 47 months, a median survival of 48 months, whereas the expected median survival for the HU group, after a median observation time of 69 months, was 90 to 100 months. Rushing et al. (36) reported, also in a retrospective study on 41 HU- and 26 busulfan-treated patients, that HU was as effective as busulfan and that HU-treated patients had some advantage in median survival (51 vs. 45 months) which, however, was not significant. It was noted that HU was associated with less serious toxicity than busulfan (Table 2).

Based on these reports and similar unpublished experience of some German centers, the German CML study group, in 1983, decided to compare in a randomized study the influence of HU vs. busulfan on the duration of the chronic phase and on survival in CML. Using a population of 371 Ph-positive patients, a significant advantage for the HU-treated patients was found (37). The median survival in the busulfan group was 45 months, and in the HU group 58 months ($p = 0.008$). A correlation with leukocyte counts as a measure of tumor burden showed that low leukocyte counts in the HU group were associated with longer survival. A similar trend was observed in the busulfan group, but this was not significant, most probably because the leukocyte counts in the busulfan arm were reduced to a lesser extent for the anticipated risk of serious busulfan toxicity.

Kolitz et al. (6) increased the HU dose to achieve a predetermined level of myelosuppression (neutrophil count $<1 \times 10^9$/L, platelets $<20 \times 10^9$/L) in order to determine cytogenetic response. Starting at a dose of 2 g/m^2/day and escalating the dose by 1 g daily every 14 days until the desired degree of myelosuppression was reached, a significant cytogenetic response (20–100% Ph negativity) was reached in 10 out of 14 patients.

INTERFERON-ALPHA

A new concept of drug treatment for CML was the application of IFN-α to CML treatment. Natural (leukocyte) IFN-α was introduced into therapy of human disease in the 1970s. Natural IFN-α consists of a mixture of several IFNs of which IFN-α2 quantitatively is the most relevant. The availability of recombinant IFN-α2 allowed its general use in studies and in hematological practice. The three commonly used recombinant IFN-α2 preparations (a, b, and c) have similar therapeutic efficacy and differ from each other in only one or two (IFN-α2c) amino acids.

The first reports on the efficacy of natural IFN-α in CML date back to 1983 and were published by Talpaz et al. (38,39), who demonstrated myeloid cytoreduction with hematologic remissions in five of seven untreated or minimally pretreated chronic-phase CML patients and control of severe, therapy-resistant thrombocytosis in nine patients with advanced CML. The IFN-α dosage was 5×10^6 IU/day, since from the few patients treated it was felt that there was a *dose-response relationship* with better response at a higher IFN-α dosage. In 1986, Talpaz et al. (40) reported not only good cytoreduction by recombinant IFN-α2a in 14 out of 17 patients, but also the *induction of complete cytogenetic remissions* in six out of 13 patients with hematological remissions.

IFN-α: Cytoreduction, Dosage

The good cytoreductive property of IFN-α in CML was rapidly confirmed by other groups. Niederle et al. (41) observed normalization of leukocyte counts in 13 out of 16 evaluable CML patients and a cytogenetic response of up to 50% Ph negativity in four patients at an IFN-α dosage of 4×10^6 IU/day. In a follow-up report (42), 64% of 71 patients obtained a cytogenetic response (13% a complete cytogenetic remission). The projected 5-year survival of cytogenetic responders was 55%, that of nonresponders only 10%. Alimena et al. (43), at a dosage of 2 or 5×10^6 IU three times per week or daily, reported partial or complete hematological remissions in 53 out of 82 patients and cytogenetic improvement in 37 of the 53 responders (70%). A complete cytogenetic remission was seen in one case. The higher and daily IFN-α dosage was found more effective, confirming a dose-response relationship. Freund et al. (44) also confirmed the dose dependence of response using IFN-α2b. A more recent Phase II study on 41 chronic Ph-positive patients (45), which claims that low doses of IFN-α are as effective as higher doses, is hard to interpret since no risk profiles of the patients were given. Probably a high percentage of good-risk patients is responsible for the reported results. Talpaz et al. (46) and Alimena et al. (43) reported that the efficacy of IFN was much less in advanced phases of CML.

IFN-α: Long-Term Phase II Observations

Talpaz et al. (47), in long-term observations of 96 IFN-α-treated patients, reported that 73% achieved hematological remissions and 19% complete cytogenetic remissions. Cytogenetic remissions were durable and long-lasting in the majority of patients (6 to >45 months; median: 30 months). Ozer and the CALGB (48) treated 107 Ph$^+$ CML patients in chronic phase with IFN-α at 5×10^6 IU/m^2 daily and found hematological remissions in 63 patients (59%; 24 complete, 39 partial); 31 patients (40% of evaluable) achieved a cytogenetic response (14 complete, 17 partial). No survival advantage of cytogenetic responders over nonresponders was found. Mahon et al. (49) treated 51 mostly good-risk patients with IFN-α 5×10^6 IU/day and observed a major cytogenetic remission rate of 50%. In patients achieving complete hematological remission within 3 months, the rate of major cytogenetic remission was >80%. Thaler et al. (50,51) treated 80 also mostly good-risk patients with IFN-α2c at an absolute dose of 3.5×10^6 IU/day and achieved hematological responses in 74% and cytogenetic responses in 28% (major in 13%) of patients. Estimated median survival is only 51 months, probably due to the low IFN-α dosage.

IFN-α: Combinations

Another group of studies analyzed the feasibility of combinations of IFN-α with other agents such as HU, ara-C, or IFN-γ. Anger et al. (52) treated nine previously untreated Ph-positive patients with IFN-α2a at 6×10^6 IU daily during the first week and 3×10^6 IU daily during the second week. At day 15 HU was started at 40 mg/kg/day and the IFN-α dosage reduced to 3×10^6 IU three times a week. The combination therapy was effective and well tolerated in all patients. The combination of IFN-α and HU has proved clinically advantageous in many clinical trials (53–55) and at present is considered standard treatment of chronic phase Ph-positive CML. Guilhot et al. (56) combined IFN-α2a with HU and low-dose ara-C (10–20 mg/m^2/day, 10–15 days/month) in 10 of 24 Ph-positive patients with lack of hematological or cytogenetic response. In five of these 10 cases a dramatic durable cytogenetic improvement was recorded. The combination was well tolerated in nine patients and had to be discontinued in one patient because of gastrointestinal side effects and fever. The combination of IFN-α with IFN-γ was analyzed by several groups (57,58), but no advantage over IFN-α monotherapy was found.

RANDOMIZED IFN-α STUDIES

Several randomized studies were started after Talpaz's report in 1986 (40) to compare IFN-α with conventional chemotherapy. In 1986, the German CML Study Group decided to expand its study and to compare IFN-α with HU and busulfan in a randomized trial. At about the same time, the Italian Cooperative Study Group started a randomized study to compare IFN-α2a with conventional chemotherapy, mostly HU. In 1987, the U.K. MRC embarked on a study that compared busulfan or HU with or without maintenance therapy with natural IFN-α. IFN-α was started only after cytoreduction had been achieved by HU or busulfan. In the same year, a Benelux group started to analyze the combination of low-dose IFN-α2b in combination with HU vs. HU monotherapy (59). In 1988, a Japanese group started a randomized study that compared IFN-α vs. busulfan. Also in 1988 a French group started a randomized study comparing IFN-α and HU with vs. without low-dose ara-C (10 mg/m^2/day) (60). In 1991, the German CML Study Group started a second study that compared standard-dose IFN-α combined with HU versus HU monotherapy (55), and in the same year, the French group began with a study that compared IFN-α combined with HU with vs. without low-dose ara-C at 20 mg/m^2/day (61). Four of these studies were published by the time this article was written (Table 4).

German Randomized IFN-α Study

Five hundred thirteen Ph-positive patients were randomized (133 for IFN-α, 186 for busulfan, 194 for HU). The median survival was 66 months for IFN-α-, 56 for HU-, and 45 for busulfan-treated patients. IFN-α-treated patients had a significant survival advantage over busulfan-treated patients ($p = 0.008$) but not over HU-treated patients ($p = 0.44$) (62). These results were recognized in all risk groups as defined by Sokal's risk grouping (63). The updated survival curves (spring 1996) of this three-arm study are shown in Figure 2. The rates of patients reaching complete or partial hematological remissions were 83% in IFN-α-treated patients and 90% in both the HU and busulfan groups. In the IFN-α arm, the time to any hematological response was approximately 2.5 months; to complete hematological remission, approximately 6.5 months. Complete hematological IFN responders had a significant survival advantage over

Table 4 Randomized Studies with IFN in CML

Studies	Therapy (Ph-positive patients)	Median survival (months)		Difference significant	Hematological remissions (partial + complete) (%)	Complete cytogenetic remissions (%)
		IFN	HU (Bu)			
Italian 1994 (53)	INF-α (n = 218) vs CHT (n = 104)	72	52 (ND)	yes	68–87	8
German 1994 (62)	IFN-α (n = 133) vs. HU (n = 194) vs. Bu (n = 186)	66	56 (45)	no (yes)	83	5
U.K.-MRC 1995 (54), 1996 (102)	IFN-α after HU or Bu (n = 273) vs. HU or Bu (n = 266)	63	43 (43)	yes (yes)	86 (A + B type response)	6
Japanese 1995 (65)	IFN-α (n = 80) vs. Bu (n = 79)	ca. 62	ND (48)	(yes)	78	9

ND = not done; Bu = busulfan.

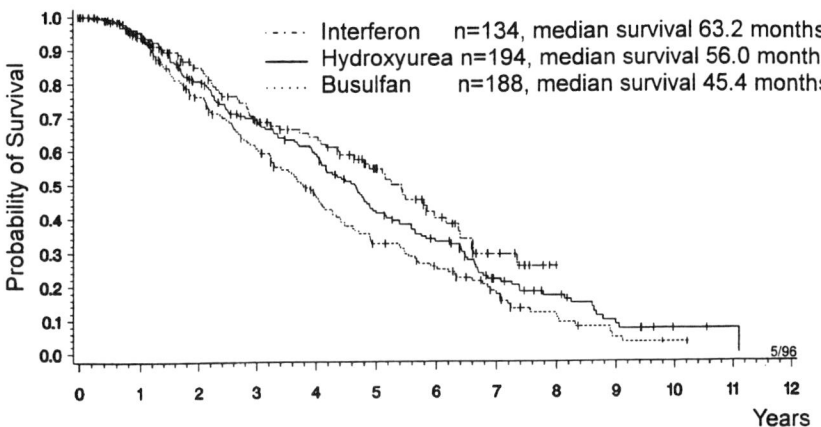

Figure 2 Survival of IFN-α vs. HU vs. busulfan update 5/96, German CML Study I. The differences IFN-α vs. busulfan ($p = 0.007$) and HU vs. busulfan ($p = 0.05$) are significant; the difference IFN-α vs. HU is not significant ($p = 0.24$).

partial or nonresponders ($p = 0.007$). Figure 3a shows the updated comparison (spring 1996).

Fifteen of 84 cytogenetically evaluable patients (18%) showed a cytogenetic response. This number probably underestimates the true response rate, since the low frequency of cytogenetic follow-up analyses (2,3/patient) would miss many transient responses. Six patients, corresponding to 7.2%, had a complete cytogenetic remission at least once in their course. A trend for a survival advantage of cytogenetic responders over nonresponders was recognized, but this was not significant ($p = 0.2$). This trend is recognized also in the 2-year update (spring 1996; $p = 0.12$) (Fig. 3b). Of special interest was the evolution of the disease in patients after IFN-α had been discontinued. The survival of the 65 IFN-α patients in whom IFN-α was discontinued when still in the chronic phase for various reasons was significantly inferior to that of the 61 patients in whom IFN had been continued ($p = 0.007$).

Analyzing the dosage of IFN-α actually administered over a 60-month period, it was found that the average IFN-α dosage declined from about 5×10^6 during the first 3 months to 3.5×10^6 IU/m²/day by 12 months to 3×10^6 IU/m²/day by 30 months and to about 2×10^6 IU/m²/day by 60 months. Since the treatment limitations were leukocytes counts of $2-4 \times 10^9$/L and tolerability, this indicates that the clinical response limits the dose of IFN-α and that the initial dosage probably is less important than hitherto thought. The impact of IFN-α dosage on cytogenetic response and long-time CML-free survival is still contro-

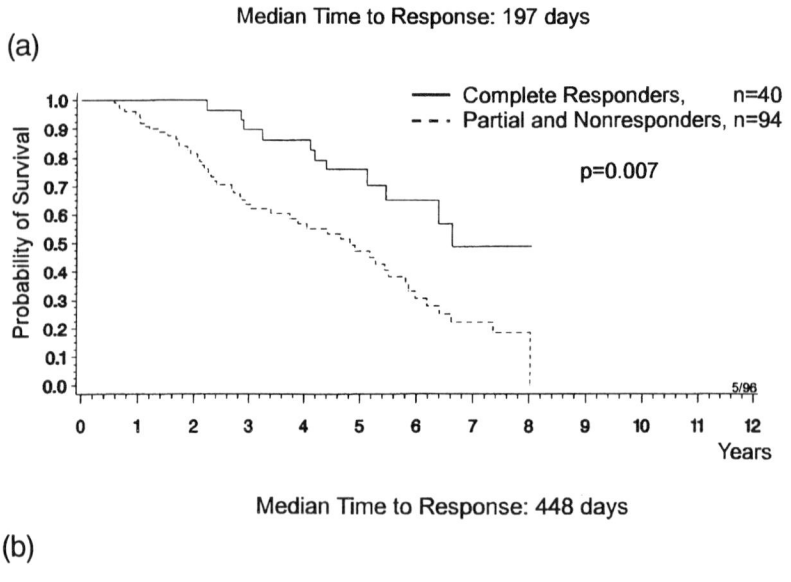

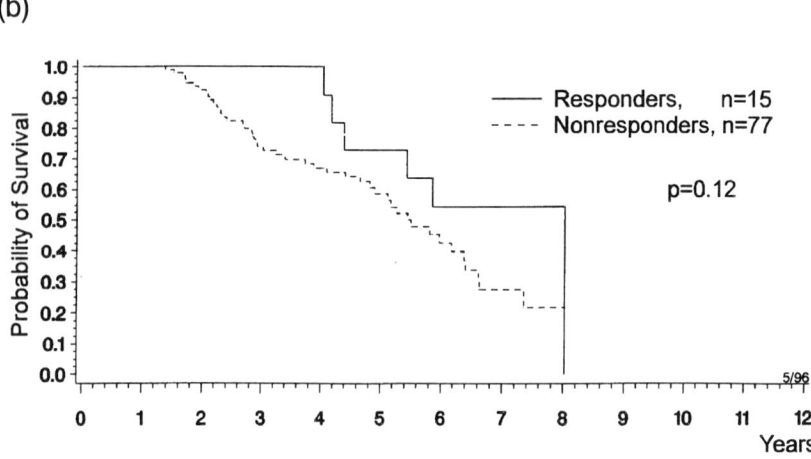

Figure 3 (a) Survival of complete hematologic IFN-α responders vs. partial and nonresponders. The difference is significant at $p = 0.007$. (b) Survival of cytogenetic IFN-α responders vs. nonresponders. The difference is not significant, but a trend is recognizable at $p = 0.12$ (update 5/96).

versially discussed. Since the discussion of this topic at the 1992 annual meeting of the German CML Study Group (64), two randomized trials comparing different IFN-α dosages have been started, but no results that would clarify the matter have been published.

Italian, British, and Japanese Randomized IFN-α Studies

An Italian study on 322 Ph-positive patients (218 randomized for IFN-α, 104 for chemotherapy, mostly HU) (53) observed a median survival time of 72 months for IFN-α-treated versus 52 months for HU-treated patients. The difference was significant at $p = 0.003$. Only major and complete cytogenetic IFN-α responders representing a group of patients with especially reduced tumor burden had a significant survival advantage over chemotherapy-treated patients.

A British study on 587 CML patients with ($n = 293$) and without IFN-α maintenance therapy ($n = 294$) (54) reported a median survival time of 63 months in 273 IFN-α-treated Ph-positive patients versus 43 months in 266 chemotherapy (busulfan or HU)-treated Ph-positive patients. This difference was also significant at $p = 0.0009$. This group found a significant survival advantage also for IFN-α-treated cytogenetic nonresponders.

A Japanese study compared the influence of IFN-α ($n = 80$) and busulfan ($n = 79$) on the duration of the chronic phase, on survival, and on hematological and cytogenetic response in Ph-positive CML (65). Predicted 5-year survival was 54% in the IFN-α group and 32% in the busulfan group ($p = 0.029$). Seven patients (8.8%) in the IFN-α arm and two patients (2.5%) in the busulfan arm reached a complete cytogenetic remission. Cytogenetic IFN-α responders had no significant survival advantage over nonresponders, but a trend was recognized ($p = 0.1065$).

Comparative Assessment of the Randomized IFN-α Studies

In comparing the four randomized and the nonrandomized IFN-α studies, the following aspects have to be considered:

1. Risk profiles: The risk profiles of the patients populations studied in the various trials differ extensively (Table 5). In the German randomized study the median survival times differ more between risk groups than between treatment groups (66) Table 6. Overall survival of a patient group may depend more on the group composition than on therapy. Therefore, the knowledge of the risk profiles of the patient populations studied is essential for the interpretation of the data. Whereas overall survival times may differ considerably among treatment studies, survival stratified according to risk profiles may be rather similar (67). As a measure of the different patient group compositions, the ratios of low- to high-risk patients according to Sokal were calculated (risk index, Table

Table 5 Risk Profiles in CML Patient Populations and Correlation with Survival (published studies on interferon-α-treated Philadelphia-positive CML patients)

Study	Patients on IFN-α n	Median survival (months)	5-year survival (%)	Risk profile (Sokal)			Risk index (n low risk/ n high risk)
				Low n (%)	Intermediate n (%)	High n (%)	
Mahon et al. 1996 (68)	81	NA	>77	39 (48%)	32 (40%)	10 (12%)	3.90
Kantarjian et al. 1995 (58)	274	89	63	124 (52%)	59 (25%)	54 (23%)	2.30
Italian group. 1994 (53)	218	72	60	94 (43%)	72 (33%)	52 (24%)	1.81
Ohnishi et al. 1995 (65)	80	NA	54	29 (37%)	26 (33%)	23 (30%)	1.26
Hehlmann et al. 1994 (62)	133	66	59	36 (27%)	47 (35%)	50 (38%)	0.72
Allan et al. 1995 (54), and Shepherd et al. 1996 (102)	267	63	54	67 (25%)	89 (33%)	111 (42%)	0.60
Kloke et al. 1993 (42)	62	NA	NA	32 (52%)	18 (29%)	12 (19%)	2.67
Alimena et al. 1988 (43)	35	NA	NA	16 (46%)	12 (34%)	7 (20%)	2.29
Guilhot et al. 1991 (56)	24	NA	NA	8 (33%)	12 (50%)	4 (17%)	2.00
Thaler et al. 1991 (50)	44	NA	NA	19 (43%)	15 (34%)	10 (23%)	1.90
Benelux study. 1996 (59)	97	NA	NA	29 (30%)	40 (41%)	28 (29%)	1.04

NA = not available.

Changing Nature of Conventional Therapy

Table 6 Median Survival (Months) According to Sokal Index[63] and Therapy: German CML Study I ($n = 490$)

	Total	Therapy groups			Maximum difference of median survival times between treatment groups (months)
		IFN-α	HU	Busulfan	
Total Risk groups (Sokal)	53	65	56	45	20
<0.8	79	>96	78	71	>25
0.8–1.2	54	65	58	45	20
>1.2	39	56	40	33	23
Difference of median survival times between low- and high-risk groups (months)	40	>40	38	38	

5). In the four randomized studies this ratio varies from 0.60 in the British study to 1.81 in the Italian study (53,54,62,65). In four nonrandomized studies (42,43,58,68), the ratios were above 2 (3.40, 2.30, 2.67, and 2.29). Study populations with higher ratios of low- to high-risk patients have a longer overall survival than those with lower ratios, as shown in Table 5.

2. Strategy of IFN-α therapy: Whereas the German protocol strictly asked for monotherapies in all therapy arms and for rerandomization to HU or busulfan after IFN-α resistance, combination of IFN-α with chemotherapy was allowed in the Italian and British studies (53,54). The British study (54) started with IFN-α only, after tumor reduction had been achieved with HU or busulfan. The combination of IFN-α with chemotherapy probably allows the continuation of IFN-α in a higher percentage of patients, which might confer some survival advantage.

3. Treatment intensity of control groups: From Table 4 it appears that whether and to what extent IFN-α is superior to HU may depend, at least in part, on the survival time of the HU control groups. The defined and more efficient reduction of WB counts by HU in the German study (62), which correlates with longer survival, is thought to be one reason (69) for not obtaining a significant survival difference between IFN and HU.

Comparison of the Italian and German Randomized IFN Studies

In order to analyze why the survival advantage of IFN-α-treated patients over HU-treated patients was significant in the Italian (53) but not significant in the

German study (62), a comparative analysis of the study protocols and the data banks was carried out (5). There were considerable differences in patients' inclusion and exclusion criteria, in treatment strategy, and in HU dosage requirement between the two studies (Table 7). The most relevant difference which almost exclusively accounted for the survival differences was the different patient populations resulting from the different inclusion and exclusion criteria of the protocols. After the patients who would not have qualified for the Italian inclusion criteria were removed from the German patient population (patients with extramedullary manifestations and >10% circulating blasts, patients older than 70 years) and after the patients who would have been excluded according to the German admission criteria were removed from the Italian study population (asymptomatic early cases), the survival differences disappeared. The adjusted IFN-α survival curves of the two studies became virtually identical. After adjustment, the survival advantage of IFN-α over HU became borderline significant in the German study ($p = 0.12$). The small remaining difference is accounted for by differences in treatment strategy (IFN-α monotherapy in the German study, combination with HU allowed in the Italian study) and by differences in HU dosage. The most important result of this comparison is the identifi-

Table 7 Differences Between Italian and German IFN Study Protocols

	Italian ($n = 218$) (53)	German ($n = 133$) (62)
Entry criteria	• Age <70 years	• No age limit
	• <10% blasts	• <30% blasts and promyelocytes
	• No extramedullary manifestations	• Early cases not requiring treatment excluded
	• No exclusion of asymptomatic early cases	
	Not fulfilling German inclusion criteria: $n = 27$[a]	Not fulfilling Italian inclusion criteria: $n = 24$[a]
IFN treatment strategies	• Combination with CHT allowed	• Strictly monotherapy
	• After IFN resistance: IFN continued at low dosage (3×3 Mill. IU/week)	• After IFN resistance: discontinuation of IFN and re-randomization to HU or Bu
HU treatment goals	• WBC <30,000/μL	• Normal WBC counts (5000–15,000/μL)

[a]Exclusion of these 51 patients yields IFN survival curves that are not significantly different.

cation of patients for whom IFN-α therapy is particularly advantageous. Evidence is emerging that IFN-α is superior in early CML whereas HU is more effective in later CML, which is in agreement with earlier observations that IFN-α is less effective in advanced CML (46,43) and with the well-known efficacy of HU even in accelerated and early blast phase (12,34).

IFN-α TREATMENT: SUMMARY AND PERSPECTIVES

Summarizing available evidence, complete or partial hematological remissions can be induced by IFN-α in 78% to 87% of cases in randomized and nonrandomized studies (Table 4). Median time to any hematological remission appears to be 2–3 months; to complete hematological remission, 6–7 months (58,68).

Complete cytogenetic remissions by IFN-α can be achieved in up to 39% of cases of Phase II studies with selected patient populations and in 5–9% of cases in randomized studies which have to follow the intention-to-treat principle. The majority of these remissions is relatively stable and longer-lasting (>1, up to 6 years and longer). The median time to complete cytogenetic remission ranges between 12 and 17 months (49,58), but complete remissions may occur 36 months after start of IFN-α therapy and even later. Due to the inherent limitations of cytogenetic analyses (bone marrow puncture and analysis of a sufficiently large number of mitoses required), the determination of the exact time when complete cytogenetic remission occurs may be difficult. Likewise, the detection of transient cytogenetic remissions may depend to a considerable extent on the frequency of cytogenetic analyses. With regard to these limitations, hematological remission probably is the more practicable prognostic and follow-up parameter. The introduction of quantitative Southern blot analysis of the BCR/ABL rearrangement (70,71) may facilitate follow up analyses in the future since it has proven clinically useful and reliable, is easy to perform, and can be done with peripheral blood not requiring bone marrow puncture.

The question which arises from the long-lasting cytogenetic remissions is whether IFN can cure CML. The analysis of 25 CML patients in complete cytogenetic remission after IFN therapy by PCR quantification of BCR/ABL transcripts (72) showed residual BCR/ABL transcripts in all cases; the number of transcripts, however, ranging over several orders of magnitude (73). Patients with high residual transcript numbers were shown to have a definite risk of relapse and sudden blast crisis (74). It can be concluded that IFN probably does not cure CML, not even in complete cytogenetic IFN responders.

Tolerability appears to limit the use of IFN-α only in a minority of patients. The observation that IFN-α is less well tolerated in patients >60 years (75) has not been confirmed in the German randomized study (62), in which the mean ages of patients who continued or discontinued IFN-α were virtually identical (47 years). Adverse effects of IFN-α, in our hands, are well controlled by the prior application of acetaminophen and/or transient dose reductions, in most cases. If the full IFN-α dosage cannot be resumed, HU is added with the goal to keep the leukocyte counts at 2000–4000/μL. Chronic neurological and immune-mediated toxicity may necessitate discontinuation in rare cases (76).

The mechanism of the life-prolonging effect of IFN-α in CML is unclear. Possible mechanisms include nonspecific inhibition of proliferation of the leukemic cell clone as well as modulation of cytokine actions and of the immune surveillance system. The different therapeutic effects of cytostatics and of IFN-α suggest that, at least in part, different modes of action may be responsible for their effects on CML. Data on intensive combination chemotherapy, HU treatment aiming at normal or low-normal white blood cell counts, and observations with relapsing patients after myeloablative chemotherapy and allogenous bone marrow transplantation as well as the low tumor burden that has to be achieved, if the life-prolonging effect of IFN-α is to be observed, all suggest that survival correlates with intensity of treatment.

NEW DRUGS

A number of new agents have been explored for CML therapy in recent years. They range from cytostatics, enzyme inhibitors, and antisense molecules to drugs that interfere with the intracellular BCR/ABL signaling pathway(s). 2-Chlorodeoxyadenosine (2-CDA), a purine analog with major activity in lymphoid neoplasms, induced complete hematological remissions in 10 of 12 patients, but lacked significant cytogenetic responses (77). Four patients experienced severe immunosuppression with opportunistic infections. Ubenimex (Bestatin), an inhibitor of aminopeptidase B and leucine aminopeptidase, was reported to have striking effects in CML (78), including induction of cytogenetic response, but no full report has followed the preliminary communication. BCR/ABL-antisense oligonucleotides were reported to have some effect in vitro and in vivo (79–81), and so were anti-myb sequences in purging CML stem cells prior to autografting (82). Effects were observed in only some patients and, apparently, were not durable. Homoharringtonine, a plant alkaloid with myelosuppressive activity and used as continuous infusion, was studied in 71 patients in late chronic phase (>12 months after diagnosis); 72% of evaluable patients achieved a complete hematologic remission and 31% a cytogenetic response (83). The substance is being further investigated in combination with other agents active in CML. Of major interest, at present, are inhibitors of tyrosine kinase. Herbimycin A, a benzoquinoid ansamycin antibiotic with tyrosine kinase-inhibiting activity, markedly inhibited the in vitro growth of Ph-positive ALL and CML cells (84), but no specificity for BCR/ABL tyrosine kinase was shown. Druker et al. (85) analyzed a 2-phenylaminopyrimidine compound (CGP 57148) designed to inhibit ABL-protein kinase and demonstrated good specificity for BCR-ABL expressing cells in vitro. Clinical studies are under way. Another approach is explored by addressing the growth factor-binding protein Grb-2 that links tyrosine kinases to ras (86). Mutant forms of Grb-2 were shown to reverse the oncogenic phenotype. An important line of ongoing research may be the development of compounds that specifically inhibit Grb-2 or other intracellular targets required for the induction or maintenance of the malignant state.

INTENSIVE CHEMOTHERAPY AND AUTOGRAFTING

If survival in CML indeed correlates with tumor burden, a further intensification of treatment would be the logical next step. This concept is currently being realized by two approaches: the combination of intensive chemotherapy with IFN-α induction and/or maintenance therapy should be able to further reduce tumor burden, since the modes of action of these therapies differ and might complement each other. One study finds some survival advantage for patients treated with this combination over historic controls with IFN-α monotherapy, but fails to reach statistical significance (87). The German CML Study Group, at present, studies the combination of idarubicine and ara-C with IFN-α induction and maintenance therapy vs. IFN-α/HU standard therapy in their CML Study III.

Another approach is treatment with high-dose chemotherapy followed by autografting either with autologous bone marrow or with peripheral blood stem cells. In a study of autologous transplants in 200 patients with CML (median age 45 years) from eight centers, survival results with a 5-year survival rate of >50% have been reported for chronic-phase patients (88). The success rate can probably be increased by purging procedures in vivo as pioneered by Carella et al. (89) and by Simonsson et al. (90), in vitro as attempted by Barnett et al. (91) with cultured marrow, or by Gewirtz et al. (82) with myb-antisense oligonucleotides.

Support for the intensive approach also comes from survival analyses of 148 patients who relapsed after allogeneic marrow transplantations (92). These patients have a significant survival advantage over 417 matched controls with conventional therapy ($p = 0.0002$).

CONCLUSION AND OUTLOOK

The impact of conventional therapy on CML has changed during the last decade from mostly palliation to an effective treatment of the disease with prolongation of life. New treatment modalities with more efficient reductions of tumor burden appear to prolong survival of chronic-phase CML and to change the natural course of CML. At present, first-line therapy for CML includes IFN-α, HU, and allogeneic bone marrow transplantation. Low-dose ara-C may increase the cytogenetic response rate and thereby survival time. The addition of intensive chemotherapy with and without autografting as a means to further prolong survival is under study in several randomized and nonrandomized trials. New drugs with specific disease-related targets may also improve therapeutic options. Forthcoming trials have to consider both conventional and new experimental treatment modalities. As an example of present study concepts with the goal of prolonging survival by intensification of treatment under consideration of adverse drug effects and quality of life, the ongoing German CML Study III is mentioned. The main goals of this study are:

1. Controlled comparison of allogeneic BMT with the best available drug treatment.
2. Randomized comparison of HU/IFN-α standard therapy vs. IFN-α with subsequent intensive chemotherapy with idarubicin, ara-C, and IFN-α maintenance.
3. Evaluation of the effect of high-dose chemotherapy followed by autografting and IFN-α maintenance on survival in CML.

Figure 4 provides an algorithm of the current treatment strategy (1996) of the German CML Study Group which considers both intensive chemotherapy and

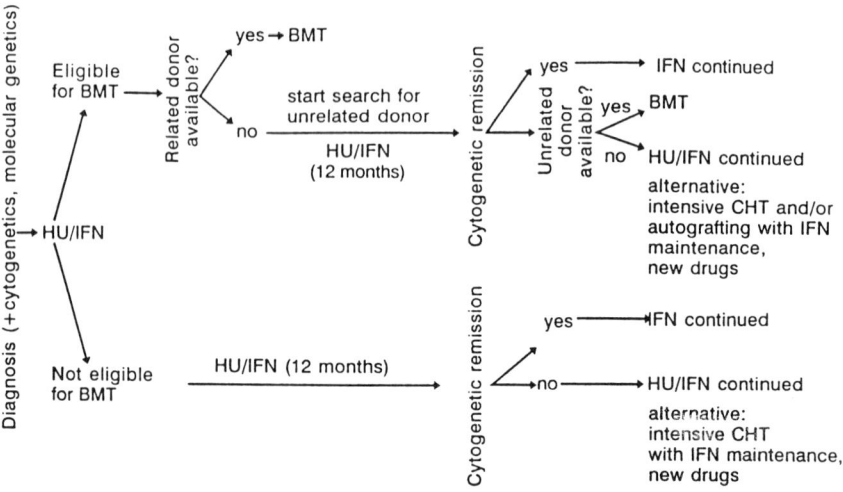

Figure 4 CML treatment strategy of the German CML Study Group 1996.

autografting as a means to further decrease tumor burden and thereby increase survival.

REFERENCES

1. Galton DAG. Chemotherapy of chronic myelocytic leukemia. Semin Hematol 1969; 6:323–343.
2. Sokal JE, Aungst CW. Snyderman M, Gomez G. Immunotherapy of chronic myelocytic leukemia: effects of different vaccination schedules. Ann NY Acad Sci 1976; 277:367–383.
3. Thomas ED, Clift RA. Indications for marrow transplantation in chronic myelogenous leukemia. Blood 1989; 73:861–864.
4. McGlave P, Bartsch G, Anasetti C, et al. Unrelated donor marrow transplantation therapy for chronic myelogenous leukemia: initial experience of the National Marrow Donor Program. Blood 1993; 81:543–550.
5. Hasford J, Baccarani M, Hehlmann R, Ansari H, Tura S, Zuffa E. Interferon-α and hydroxyurea in early chronic myeloid leukemia: a comparative analysis of the Italian and German chronic myeloid leukemia trials with interferon-α. Blood 1996; 88:5384–5391.
6. Kolitz JE, Kempin SJ, Schluger A, et al. A phase II pilot trial of high-dose hydroxyurea in chronic myelogenous leukemia. Semin Oncol 1992; 19:27–33.
7. Goldman JM, Szydlo R, Horowitz MM, et al. Choice of pretransplant treatment and timing of transplants for chronic myelogenous leukemia in chronic phase [see comments]. Blood 1993; 82:2235–2238.
8. Carella AM, Chimirri F, Podesta M, et al. High-dose chemoradiotherapy followed by autologous Philadelphia chromosome-negative blood progenitor cell transplantation in patients with chronic myelogenous leukemia. Bone Marrow Transplant 1996; 17:201–205.
9. Minot GR, Buckman TE. Isaacs R. Chronic myelogenous leukemia. JAMA 1924; 82:1489–1494.
10. Medical Research Council's Working Party for Therapeutic Trials in Leukaemia. Chronic granulocytic leukemia: comparison of radiotherapy and busulphan therapy. Br Med J 1968; 1:201–208.
11. Haut A, Abbott WS, Wintrobe MM, Cartwright GE. Busulfan in the treatment of chronic myelocytic leukemia. The effect of long term intermittent therapy. Blood 1961; 17:1–19.
12. Kennedy BJ. Hydroxyurea therapy in chronic myelogenous leukemia. Cancer 1972; 29:1052–1056.
13. Rundles RW, Grizzle J, Bell WN, et al. Comparison of chlorambucil and myleran in chronic lymphocytic and granulocytic leukemia. Am J Med 1959; 27:424–432.
14. Southeastern Cancer Chemotherapy Cooperative Study Group. Comparison of 6-mercaptopurine and busulfan in chronic granulocytic leukemia. Blood 1963; 21: 89–100.
15. Kaung DT, Close HP, Whittington RM, Patno ME. Comparison of busulfan and

cyclophosphamide in the treatment of chronic myelocytic leukemia. Cancer 1971; 27:608–612.
16. Musshoff K, Boutis L, Obrecht P, Karsch T. Die Lebenserwartung der chronischen myeloischen Leukaemie in Abhaengigkeit von individuellen und krankheitsspezifischen Faktoren und der Therapie. Klin Wochenschr 1969; 47:179–183.
17. Gollerkerl MP, Shah GB. Management of chronic myeloid leukemia: a five year survey with a comparison of oral busulfan and splenic irradiation. Cancer 1971; 27:596–601.
18. Conrad CFG. Survival in chronic granulocytic leukemia. Arch Intern Med 1973; 131:684–685.
19. Spiers ASD, Galton DAG, Kaur J, Goldman JM. Thioguanine as primary treatment for chronic granulocytic leukaemia. Lancet 1975; 1:829–832.
20. Dibromomannitol Cooperative Study Group. Survival of chronic myeloid leukaemia patients treated by dibromomannitol. Eur J Cancer 1973; 9:583–589.
21. Hauch T, Logue G, Laszlo J, Cox E, Rundles W. Treatment of chronic granulocytic leukemia with melphalan. Blood 1978; 51:571–577.
22. Canellos GP, Young RC, Nieman PE, DeVita VT. Dibromomannitol in the treatment of chronic granulocytic leukemia: a prospective randomized comparison with busulfan. Blood 1975; 45:197–203.
23. Vallejos CS, McCredie KB, Brittin GM, Freireich EJ. Biological effects of repeated leukapheresis of patients with chronic myelogenous leukemia. Blood 1973; 42:925–933.
24. Hadlock DC, Fortuny IE, McCullough J, Kennedy BJ. Continuous flow centrifuge leucapheresis in the management of chronic myelogenous leukaemia. Br J Haematol 1975; 29:443–453.
25. Hehlmann R, Heimpel H. Current aspects of drug therapy in Philadelphia-positive CML: correlation of tumor burden with survival. Leuk Lymph 1996; 22:161–167.
26. Finney R, McDonald GA, Baikie AG, Douglas AS. Chronic granulocytoc leukaemia with Ph^1 negative cells in bone marrow and a ten year remission after busulphan hypoplasia. Br J Haematol 1972; 23:283–288.
27. Golde DW, Bersch NL, Sparkes RS. Chromosomal mosaicism associated with prolonged remission in chronic myelogenous leukemia. Cancer 1976; 37:1849–1852.
28. Brandt L, Mitelman F, Panani A, Lenner HC. Extremely long duration of chronic myeloid leukaemia with Ph1 negative and Ph1 positive bone marrow cells. Scand J Haematol 1976; 16:321–325.
29. Mueller L, Hehlmann R. 24 Jahre Überlebenszeit bei chronisch myeloischer Leukämie. Klin Wochenschr 1987; 65:673–676.
30. Lengfelder E, Hehlmann R. Intensive combination chemotherapy in treatment of CML. Bone Marrow Transplant 1996; 17(suppl 3):S55–S57.
31. Kantarjian HM, Talpaz M, Kurzrock R, et al. Intensive combination chemotherapy and interferons in the management of chronic myelogenous leukemia. Acta Haematol 1987; 78:70–74.
32. Kennedy BJ. The evolution of hydroxyurea therapy in chronic myelogenous leukemia. Semin Oncol 1992; 19(suppl 9):21–26.

33. Schwarzenberg L, Mathe G, Pouillart P, et al. Br Med J 1973; 1:700–703.
34. Schwartz JH, Canellos GP. Hydroxyurea in the management of the hematologic complications of chronic granulocytic leukemia. Blood 1975; 46:11–16.
35. Bolin RW, Robinson WA, Sutherland J, Hamman RF. Busulfan versus hydroxyurea in long-term therapy of chronic myelogenous leukemia. Cancer 1982; 50: 1683–1686.
36. Rushing D, Goldman A, Gibbs G, Howe R, Kennedy BJ. Hydroxyurea versus busulfan in the treatment of chronic myelogenous leukemia. Am J Clin Oncol 1982; 5:307–313.
37. Hehlmann R, Heimpel H, Hasford J, et al. Randomized comparison of busulfan and hydroxyurea in chronic myelogenous leukemia: prolongation of survival by hydroxyurea. The German CML Study Group. Blood 1993; 82:398–407.
38. Talpaz M, Mavligit G, Keating M, Walters RS, Gutterman JU. Human leukocyte interferon to control thrombocytosis in chronic myelogenous leukemia. Ann Intern Med 1983; 99:789–792.
39. Talpaz M, McCredie KB, Mavligit GM, Gutterman JU. Leukocyte interferon-induced myeloid cytoreduction in chronic myelogenous leukemia. Blood 1983; 62: 689–692.
40. Talpaz M, Kantarjian HM, McCredie K, Trujillo JM, Keating MJ, Gutterman JU. Hematologic remission and cytogenetic improvement induced by recombinant human interferon alpha$_{2a}$ in chronic myelogenous leukemia. N Engl J Med 1986; 314:1065–1069.
41. Niederle N, Kloke O, Doberauer C, Becher R, Beelen DW, Schmidt CG. Alpha 2-interferon: preliminary treatment results in chronic myeloid leukemia. Dtsch Med Wochenschr 1986; 111:767–772.
42. Kloke O, Niederle N, Qiu MY, et al. Impact of interferon alpha-induced cytogenetic improvement on survival in chronic myelogenous leukaemia. Br J Haematol 1993; 83:399–403.
43. Alimena G, Morra E, Lazzarino M, et al. Interferon alpha-2b as therapy for Ph^1-positive chronic myelogenous leukemia: a study of 82 patients treated with intermittent or daily administration. Blood 1988; 72:642–647.
44. Freund M, von Wussow P, Diedrich H, et al. Recombinant human interferon (IFN) alpha-2b in chronic myelogenous leukaemia: dose dependency of response and frequency of neutralizing anti-interferon antibodies. Br J Haematol 1989; 72:350–356.
45. Schofield JR, Robinson WA, Murphy JR, Rovira DK. Low doses of interferon-a are as effective as higher doses in inducing remissions and prolonging survival in chronic myeloid leukemia. Ann Intern Med 1994; 121:736–744.
46. Talpaz M, Kantarjian HM, McCredie KB, Keating MJ, Trujillo J, Gutterman J. Clinical investigation of human alpha interferon in chronic myelogenous leukemia. Blood 1987; 69:1280–1288.
47. Talpaz M, Kantarjian H, Kurzrock R, Trujillo JM, Gutterman JU. Interferon-alpha produces sustained cytogenetic responses in chronic myelogenous leukemia. Ann Intern Med 1991; 114:532–538.
48. Ozer H, George SL, Schiffer CA, et al. Prolonged subcutaneous administration of recombinant alpha 2b interferon in patients with previously untreated Philadelphia

chromosome-positive chronic-phase chronic myelogenous leukemia: effect on remission duration and survival: Cancer and Leukemia Group B study 8583. Blood 1993; 82:2975–2984.
49. Mahon FX, Montastruc M, Faberes C, Reiffers J. Predicting complete cytogenetic response in chronic myelogenous leukemia patients treated with recombinant interferon α. Blood 1994; 84:3592–3594.
50. Thaler J, Kuhr T, Gastl G, et al. Rekombinantes Interferon α-2c bei Ph-positiver chronischer myeloischer Leukaemie. Dtsch Med Wochenschr 1991; 116:721–728.
51. Thaler J, Gastl G, Fluckinger T, et al. Interferon alpha-2c therapy of patients with chronic myelogenous leukemia: long term results of a multicenter phase-II study. Ann Hematol 1996; 72:349–355.
52. Anger B, Porzsolt F, Leichtle R, Heinze B, Bartram C, Heimpel H. A phase I/II study of recombinant interferon alpha 2a and hydroxyurea for chronic myelocytic leukemia. Blut 1989; 58:275–278.
53. Italian Cooperative Study Group on Chronic Myeloid Leukemia. Interferon alfa-2a as compared with conventional chemotherapy for the treatment of chronic myeloid leukemia. N Engl J Med 1994; 330:820–825.
54. Allan NC, Richards SM, Shepherd PC. UK Medical Research Council randomised, multicentre trial of interferon-alpha n1 for chronic myeloid leukaemia: improved survival irrespective of cytogenetic response. UK Medical Research Council's Working Parties for Therapeutic Trials in Adult Leukaemia. Lancet 1995; 345:1392–1397.
55. Hehlmann R, Heimpel H, Hossfeld DK, et al. Randomized study of the combination of hydroxyurea and interferon alpha versus hydroxyurea monotherapy during the chronic phase of chronic myelogenous leukemia (CML Study II). Bone Marrow Transplant 1996; 17(suppl 3):S21–S24.
56. Guilhot F, Dreyfus B, Brizard A, Huret JL, Tanzer J. Cytogenetic remissions in chronic myelogenous leukemia using interferon alpha-2a and hydroxyurea with or without low-dose cytosine arabinoside. Leuk Lymph 1991; 4:49–55.
57. Wandl UB, Niederle N, Kranzhoff M, Seeber S. Clonogenic assay is not predictive but reflects therapeutic efficacy of interferons in the treatment of chronic myelogenous leukemia. Int J Cell Cloning 1992; 10:292–298.
58. Kantarjian HM, Smith TL, O'Brien S, et al. Prolonged survival in chronic myelogenous leukemia after cytogenetic response to interferon-α therapy. Ann Intern Med 1995; 122:254–261.
59. Benelux CML Study Group. Low-dose interferon-alpha 2b combined with hydroxyurea versus hydroxyurea alone for chronic myelogenous leukemia. Bone Marrow Transplant 1996; 17(suppl 3):S19–S20.
60. Guilhot F, Abgrall JF, Harousseau JL, et al. A multicentric randomised study of alpha 2b interferon (IFN) and hydroxyurea (HU) with or without cytosine-arabinoside (Ara-c) in previously untreated patients with Ph+ chronic myelocytic leukemia (CML): preliminary cytogenetic results. Leuk Lymph 1993; 11(suppl 1):181–183.
61. Guilhot F, Guerci A, Fiere D, et al. The treatment of chronic myelogenous leukemia by interferon and cytosine-arabinoside: rationale and design of the French trials. Bone Marrow Transplant 1996; 17(suppl 3):S29–S31.

62. Hehlmann R, Heimpel H, Hasford J, et al. Randomized comparison of interferon-alpha with busulfan and hydroxyurea in chronic myelogenous leukemia. German CML Study Group. Blood 1994; 84:4064–4077.
63. Sokal JE, Cox EB, Baccarani M, et al. Prognostic discrimination in "good-risk" chronic granulocytic leukemia. Blood 1984; 63:789–799.
64. Griesshammer M, Hehlmann R, Hochhaus A, et al. Interferon in chronic myeloid leukemia. A workshop report. Ann Hematol 1993; 67:101–106.
65. Ohnishi K, Ohno R, Tomonaga M, et al. A randomized trial comparing interferon-alpha with busulfan for newly diagnosed chronic myelogenous leukemia in chronic phase. Blood 1995; 86:906–916.
66. Hehlmann R, Ansari H, Hasford J, et al. Comparative analysis of the impact of risk profile and of drug therapy on survival in CML using Sokal's index and a new score. Br J Hematol 1997; 97:76–85.
67. Hehlmann R, Heimpel H, Hasford J. Randomized comparison of interferon-α, hydroxyurea, and busulfan in chronic myeloid leukemia: response to Kantarjian and Talpaz and to Tura and Baccarani. Blood 1995; 85:3000–3002.
68. Mahon FX, Faberes C, Montastruc M, et al. High response rate using recombinant interferon-alpha in patients with newly diagnosed chronic myeloid leukemia. Bone Marrow Transplant 1996; 17(suppl 3):S33–S37.
69. Hehlmann R. Chronic myelogenous leukemia: does interferon alpha prolong life? Leukemia 1996; 10:193–196.
70. Verschraegen CF, Talpaz M, Hirsch Ginsberg CF, et al. Quantification of the breakpoint cluster region rearrangement for clinical monitoring in Philadelphia chromosome-positive myeloid leukemia. Blood 1995; 85:2705–2710.
71. Reiter A, Skladny H, Hochhaus A, et al. Molecular response of CML patients treated with interferon-α monitored by quantitative Southern blot analysis. Br J Haematol 1997; 97:86–93.
72. Cross NCP, Feng L, Chase A, Bungey J, Hughes TP. Goldman JM. Competitive polymerase chain reaction to estimate the number of BCR-ABL transcripts in chronic myeloid leukemia patients after bone marrow transplantation. Blood 1993; 82:1929–1936.
73. Hochhaus A, Lin F, Reiter A, et al. Variable numbers of BCR-ABL transcripts persist in CML patients who achieve complete cytogenetic remission with interferon-α. Br J Haematol 1995; 91:126–131.
74. Hochhaus A, Reiter A, Skladny H, et al.: Molecular heterogeneity in complete cytogenetic responders after interferon-α-therapy of chronic myelogenous leukemia: Levels of minimal residual disease predict risk of relapse. Blood 1996; 88(Suppl 1):664a.
75. Cortes J, Kantarjian H, O'Brien S, Robertson LE, Pierce S, Talpaz M. Results of interferon-alpha therapy in patients with chronic myelogenous leukemia 60 years of age and older. Am J Med 1996; 100:452–455.
76. Sacchi S, Kantarjian H, O'Brien S, Cohen PR, Pierce S, Talpaz M. Immune-mediated and unusual complications during interferon alfa therapy in chronic myelogenous leukemia. J Clin Oncol 1995; 13:2401–2407.
77. Saven A, Piro LD, Lemon RH, et al. Complete hematologic remissions in chronic-

phase, Philadelphia-chromosome-positive, chronic myelogenous leukemia after 2-chlorodeoxyadenosine. Cancer 1994; 73:2953–2963.
78. Murata M, Kubota Y, Tanaka T, Iida-Tanaka K, Takahara J, Irino S. Effect of ubenimex on the proliferation and differentiation of U937 human histiocytic lymphoma cells. Leukemia 1994; 8:2188–2193.
79. Szczylik C, Skorski T, Nicolaides NC, et al. Selective inhibition of leukemia cell proliferation by BCR-ABL antisense oligodeoxynucleotides. Science 1991; 253: 562–565.
80. Martiat P, Lewalle P, Taj AS, et al. Retrovirally transduced antisense sequences stably suppress P210BCR-ABL expression and inhibit the proliferation of BCR/ABL-containing cell lines. Blood 1993; 81:502–509.
81. Skorski T, Nieborowska Skorska M, et al. Suppression of Philadelphia-1 leukemia cell growth in mice by BCR-ABL antisense oligodeoxynucleotides. XVI Symposium of the International Association for Comparative Research on Leukemia and Related Diseases 1992; 1993:48.
82. Gewirtz AM. Treatment of chronic myelogenous leukemia (CML) with c-myb antisense oligodeoxynucleotides. Bone Marrow Transplant 1994; 14(suppl 3): S57–S61.
83. O'Brien S, Kantarjian H, Keating M, et al. Homoharringtonine therapy induces responses in patients with chronic myelogenous leukemia in late chronic phase. Blood 1995; 86:3322–3326.
84. Okabe M, Uehara Y, Miyagishima T, et al. Effect of herbimycin A, an antagonist of tyrosine kinase, on bcr/abl oncoprotein-associated cell proliferations: abrogative effect on the transformation of murine hematopoietic cells by transfection of a retroviral vector expressing oncoprotein P210bcr/abl and preferential inhibition on Ph1-positive leukemia cell growth. Blood 1992; 80:1330–1338.
85. Druker BJ, Tamura S, Buchdunger E, et al. Effects of a selective inhibitor of the Abl tyrosine kinase on the growth of Bcr-Abl positive cells. Nat Med 1996; 2: 561–566.
86. Gishizky ML, Cortez D, Pendergast AM. Mutant forms of growth factor-binding protein-2 reverse BCR-ABL-induced transformation. Proc Natl Acad Sci USA 1995; 92:10889–10893.
87. Kantarjian HM, Talpaz M, Keating MJ, et al. Intensive chemotherapy induction followed by interferon-alpha maintenance in patients with Philadelphia chromosome-positive chronic myelogenous leukemia. Cancer 1991; 68:1201–1207.
88. McGlave PB, De Fabritiis P, Deisseroth A, et al. Autologous transplants for chronic myelogenous leukaemia: results from eight transplant groups. Lancet 1994; 343:1486–1488.
89. Carella AM, Podesta M, Frassoni F, et al. Collection of 'normal' blood repopulating cells during early hemopoietic recovery after intensive conventional chemotherapy in chronic myelogenous leukemia. Bone Marrow Transplant 1993; 12: 267–271.
90. Simonsson B, Oberg G, Killander A, et al. Intensive treatment in order to minimize the Ph-positive clone in chronic myelogenic leukemia. Stem Cells Dayt 1993; 11(suppl 3):73–76.

91. Barnett MJ, Eaves CJ, Phillips GL, et al. Autografting with cultured marrow in chronic myeloid leukemia: results of a pilot study [see comments]. Blood 1994; 84:724–732.
92. Gale RP, Baccarani M, Horowitz MM, Zhang MJ. Is the course of chronic myelogenous leukemia affected by bone marrow transplantation? An analysis in patients relapsing after bone marrow transplants. Blood 1993; 92:167. Abstract.
93. Cunningham I, Gee T, Dowling M, et al. Results of treatment of Ph^1+ chronic myelogenous leukemia with an intensive treatment regimen (L-5 protocol). Blood 1979; 53:375–395.
94. Kantarjian HM, Vellekoop L, McCredie KB, et al. Intensive combination chemotherapy (ROAP 10) and splenectomy in the management of chronic myelogenous leukemia. J Clin Oncol 1985; 3:192–200.
95. Gratwohl A, Hermans J. Allogeneic bone marrow transplantation for chronic myeloid leukemia. Bone Marrow Transplant 1996; 17(suppl 3):S7–S9.
96. Horowitz MM, Rowlings PA, Passweg JR. Allogeneic bone marrow transplantation for CML: a report from the International Bone Marrow Transplant Registry. Bone Marrow Transplant 1996; 17(suppl 3):S5–S6.
97. Clift RA, Storb R. Marrow transplantation for CML: the Seattle experience. Bone Marrow Transplant 1996; 17(suppl 3):S1–S3.
98. Haut A, Abbott WS, Wintrobe MM, Cartwright GE. Busulfan in the treatment of chronic myelocytic leukemia. The effect of long term intermittent therapy. Blood 1996; 17:1–19.
99. Brodsky I, Fuscaldo KE, Kahn SB, Conroy JF. Myeloproliferative disorders. II. CML: clonal evolution and its role in management. Leuk Res 1979; 3:379–393.
100. Sharp JC, Joyner MV, Wayne AW, et al. Karyotypic conversion in Ph^1-positive chronic myeloid leukaemia with combination chemotherapy. Lancet 1979; 1:1370–1372.
101. Goto T, Nishikori M, Arlin Z, et al. Growth characteristics of leukemic and normal hematopoietic cells in Ph^1+ chronic myelogenous leukemia and effects of intensive treatment. Blood 1982; 59:793–808.
102. Shepherd PCA, Richards SM, Allan NC. Progress with interferon in CML. Results of the MRC UK CML III Study. Bone Marrow Transplant 1996; 17(suppl 3):S15–S18.

6
Interferon Therapy: Is It the Standard of Care?

Sante Tura
University of Bologna, Bologna, Italy

Michele Baccarani
Udine University, Udine, Italy

INTRODUCTION

From the beginning of the century, the management of chronic myeloid leukemia (CML) was based on the use of a moderate amount of cytotoxic agents, either radiation or drugs, with the aim of controlling leukemic cell mass with minimum discomfort or risk to the patient. That so-called conventional treatment helped to improve and even to normalize quality of life and, possibly, survival at a low cost, but failed to achieve any remission and to modify the progression of the disease toward accelerated and blastic phase (1–7). Several attempts that were based on nonconventional chemotherapy, sometimes including splenectomy, showed that it was possible to obtain better remission but not to modify the natural progression of the disease and prolong survival (5,7,8). At that time, when the median survival by conventional chemotherapy was less than 4 years and 10-year survivors were less than 10%, syngeneic and allogeneic bone marrow transplantation (BMT) were shown to be effective and to have the potential of curing some of the eligible patients (9–12). Therefore, BMT soon became the treatment of choice for CML, and a number of attempts are being made to raise the age limit beyond 50, to use alternative donors, and to limit the mortality and morbidity of the transplant procedure and its immunological sequelae (12–20). For some years, the management of CML remained frozen between the pole of conventional and conservative chemotherapy and the pole of allogeneic BMT. Within this scenario, human natural interferon-α (IFN-α) was reported to have antileukemic activity in Ph-positive CML and to induce cytogenetic responses (21,22), a distinct feature that was unusual with conventional chemotherapy (5,7). These findings provided a powerful stimulus and interest to the application of IFN-α to the management of CML that was made possible by the availability of larger amounts of IFN-α thanks to recombinant DNA technology and other techniques (8,23,24).

RESPONSE TO IFN-α TREATMENT

IFN-α was first reported to be effective for the treatment of CML and to induce cytogenetic response in 1983 and 1985, respectively (21,22). Subsequent studies provided independent confirmation (25–30). The results of 10 studies published between 1993 and 1996 are summarized in Table 1, where the data are sequenced not according to the date of reporting but according to the cytogenetic response rate. The complete + major (or partial) cytogenetic response rate (Ph-negative ≥65%) ranged between 6% and 19% in four multicenter randomized studies (31–36). It was 12% and 26%, respectively, in two other multicenter but not randomized studies (37,38). In single-center, nonrandomized studies the cytogenetic response rate was consistently higher, ranging between 26% and 44% (39–43). The median survival of patients who were assigned to IFN-α treatment, as it was calculated based on the intention to treat, ranged between 61 and 89 months, and again survival was consistently longer in single-center, nonrandomized studies than in multicenter randomized ones.

A relationship between cytogenetic response to IFN-α and survival was investigated in 9 of 10 studies. It was not found in one (37), was of borderline statistical significance in three (33,35,41), and was statistically significant in five (32,34,38–40,42). The cytogenetic response rate to IFN-α was likely to be lower in the two studies with the lowest proportion of patients with a low relative risk, as defined by Sokal et al. (44). As a matter of fact, the cytogenetic response rate was 6% and 10%, respectively, in the German and in the British studies (where low-risk patients were 27% and 24%), and it was 19% in the Italian study (where low-risk patients were 43%). In single-center nonrandomized studies the proportion of low-risk patients was even higher, close to 50% (39–43).

Apart from differences in patients' recruitment and features, there were differences in IFN-α type, dose, schedule, and duration, as well as in the criteria required to define the response, to evaluate the toxicity, and to decide on treatment continuation or discontinuation. Moreover, it should not be overlooked that the majority of the patients included in these reports were treated at a time when IFN-α was very experimental and many doctors either lacked specific

Table 1 Summary of the Main Studies of IFN-α in Previously Untreated or Minimally Pretreated Patients with Early-Phase Ph-Positive CML

Reference	Study type	No. pts	Low-risk pts	Cytogenetic response	Median survival (months)	Relationship between cytogenetic response and survival
Hehlmann et al. 1985	multicenter randomized	133	27%	6%	66	Trend, $p = 0.2$
Allan et al. 1995	multicenter randomized	293	24%	10%	61	Yes
Thaler et al. 1996	multicenter not randomized	80	NR	12%	61	Yes
Ohnishi et al. 1995	multicenter randomized	80	36%	16%	>60	Trend, $p = 0.1$
ICSG on CML 1994	multicenter randomized	218	43%	19%	72	Yes
Ozer et al. 1993	multicenter not randomized	112	NR	26%	66	No
Kloke et al. 1993	single-center not randomized	71	48%	26%	>72	Yes
Schofield et al. 1994	single-center not randomized	41	NR	27%	84	Trend, p NR
Kantarjian et al. 1995	single-center not randomized	274	52%	38%	89	Yes
Montastruc et al. 1995	single-center not randomized	52	46%	44%	NR	NR

The data are ordered by cytogenetic response. Cytogenetic response is defined by a proportion of Ph negative metaphases more than 65%, with the exception of the study by Ozer et al (37) (Ph neg more than 50%). Low risk patients were identified by a relative risk lower than 0.8, according to Sokal et al (44). NR = not reported.

experience or were skeptical about the efficacy of that specific treatment. Although there was an appreciable effort to preestablish and to maintain the same treatment guidelines, there is no doubt that all treatment policies underwent several changes over the years. Also for these reasons, it is difficult to evaluate retrospectively if different results could be related to different treatment policies.

Two points are worth mentioning. The first point concerns the association between IFN-α and chemotherapy, as required for better disease control. That association was discouraged but was actually allowed in all the studies, with the exception of the German one, where the patients who did not achieve hematological response to IFN-α alone in 4 months were counted as failures and were removed from the IFN-α arm (33). In the German study, the cytogenetic response rate was the lowest (6%). The second point concerns the dose. The dose that was scheduled at the beginning of the treatment was in the range of 4–5 MIU/m^2/day in eight studies (31–33,35–40,42,43). The dose was consistently lower, averaging 3 MIU three times a week only in the British study (34), where the cytogenetic response rate was low (10%), and in Schofield's study (41), where the cytogenetic response rate was 27%. However, this study was monocentric, was not randomized, and included only 41 cases.

IFN-α VS. CONVENTIONAL CHEMOTHERAPY: RANDOMIZED STUDIES

All the reports on the treatment of Ph-positive CML with IFN-α showed that IFN-α was effective and that a substantial number of patients could also achieve a significant and a sustained cytogenetic response. As previously noticed, that distinct feature was unusual with conventional chemotherapy and also with experimental chemotherapy (where cytogenetic responses may be frequent but have a short duration) (reviewed in Refs. 5–7). Accordingly, several studies addressed the issue of the effect of IFN-α on survival by comparison with chemotherapy. Four of the studies were completed and published so far (Table 2). Basically, all four studies were similar in that they were multicentric, they included only Ph-positive patients in early chronic phase, and the patients were assigned to receive either IFN-α or a regimen of conventional chemotherapy (32–35). However, there were also many differences, concerning either IFN-α (type, dose, dose adjustment, schedule, treatment duration) or chemotherapy (drug, dose, schedule, treatment intensity). Also patients' inclusion and exclusion criteria were different in the four studies, as well as patients' distribution by risk. For example, low-risk patients, as defined according to Sokal et al. (44), were 45% in the Italian study, 28% in the German study, 23% in the British study, and 37% in the Japanese study. The frequency of complete and major (or partial) cytogenetic responses (Ph-neg ≥65%) was also different, ranging from

Table 2 Summary of Four Prospective Randomized Studies Comparing IFN-α with Chemotherapy

Reference	Recruitment period	Median observation time of living pts (months)	No. randomized pts				Median survival (months)				p
			IFN	HU + BUS	HU	BUS	IFN	HU + BUS	HU	BUS	
ICSG on CML 1994	7/84–7/86 24 mo.	68	218	104	/	/	72	52	/	/	0.002
Hehlmann et al. 1994	7/83–1/91 90 mo.	53	133	/	194	186	66	/	56	45	0.008 vs. BUS 0.44 vs. HU
Allan et al. 1995	9/86–4/94 92 mo.	52	293	294	/	/	61	41	/	/	0.0009
Ohnishi et al. 1995	10/88–10/91 36 mo.	50	80	/	/	79	>60	/	/	50	0.02

HU = hydroxyurea; BUS = busulfan.

19% and 16% in the Italian and Japanese studies, to 10% and 6%, respectively, in the British and the German ones. The possible reasons for these apparent differences in the cytogenetic response rate were discussed in the prior section. Moreover, they could also merely reflect a difference in the number and the frequency of cytogenetic examinations, which was highest in the Italian and lowest in the German study. In spite of these many differences, all four studies showed that the survival of the patients who were assigned to receive IFN-α was longer than the survival of the patients who were assigned to receive chemotherapy (Table 2). The crude advantage was of about 20 months in all four studies as far as median survival was concerned. The long-term benefit could not yet be assessed.

In the German study, IFN-α was found to be better than busulfan (BUS) and hydroxyurea (HU), but the difference was significant only for BUS ($p = 0.008$) and not for HU ($p = 0.44$). These results raised some concern about the interpretation of the Italian study, where the patients who were assigned to receive chemotherapy could be treated with different HU dose and schedule and could also receive BUS (21,32,36). That concern prompted a collaborative study of the Italian and the German groups to establish the reason for the apparent discrepancies (45). When the two databases were examined by the same statistical team, it was found that the apparent discrepancy was accounted for by different inclusion and exclusion criteria. The German protocol required that all patients be symptomatic and allowed for the inclusion of patients with >10% blast cells in peripheral blood or with extramedullary manifestations, whereas the Italian protocol allowed for the inclusion of nonsymptomatic patients and required that all the patients have less than 10% blast cells in peripheral blood and no extramedullary manifestations.

These inclusion-exclusion criteria were clearly stated in both original reports, but it was overlooked that a substantial proportion of Italian patients (13%) would not have been eligible for the German trial and that an even higher proportion of German patients (16%) would not have been eligible for the Italian trial. When these patients were excluded, the results of the Italian and the German studies became more similar, with a p value for IFN-α vs. chemotherapy of 0.001 for Italian patients and 0.12 for German ones. Median survival of IFN-α-treated patients was calculated to be 76 months for the former and 72 months for the latter (45). Moreover, it should not be overlooked that between the Italian and the German protocols there was a potentially important difference, because the Italian protocol required that all patients who were assigned to receive IFN-α be treated at maximum tolerated dose for a minimum of 14 months, and indefinitely in case of response. In contrast, the German protocol required treatment at maximum tolerated does only for a much shorter period (4 months) and allowed for dose downmodulation in case of response. It may also be important to notice that the Italian protocol allowed for the addition of chemotherapy at any time, whenever it was felt that chemotherapy was useful to help control leukemia, while the German protocol did not because it was essentially a trial of IFN-α strictly as monotherapy.

SHOULD IFN-α TREATMENT BE BASED ON RESPONSE?

It is not clear if one should continue the administration of IFN-α independently of the response. That is very important, because IFN-α is expensive and may have several unpleasant side effects resulting in a decrease in the quality of life and also because continuing with IFN-α would prevent offering the patient other potentially useful treatment modalities. Many studies found a positive relationship between cytogenetic response to IFN-α and overall survival (Table 1). In the same and other studies it was also found that hematological response to IFN-α was associated with a longer survival. Hematological response is a prerequisite of cytogenetic response, but not all hematological responders also become cytogenetic responders. The cytogenetic response rate in patients who achieved a hematological response is shown it Table 3.

With the exception of the German and the British studies already commented upon, the cytogenetic response rate ranged between 18% and 45% for all hematological responders (partial and complete) and between 34% and 64%

Table 3 Cytogenetic Response to IFN-α, as Calculated on All Cases (% of total), on Patients Who Achieved Hematological Response, Either Partial or Complete, and on Patients Who Achieved a Complete Hematological Response

			Cytogenetic response	
Reference	No. cases	% Total	% Partial and complete hematological responses	% Complete hematological responses
Hehlmann et al. 1995	133	6	7	19
Allan et al. 1995	293	10	16	21
Thaler et al. 1996	80	12	18	34
Ohnishi et al. 1995	80	16	21	42
ICSG on CML 1994	218	19	40	64
Ozer et al. 1993	112	26	NR	49
Kloke et al. 1993	71	26	NR	NR
Schofield et al. 1994	41	26	33	44
Kantarjian et al. 1995	274	38	44	47
Montastruc et al. 1995	52	44	45	55

(median 47%) for complete hematological responders. That difference between the hematological and the cytogenetic response rate highlights some very important questions that are still unanswered—namely, if the primary target of treatment is cytogenetic response, should that target be pursued and should the response be maintained at any cost; and if hematological response in the absence of cytogenetic response is beneficial enough to warrant the cost and side effects of treatment.

These points will be developed in a subsequent section, but it is important to recall that, although much attention was obviously focused on cytogenetic response as a prerequisite of a true complete remission, all the reports published so far showed that hematological response was also associated with a longer survival. Moreover, in the British study, the survival of a subset of patients who were assigned to IFN-α and were poorly responsive to IFN-α, was longer than the survival of the patients who were assigned to chemotherapy (34).

IFN-α, CONVENTIONAL CHEMOTHERAPY, AND BONE MARROW TRANSPLANTATION (BMT)

When allogeneic BMT was applied to the treatment of CML, median survival was 4 years or less with conventional chemotherapy and there was no convincing evidence that nonconventional chemotherapy could lead to prolongation of survival. Therefore, allogeneic BMT quickly became the first option in patients who where <50 years old and had an HLA-compatible sib (13–20). Soon after, an experimental option was opened to patients who were >50 years, as well as for transplants from unrelated matched donors. At that time, not much attention was paid to the existence of different prognostic groups with a different life expectancy, because even in the best group median survival with conventional chemotherapy was <6 years and 10-year survival was <10% (5,6).

Conventional chemotherapy has several important advantages over IFN-α and allogeneic BMT. It can be used at any age, it is cheap, well tolerated, and allows moving to another treatment modality at any time. However, conventional chemotherapy is significantly inferior to both IFN-α and allogeneic BMT as far as overall survival (18,46) and does not lead to any cure. Therefore, conventional chemotherapy can be the treatment of choice only in the elderly or in particular clinical situations where other treatment modalities cannot be applied. Otherwise, conventional chemotherapy can be considered only as an ancillary measure to control leukemia temporarily, prior to or after BMT, IFN-α, or other treatments.

A choice between allogeneic BMT and IFN-α is more difficult. The decision should depend on several variables and would require a comparative analysis of the survival with IFN-α and with BMT. There are no prospective studies comparing IFN-α with allogeneic BMT, but it can be useful to trace back the fate of the patients who were assigned to either treatment during the last decade. This kind of information is currently available at the Italian Cooperative Study Group of CML, which registered and followed up all the patients <55 years old who were first seen during the period 1984–1991 (46). Four hundred thirty of these patients were assigned to receive IFN-α, and 120 of them (28%) were transplanted in first chronic phase from an identical sib and without T-depletion, a "standard" transplant procedure. The comparison is shown in Table 4.

When patients were considered overall BMT was likely to be better than IFN-α, but with a median follow-up of 8 years p value was not yet significant (0.27). When patients were divided by age (±32 years, which was the median age at transplant), BMT was again likely to be better than IFN-α in the younger patients ($p = 0.17$), but not in those who were between 33–55 years of age ($p = 0.68$). When patients were divided by risk, BMT was better than IFN-α in intermediate and high-risk patients ($p = 0.11$) but was identical to IFN-α in low-risk patients (10-year survival 55% and 53%, $p = 0.83$). It may be important to point out that today about 50% of all patients fall in the low-risk group. These data should not be taken and used as a proof for or against either treatment for a number of reasons, including the retrospective nature of the observation and methodological problems (in the transplant group, survival was not adjusted for the time lapsed from diagnosis to transplant, a median of 1 year). Moreover, these data cannot tell us what will happen in the next few years. However, this prospective and continuous surveillance can help us to understand what happened in the last decade and also to plan future interventions.

We think that the main message that can be obtained from Table 1 is that survival of CML improved substantially but that almost 50% of cases failed with either treatment. Therefore, the main issue is not comparing the present transplantation methodology with the current policy of IFN-α treatment, but to improve both treatment modalities. For IFN-α it is necessary to increase the response rate and to prolong and maintain the response. For allogeneic BMT it is necessary to reduce morbidity and mortality and to increase the number of those who are eligible for a "safe" transplant. Both issues are discussed in other chapters.

DECIDING ON THE TREATMENT

Based on present knowledge, a patient with Ph-positive CML in chronic phase, previously untreated or minimally pretreated, can be advised depending on age and risk. A young patient with an HLA-identical sib should be offered the transplant immediately. A young patient without a matched family donor could be treated initially with IFN-α and would be moved to other experimental proce-

Table 4 Comparison of Overall Survival by Age and Risk, Italian Cooperative Study Group on CML

	No. pts		Median survival		Projected 10-year survival		
	IFN-α	BMT	IFN-α	BMT	IFN-α	BMT	p
All patients	310	120	6 yr	>10 yr	40%	53%	0.27
Age ≤32 yr	85	66	7 yr	>10 yr	42%	58%	0.17
Age >32 yr	225	54	6.5 yr	5.5 yr	38%	45%	0.68
High + int. Sokal's risk	157	60	5 yr	9 yr	25%	49%	0.11
Low Sokal's risk	153	60	>10 yr	>10 yr	53%	55%	0.83

Between 1986 and 1991 430 patients <55 years old were registered at the Italian Cooperative Study Group on CML with newly diagnosed and previously untreated Ph+ CML and were assigned to treatment with IFN-α; 120 of them were transplanted in first chronic phase, from an HLA-identical sib and without T-depletion. Survival was calculated from diagnosis by the method of Kaplan and Meyer (47), without any adjustment for the time lapsed between diagnosis and transplant. Comparison was made by the log-rank method (48). Risk was defined according to Sokal et al. (44) (low risk <0.8, intermediate + high risk ≥0.8). Follow-up of living patients ranged between 5 and 13 years (median 8 years). By courtesy of the Italian Cooperative Study Group on CML.

dures, namely, transplant from a matched unrelated donor if IFN-α fails. An older patient (35–55 years old) with an HLA-identical sib could be offered a transplant immediately if its (Sokal's) risk was high or intermediate, but could be treated with IFN-α if the risk was low. A middle-aged patient without a matched family donor would be a candidate for IFN-α, and hence for experimental therapeutic procedures if IFN-α failed. These guidelines should be adapted to each individual patient, depending on clinical conditions and on the patient's willingness. The latter is very important because a patient should be informed that with IFN-α the risk of dying of treatment is minimal and the probability of a cure is hypothetical, while with allogeneic BMT both the risk of dying from treatment and the probability of a cure are substantial. In that setting, personal, family, and economic reasons may contribute in very different ways to a decision. Patients >55 years old, who account for about 50% of all the cases of CML (median age is around 55 years), are obvious candidates for IFN-α, depending on the age and tolerance. As discussed elsewhere, IFN-α is not well tolerated in the elderly, but that is not true for all patients and there is no point in excluding a patient from treatment a priori, if the only contraindication is age.

The advantage of a balanced policy of allogeneic BMT and IFN-α is that standard BMT is offered as first-line treatment to patients who are expected to get the maximum benefit with the lowest risk (young age and HLA-identical sib) and to patients who are expected to be less responsive to IFN-α (any intermediate and high-risk patients). For all other patients, treating with IFN-α first can have the disadvantage of delaying the transplant, and delaying the transplant can worsen transplant results (13,14,16,17). However, even if the time to complete cytogenetic response can be as long as 2 or 3 years and even more, the time that is required to judge if a patient is responsive (hematological response) ranges between 3 and 6 months, and the time that is required to decide if a patient will get a cytogenetic response rarely exceeds 1 year. We estimate that within 1 year it is possible to identify >90% of the patients who are responsive to IFN-α and >70% of the patients who will become long survivors with IFN-α.

During 1 year <10% of the patients would progress to accelerated phase and could actually miss the opportunity of an early transplant. There may be some concern about the effect of IFN-α pretreatment on the outcome of allogeneic BMT (49). However, prior treatment with IFN-α did not adversely affect transplant outcome in 77 patients who were treated at M.D. Anderson Cancer Center in Houston, Texas (50). Moreover, at a recent meeting of the European investigators of IFN-α in CML that was held in Seville in March 1996, that point was carefully reviewed by representatives of several national committees (Italy, Germany, Spain, and U.K.) who did not report any adverse effects, either early or late, of IFN-α pretreatment on the outcome of allogeneic BMT (51). The fact that treatment with IFN-α does not prevent resorting to other treatments with a curative potential may be an important advantage of IFN-α over some other experimental and toxic procedures that could increase substantially the risk of a subsequent procedure of allogeneic BMT, like intensive treatment with autologous stem-cell rescue (19,52,53).

PREDICTING RESPONSE

To put IFN-α in a proper place in the management of CML would require the capacity first to predict the response to IFN-α and second to predict the benefit that can be obtained with IFN-α, as it concerns survival. This issue was discussed in several reports and, in spite of several minor differences, there was a general trend toward a relationship between response, survival, and any features that may identify a case of leukemia at a low risk or of a small size. This is exemplified in Table 5, where the main data are reported of 274 patients who were treated at the M.D. Anderson Cancer Center (42). A candidate for a good response and long survival is defined by absence of symptoms, small spleen,

Table 5 Association Between Patients' Characteristics, Cytogenetic Response Rate (complete + major or partial, Ph-neg ≥65%), and Survival

	p values for:	
	Cytogenetic response rate	Survival
Performance status	0.01	0.02
Symptoms	<0.01	0.18
Spleen size	<0.01	<0.01
Hb level	<0.01	0.01
Platelet count	0.06	0.02
Leukocyte count	<0.01	0.02
Peripheral blast cells (%)	<0.01	0.01
Peripheral nucleated red cells (%)	>0.20	<0.01
Marrow basophils (%)	0.11	<0.01
Prognostic model-MDACC	<0.01	<0.01
-SOKAL's	<0.01	0.10
-SYNTHESIS	<0.01	<0.01

Data are taken from a review of 274 Ph+ early-phase CML patients who were treated with IFN-α at M.D. Anderson Cancer Center (MDACC), Houston (42). Numbers are p values that refer either to a chi-square test (for cytogenetic response rate) or to a log-rank test (for survival). Prognostic models are described in Refs. 44, 54, and 55.

normal Hb level and platelet count, relatively normal leukocyte count, and no blast cells in the peripheral blood—a complex of features that identify low-risk patients in all the prognostic models developed so far (44,54,55).

As a matter of fact, from all studies it appears that the higher the proportion of low-risk cases, the higher the cytogenetic response rate (Table 1). The relationship is quite obvious and in fact is valid for many diseases and for many treatments. The point is not to acknowledge that a low-risk patient can have a long survival with any treatment, whether it is IFN-α or conventional chemotherapy, but to establish if IFN-α is better, risks being equal. That is shown in Figures 1 and 2, where the survival data of the Italian study are updated and presented by risk. Low-risk patients survived longer with IFN-α than with chemotherapy (Fig. 1), as did high-risk patients (Fig. 2).

PLANNING IFN-α TREATMENT

Low-risk patients respond to IFN-α better than high-risk ones, but present risk classifications cannot establish whether or not a patient should receive IFN-α. Achieving a hematological response, whether it is partial or complete, within 3 to a maximum of 6 months is the first target. A cytogenetic response begins to be detectable from the sixth month on, sometimes even earlier, and is usually easily found within 12 months in all responsive patients. To become complete, it can take more time and even years, but achieving a cytogenetic response, even

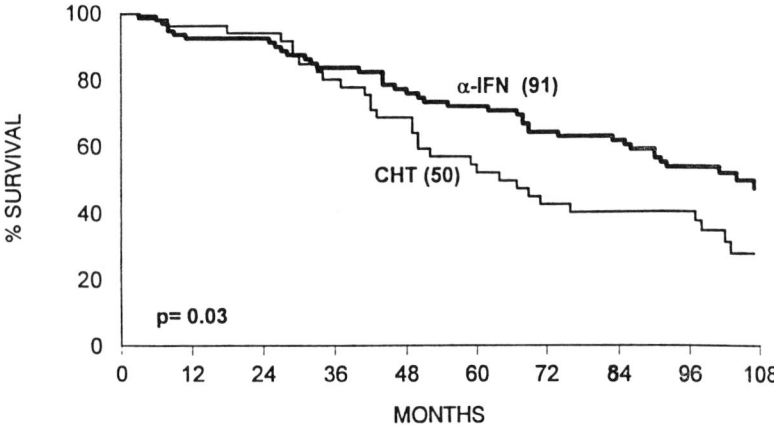

Figure 1 Italian study (31,32). Overall survival of Sokal's low-risk patients who were assigned to treatment with IFN-α or with chemotherapy (CHT). Kaplan-Meyer (47). Log-rank test (48). By courtesy of the Italian Cooperative Study Group on CML.

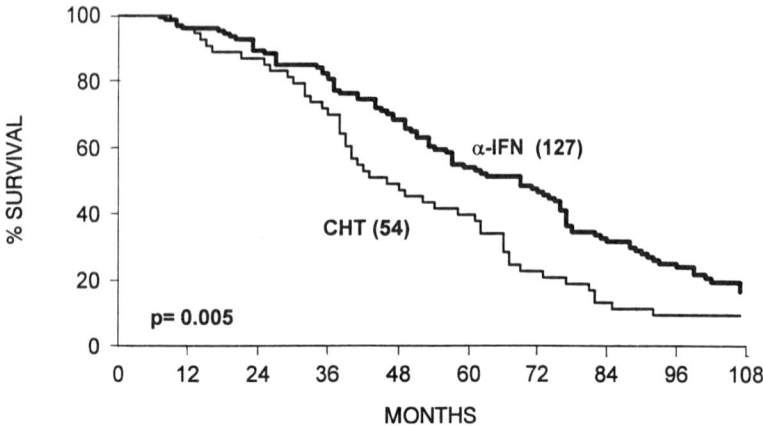

Figure 2 Italian Study (31,32). Overall survival of Sokal's high- and intermediate-risk patients who were assigned to treatment with IFN-α or with chemotherapy (CHT). Kaplan-Meyer (47). Log-rank test (48). By courtesy of the Italian Cooperative Study Group on CML.

minor (Ph-neg 33–65%), within the first year is the second important target. To achieve both targets, a policy of "maximum tolerated dose" (5 MIU/m^2/day) can be recommended, where "maximum" can mean a performance status ≥80, Hb ≥100 g/L, platelet ≥50 × 10^9/L, and WBC ≥2 × 10^9/L.

However, it was shown that some patients can respond as well to much smaller doses of IFN-α (34,41). Once the maximum response (complete cytogenetic response) is obtained or once the best response (whether it is cytogenetic or hematological) has become stable, it is not known if treatment should be maintained at maximum tolerated dose, should be kept at minimum effective dose, or should even be discontinued. As time goes by, a dose reduction becomes unavoidable, leading sooner or later to treatment discontinuation. Losing cytogenetic response does not herald progression to accelerated or blastic phase, and a very long survival may be possible as well. However, losing hematological response is usually a marker of a poor prognosis in the short term, and in such a case IFN-α continuation becomes unacceptable. As already discussed, there is a logical trend to use IFN-α only if it proves to be effective and only until it is effective. However, the concept of effectiveness may be quite broad and may range from only partial hematological response to complete cytogenetic response. It should not be overlooked that in the British study a survival benefit, by comparison with conventional chemotherapy, was also found in patients who responded poorly to IFN-α (34). Treatment with IFN-α is much more expensive than conventional chemotherapy, but it can become cheaper and more cost effective if it is limited to responding patients. Moreover, IFN-α discontinuation in the patients who do not respond or who lose the response can allow these patients to profit by other experimental treatments, with special reference to allogeneic BMT from matched unrelated donors.

CONCLUSIONS

Treatment with IFN-α has several drawbacks including the cost and the side effects of IFN-α. The cost can be reduced and substantial efforts should be made to control the side effects, as they were made in other settings, like for drug-induced emesis. Several important questions are unanswered, including the dose, the best target to which the dose should be adapted, and the duration. The response rate can be improved by combination with other drugs or treatment modalities. However, IFN-α is presently the treatment of choice for all patients who cannot be transplanted from an HLA-identical sib, and in middle-aged patients IFN-α may even be preferred to allogeneic BMT.

The apparent competition between IFN-α and allogeneic BMT is artificial, transitory, and probably short-sighted. The main problem is not to establish which treatment is better or can be better adapted in different clinical situations, but to improve treatment results. Although the management of Ph-positive CML has improved substantially, it is not yet satisfactory. Even in the best situation, the 10-year failure rate is still as high as 50%. The best treatments still carry a substantial risk of morbidity or mortality and are very expensive. Accordingly, the management of CML should remain investigational, either in the field of IFN-α or in the area of allogeneic or autologous BMT. The attempts at optimizing the treatment and tracing algorithms (19) are inviting, but they may be dangerous because optimizing implies knowing what is the best treatment for any patients and following an algorithm can delay treatment improvements.

REFERENCES

1. Galton DAG. Chemotherapy of chronic myelocytic leukemia. Semin Hematol 1969; 6:323–343.
2. Stryckmans PA. Current concepts in chronic myelogenous leukemia. Semin Hematol 1974; 11:101–127.
3. Goldman JM. Modern approaches to the management of chronic granulocytic leukemia. Semin Hematol 1978; 15:420–430.
4. Koeffler HP, Golde DW. Chronic myelogenous leukemia—new concepts. N Engl J Med 1981; 304:1201–1209, 1269–1274.
5. Tura S, Baccarani M, Zaccaria A. Chronic myeloid leukemia. Haematologica 1986; 71:169–176.

6. Sokal JE, Baccarani M, Russo D, et al. Staging and prognosis in chronic myeloid leukemia. Semin Hematol 1988; 25:49–61.
7. Kantarjian HM, O'Brien S, Anderlini P, et al. Treatment of chronic myelogenous leukemia: current status and investigational options. Blood 1996; 87:3069–3081.
8. Talpaz M, Kantarjian HM, Kurzrock R, et al. Therapy of chronic myelogenous leukemia: chemotherapy and interferons. Semin Hematol 1988; 25:62–73.
9. Fefer A, Cheever MA, Thomas ED, et al. Disappearance of Ph-positive cells in four patients with chronic granulocytic leukemia after chemotherapy, irradiation and marrow transplantation from an identical twin. N Engl J Med 1979; 300:333–337.
10. Doney KC, Buckner CD, Thomas ED, et al. Allogeneic bone marrow transplantation for chronic granulocytic leukemia. Exp Hematol 1978; 6:738–747.
11. Goldman JM, Baughan AS, McCarthy DM, et al. Marrow transplantation for patients in the chronic phase of chronic granulocytic leukaemia. Lancet 1982; 2:623–625.
12. Thomas ED, Clift RA, Fefer A, et al. Marrow transplantation for the treatment of chronic myelogenous leukemia. Ann Intern Med 1986; 104:155–163.
13. Goldman JM, Gale RP, Horowitz MM, et al. Bone marrow transplantation for chronic myelogenous leukemia in chronic phase. Ann Intern Med 1988; 108:806–814.
14. Thomas ED, Clift RA. Indications for marrow transplantation in chronic myelogenous leukemia. Blood 1989; 73:861–864.
15. Clift RA, Buckner CD, Appelbaum FR, et al. Allogeneic marrow transplantation in patients with chronic myeloid leukemia in the chronic phase: a randomized trial of two irradiation regimens. Blood 1991; 77:1660–1665.
16. Clift RA, Appelbaum FR, Thomas ED. Treatment of chronic myeloid leukemia by marrow transplantation. Blood 1993; 82:1954–1956.
17. Goldman JM, Szydlo R, Horowitz MM, et al. Choice of pretransplant treatment and timing of transplant for chronic myelogenous leukemia in chronic phase. Blood 1993; 82:2235–2238.
18. Italian Cooperative Study Group on Chronic Myeloid Leukemia. Evaluating survival after allogeneic bone marrow transplant for chronic myeloid leukaemia in chronic phase: a comparison of transplant versus no-transplant in a cohort of 258 patients first seen in Italy between 1984 and 1986. Br J Haematol 1993; 85:292–299.
19. Goldman JM. Management of chronic myeloid leukaemia. Blood Rev 1994; 8:21–29.
20. Devergie A, Blaise D, Attal M, et al. Allogeneic bone marrow transplantation for chronic myeloid leukemia in first chronic phase: a randomized trial of busulfan-cytoxan versus cytoxan-total body irradiation as preparative regimen: a report from the French society of bone marrow graft (SFGM). Blood 1995; 85:2263–2268.
21. Talpaz M, McCredie K, Mavligit GM, et al. Leukocyte interferon-induced myeloid cytoreduction in chronic myelogenous leukemia. Blood 1983; 62:689–692.
22. Talpaz M, Kantarjian HM, McCredie K, et al. Hematologic remission and cytogenetic improvement induced by recombinant human interferon alpha in chronic myelogenous leukemia. N Engl J Med 1986; 314:1065–1069.

23. Aulitzky WE, Peschel C, Schneller F, et al. Biotherapy of chronic myelogenous leukemia. Ann Hematol 1995; 70:113–120.
24. Wetzler M, Kantarjian H, Kurzrock R, et al. Interferon-α therapy for chronic myelogenous leukemia. Am J Med 1995; 99:402–411.
25. Alimena G, Morra E, Lazzarino M, et al. Interferon alpha-2b as therapy for Ph-positive chronic myelogenous leukemia: a study of 82 patients treated with intermittent or daily administration. Blood 1988; 72:642–647.
26. Guilhot F, Dreyfus B, Brizard A, et al. Cytogenetic remission in chronic myelogenous leukemia using interferon alpha-2a and hydroxyurea with or without low-dose cytosine arabinoside. Leuk Lymph 1991; 4:49–55.
27. Opalka B, Wandl UB, Becher R, et al. Minimal residual disease in patients with chronic myelogenous leukemia undergoing long-term treatment with recombinant interferon α-2b alone or in combination with interferon γ. Blood 1991; 78:2188–2193.
28. Bilhou-Nabera C, Viard F, Marit G, et al. Complete cytogenetic conversion in chronic myelocytic leukemia patients undergoing interferon-α therapy: follow-up with reverse polymerase chain reaction. Leukemia 1992; 6:595–598.
29. Fernandez-Rañada JM, Lavilla E, Odriozola J, et al. Interferon alpha 2A in the treatment of chronic myelogenous leukemia in chronic phase. Results of the Spanish Group. Leuk Lymph 1993; 11(suppl 1):175–179.
30. Shtalrid M, Lugassy G, Rosensaft J, et al. Treatment of chronic myeloid leukemia with interferon alpha (Roferon): results of the Israeli Study Group on CML. Leuk Lymph 1993; 11(suppl 1):193–197.
31. Italian Cooperative Study Group on Chronic Myeloid Leukemia. A prospective comparison of α-IFN and conventional chemotherapy in Ph+ chronic myeloid leukemia. Clinical and cytogenetic results at 2 years in 322 patients. Haematologica 1992; 77:204–214.
32. Italian Cooperative Study Group on Chronic Myeloid Leukemia. Interferon alfa-2a as compared with conventional chemotherapy for the treatment of chronic myeloid leukemia. N Engl J Med 1994; 330:820–825.
33. Hehlmann R, Heimpel H, Hasford J, et al. Randomized comparison of interferon-α with busulfan and hydroxyurea in chronic myelogenous leukemia. Blood 1994; 84:4064–4077.
34. Allan NC, Richards SM, Shepherd PAC, et al. UK medical research council randomised, multicentre trial of interferon-αn1 for chronic myeloid leukemia: improved survival irrespective of cytogenetic response. Lancet 1995; 345:1392–1397.
35. Ohnishi K, Ohno R, Tomonaga M, et al. A randomized trial comparing interferon-α with busulfan for newly diagnosed chronic myelogenous leukemia in chronic phase. Blood 1995; 86:906–916.
36. Rosti G, De Vivo A, Zuffa E, et al. Interferon-α in the treatment of chronic myeloid leukemia. A summary and an update of the Italian studies. Bone Marrow Transplant 1996; 17(suppl 3):S11–S13.
37. Ozer H, George SL, Schiffer CA, et al. Prolonged subcutaneous administration of recombinant α2b interferon in patients with previously untreated Philadelphia chromosome-positive chronic-phase chronic myelogenous leukemia: effect on remission duration and survival: cancer and leukemia Group B Study 8583. Blood 1993; 82:2975–2984.

38. Thaler J, Gastl G, Fluckinger T, et al. Interferon alpha-2c therapy of patients with chronic myelogenous leukemia: long-term results of a multicenter phase-II study. Ann Hematol 1996; 72:349–355.
39. Talpaz M, Kantarjian H, Kurzrock R, et al. Interferon-alpha produces sustained cytogenetic responses in chronic myelogenous leukemia. Ann Intern Med 1991; 114:532–538.
40. Kloke O, Niederle N, Qiu JY, et al. Impact of interferon alpha-induced cytogenetic improvement on survival in chronic myelogenous leukaemia. Br J Haematol 1993; 83:399–403.
41. Schoffield JR, Robinson WA, Murphy JR, et al. Low doses of interferon-α are as effective as higher doses in inducing remissions and prolonging survival in chronic myeloid leukemia. Ann Intern Med 1994; 121:736–744.
42. Kantarjian HM, Smith TL, O'Brien S, et al. Prolonged survival in chronic myelogenous leukemia after cytogenetic response to interferon-α therapy. Ann Intern Med 1995; 122:254–261.
43. Montastruc M, Mahon FX, Faberes C, et al. Response to recombinant interferon alpha in patients with chronic myelogenous leukemia in a single centre: results and analysis of predictive factors. Leukemia 1995; 9:1997–2002.
44. Sokal JE, Cox EB, Baccarani M, et al. Prognostic discrimination in "good risk" chronic granulocytic leukemia. Blood 1984; 63:789–799.
45. German and Italian Chronic Myeloid Leukemia Study Groups. Interferon-α and hydroxyurea in early chronic myeloid leukemia: a comparative analysis of the Italian and German chronic myeloid leukemia trials with interferon-α. Blood 1996; 87:5384–5391.
46. Baccarani M, Bandini G, Arcese W, et al. The influence of allogeneic bone marrow transplantation (BMT) on survival in chronic myeloid leukemia (CML). A national survey in Italy. 25th Annual Meeting Intern Soc Exp Hematol, New York, 1996, Exp Hematol 1996; 24(suppl):1145. Abstract 660.
47. Kaplan EL, Meier P. Nonparametric estimation from incomplete observations. J Am Stat Assoc 1958; 53:475–481.
48. Peto R, Pike MC, Armitage P, et al. Design and analysis of randomized clinical trials requiring prolonged observation of each patient. II. Analysis and examples. Br J Cancer 1977; 35:1–39.
49. Beelen DW, Graeven U, Elmaagacli AH, et al. Prolonged administration of interferon-α in patients with chronic-phase Philadelphia chromosome-positive chronic myelogenous leukemia before allogeneic bone marrow transplantation may adversely affect transplant outcome. Blood 1995; 85:2981–2990.
50. Giralt SA, Kantarjian TM, Talpaz M, et al. Effect of prior interferon alfa therapy on the outcome of allogeneic bone marrow transplantation for chronic myelogenous leukemia. J Clin Oncol 1993; 11:1055–1061.
51. Fourth Meeting of the European Investigators of Interferon in Chronic Myeloid Leukemia, Sevilla, 22–23 March, 1996.
52. Butturini A, Keating A, Goldman J, et al. Autotransplants in chronic myelogenous leukaemia: strategies and results. Lancet 1990; 335:1255–1258.
53. McGlave PB, de Fabritiis P, Deisseroth A, et al. Autologous transplants for chronic

myelogenous leukaemia: results from eight transplant groups. Lancet 1994; 343: 1486–1488.
54. Kantarjian HM, Smith TL, McCredie KB, et al. Chronic myelogenous leukemia: a multivariate analysis of the associations of patients' characteristics and therapy with survival. Blood 1985; 66:1326–1335.
55. Kantarjian HM, Keating MJ, Smith TL, et al. Proposal for a simple synthesis prognostic staging system in chronic myelogenous leukemia. Am J Med 1990; 88:1–8.

7
Practical Management of Interferon Therapy and Side Effects

Susan O'Brien, Hagop M. Kantarjian, and Moshe Talpaz
M.D. Anderson Cancer Center, Houston, Texas

INTRODUCTION

Interferon-α has become the standard of care in the management of chronic myelogenous leukemia (CML). Complete hematological remissions (CHR) occur in 70–80% of patients with newly diagnosed CML, and the number of cells containing the Philadelphia (Ph) chromosome is reduced in about 50% of hematological responders (1,2). A major cytogenetic (CG) response (defined as a Ph-positive cell count of <35%) is associated with delayed time to blastic transformation and with prolonged survival, although this response varies in different series from <10% to 38% (Table 1). This wide variance has been attributed to (1) different population characteristics, (2) different dose schedules for IFN-α, and (3) the relative expertise of investigators (1–10).

Though the importance of dose is controversial, it appears that higher doses of IFN-α usually result in higher response rates. This is supported by the disparate results of two groups of studies. There are several trials that used lower doses of IFN-α and had lower response rates. Five of them report daily doses of 2–4 million units (MU)/m^2 and CG response rates of 18–44% (5–9). Other small studies report two or three weekly doses of 2–5 MU, CG response rates of 0–20%, and no complete CG remissions (10–12). In contrast are studies by groups that used higher IFN-α doses of >4 MU/m^2 and report CG response rates of >50% (2–4).

The five largest trials to use IFN-α in treating CML include the collected M.D. Anderson experience, randomized trials conducted by the Italian Cooperative Study Group on CML (ICSG-CML) and German, British, and Japanese

Table 1 Dose Response and Survival with IFN-α Therapy in CML

Study (reference)	Dose/schedule	No. pts	CHR	Percent CG response Any	Percent CG response Major	Median survival[a] (months)
MDACC (2)	5 MU/m^2/D	274	80	58	38	89
Montastruc et al. (3)	5 MU/m^2/D	52	81	69	44	—
ICSG-CML (4)	4.3 MU/m^2/D[b]	218	>68	55	19	72
Ohnishi et al. (5)	3.6–4 MU/m^2/D	170	39	44	16	—
Allan et al. (6)	3.2 MU/D[c]	293	69	22[d]	11	61
CALGB (7)	3 MU/m^2/D[b]	107	59	29[e]	—	66
Hehlmann et al. (8)	2 MU/m^2/D[b]	133	31	18	8	66
Schofield et al. (9)	2 MU/m^2/D	27	71	34	22	84
Alimena et al. (10)	2 MU/m^2/TIW	33	24	—	—	—
	5 MU/m^2/TIW	30	47	—	—	—
Freund et al. (11)	5 MU/TIW	14	29	20	0	—
Anger et al. (12)	3 MU/TIW	9	22	0	0	—

MDACC = MD Anderson Cancer Center; CALGB = Cancer and Leukemia Group B; ICSG = Italian Cooperative Study Group; MU = million units; D = day; TIW = three times weekly; CHR = complete hematologic response; CG = cytogenetic.
[a]Refers only to the IFN-α arm in trials that are randomized.
[b]Median dose delivered.
[c]Mean dose delivered.
[d]≤80% Ph-positive cells.
[e]Only ≥50% reduction in Ph chromosome considered.

study groups, and a single-arm study by the Cancer and Leukemia Group B (CALGB) (2,5–8). In the M.D. Anderson trials, the median daily dose of IFN-α was 5 MU/m^2, resulting in overall and major CG response rates of 58% and 38%, respectively. Landmark and multivariate analyses showed a significant correlation between a major CG response anytime after 12 months and prolonged survival (2). With a similar median dose of 4.3 MU/m^2, the ICSG-CML also demonstrated a correlation between survival and a major CG response (4). The Japanese group used an average daily IFN-α dose of 6.5–8.1 MU. Patients with a CG response had a longer duration of chronic phase and increased survival (5). Allan et al., in the largest study, treated 293 patients with a mean daily dose of IFN of 3.2 MU (6). Major CG responses were noted in only 11% of patients. However, those patients survived significantly longer, even when analysis was done allowing for time to response bias (6). The German group found no improvement in survival for patients treated with IFN-α versus hydroxyurea; however, they reported a median daily IFN-α dose of only 2 MU/m^2 and a low major CG response rate of 8% (8).

In the CALGB trial, 29% of the patients had major CG responses, and these showed similar survival durations to those who did not achieve a cytogenetic response. However, the CALGB trial differed from the above trials in how it defined a major cytogenetic response: for the CALGB, it was <50% Ph-positive cells (7); for the others, it was <35%. Thus, some of the patients the CALGB considered major responders would be considered minor responders in the other trials.

Overall, the data from the aforementioned trials suggest (1) a correlation between IFN-α dose and a major CG response, and (2) a survival advantage for patients who achieve a major CG response. IFN-α treatment at a dose of 5 MU/m^2 is associated with significant side effects that may limit therapy in patients who would most benefit. Thus, it is important to establish guidelines for using IFN-α in CML patients in order to minimize toxicity, improve patient compliance, and increase response rates. Such approaches are empirical and not often described in detail in published trials; they are elaborated upon in this chapter.

INITIATION OF IFN-α THERAPY IN CML

In the early studies, IFN-α was used as a single agent to establish its anti-CML efficacy in achieving hematological remissions. However, initial tumor reduction can be achieved faster, less expensively, and with less toxicity with hydroxyurea. The current focus of IFN-α therapy is to induce reduction in disease burden (from hematological to cytogenetic response) to further improve prognosis.

Acute toxicities with IFN-α are related to flulike side effects including fever, malaise, and muscle and bone aches. An increased white blood cell (WBC) count is associated with increased severity of these initial effects. This may be related to the release of cytokines from the circulating hematopoietic cells, with high tumor burden resulting in more acute side effects. CML cells have high levels of leukotriene C4, which may induce an inflammatory response (13). Thus, IFN-α therapy should not be initiated immediately at diagnosis when WBC counts are elevated, often to >100 × 10^3/μL.

Hydroxyurea is the drug of choice to lower WBC counts to <20 × 10^3/μL, at which point INF-α can more easily be administered. Importantly, the hematological response to IFN-α therapy is delayed (weeks) as compared to the time to response with hydroxyurea (days) so that hydroxyurea therapy should be continued during the initial phase of IFN-α therapy to prevent rebound leukocytosis and its concomitant toxicity. Hydroxyurea doses should be adjusted according to the WBC count exactly as if IFN-α were not being used. In patients taking full dose IFN-α (5 MU/m^2 daily), the need for hydroxyurea (to control blood counts) for >6 months is a poor prognostic sign and indicates a group of patients unlikely to achieve a major CG response.

When the WBC count is $<20 \times 10^3/\mu L$, IFN-α can be started. Tolerance to IFN-α is improved if the drug is started at 25% of the target dose (about 3 MU daily) and gradually increased. In patients whose side effects are grade 2 or lower, IFN-α can be escalated in 50–100% increments every 7 days. Thus, full-dose IFN-α may be administered within 2–4 weeks after starting therapy. A useful approach is to start with 3 MU daily for 3–7 days, then increase to 5–6 MU daily for 3–7 days, and to the full dose of 5 MU/m^2 daily or the maximally tolerated individual dose (not to exceed 5 MU/m^2 daily).

Dose Modifications

For patients experiencing severe (grade 3–4) toxicity (NCI criteria), IFN-α should be withheld. When the toxicity is resolved, therapy can be restarted at 50% of the dose and escalated to 75% if side effects are tolerable. Chronic grade 2 toxicities can be ameliorated by a 25% dose reduction; alternatively, patients may be enrolled in a program aimed at counteracting toxicities.

Myelosuppression is desirable to a certain extent. Although a WBC count of $<10 \times 10^3/\mu L$ is indicative of CHR, the incidence of CG response is higher in patients who achieve low-normal blood counts. The common practice of holding or reducing the dose of IFN-α when the WBC count reaches 5–$10 \times 10^3/\mu L$ may preclude the maximum benefit of IFN-α therapy occurring—i.e., the achievement of a CG response. The dose of IFN-α should not be decreased in patients achieving CHR, unless the WBC count is $<2 \times 10^3/\mu L$ and/or the platelet count is $<50 \times 10^3/\mu L$. If the latter occurs, dose reductions of 25% are initiated and the dose is adjusted to keep the WBC count at 2–$3 \times 10^3/\mu L$.

Defining Specific Endpoints

The survival advantage associated with a major CG response to IFN-α has been documented by several trials. A more controversial issue is whether IFN-α prolongs survival in patients not achieving a CG response. Although this may occur, the prolongation in survival is significantly less than that associated with a major CG response. A recent update of our IFN-α trials demonstrated a survival rate of >80% at 6–8 years for patients with a major CG response (2). It has been suggested that these results may reflect a population with a better prognosis. However, multivariate analysis revealed CG response to be an independent prognostic factor, after accounting for pretreatment prognostic factors (2). CG response was also associated with better survival as determined by landmark analysis, and with improved survival within each prognostic subgroup. The ICSG-CML found an 85% survival at 6 years for patients with a reduction in Ph-positive cells to <66% (4). Similarly, the Japanese group reported 100% of major CG responders to IFN-α to be alive without disease progression at 5 years

Interferon Therapy

(5). In the German trial, which reported a low CG response rate and consequent lack of statistical significance when analyzing survival, the authors noted that no patients with a major CG response (Ph <35%) had died, "suggesting that the patients in this subgroup have a survival advantage" (8). Therefore, attainment of a major CG response is an important therapeutic target. Given the cost and toxicity of IFN-α, it is reasonable to consider changing therapy when the likelihood of achieving a major CG response becomes low (*vide infra*).

Patient Selection

There may be reluctance to initiate treatment with IFN-α, a relatively cumbersome and expensive therapy, in all patients, when only a fraction will achieve a major CG response. However, it is difficult to identify the responders initially, and no subset does poorly enough with IFN-α therapy to be denied the option. Several published models allocate CML patients into prognostic groups based on pretreatment characteristics (14–18). Some common prognostic parameters are age, splenomegaly, thrombocytosis, and blast and basophil count. However, even patients with the worst prognosis ("poor-risk" group) may achieve a major CG response (Table 2) (19), although at a lower rate than patients with a good prognosis. As such, all eligible patients should have the option of IFN-α ther-

Table 2 Response to IFN-α in CML According to Risk Groups

Risk category	Percent with CHR	
	Morra et al.	MDACC[a]
Low	87	80–90
Intermediate	58	50–60
High	14	20–60

Risk category	Percent with CG response		
	Allan et al.[b]	MDACC[a]	
	Any	Any	Major
Low	34	60	40
Intermediate	20	40	20–30
High	7	10–20	5–10

CHR, complete hematologic response; MDACC, M.D. Anderson Cancer Center.
[a]Risk groups defined using Kantarjian model (Blood 1985; 66:1326).
[b]Risk groups defined using Sokal model (Blood 1984; 63:789).

apy, provided that they achieve specific responses by defined time points. This would allow stopping IFN-α therapy in patients who appear unlikely to attain a major CG response.

Patients who do not achieve a CHR by 6 months have little chance (<5%) of obtaining a major CG remission and are candidates for alternative therapy. After achieving a CHR, the next endpoint is any CG response after 12 months on IFN-α therapy (at the maximally tolerated dose). Patients not achieving this are unlikely to obtain a major CG response (<5%). If a CG response is observed after 12 months of IFN-α therapy, patients should continue on the treatment. Using such a schema, 60% of patients who would not achieve a major CG response will not require treatment with IFN-α for >1 year.

Communicating Endpoints to the Patient

The flu-like side effects of IFN-α therapy are the first ones encountered, but are usually short-lived as tachyphylaxis develops. The toxicities that are most likely to be dose-limiting during long-term therapy are those related to fatigue, malaise, and neurotoxicity, usually manifested by anhedonia or depression. These side effects are often exacerbated by the patient's perception that the therapy is indefinite. When the specified endpoints are described (initially and at regular intervals) and therapeutic goals are established, a sense of rational direction in the treatment is formed. Achievement of each endpoint (e.g., CHR, minor CG response) should be clearly communicated to the patient, who in turn may be encouraged and more accepting of side effects when they feel the therapy is improving their outcome.

Managing Neurotoxicity

Although reinforcement of a continued good response to therapy is important for patient well-being, depression, and fatigue may continue to be problems, especially in older patients. Small doses of antidepressants can be helpful in this setting, especially in patients with disturbed sleep patterns. Varying the time of the daily IFN-α injection may ameliorate symptoms. Patients experiencing fatigue shortly after the daily injection may benefit from receiving their IFN-α dose at bedtime. A triad of depression, fatigue, and insomnia (which resembles "jet lag") is common and can be improved with amitriptyline 25–50 mg at bedtime. Patients sleep excessively in the first few days after this therapy is started before the response is noted, and beginning this treatment on weekends may allow the patient to continue normal week-time activities. Some patients respond better to other antidepressants (e.g., fluoxetine, sertraline) if one component of the triad is more prominent; in such cases a neuropsychiatric consult is helpful.

Patients with significant fatigue should be evaluated for hypothyroidism, which is part of a spectrum of autoimmune phenomena that may be induced by IFN-α and has been reported in 5% of patients in a large series (20). This side effect can be readily reversed by initiating thyroid hormone replacement and requires no interruption of IFN-α therapy.

DURATION OF THERAPY

Although complete or major CG remissions on IFN-α therapy are durable, it is uncertain how long they can last after IFN-α therapy is stopped. One policy has been to continue therapy until a CG CR had been documented for 3 years. At that point the decision whether to continue treatment was left to the individual investigator and patient team. Of 34 patients, 18 were continued on IFN-α therapy, sometimes with a dose reduction. All of these patients continued in CG CR. Sixteen patients had their therapy discontinued because of toxicity (five patients) or patient or physician choice (11 patients). Seven patients continued in CR at a median of 34 months off therapy (range, 12+ to 56+ months); nine patients showed increase in Ph-positive cells. IFN-α therapy was reinstituted in six patients, three of whom showed only normal diploid cells after reinitiation of therapy and three of whom showed reduction of Ph-positive cells to <35%. Three patients with recurrent Ph-positive cells remain without treatment in continued hematological remission (1).

Sensitive techniques such as the polymerase chain reaction (PCR) detect occasional cells with a breakpoint cluster region (BCR) rearrangement in many patients with CML in remission after IFN-α therapy (21,22). However, these patients may remain in remission (sometimes even after discontinuing therapy), do not develop blastic-phase CML, and have prolonged survival. The PCR technique may be detecting nonclonogenic cells; alternatively, minimal residual disease may be controlled effectively by the immune system. The PCR procedure is not useful for making treatment decisions since its results are not easily quantifiable and since, more importantly, the clinical relevance of PCR positivity is unknown. A new technique may be more useful for deciding if patients in remission may discontinue therapy. Hypermetaphase fluorescent in situ hybridization (FISH) allows rapid screening of a large number of cells (500) for the presence of the Ph chromosome using a fluorescent probe that overlaps the region of the translocation at chromosome 9q34 (23). In individuals with normal chromosomes, only two fluorescent spots will be seen, corresponding to the two normal 9 chromosomes. Translocations between chromosomes 9 and 22 result in detection of a third signal representing a small piece of chromosome 9 now present on chromosome 22. The ability to screen a much large number of cells than is possible with conventional cytogenetics may allow more informed decisions on the need to continue therapy. Patients in CG CR for 3 years and with no evidence of Ph-positive cells by hypermetaphase FISH may have their treatment tapered or discontinued. Reappearance of even 2% Ph-positive cells (10 of 500) would be a statistically significant change and would suggest the need for treatment resumption.

Currently, the options of continuing treatment, lowering the dose for patients with significant side effects, or stopping therapy are all possibilities. Stopping therapy necessitates careful follow-up and regular CG analysis to ensure that IFN-α is restarted early if disease recurrence is noted. Frequently, physicians may stop IFN-α therapy at the first sign of a CG response. Such an approach jeopardizes the treatment goals.

DIFFICULTY WITH BONE MARROW ASPIRATION

Patients on continuous IFN-α therapy may have CG analyses showing insufficient metaphases resulting from a poor-quality sample. This phenomenon is frequently associated with difficulty in aspirating the bone marrow and may preclude efficient decision making regarding further therapy. A common perception is that poor aspirations must be due to marrow fibrosis. A review of bone marrow samples from 41 CML patients obtained during IFN-α treatment at M.D. Anderson showed no evidence of increasing fibrosis above that detected at baseline in patients with CML (24). In fact, 8 of 18 (44%) patients with grade 3–4 fibrosis pretreatment had a decline in this level after a median of 25 months of IFN-α therapy. It is known that colony-forming cells from patients with CML are defective in their attachment to bone marrow stromal cells (26). In vitro use of IFN-α can increase the adherence of primitive CML cells to bone marrow stroma by reducing the amount of neuraminic acid on the stromal cells (26). Thus, IFN-α may affect the marrow microenvironment so that CML progenitors are subject to local control and change the extracellular matrix to make aspiration of the marrow more difficult.

The lack of significant fibrosis in IFN-α-treated patients is corroborated by the fact that patients receiving allogeneic bone marrow transplants after prior IFN-α therapy showed no significant difference in the time to neutrophil or platelet recovery, or in survival, compared with similar patients who had not received IFN-α treatment (27). Recently the International Bone Marrow Transplant Registry evaluated 882 recipients of HLA-identical sibling bone marrow transplants for CML in chronic phase reported between 1987 and 1994 (28). Three-year survival rates for patients treated with hydroxyurea and transplanted either within 1 year or >1 year from diagnosis were $68 \pm 5\%$ and $67 \pm 7\%$, respectively (28). For patients with a similar time from diagnosis who had received IFN-α therapy, the 3-year survival rates were $70 \pm 10\%$ and $72 \pm 10\%$.

The authors noted that "leukemia recurrence rates were somewhat lower in persons receiving α-interferon pretransplant" (28). Stopping IFN-α therapy 1–2 weeks before obtaining the bone marrow sample increases the yield of adequate metaphases for cytogenetic analysis. Patients with long-standing remissions evidence no change in peripheral WBC counts over this period of time. Reinitiation of IFN-α after such a short interval is not associated with significant side effects. The need for a large number of cells, such as a bone marrow harvest, requires discontinuation of IFN-α for 4–6 weeks in order to obtain adequate cells for engraftment.

SUMMARY

Patients with CML who are treated with IFN-α may achieve a minimal tumor burden as manifested by a CG response and prolonged survival. However, the use of IFN-α therapy may be associated with both acute and chronic toxicities. Strategies to minimize these toxicities have been described. A physician's familiarity with these strategies results in enhanced patient compliance and increases the therapeutic benefit of this modality.

REFERENCES

1. Kantarjian H, Deisseroth A, Kurzrock R, Estrov Z, Talpaz M. Chronic myelogenous leukemia: a concise update. Blood 1993; 82(3):691–703.
2. Kantarjian H, Smith TL, O'Brien S, et al. Prolonged survival in chronic myelogenous leukemia after cytogenetic response to interferon-α therapy. Ann Intern Med 1995; 122:254–261.
3. Montastruc M, Mahon FX, Fabères C, et al. Response to recombinant interferon alpha in patients with chronic myelogenous leukemia in a single center: results and analysis of predictive factors. Leukemia 1995; 9:1997–2002.
4. Italian Cooperative Study Group on Chronic Myeloid Leukemia. Interferon alfa-2a as compared with conventional chemotherapy for the treatment of chronic myeloid leukemia. N Engl J Med 1994; 330:820–825.
5. Ohnishi K, Ohno R, Tomonaga M, et al. A randomized trial comparing interferon-α with busulfan for newly diagnosed chronic myelogenous leukemia in chronic phase. Blood 1995; 86(3):906–916.
6. Allan NC, Richards SM, Shepherd PCA. UK Medical Research Council randomized, multicentre trial of interferon-αn1 for chronic myeloid leukaemia: improved survival irrespective of cytogenetic response. Lancet 1995; 345:1392–1397.
7. Ozer H, George SL, Schiffer CA, et al. Prolonged subcutaneous administration of recombinant α2b interferon in patients with previously untreated Philadelphia chromosome-positive chronic-phase chronic myelogenous leukemia: effect on remission duration and survival: Cancer and Leukemia Group B study 8583. Blood 1993; 10(15):2975–2984.

8. Helmann R, Heimpel H, Hasford J, et al. Randomized comparison of interferon-α with busulfan and hydroxyurea in chronic myelogenous leukemia. Blood 1994; 84(12):4064–4077.
9. Schofield JR, Robinson WA, Murphy JR, Rovira DK. Low doses of interferon-α are as effective as higher doses in inducing remissions and prolonging survival in chronic myeloid leukemia. Ann Intern Med 1994; 121:736–744.
10. Alimena G, Morra E, Lazzarino M, et al. Interferon alpha-2b as therapy for Ph^1-positive chronic myelogenous leukemia: a study of 82 patients treated with intermittent or daily administration. Blood 1988; 72(2):642–647.
11. Freund M, Von Wussow P, Diedrich H, et al. Recombinant human interferon (IFN) alpha-2b in chronic myelogenous leukemia: dose dependency of response and frequency of neutralizing anti-interferon antibodies. Br J Haematol 1989; 72:350–356.
12. Anger B, Porzsolt F, Leichtle R, Heinze B, Bartram C, Heimpel H. A phase I/II study of recombinant interferon alpha-2a and hydroxyurea for chronic myelocytic leukemia. Blut 1989; 58:275–278.
13. Stenke L, Samuelsson J, Palmblad J, Dabrowski L, Reizenstein P, Lindgren JA. Elevated white blood cell synthesis of leukotriene C4 in chronic myelogenous leukemia but not in polycythemia vera. Br J Haematol 1990; 74:257–263.
14. Tura S, Baccarani M, Corbelli G, et al. Staging of chronic myeloid leukemia. Br J Haematol 1981; 47:105–119.
15. Cervantes F, Rozman C. A multivariate analysis of prognostic factors in chronic myeloid leukemia. Blood 1982; 60:1298–1304.
16. Sokal JE, Cox EB, Baccarani M, et al. Prognostic discrimination in "good-risk" chronic granulocytic leukemia. Blood 1984; 63:789–799.
17. Kantarjian HM, Smith TL, McCredie KB, et al. Chronic myelogenous leukemia: a multivariate analysis of the association of patient characteristics and therapy with survival. Blood 1985; 66:1326–1335.
18. Kantarjian H, Keating MJ, Smith T, Talpaz M, McCredie KB. Proposal for a simple synthesis prognostic staging system in chronic myelogenous leukemia. Am J Med 1990; 88:1–8.
19. Morra E, Alimena G, Lazzarino M, et al. Evolving modalities of treatment with interferon alfa-2b for Ph^1-positive chronic myelogenous leukemia. Eur J Cancer 27(suppl 4):S14–S17.
20. Sacchi S, Kantarjian H, Cohen P, Pierce S, Talpaz M. Immune-mediated and unusual complications during alpha interferon therapy in chronic myelogenous leukemia (CML). Blood 1992; 84(10):150a, No. 587.
21. Lee MS, Kantarjian H, Talpaz M, et al. Detection of minimal residual disease by polymerase chain reaction in Philadelphia chromosome-positive chronic myelogenous leukemia following interferon therapy. Blood 1992; 79(8):1920–1923.
22. Dhingra K, Kurzrock R, Kantarjian H, et al. Minimal residual disease in interferon-treated chronic myelogenous leukemia: results and pitfalls of analysis based on polymerase chain reaction. Leukemia (1992; 6(8):754–760.
23. Seong DC, Kantarjian HM, Ro JY, et al. Hypermetaphase FISH for quantitative monitoring of Philadelphia chromosome positive cells in chronic myelogenous leukemia patients during treatment. Blood 1995; 86:2343–2349.
24. Wilhelm M, Ramos CM, O'Brien S, et al. Effect of interferon-alpha (IFN-A) ther-

apy on bone marrow (BM) fibrosis in chronic myelogenous leukemia (CML). Blood 1996; 88:10(suppl 1):#3537.
25. Gordon MY, Dowding CR, Riley GP, Goldman JM, Greaves JM. Altered adhesive interactions with marrow stroma of haematopoietic progenitor cells in chronic myeloid leukemia. Nature 1987; 328:342–344.
26. Dowding C, Guo AP, Osterholz J, Siczkowski M, Goldman J, Gordon M. Interferon-α overrides the deficient adhesion of chronic myeloid leukemia primitive progenitor cells to bone marrow stromal cells. Blood 1991; 78:499–505.
27. Giralt SA, Kantarjian HM, Talpaz M, et al. Effect of prior interferon alfa therapy on the outcome of allogeneic bone marrow transplantation for chronic myelogenous leukemia. J Clin Oncol 1993; 11(6):1055–1061.
28. Horowitz MM, Giralt S, Szydlo R, Goldman J, Veum-Stone J. Effect of prior interferon therapy on outcome of HLA-Identical sibling bone marrow transplants for chronic myelogenous leukemia (CML) in first chronic phase. Blood 1996; 88: 10(supp 1):#2716.

8
Treatment of Chronic Myelogenous Leukemia by Interferon and Cytarabine

François Guilhot
Centre Hospitalier Universitaire de Poitiers, Poitiers, France

INTRODUCTION

The value of interferon (IFN) alpha 2a or 2b for the treatment of chronic myelogenous leukemia (CML) during the chronic phase has been amply demonstrated. Several reports have shown that this cytokine produces hematologic remission in 60–80% of patients in chronic-phase CML (1). In some studies the achievement of complete hematologic response within 3 months is the most significant factor correlated with a cytogenetic response (2). Also, the treatment with IFN resulted in suppression of the Ph-positive cells population which was complete in 7–25% of the patients (3,4). A major cytogenetic response (i.e., <35% Ph-positive cells) was noted in 35–45% of the patients. Such cytogenetic response was not only complete but also prolonged for periods ranging between 2 and 8 years (5). This prolonged effect is certainly the most important and most original since it is never observed using conventional single-drug therapy.

Several groups have also shown that survival was improved in patients receiving IFN. The survival was improved mostly in patients with major (i.e., Ph+ cells <35%) or complete cytogenetic response but also in patients without any cytogenetic response. This latest result was reported by the U.K. Medical Research Council trial (6). However, it is generally assumed that achieving major or complete cytogenetic response prolongs survival. Moreover, it would appear that IFN also delays the appearance of blast crisis. The incidence of major and complete cytogenetic responses fluctuates from study to study (for example, 7–25% for the complete response). This discrepancy between trials may partially explain the differences in survival rates. However, the cytogenetic response rates obtained with IFN alone remain low. Accordingly, new strategies combining IFN and other cytotoxic agents in order to improve the cytogenetic response rates are warranted.

RATIONALE FOR USE OF CYTOSINE-ARABINOSIDE IN CML

In leukemic patients the aim of cytotoxic therapy is eradication of the leukemic stem cells with relative sparing of the normal bone marrow stem cells. Cytarabine (1-β-D-arabinofuranosylcytosine) is a pyrimidine nucleoside analog with a configuration similar to that of cytidine and deoxycytidine, but differing in that the sugar moiety is arabinose rather than ribose or deoxyribose. The cytotoxic effect of ara-C is thought to be determined mainly by the intracellular synthesis and retention of ara-C triphosphate (ara-C-CTP), which interferes with DNA synthesis. For that reason ara-C is preferentially cytotoxic to proliferating cells. In vivo, ara-C is rapidly inactivated to uracil-arabinoside (ara-U), so that ara-C chemotherapy consisting of push injection or a few hours of infusion only results in short-term exposure of the cells to ara-C. A comparison of pharmacokinetics of continuous intravenous and subcutaneous infusion of ara-C demonstrated that steady-state serum ara-C levels were similar with both routes of administration (7). Because of its short half-life after a single intravenous or subcutaneous injection and its S phase activity, prolonged intravenous infusion of ara-C has been administered to patients with AML. The administration of ara-C by continuous IV infusion results in plasma ara-C levels ranging between 10^{-8} and 10^{-7} mol/L. In contrast, peak plasma level is approximately 10^{-6} mol/L after a subcutaneous single injection. Furthermore, plasma ara-C levels are undetectable 6 hours after bolus injection. Thus, using a dose schedule of daily injection of ara-C could result in an 18-hour interval with no detectable drug before the next injection (8).

Cytosine-arabinoside (ara-C) is an attractive chemotherapy for the treatment of CML. In vitro studies and preliminary clinical experience suggest that ara-C can selectively inhibit the growth of neoplastic Ph-positive progenitors. In vitro studies demonstrated a preferential inhibition by ara-C of granulocyte-macrophage colony-forming cells (CFU-GM) from patients with CML compared to CFU-GM from normal subjects. Two groups found that CFU-GM from patients in the chronic-phase CML were inhibited by significantly lower concentration of ara-C than were CFU-GM from normal subjects (9,10). This effect was seen in experiments involving prolonged exposure of CFU to low concentrations of the drug. In one study, the median 50% inhibitory concentration of ara-C from CFU-GM from patients in CML chronic phase was 3.4 ng/mL (range 0.6–9.4 ng/mL) versus a median of 11.8 ng/mL for cells from normal subjects.

An ara-C concentration of 10 ng/mL, at which considerably more inhibition of leukemic than normal colony growth was seen, is below the plasma concentration maintained during conventional therapy with intravenous infusion of cytarabine. It is also within the range achieved with schedules of low dose subcutaneous injection of ara-C. Because of this in vitro activity, ara-C has been tested in vivo for the treatment, as single agent, of patients with CML in chronic phase. Treatment of two patients in chronic-phase CML with low-dose ara-C (SC continuous infusion) resulted in a significant reduction of Ph+ metaphases (11). These patients were in chronic-phase CML, diagnosed <6 months before and in good clinical control on HU. Ara-C was administered by subcutaneous infusion at a dose rate of 20 mg/m^2/day with the aim to induce and maintain a granulocyte count of <2000/μL for at least 10 days. Ara-C was administered for 17–31 days, either continuously or with interruptions of 2–7 days because of hematological toxicity or side effects. Plasma ara-C levels ranged from 5 to 22 ng/mL. Cytogenetic analyses were performed 4–9 days after the end of the ara-C infusion. After two or three successive cycles, Ph+ metaphases decreased from 100% to 2/27 and 3/26 Ph+ metaphases in patients 1 and 2, respectively.

In contrast, subsequent intensive chemotherapy with high-dose hydroxyurea in dosage sufficient to maintain granulocytopenia and normal serum B_{12} levels reduced the Ph positivity to only 46% and 72%. Thus it was concluded that a selective antileukemic effect has been seen with ara-C but not with hydroxyurea. Also it was assumed that ara-C exhibits significant antileukemic selectivity while hydroxyurea is a nonspecific inhibitor of granulopoiesis. More recently, subcutaneous cycles of ara-C were administered to five patients in the chronic phase (12). Ara-C was started at a dose of 15 mg/m^2/day. This dose was increased by increments of 5 mg/m^2/day every 2 weeks to a maximum dose of 30 mg/m^2/day. Ara-C was discontinued for a white cell count below 2500/μm or a platelet count below 75,000/μL. Four cycles of ara-C were administered to all patients and the treatment was continued in case of cytogenetic response with <30% of Ph-positive cells. The dose of ara-C required to achieve a leukocyte count ≤2500/μL or a platelet count ≤75,000/μL was between 15 and 30 mg/m^2/day. The median duration of the ara-C courses was 29 days per cycle (range 15–72). Hematological remission was consistently observed, and, in addition, four patients had a cytogenetic response. Overall, 21 cycles resulted in a reduction of Ph-positive cells to <50% of metaphases. One cycle resulted in complete cytogenetic response, and nine cycles resulted in partial response (1–34% Ph+ metaphases). These results also indicate that prolonged continuous administration of ara-C can inhibit Ph-positive hematopoiesis. However, this inhibition was always transient and there is at the present time no evidence that such treatment could prolong the survival.

One of the mechanisms by which IFN acts as an antitumor agent is that IFN blocks cell cycle progression in the G0/G1 phase (13). The effects of IFN alone and in combination with ara-C on normal and leukemic human hematopoietic progenitor cells have been investigated in vitro. Mononuclear cells from normal bone marrow, peripheral blood of patients with chronic-phase CML, or the cell line HL-60 were incubated with various types of interferons followed by the addition of ara-C. The survival of normal CFU-GM was significantly increased if the cells were incubated with IFN 1 hour before ara-C exposure. These in vitro studies suggest that IFN and ara-C act synergistically. It is assumed that normal cells are blocked in phase G0/G1 by IFN and are, hence, protected from the cytotoxic effect of ara-C which acts in S phase, whereas leukemic cells, which are more autonomous in their division, are destroyed by ara-C (14). Because of these mechanisms of action, one could suggest that the treatment of patients with CML CP using these two agents could result in more cytogenetic responses and better survival.

Thus, the combination of IFN-α and low-dose ara-C was studied by several investigators. In 1986, we initiated a pilot study by using such a combined approach. Twenty-four patients (12 previously treated by standard chemotherapy and 12 previously untreated) received hydroxyurea 50 mg/kg/day orally and IFN-α2a at a starting dose of 5×10^6 IU/m^2/d subcutaneously. Courses of low-dose ara-C were given to 11 patients. Ara-C was administered once a day 10–15 days per month at a dose of 10–20 mg/m^2/d. A CHR was obtained in 18 to 24 patients. Eight out of 24 patients obtained a major cytogenetic response. Furthermore, a rapid cytogenetic improvement was recorded in six out of 11 patients receiving courses of low-dose ara-C, with a complete Ph chromosome suppression in four (15). Summarizing, IFN improves survival in the fraction of patients in which it induces a cytogenetic response. The combination of IFN and ara-C should make it possible to increase the cytogenetic response rate and improve survival even further. The two French multicenter trials, the CML 88 and the CML 91 studies, were initiated to explore further this hypothesis.

DESIGN AND RESULTS OF THE FRENCH TRIALS

CML 88 Trial

The CML 88 protocol was worked out and accomplished in order to show the advantage of using an IFN plus ara-C combination.

Design of the Trial

The principal assessment criterion was the study of the cytogenetic response rate in the experimental group (IFN + ara-C) compared with the cytogenetic response rate in the reference group (IFN alone). Secondary criteria consisted of patient tolerance of the treatment, and survival. Inclusion criteria were as follows

Diagnosis of CML based on cytogenetic analysis (complex translocations and certain additional cytogenetic anomalies were not considered as exclusion criteria, but anomalies such as iso 17q, duplication of Ph1 or trisomy 8 were regarded as exclusion criteria since they indicated and accelerated phase of the disease)

CML in the chronic phase, aged between 15 and 70 years, WHO score, 0, 1, 2, without visceral impairment or renal, hepatocellular, or heart failure

No treatment or conventional chemotherapy of <6 months' duration following diagnosis

Patients were randomized by telephone (to the coordination center) and included in one of the two maintenance therapy arms. The maintenance therapy had to be initiated in the third month of induction treatment in a patient in stable hematological remission and no longer receiving HU.

In the induction phase, all patients received IFN-α2b starting at 5×10^6 U subcutaneously plus hydroxyurea (HU) 50 mg/kg/d orally until stable hematological remission was achieved. The maintenance treatment was scheduled to begin during the third month in a patient in stable hematological remission no longer receiving HU. Patients were randomized to receive either IFN-α2b alone (5.10^6 IU/m^2) or the same dose of IFN plus low-dose ara-C 10 mg/m^2/d subcutaneously 10 days each month. The protocol was stopped in the following situations

If a related or unrelated compatible HLA donor was found, and if a bone marrow allograft appeared possible, given the patient's age and condition, or if severe toxicity required the discontinuation of treatment

If complete hematological remission was not obtained after 3 months of induction treatment

If a hematologic relapse occurred, in spite of the correct administration of interferon

If a cytogenetic relapse occurred (Table 1).

Results

Two hundred thirty-seven patients were registered (centralized registration in Poitiers) over a 33-month period from April 1988 to January 1991. Patient registration was carried out by 36 French hematology centers and was stopped on 16/01/1991. An analysis of this trial was performed on July 1994 with 207 evaluable patients after a median follow-up of 50 months. In this trial, 31 patients are not available for the analysis. Of these, data are still expected for five patients, two patients refused treatment and follow-up, while six others were wrongly diagnosed. In addition, 17 patients were not evaluable per protocol

Table 1 CML 88: Treatment Plan

INDUCTION	HYDROXYUREA 50 mg/kg/day
Same for all patients	+
	INTERFERON 5.10^6 IU/m^2/day

⇓

MAINTENANCE TREATMENT	3 MONTHS	
for patients in hematological remission	↙ IFN alone	↘ IFN + low-dose ara-C 10 mg/m^2/day 10 days each month

because of exclusion criteria; i.e., the interval with respect to diagnosis was excessive in the case of two patients, blast crisis occurred right away in three patients, an allograft was directly performed in four patients, seven patients had chronic myelocytic leukemia without Philadelphia chromosome but with a bcr/abl rearrangement, and one patient committed suicide a few days after randomization. The number and distribution of nonanalyzable patients are similar in the two groups and do not impede the analysis.

The distribution of clinical and laboratory parameters was identical in the two groups. Each risk category (low, intermediate, or high), based on the Sokal score, was evenly distributed in the two groups. Complete hematological remission was observed in 83% of patients, without a difference between the two arms. Statistical analysis of the cytogenetic response does not demonstrate a superiority of the IFN + ara-C arm in terms of achieving major cytogenetic responses. However, in the IFN + ara-C group, 24 of 103 patients (23%) were in CCR, whereas in the IFN-alone group, 16 of 104 (15%) patients obtained this result. Thus in the CML 88 study, the rate of complete cytogenetic responses seems higher in the IFN + ara-C arm, but this is only a trend.

Side Effects

The side effects of IFN-α are not trivial and include fever, chills, malaise, headaches, anorexia, joint pain, vomiting, low backache, myalgia, various types of neuropathy, changes in mood and concentration, abnormalities of liver enzymes, leukopenia, and thrombocytopenia. Sufficient dosage is important because it is necessary to induce leukopenia and thrombocytopenia in order to obtain cytogenetic responses. It is wise to explain in advance to patients with CML the need to anticipate and hopefully to tolerate the effects of r-IFN-α. In some patients, serious late side effects are dose-limiting, and for some of them treatment must be interrupted. These include neurotoxicity with frontal lobe signs (depression) and immune-mediated events. A triad of depression, fatigue, and insomnia is frequently observed in some patients. A poor neuropsychiatric tolerance must be recognized early with the need to stop interferon treatment in case of neuropsychiatric symptoms and in particular in case of suicidal tendencies. The objective of CML 88 trial was to assess patients' tolerance of IFN when administered during the chronic phase of chronic myelocytic leukemia. It sought to demonstrate the possible effect of adding courses of treatment with cytosine-arabinoside to maintenance therapy with IFN in order to increase the cytogenetic response rate. The combination of hydroxyurea-IFN given as induction treatment produced a satisfactory hematological remission rate.

Hematological Toxicity

Evolution of leukocyte and platelet counts and medullary cellularity during treatment are presented in Tables 2 and 3. In patients maintained in complete hematological remission by the treatment, the evolution of the mean leukocyte and platelet counts was compared. Table 2 shows that there was no difference with regard to these parameters between the two groups for patients maintained in complete hematological remission.

Medullary cellularity was evaluated every 3 months by a marrow puncture and graded as hypercellular (4), normal cellularity (3), hypocellularity (2), extremely low cellularity (1). Medullary cellularity was studied over a 2-year period. Table 2 shows that there were no significant differences in this parameter between the two treatment groups: the percentage of patients with hypocellularity or very low cellularity is the same in both groups.

In conclusion, in this trial patients who achieved a major or a complete cytogenetic response had a significantly better survival than those with minor or no response. The probability of obtaining complete cytogenetic remission was greater in the interferon + ara-C group, but this was only a tendency and global curves were identical for the two groups. Median survival is approximately 64 months in the IFN group and 67 months in the IFN + ara-C group; this corresponds to data published in the literature.

CML 91 Trial

The CML 91 trial is based on CML 88. The objectives of the CML 91 trial are to treat patients on the basis of prognostic scores derived from Sokal criteria and to try to conclusively demonstrate the advantage of combining interferon with ara-C. In the CML 91 study, patients for induction are randomized between two regimens, HU + IFN (same doses as in the CML 88 study) or HU + IFN + courses of low-dose ara-C, which is administered at a dose of 20 mg/m^2/10 d for 2 weeks after the beginning of the induction regimen. Moreover, patients

Table 2 Evolution of Leukocyte and Platelet Counts

	\multicolumn{9}{c}{Month}								
	3	6	9	12	15	18	21	24	27
IFN + ara-C									
No. in CHR	50	54	51	38	26	26	16	15	8
WBC min-max	2.1–9.8	2.5–8.3	2.5–9.8	2–7.6	1.9–8.8	2.4–8	2.3–8.2	2.5–8.7	2.7–6.8
mean	5	4.1	4.3	4.2	4.5	4.4	3.8	4.5	4.1
Platelets min-max	14–386	57–406	34–441	33–416	74–430	73–377	73–441	79–306	104–269
mean	166	167	176	176	189	184	184	183	201
IFN									
No. in CHR	64	60	45	40	19	18	13	11	3
WBC min-max	2–9.8	1.3–9.7	1.9–9.6	2.2–8.9	1.8–9.6	1.9–6.1	2.3–9.4	2–5.3	3.5–5.7
mean	4.8	4.7	4.5	4.9	4.1	4.3	4.7	3.8	4.3
Platelets min-max	16–425	59–398	87–368	27–441	100–313	83–320	87–345	62–269	171–341
mean	189	187	193	206	209	216	216	154	234

Interferon and Cytarabine

Table 3 Evolution of Medullary Cellularity

					Grade				
	Dg UA	3	6	9	12	15	18	21	24
IFN + ara C									
1	0	12	12	14	10	13	7	4	0
	0%	21%	29%	31%	26%	50%	33%	33%	0%
2	1	7	9	10	9	4	4	2	7
	1%	13%	21%	22%	23%	15%	19%	17%	29%
3	11	33	20	19	19	8	9	5	8
	15%	59%	48%	45%	49%	30%	43%	41%	33%
4	59	4	1	2	1	1	1	1	0
	89%	71%	2%	4%	3%	4%	5%	8%	0%
Total	71	56	42	45	39	26	21	12	15
IFN									
1	1	13	19	10	7	4	6	0	4
	1%	20%	34%	24%	18%	21%	35%	0%	40%
2	2	11	13	10	9	7	2	3	2
	2%	17%	23%	24%	23%	37%	12%	43%	20%
3	12	31	17	15	19	5	7	4	3
	14%	48%	30%	36%	49%	26%	41%	57%	30%
4	73	10	7	7	4	3	2	0	1
	82%	15%	13%	17%	10%	16%	12%	0%	10%
Total	88	65	56	42	39	19	17	7	10

are treated according to their age and Sokal score (Table 4). From January 1991 to May 1996, 745 pts (age ≤ 70 yr) with a CML Ph+ chronic phase were included. All patients were simultaneously given HU at a daily dose of 50 mg/kg and IFN-α2b at a starting dose of 5×10^6 IU/m^2/day for induction. HU was discontinued when a complete hematologic remission (CHR) was achieved. Patients randomized in the IFN + ara-C group received the same regimen plus monthly courses of ara-C, 20 mg/m^2/day, 10 days. The endpoints were overall survival, CHR at 6 months, major cytogenetic response (i.e., <35% Ph+ cells) at 12 months. A preliminary analysis was performed on 646 randomized patients, 324 in the IFN group and 322 in the IFN + ara-C group. Risk categories based on the Sokal score were evenly distributed in the two groups: 48% (low), 40% (intermediate), 12% (high) in the IFN + ara-C group and 41%, 42%, 17% in the IFN group. At 6 months, the CHR rate was higher in the IFN + ara-C group (67%) than in the IFN group (54%) ($p = 0.002$), but time to response was similar in the two groups. At 12 months, a major cytogenetic response was

Table 4 CML 91: Design of the Study

Age	Sokal's index	Treatment
<35 years	Any	HU until BMT allo if sib donor or randomization (R)
35–50	>1, 2	Same as above
	<1, 2	Randomization (R) even if sib donor
50–70	Any	Randomization (R)

R
↙ ↘

IFN + HU   IFN + HU + ara-C
↓
6 months (HU stopped)
↙ ↘

Complete hematologic remission	No CHR = failure
Each arm Continued	<50 years: BMT allo
	50–60 years: BMT auto
	Otherwise:
	IFN → + ara-C
	IFN + ara-C → chemotherapy

↓
12 months
Cytogenetic response
↙ ↘

<or = 35% Ph1 + cells	>35% Ph1 + cells = failure
Each arm Continued	⇒ same as above
Evaluation every 4 months	

obtained in 96 (39%) out of 248 patients with ara-C and 55 (22%) out of 249 patients without ara-C ($p < 0.001$). Survival of patients in the IFN + ara-C group was improved ($p = 0.006$). The 3-year survival rate was 88% (95% CI: 83–93) with IFN + ara-C and 76% with IFN (95% CI: 69–83). During the first 12 months, the mean daily dose of IFN was 5×10^6/day in both groups, the median number of courses of ara-C was 7 with a median daily dose of 31 mg. Adverse events were responsible for discontinuation of treatment in 71 patients included in the IFN + ara-C group and in 75 patients in the IFN group. Main side effects with ara-C were gastrointestinal disorders and thrombocytopenia (16).

This preliminary analysis of this CML 91 trial shows that patients who received IFN and ara-C had a better survival than those who received IFN alone.

The cytogenetic response rate was also significantly improved with the combination of ara-C and IFN.

REFERENCES

1. Talpaz M, Kantarjian HM, McCredie K, Trujillo JM, Keating MJ, Gutterman JU. Hematologic remission and cytogenetic improvement induced by recombinant human interferon alpha, in chronic myelogenous leukemia. N Engl J Med 1986; 314: 1065–1069.
2. Montastruc M, Mahon FX, Faberes C, et al. Response to recombinant interferon alpha in patients with chronic myelogenous leukemia in a single center: results and analysis of predictive factors. Leukemia 1995; 9:1997–2002.
3. Talpaz M, Kantarjian H, Kurzrock R, Trujillo JM, Gutterman JU. Interferon-alpha produces sustained cytogenetic responses in chronic myelogenous leukemia: Philadelphia chromosome-positive patients. Ann Intern Med 1991; 114:532–538.
4. Italian Cooperative Study Group on Chronic Myeloid Leukemia. Interferon alfa-2a as compared with conventional chemotherapy for the treatment of chronic myeloid leukemia. N Engl J Med 1994; 330:825–825.
5. Kantarjian HM, Smith TL, O'Brien S, Beran M, Pierce S, Talpaz M. Prolonged survival in chronic myelogenous leukemia after cytogenetic response to interferon therapy. Ann Intern Med 1995; 122:254–261.
6. Allan NC, Richards SM, Shepherd PCA. UK Medical Research Council randomised, multicentric trial of interferon-n1 chronic myeloid leukaemia: improved survival irrespective of cytogenetic response. Lancet 1995; 345:1392–1397.
7. Weinstein HJ, Griffin TW, Feeney J, Cohen HJ, Propper RD, Sallan SE. Pharmacokinetics of continuous intravenous and subcutaneous infusions of cytosine-arabinoside. Blood 1982; 59:1351–1353.
8. Spriggs D, Griffin J, Wisch J, Kufe D. Clinical pharmacology of low dose cytosine-arabinoside. Blood 1985; 65:1087–1089.
9. Spiro TE, Mattelear MA, Efira A, Strychmans P. Sensitivity of myeloid progenitors cells in healthy subjects and patients with chronic myeloid leukemia to chemotherapeutic agents. J Natl Cancer Inst 1979; 66:1053–1059.
10. Sokal JE, Leong SS, Gomez GA. Preferential inhibition by cytarabine of CFU-GM from patients with chronic granulocytic leukemia. Cancer 1987; 59:197–202.
11. Sokal JE, Gockerman JP, Bigner SH. Evidence for a selective anti-leukemic effect of cytosine arabinoside in chronic granulocytic leukemia. Leukemia Res 1988; 12: 453–458.
12. Robertson MJ, Tantravahi R, Griffin JD, Canellos GP, Cannistra SA. Hematologic remission and cytogenetic improvement after treatment of stable-phase chronic myelogenous leukemia with continuous infusion of low-dose cytarabine. Am J Hematol 1993; 43:95–102.
13. Imanishi J, Tanaka A. Experimental research from clinical applications of interferon. Jpn J Cancer Chemother 1984; 11:53–59.

14. Richman CM, Slapak CA, Toh B. Interferon protects normal human granulocyte, macrophage colony forming cells from ara-C toxicity. J Biol Response Mol 1990; 9:570–575.
15. Guilhot F, Dreyfus B, Brizard A, Huret JL, Tanzer J. Cytogenetic remissions in chronic myelogenous leukemia using interferon alpha 2a and hydroxyurea with or without low-dose cytosine arabinoside. Leuk Lymph 1991; 4:49–55.
16. Guilhot F, Chastang C, Guerci A, et al. Interferon alpha 2b and cytarabine increase survival and cytogenetic response in chronic myeloid leukemia. Results of a randomized trial. Blood 1996; 88(suppl 1). Abstract 551.

9
Chronic Myeloid Leukemia: Australian Experience with Interferon Combinations and High-Dose Interferon

Christopher K. Arthur
Royal North Shore Hospital, Sydney, Australia

INTRODUCTION AND BACKGROUND

Recent experience with the use of interferon (IFN) in chronic myeloid leukemia shows that IFN can reduce the risk of blastic transformation in this disease. The reduction in blastic transformation has resulted in improved survival (1–3). The mechanism by which IFN can achieve this result, however, is not clear. IFN has pleiotropic effects on cell function with antiproliferative and immunomodulatory activity (4,5). The antitumor effect in chronic myeloid leukemia (CML) may be mediated by several possible mechanisms including suppression of oncogenes (6,7), restoration of normal control mechanisms (8–10), or simply a reduction in the population of leukemic cells at risk of further genetic mutation (11).

There is a correlation between the risk of blast transformation and the proportion of Philadelphia-positive cells in bone marrow samples (2,3,12) which may reflect the degree of reduction of the leukemic clone and therefore the risk of random genetic mutation. It is hypothesized that the reduction of Ph-positive cells is intrinsically related to the reduced blast transformation rate rather than simply being a surrogate marker for low-risk patients. The achievement of the Philadelphia-negative state or "cytogenetic remission" has therefore been a goal of CML treatment. Based on this hypothesis, new treatment strategies are being designed to achieve cytogenetic remissions in a greater proportion of patients and in individual patients a more complete cytogenetic response. Currently, cytogenetic responses are achieved in approximately 50% of patients treated with IFN but in only 5–20% are these complete remissions (1).

Attempts to improve the rate of cytogenetic responses have included intensive chemotherapy (13), combination of alpha IFN with IFN-γ (14), high-dose chemotherapy followed by autologous marrow or peripheral blood stem cell transplantation (15,16), and combination of IFN with chemotherapy (11,17,18). Australian investigators have focused on the use of IFN in combination with chemotherapy. The aim of these studies was to improve the cytogenetic responses in chronic-phase CML. Two studies used a combination of IFN (one with high-dose IFN) and cytosine arabinoside (ara-C) (11,19), and one study investigated IFN plus hydroxyurea (20,21). The most recent study examines the use of IFN in combination with all-*trans* retinoic acid (ATRA) (22).

The rationale for combination of IFN with chemotherapy is based on in vitro synergy against tumor cells in vitro (23,24). Ara-C is particularly interesting for study in combination since it has a selective suppressive effect on CML cells in culture (25). Ara-C used in low dose as a single agent can induce partial cytogenetic remissions in chronic-phase CML (26,27). Ara-C plus IFN has demonstrated synergy against tumors in animal models (28). Hydroxyurea (HU) in high doses can also result in partial cytogenetic remissions, but such responses are transient (29). The history of cancer chemotherapy has many examples of success with chemotherapy combinations when active agents used alone are unable to reliably induce complete remissions. It is therefore logical to test IFN in combination with chemotherapy.

Since 1987 a series of clinical trials in Australia have tested the use of IFN in combination with other agents. These clinical trials are ongoing and the results to date are presented. The first clinical trial evaluated the combination of IFN with low-dose intermittent cytosine arabinoside in early chronic-phase CML. This was followed by a study of IFN dose escalation in early chronic-phase CML. In this study good-risk patients who failed IFN-ara-C combination therapy crossed over to high-dose IFN at 18 million units (MU) daily for 3 months, while poor-risk patients were treated initially with high-dose IFN. Another study evaluated a combination of IFN and hydroxyurea. The most recent study is testing the addition of ATRA to IFN. The long-term follow-up of the initial study and the interim results of the later studies are presented in this review.

IFN COMBINED WITH LOW-DOSE CYTOSINE ARABINOSIDE

Introduction

The aim of this first study was to test the tolerability and efficacy of IFN when combined with low-dose ara-C given daily for 21 days every 42 days. The rationale for combining IFN with ara-C was based on the evidence of synergy between these two agents in vitro and the evidence for independent activity of ara-C against CML both in vitro and in small clinical studies (23–28). Low-dose ara-C was used in small patient series and achieved partial cytogenetic responses (26,27). A number of clinical studies have now supported the benefit of adding ara-C to IFN (30–35).

Patients and Methods

This study commenced in October 1987 and completed patient accrual in May 1991. It was designed as a phase I/II study to test the efficacy and tolerance of adding low-dose ara-C to IFN. Patients were recruited from patients referred to members of the study group. Thirty patients from eight participating centers were entered. Patient characteristics are listed in Table 1. All clinical trials were approved by the institutional medical ethics review committee.

Inclusion criteria: Ph-positive CML, age <65 years, CML in chronic phase (according to criteria of the international bone marrow transplant registry), diagnosis of CML <1 year.

Exclusion criteria: Patients were excluded if they received previous IFN therapy or previous cytotoxic therapy (except in the case of busulfan if <7 days' duration or HU for <12 months).

Treatment: Initial treatment consisted of hydroxyurea until the white cell count (WCC) was normalized and interferon-α2a (Roferon-A, Hoffman-La Roche Pharmaceuticals) was then started with dose escalation over 9 days starting from 3 MU daily up to 9 MU daily. Hydroxyurea was stopped but if the WCC rose above 4×10^9/L then hydroxyurea was restarted and the dose adjusted to keep the WCC between 1 and 4×10^9L.

Table 1 IFN Plus Ara-C Trial: Patient Characteristics

Patient number = 30	Range	(median)
Age	6–63	(44)
Sex M : F	2.75 : 1	
WCC ($\times 10^9$/L)	8.6–476	(141)
Hemoglobin (g/L)	64–150	(112)
Platelets ($\times 10^9$/L)	115–1908	(410)
Blasts (%)	0–6	(0)
Spleen (cm)	0–20	(3)
Sokal index	0.5–2.2	(0.84)
Sokal index: <0.8	14	
0.8–1.19	12	
≥1.2	4	

Ara-C was commenced as soon as the patient was stabilized on the maximally tolerated dose of IFN or after 4 weeks of IFN, whichever was the shorter. The intention was to avoid long delays in the commencement of ara-C. Ara-C was given at 20 mg/M^2 once daily by deep subcutaneous injection for 21 days, and this course was repeated every 42 days. Repeated cycles of ara-C were given for 12 months, after which IFN alone was continued.

Toxicity due to IFN or ara-C was managed by temporary cessation or dose reduction, and once the problem resolved, an attempt was made to escalate the dose or reintroduce the drug.

Assessment of response: Hematological and cytogenetic response was defined according to the criteria used by Talpaz (36). Complete cytogenetic response (CCR) if Ph-positive metaphases are <1%, partial cytogenetic response (PCR) if Ph-positive cells are 1–34%, minor cytogenetic response (MCR) if Ph-positive cells are 35–95%, No cytogenetic response (NCR) if Ph-positive cells are >95%. The group of complete plus partial cytogenetic responses are referred to as major cytogenetic responses. The classification of cytogenetic response was based on the best result achieved.

Cytogenetic studies were done at the start of the study, just prior to starting ara-C, and then at 6 weekly intervals just prior to each cycle of ara-C. Patients stopped the IFN 2 days before each bone marrow examination since it was our experience that adequate metaphases were more reliably obtained. Forty metaphases were examined if possible.

The date of starting IFN was used for calculation of the time to hematological and cytogenetic responses. Survival times were calculated from the time of diagnosis, but time to response and follow-up times are from the start of IFN. Survival curves were constructed using the methods of Kaplan and Meier. Differences between survival curves were compared by the log-rank test. Comparison of Sokal index between groups of responders and nonresponders was performed using a two-sample unpaired t-test.

Results

The median follow-up of living patients is 75 months (range 61–101 months). Twenty-eight patients achieved a complete hematological response (CHR), and two achieved partial hematological response (PHR). However, this includes six patients treated with hydroxyurea since it was a predetermined objective of the study to achieve hematological response in all patients even if this required the addition of hydroxyurea.

A complete cytogenetic response (CCR) occurred in 10/30 (33%) patients, and a partial cytogenetic response (PCR) occurred in 6/30 (20%) patients. Hence 16/30 (53%) patients achieved a major (complete + partial) cytogenetic response. A further 4/30 (13%) achieved a minimal response.

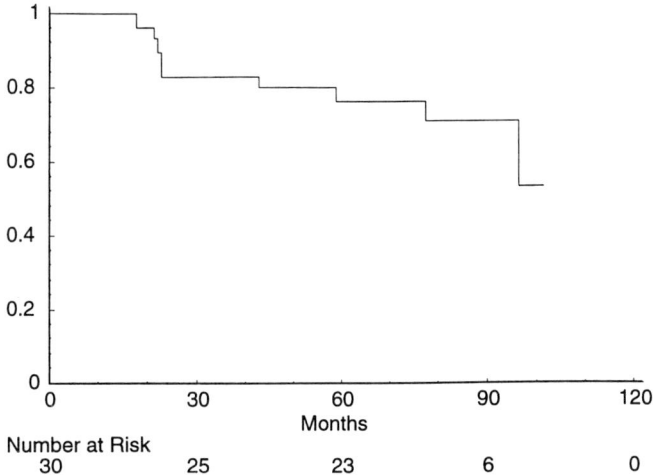

Figure 1 Survival of 30 patients in early chronic-phase CML treated with IFN plus ara-C.

At the time of the latest analysis in June 1996, 9/30 patients remain on IFN alone and in first chronic phase, with 4/9 in CCR, 4/9 in PCR, and one patient no cytogenetic response. Transplantation was performed in 14/30 patients (10 allogeneic, one matched unrelated donor, three autologous). Of the remaining 7/30 patients, three patients are deceased following disease progression and four are on alternative treatments.

Transformation to accelerated or blastic phase has occurred in 9 patients. Death has occurred in nine patients—6/9 from transplant-related complications, and 3/9 from disease progression. Median survival is not yet reached, and at the time of median follow-up of 6 years the projected survival is 76% (Fig. 1).

We were interested to see if the combination of IFN and ara-C led to a rapid cytogenetic response. Response times were quite variable, but five patients achieved cytogenetic responses in 3–6 months. The median time to reach the first PCR was 8 months (2–12 months), and in the 10 complete responders the median time to reach CCR was 12 months (3–28 months). The median time to reach the best response in all responding patients was 10 months (2–38 months).

Adverse reactions to the combination were common (Table 2); however, they were tolerable in the majority of patients. Only one patient permanently discontinued treatment due to toxicity. The toxicity from ara-C could be distinguished by the temporal relationship to treatment courses.

The expected toxicity of IFN included influenza-like symptoms that were controlled by paracetamol or dose reduction. The main toxicities of ara-C were

Table 2 IFN Plus Ara-C Trial: Toxicity

Side effect	Frequency
Thrombocytopenia (<150 × 10^9/L)	83%
Nausea	56%
Mucositis	53%
Neutropenia (<1.0 × 10^9/L)	50%
Lethargy	46%
Flu-like symptoms	30%
Vomiting	23%
Depression	20%
Diarrhea	20%
Skin rash	20%
Fever	20%
Weight loss	16%
Anemia requiring transfusion	10%
Hypothyroidism	1 pt
Pernicious anemia	1 pt
Gynecomastia	1 pt

painful mouth ulceration occurring 5–10 days after each course, nausea, and cytopenia. The mouth ulceration was not due to severe neutropenia (neutrophils <0.5 × 10^9/L) since it occurred without severe neutropenia. Interestingly, the severity of the mouth ulceration lessened in subsequent courses even if the dose of ara-C was not changed.

Cytopenia was encountered in most patients, but it was noted that despite moderate neutropenia and/or thrombocytopenia the marrow frequently remained hypercellular, suggesting that there was significant marrow reserve and dose adjustment according to peripheral blood counts needs to consider this factor.

Response was correlated with the Sokal index. In the cytogenetic responding patients (Ph+ < 95%) the mean Sokal index was 0.76 (range 0.5–1.16), and in nonresponders mean 1.16 (range 0.56–2.24) ($p < 0.001$).

An analysis of molecular predictors of response in this group of patients has been reported (37). The technique of two-step reverse transcriptase polymerase chain reaction (RT-PCR) was used to examine the transcript of chimeric ABL/BCR and BCR/ABL genes in 24 patient samples. No correlation was found between response and the expression of the b2a2, b3a2 or coexpressed b2a2 + b3a2 transcripts. We were interested in the expression of the reciprocal ABL/BCR gene which has been identified in up to 70% of CML patients (38). In the 24 patients, 10 expressed ABL/BCR, and of the four possible types of mRNA, only a1B/b4 was identified. Seven of 10 patients expressing ABL/BCR showed a major cytogenetic response, compared with only two of 11 who did not express ABL/BCR ($p = 0.013$). A larger cohort of patients is needed, however, before these results can be confirmed.

Conclusion

The combination of IFN with intermittent low-dose ara-C is tolerable; however, there is increased toxicity due to the addition of ara-C, particularly manifested by mouth ulcers, nausea, and cytopenia. In this Phase I/II study the hematological and cytogenetic response rates are very encouraging and suggest that the addition of ara-C could double the cytogenetic response rate achieved by the use of IFN alone. These results provide a basis for further clinical studies with ara-C and with other IFN-cytotoxic drug combinations. The optimal dose of ara-C and the optimal schedule remain unclear. It is possible that a lower dose or a different schedule of administration could be more effective and/or less toxic.

Although the major cytogenetic response reached approximately 50%, there are still many patients who do not respond. In the light of these results we used the combination of IFN and ara-C as our initial therapy in newly diagnosed patients with CML and proceeded in a subsequent study to evaluate the dose response of IFN.

DOSE ESCALATION OF IFN IN CHRONIC MYELOID LEUKEMIA

Introduction

Following completion of the study of IFN with ara-C, several strategies were being explored by various investigators to improve the remission rate in CML. It was clear that remissions could be achieved, and several studies indicated a survival benefit for IFN-treated patients which was most marked if a major cytogenetic response was achieved (2,3,12).

Our group pursued therapies to increase the cytogenetic response rate; however, rather than study new drug combinations, we believed that the optimal dose of IFN had not yet been evaluated. Specifically, it was important to know if there is a clinically significant dose response above the commonly used dose of up to 9 MU daily (or approximately 5×10^6 U/M^2). Apart from case reports there was no prospective study to evaluate dose response above 5×10^6 U/M^2 daily.

Randomized and nonrandomized studies showed an association with dose in the dose range 2×10^6 U/m^2 thrice weekly to 5×10^6 U/m^2 daily (39–41). Dose escalation above 9×10^6 U daily has been associated with suppression of transformed clones (42). Other studies, however, have disputed the importance of dose response achieving similar hematological and cytogenetic responses with IFN doses of only 2×10^6 U/m² daily for 1 month and then thrice weekly (43). The precise mechanism of action of IFN in CML is unknown, but it is logical to postulate that whatever the mechanism, the dose-response curve may continue to rise at doses $>5 \times 10^6$ U/m². In vitro there is a dose-response effect of IFN in suppression of hemopoietic progenitor cell growth (44,45). Pharmacodynamic studies in volunteers have shown increasing expression of IFN-induced gene products over a dose range from 0.9×10^6 U to 45×10^6 U (46). Since IFN appears to be one of the most active single agents in CML, it is logical to test this agent in a dose escalation study. We aimed to reach a dose of 18×10^6 daily, which was a doubling of the highest commonly recommended dose and from personal observations and experience in other malignancies appeared to be tolerable.

A concern about the dose escalation study was that some patients would be overtreated if they otherwise would have responded to standard doses of IFN. A strategy was needed to avoid overtreating good responders. Studies using IFN alone or with ara-C show marked heterogeneity in the response. Some patients respond rapidly and completely and appear very sensitive to relatively small doses of IFN, whereas others respond slowly and incompletely. Patients with poor prognostic factors as defined by the Sokal Index tend to respond poorly to IFN (1–3,11), and so high-risk patients (Sokal ≥1.2) were treated with high-dose IFN from the start. Low-risk patients were treated according to the previous study of IFN plus ara-C, but if cytogenetic response was >50% Ph+ after 8 months (equivalent to five courses of ara-C), then they were changed to high-dose IFN. Any further response thereafter could suggest a response to high-dose IFN. Eight months and 50% Ph+ were chosen as useful cutoff points to predict those who would ultimately become responders if given more time on the standard therapy since in our previous study 13/16 major cytogenetic responders achieved <50% Ph+ within 8 months of IFN.

The objective of this study was to determine, first, if dose escalation of IFN from 9×10^6 U daily to 18×10^6 U daily is tolerable in CML patients, and secondly, if dose escalation will increase the cytogenetic remission rate. An interim analysis of this study has been presented (19) and is presented in this review.

Patients and Methods

This is a phase I/II study testing the efficacy and tolerance of IFN dose escalation in early chronic-phase CML. The study has two arms stratified according to Sokal prognostic index. The low-risk arm receive IFN 9×10^6 U daily with five courses of ara-C and crossover onto IFN at 18×10^6 U daily for 12 weeks if they are cytogenetic nonresponders (Ph+ >50%). The high-risk arm received

Australian Experience

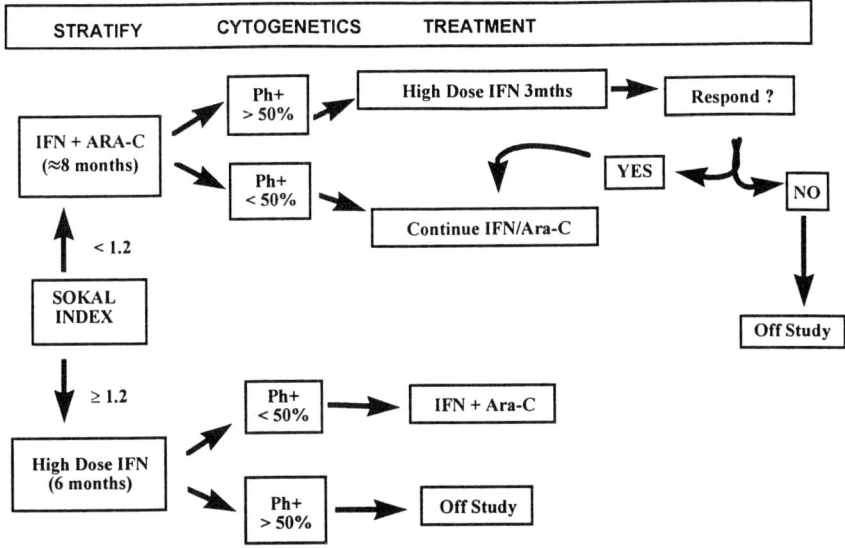

Figure 2 Protocol for high-dose interferon. Flow diagram of treatment schedule for IFN dose escalation study.

treatment with IFN 18×10^6 U daily after initial cytoreduction with hydroxyurea (see Fig. 2).

The inclusion and exclusion criteria are identical to the first study (see above). Patients were stratified into high and low risk according to the formula of Sokal. Low risk was defined as Sokal index <1.2, and high risk as Sokal Index ≥1.2.

Between April 1991 and March 1996, 34 patients with newly diagnosed CML patients were enrolled in this study. Patient characteristics are given in Table 3. The study closed to enrollment in March 1996. Six centers participated in the trial (see Appendix).

Treatment

Low-Risk Patients

Low-risk patients were treated according to our previous protocol using IFN and low-dose ara-C. The initial hydroxyurea, however, was more intense since it was clear from previous experience that the marrow remained markedly hypercellular despite normalization of peripheral blood counts. If IFN is most active in a state of minimal disease, then achieving cytoreduction in the marrow

Table 3 IFN Dose Escalation Trial: Patient Characteristics

	Low-risk patients ($n = 23$)	High-risk patients ($n = 9$)
Age (yr)	4–54	14–62
Sex: M : F	13 : 10	4 : 5
Hb (g/L)	6.0–15.3	7.5–13.7
WCC ($\times 10^9$/L)	20–430	53.2–439
Platelets ($\times 10^9$/L)	162–594	150–1676
Blasts (%)	0–3	1–8
Spleen size (cm)	0–16	5–22
Sokal index: <0.8	14 (range 0.5–0.7)	—
0.8–1.19	9 (range 0.8–1.0)	—
≥1.2	—	9 (range 1.2–2.6)

early might improve the response. Therefore, the initial leukocytosis was controlled by hydroxyurea 2 g daily with dose adjustment until neutrophils $<1.5 \times 10^9$/L and/or platelets $<50 \times 10^9$/L. At this point HU was stopped, a bone marrow examination was performed, and IFN commenced immediately. Hydroxyurea was restarted if the neutrophil count rose above 4.0 or the platelet count rose above 450×10^9/L.

Ara-C was commenced 4 weeks after starting IFN and then the treatment was reviewed after five cycles of ara-C. If the marrow cytogenetics showed a response to <50% Ph+ cells, then the current treatment continued as in the previous study. Ara-C was given for another four cycles and then stopped. IFN was continued for at least 3 years, but once a major cytogenetic response occurred the dose was reduced at the investigator's discretion as long as a major cytogenetic response was maintained. In this way good responders received the minimum necessary treatment.

Patients who had >50% Ph+ cells when assessed after five courses of ara-C then received high-dose IFN—18×10^6 U daily for 12 weeks. It was anticipated that the concurrent administration of ara-C during this time would be intolerable and so ara-C was stopped while on high-dose IFN. If patients responded with reduction of Ph+ chromosomes to <50%, then they went back to IFN at 9×10^6 U daily and received a further four courses of ara-C according to the protocol.

High-Risk Patients

Hydroxyurea was given in the same schedule as for low-risk patients in order to achieve moderate neutropenia and/or thrombocytopenia. IFN was commenced in a dose escalation schedule starting at 3×10^6 U daily 2 days, then 6×10^6 U daily for 2 days, then increased to 9×10^6 U daily for 2 weeks. Patients who were tolerating IFN satisfactorily at this dose then increased the daily dose by 3×10^6 U daily each week until they reach a daily dose of 18×10^6 U. At any dose level if the patient experienced side effects that were interfering with normal daily activities or in the investigator's opinion were intolerable, prednisolone 25 mg daily was started. The intention of adding prednisolone rather than IFN dose reduction was to minimize the possibility that patients would not receive the intended dose escalation, thereby making assessment of efficacy unreliable.

Hydroxyurea was added for WCC >4.0×10^9/L or platelets >450×10^9/L.

After IFN at 18×10^6 U daily had been reached, it was continued for a maximum of 6 months. At this time the following treatment decisions were made:

1. Bone marrow <50% Ph+ cells then the IFN was reduced to 9×10^6 U daily and continued for a total of 3 years from the commencement of IFN.

2. If the Ph+ cells are >50%, then the treatment is considered a failure and the patient is taken off the study.

Response: Response criteria were identical to those used in our previous study (see above).

Results

Thirty-two patients are currently evaluable (1/34 no information available, 1/34 withdrawn prior to commencing IFN). Median follow-up is 28 months (6–50 months).

There were 23 evaluable patients in the low-risk group and nine in the high-risk group. Two patients in the low-risk group did not proceed to ara-C because of cytopenia on IFN alone.

Complete hematological remission occurred in 27/32 (84%). Overall, 12 (37%) patients achieved CCR or PCR, 10 in the low-risk and 2 in the high-risk groups (Table 4).

Table 4 IFN Dose Escalation Trial: Response

	Low-risk patients ($n = 23$)	High-risk patients ($n = 9$)
CCR	3 (13%)	0
PCR	7 (30%)	2 (22%)
MR	6 (27%)	0
NR	7 (30%)	7 (78%)

Table 5 IFN Dose Escalation Trial: Toxicity

Side effect	Low-dose IFN and ara-C ($n = 23$)	High-dose IFN ($n = 19$)
Mucositis	15 (65%)	4 (21%)
Fatigue	12 (52%)	8 (42%)
Nausea	12 (52%)	5 (26%)
Anorexia	9 (39%)	4 (21%)
Infection	7 (30%)	5 (26%)
Flu-like symptoms	7 (30%)	3 (16%)
Fever	7 (30%)	2 (11%)
Myalgia	6 (26%)	3 (16%)
Weight loss	5 (22%)	5 (26%)
Headache	5 (22%)	2 (11%)
Diarrhea	4 (17%)	4 (21%)
Thrombocytopenia ($<150 \times 10^9$/L)	4 (17%)	3 (16%)
Arthralgia	4 (17%)	3 (16%)
Depression	4 (17%)	2 (11%)
Alopecia	2 (8%)	5 (26%)
Neutropenia ($<1.0 \times 10^9$/L)	2 (8%)	0
Raised LFTs	2 (8%)	4 (21%)

In the low-risk group, results of treatment were similar to our previous experience with IFN plus Ara-C. Similar toxicity was encountered. One patient ceased IFN due to toxicity; however, four patients ceased ara-C after two to four courses due to toxicity, and a further two patients never received ara-C due to IFN-related cytopenia. Toxicity is summarized in Table 5. Ten patients showed major cytogenetic responses, three CCR and seven PCR giving a major cytogenetic response of 43% in low-risk patients.

Ten patients in the low-risk group who failed to achieve <50% Ph+ cells after five courses of ara-C entered the IFN dose escalation arm. Nine of 10 completed 12 weeks of high-dose IFN, and one stopped after developing a cardiomyopathy. Three of 10 patients required temporary dose reductions for thrombocytopenia. High-dose IFN was generally well tolerated, and some patients commented that it proved to be more tolerable than the combination of IFN (at 9×10^6 U/d) plus ara-C. None of the patients who escalated from low-dose IFN to high-dose IFN patients showed a cytogenetic response after 12 weeks on high-dose IFN.

Results of high-dose IFN in the high-risk group were also disappointing. Four patients did not complete the 6-month course of therapy, three due to blast transformation and one due to abnormal liver enzymes requiring dose reduction

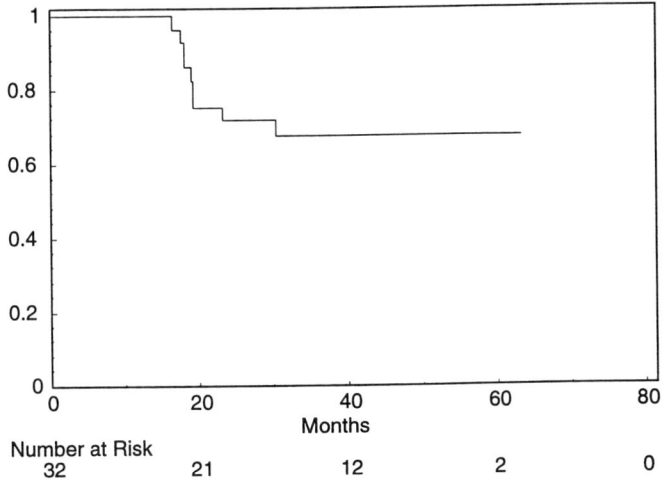

Figure 3 Survival of 32 patients in early chronic-phase CML treated on IFN dose escalation study.

back to 9×10^6 U/d. Two patients achieved a transient partial cytogenetic response (Ph+ 5% and 17%).

Overall, 19 patients received high-dose IFN (10 low risk and 9 high risk). Only three patients did not complete the planned course due to side effects; however, none showed a sustained cytogenetic response. Eight of the 19 received short courses of prednisolone 5–25 mg/day to ameliorate side effects.

Disease progression to accelerated or blastic phase has occurred in nine patients. Ten patients have undergone bone marrow transplantation. Ten patients have died, five from disease progression and five from transplant related complications. Projected survival at 3 years is 68% (Fig. 3).

Addition of Ara-C in Patients Failing High-Dose IFN

The study design did not allow for patients who failed to respond to high-dose IFN to cross over onto a combination IFN plus ara-C. In retrospect it would have been ideal to test if ara-C provides an additional therapeutic benefit in the high-risk patients. Although not part of the original study design, three high-risk patients failing high-dose IFN have now been treated with combined IFN (at 9×10^6 U daily) and ara-C 20 mg/m^2 daily for 21 days every 42 days. One patient achieved a major cytogenetic remission after four courses of ara-C (Fig. 4). It is possible that a cytogenetic response would have occurred by continuing IFN alone; however, the chronological association supports an effect of Ara-C.

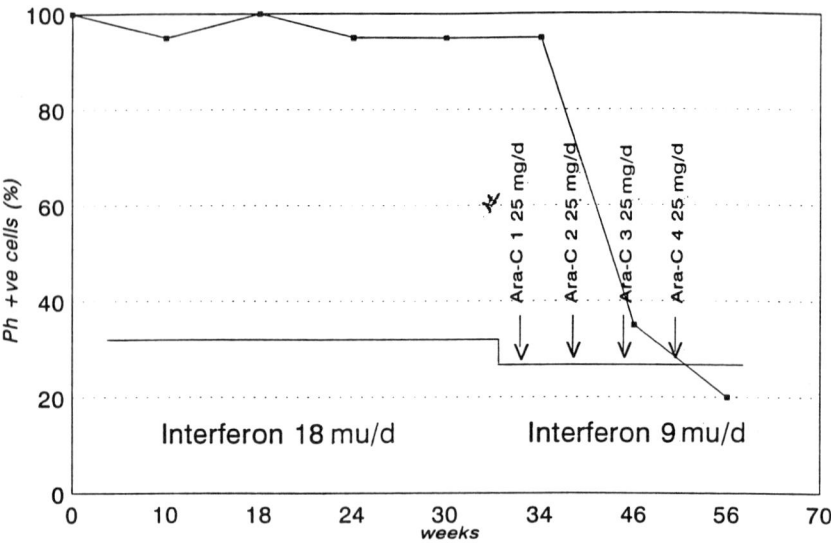

Figure 4 Addition of ara-C. Graph of cytogenetic response in a patient failing high-dose IFN (18×10^6 U daily) after treatment with four courses of ara-C 25 mg daily for 21 days every 42 days.

Combined Results of IFN/Ara-C and IFN Dose Escalation Study

The results of the 62 patients treated on the two studies of IFN/ara-C and IFN dose escalation have been combined to assess the effect of Sokal index and cytogenetic response. There is a significantly poorer survival in patients with a Sokal index ≥1.2 compared with <1.2 (Fig. 5), and survival appears worse in patients without a major cytogenetic response (Fig. 6).

Conclusion

The results of this second study evaluating dose escalation of IFN up to 18×10^6 U daily indicate that most patients can tolerate IFN at this dose. The results of dose escalation are disappointing, however, and no significant sustained responses were seen. The patient population selected for testing high-dose IFN, however, was a very poor risk group and had already selected themselves for poor response to the standard doses of IFN. The results cannot be extrapolated to all patients with early chronic-phase CML in which the optimal dose of IFN is still unknown. Some investigators claim that good hematological and cytoge-

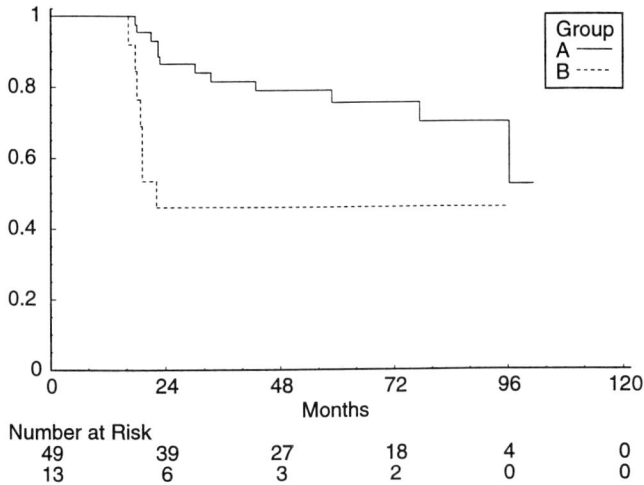

Figure 5 Survival estimates of 62 patients in the two studies of IFN/ara-C and IFN dose escalation according to Sokal index. Group A (———) are patients with Sokal index <1.2. Group B(--------) are patients with Sokal index ≥1.2. The difference between the curves is significant, $p = 0.004$.

netic responses can be obtained with low doses of IFN (43), but most studies show superior hematological and cytogenetic responses to higher doses of IFN (1,39,40). It is possible that some low-risk patients failing IFN at 9×10^6 U daily as a single agent could respond to dose escalation. The current study, however, was designed to see if patients failing combined IFN plus ara-C would benefit from high-dose IFN or if poor-prognosis patients would benefit from high-dose IFN as initial therapy. There are very few studies regarding dose escalation above 9×10^6 U daily; however, Allan et al. were also unable to increase the complete response rate in patients pretreated with busulphan by IFN dose escalation from 3×10^6 U daily to 15×10^6 U daily (47). At present it does not seem that dose escalation above 9×10^6 U daily will improve response rates in these selected groups of patients.

INTERFERON PLUS HYDROXYUREA

The combination of IFN plus HU was studied by Taylor and colleagues (20,21). In this study 31 patients in early chronic phase CML (diagnosis <1 year from start of IFN and with no or minimal pretreatment) received IFN-α2a (Roferon-A; Hoffmann-La Roche) 9×10^6 U daily and hydroxyurea with dose adjusted to

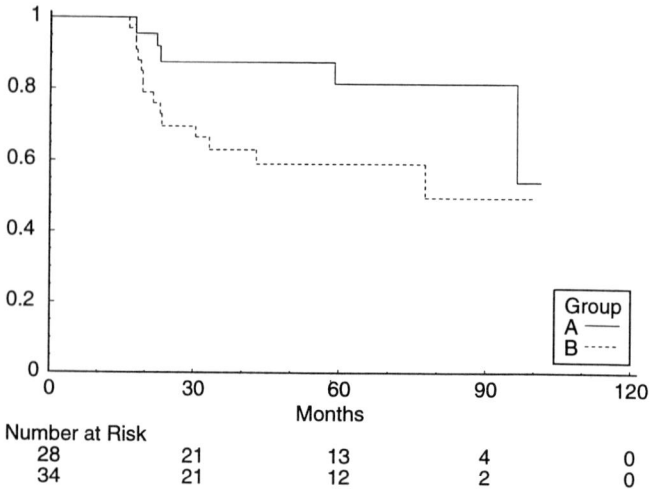

Figure 6 Survival estimates of 62 patients in the two studies of IFN/ara-C and IFN dose escalation according to cytogenetic response. Group A(———) are patients with major cytogenetic responses (Ph+ <35%) and Group B (-------) are patients with minimal or no cytogenetic response. The difference between the curves is significant, $p = 0.044$.

maintain the granulocyte count at $1.0–2.0 \times 10^9$/L. The median age of patients was 37 years (range 22–65). Patients had received treatment for a median of 24 months (range 9–50).

Cytogenetic responses were classified according to the criteria of Talpaz (36). The Sokal index was used to classify patients into low-, intermediate-, and high-risk categories (Sokal <0.8, 0.8–1.2, and >1.2). An interesting feature of this study was the evaluation of response according to the location of the breakpoint in the M-bcr region of the BCR gene on chromosome 22. The analysis of the breakpoint was done by Southern hybridization and reverse transcriptase polymerase chain reaction (RT-PCR). Major cytogenetic responses (Ph+ cells <35%) occurred in 12/31 (39%) patients, and complete remission occurred in 9/31 (29%).

The response in different Sokal groups was not significantly different, but there were only five patients in the high-risk subgroup and significant differences may have been missed due to the small numbers.

There was a significant correlation between response and the breakpoint in M-bcr. Using the RT-PCR technique 29 patients were analyzed. Thirteen of 29 (45%) with a 5′ breakpoint showed a major cytogenetic response, compared with only three of 16 (19%) with a 3′ breakpoint ($p = 0.014$). The results of studies correlating breakpoint locations with response have been conflicting. In the initial study of IFN plus ara-C our group found no correlation between the location of the breakpoint and major cytogenetic response (37). Inoue et al. (48) did not confirm a correlation between cytogenetic response and breakpoint location. Fioretos et al. (49) found no difference between breakpoint position and any clinical parameters. In contrast, however, the study by Lee et al. (50) showed a significantly better cytogenetic response to IFN in patients with the b2a2 breakpoint. The differences between these studies may be explained by differences in methodology and/or differences in the patient population and therapy. If a true difference does exist, then perhaps it may be overcome by a more intensive therapy such as with combined IFN plus ara-C, and this might explain why we have not seen a correlation.

A recent follow-up report of this group of patients has revealed a high rate of delayed toxicity in responding patients (21). Favorable cytogenetic responses were seen in 12/31 (39%) patients (10 CCR and two MRC). However, only four patients remain on IFN in CCR, and two of these have required dose reduction due to polymyositis (1) or fatigue and lethargy (1). Four patients ceased IFN due to toxicity, vasculitis in three and encephalopathy in one. Another disturbing result was the rapid evolution to myeloid blast crisis in two patients despite documentation of CCR only 1 and 3 months prior to the onset of blast crisis. This report reminds investigators of the importance of careful long-term monitoring even in patients apparently stable in CCR on long-term maintenance IFN. Since a good proportion of patients in CCR develop problems after prolonged follow-up, it is suggested that alternative strategies should be considered for treatment even in this group of patients generally regarded as very low risk. One option being considered is the collection of stem cells whilst in CCR or MCR (51).

INTERFERON PLUS ALL-*TRANS* RETINOIC ACID (ATRA)

Introduction

After completion of the earlier Australian studies it was evident that innovative therapies were required for the large proportion of patients who had inadequate responses to IFN or a combination of IFN and ara-C. There was general interest in combinations of IFN and either cytotoxic agents or other biological response modifiers. Spectacular results were being seen with the use of all-*trans* retinoic acid (ATRA) in promyelocytic leukemia (52,53), and this renewed interest in antileukemic therapies focused on cell differentiation and antiproliferative actions. CML cells appear to have defects in maturation and proliferation as well as failure to undergo apoptosis (54–56). Since interferons and retinoids have activity as antiproliferative and maturation-inducing agents, the combination of IFN with ATRA could lead to a synergistic response against CML.

There are many retinoid compounds with antitumor activity. We chose to investigate ATRA, which is a natural metabolite of vitamin A. Retinoid compounds have an antitumor activity via various mechanisms. They induce differentiation in a series of human and murine transformed cell lines and also have a direct antiproliferative effect without differentiating effect on lung, testicular, breast, or prostate cancer cell lines (57–60). Clinical studies of retinoids are in progress for cancer prevention and treatment and include CML. The South West Oncology Group randomized 153 patients with early chronic-phase CML to receive oral pulse busulfan with our without continuous oral vitamin A (61). Nonsignificant prolongation of overall survival was seen in the vitamin A group (51 months v. 44 months; $p = 0.081$). After adjustment for differences in significant risk factors between the groups, there was a 53% greater risk of clinical disease progression or death among patients not receiving vitamin A ($p = 0.022$).

Retinoids are likely to find a place as adjunctive therapy, and interestingly, preclinical and clinical data support the study of a combination of ATRA and IFN. Both IFN and ATRA have antiproliferative, differentiating, and immunomodulatory properties. Particularly interesting is that both agents may promote programmed cell death, which may be a significant defect in CML cells (56). There is evidence that simultaneous exposure to both IFN and retinoids can enhance the antiproliferative and differentiating effects compared to either agent alone (57,62,63).

In vitro, Zheng et al. (64) showed a significant inhibitory effect on CML CFU-GM when both ATRA and IFN were added to cell cultures, but either agent alone showed only insignificant inhibition of colony growth. Interestingly normal CFU-GM from healthy controls and in other myeloproliferative disorders did not show an inhibitory effect of the ATRA + IFN combination. This suggests that the combination may have a selective inhibitory effect on CML in vivo.

Preisler et al. have used *cis*-retinoic acid plus IFN alternating with ara-c + HU in 15 patients with CML (65). Complete hematological response occurred in 14 patients, and seven have achieved a partial cytogenetic response; however, follow-up is <6 months in the majority of patients. An earlier report from this group showed the addition of *cis*-retinoic acid was associated with a reduction in the percentage of cells in S phase, and reduced expression of c-myc oncogene in the myeloid cells (66). These results suggest that *cis*-retinoic acid can facilitate differentiation of CML cells, and it is anticipated that ATRA would show a similar effect.

There are several groups of CML patients in which the combination of ATRA and IFN might be usefully tested. Patients who fail to achieve any cytogenetic response to IFN have a poor survival and those who achieve minor cytogenetic responses have intermediate survival (1–3). Patients who present with accelerated-phase CML or develop this during the course of the disease

Australian Experience

rarely achieve good responses to IFN and have poor survival (1). Some CML patients are treated with autologous bone marrow or peripheral blood stem cell transplants, but most patients eventually relapse (67). The relapse after autologous transplant may be detected early, when the disease is still minimal, a situation when IFN and ATRA may be most effective.

The three treatment groups noted above will test various aspects of the study hypothesis. The group of IFN failures who remain in chronic phase will be ideal to test the efficacy of the addition of ATRA to IFN. A response in this group would be strong evidence for an additive or synergistic effect. The group of accelerated-phase patients may provide evidence that the combination of ATRA and IFN is effective in this phase of the disease, in contrast to the use of IFN alone, which is rarely effective. The group of patients relapsing after autologous bone marrow transplants will provide an opportunity to test the activity of the combination in minimal residual disease. These three groups, therefore, will allow a more complete assessment of the potential advantages of the combination in the one study design.

Patients and Methods

This study is ongoing and an interim analysis has been reported (22). The results of this interim analysis are presented here. Patient details are given in Table 6. The aim of the study is, first, to evaluate the safety and tolerability of ATRA plus IFN, and, second, to evaluate efficacy in terms of hematological and cytogenetic response by the addition of oral ATRA to IFN in patients with CML in any of the following groups:

Table 6 IFN Plus ATRA in CML: Patient Details

Characteristics	Patients ($n = 16$)
Age range	30–64 (median 50)
Sex: M : F	1 : 1
Subgroups	
Chronic phase—failed IFN	9
Accelerated phase	3
Relapsed postautograft	4
Hematology at study entry	
WCC ($\times 10^9$/L)	1.8–80.0
Platelets ($\times 10^9$/L)	45–807
Blasts (%)	0–3
Spleen size (cm)	0–3

1. Have failed to show a cytogenetic response (Ph+ >50%) to a 12-month treatment course with IFN
2. Are in accelerated phase of the disease
3. Relapsed following an autologous bone marrow or peripheral blood stem cell transplant and have failed to achieve a cytogenetic response after 3 months of IFN.

This study also used a dosing regimen to avoid the decreasing bioavailability of continuous daily ATRA administration. After several days of ATRA administration the plasma concentration falls markedly and is due to increased clearance. This effect can be minimized by an alternate-week dosing schedule (68,69).

Treatment

Patients are stabilized on the maximum tolerated dose of IFN and then commence ATRA 45 mg/m^2 daily in divided doses (bid) for 7 days every 14 days. Treatment is continued for 6 months and if a hematological response is not achieved then subjects are withdrawn. Patients in a state of hematological remission continue ATRA for a maximum of 12 months. Grade 3–4 toxicity is managed with temporary cessation of ATRA and restarting at a lower dose according to specified protocol guidelines.

Results

Sixteen patients have entered this study. Nine chronic-phase patients failing IFN, three accelerated-phase, and four relapsed after autologous bone marrow/pbsc transplant. Three have completed therapy, three are still on treatment, and 10 have withdrawn. Three patients have completed therapy, of whom one has achieved complete cytogenetic response and two have complete hematological responses (Ph+ 100% and 90%).

Three patients are currently continuing on study treatment of whom one patient in accelerated phase with an chromosomal abnormality, der(17) clone, has achieved suppression of Ph+ cells from 100% to 62% with a proportional reduction in the transformed clone. Ten patients have withdrawn from the study. Three had no response after 24 weeks, one had disease progression after 8 weeks, and six withdrew due to adverse events. Five of the adverse-event withdrawals were considered due to side effects of ATRA. These included severe headaches in two, mucositis lethargy and fever in two, bleeding in one, and transient cerebral ischemic attack in one. Although most patients developed ATRA-related side effects, they tended to diminish with each successive course of therapy.

Australian Experience

Table 7 IFN Plus ATRA in CML: Toxicity

Side effect	Frequency grade 1–2	Frequency grade 3–4
Dry lips	11 (73%)	
Headache	9 (60%)	5 (33%)
Dry skin	8 (53%)	
Nausea and vomiting	4 (26%)	1 (6%)
Anemia	4 (26%)	
Fatigue and lethargy	4 (26%)	
Skin rash	4 (26%)	
Dry eyes	3 (20%)	
Sweats	3 (20%)	
Thrombocytopenia	3 (20%)	
Myalgia	3 (20%)	
Mucositis	2 (13%)	1 (6%)
Arthralgia	2 (13%)	
Fevers	2 (13%)	
Bleeding (PV)	1 (6%)	
Pericarditis		1 (6%)
Raised LFTs	1 (6%)	
Visual disturbances/vertigo	1 (6%)	

Grade 3 and 4 toxicity included headache, dry skin, mucositis, nausea and vomiting, pericarditis, and fatigue (Table 7).

Conclusion

A preliminary analysis of this study shows that the combination of IFN and ATRA has significant toxicity related to the known side effects of ATRA; however, these side effects are more pronounced than those seen with the same dose of ATRA used in studies of promyelocytic leukemia. The possible potentiation of ATRA side effects by IFN could be related to altered pharmacokinetics and drug levels of IFN. A recent study of two patients receiving alternating IFN and ATRA for promyelocytic leukemia showed significantly higher ATRA levels during IFN + ATRA treatment compared with levels observed in patients receiving ATRA alone (70). The dose schedule of ATRA used, for example, in promyelocytic leukemia, may be inappropriate when combined with IFN, and further studies need to explore the maximally tolerated dose when the combination is used.

The efficacy of combined IFN plus ATRA is still in doubt. All the patients in this study were already in a poor prognostic group, so even a 10% major response rate would be encouraging. The one complete cytogenetic responder in this group had already failed a combination of IFN plus ara-C and autologous marrow transplantation in chronic phase, so a CCR temporally related to ATRA therapy is suggestive of an ATRA effect. The second patient showing an interesting cytogenetic response (currently Ph+ 62%) was in accelerated phase with an additional cytogenetic abnormality and had progressed from chronic phase after receiving high-dose IFN (18×10^6 U daily). Prior to study entry, only small doses of IFN were tolerated ($3-6 \times 10^6$ U daily), yet despite remaining on the low dose, the Ph+ clone and the additional transformed clone have reduced after 10 months on the combination therapy.

This study continues, but it is possible that a small proportion of responses will be seen in this group of relatively poor prognosis patients. The problem of toxicity needs to be evaluated with further dose-finding studies.

DISCUSSION AND SUMMARY

The management of CML by investigators in Australia has followed the trends in America and Europe. Allogeneic bone marrow transplantation is offered to patients under the age of 50–55 years with HLA-compatible siblings. In the majority, however, who do not fit into this group, a variety of treatments may be offered, but with the wider availability of IFN most patients <60–65 years would be considered for this therapy.

The relatively small population of Australia has made it difficult to conduct large randomized studies in CML, but other factors have allowed the formation of cooperative study groups that have linked the majority of clinically active hematologists and made the clinical protocols available to most hematologists. Since large randomized trials have been impractical in CML, local investigators have focused on novel strategies in Phase I/II studies. These studies have been linked with molecular and biological studies such as the assessment of the BCR/ABL breakpoint and response to treatment. The main interest in early chronic-phase CML has centered around combinations of IFN with cytotoxic agents such as hydroxyurea or ara-C, or more recently the combination of ATRA plus IFN. If combinations are found to be useful, then the next phase is to try multiple combinations. Already Preisler et al. (65,66) have been investigating such an approach.

The combination of ara-C and IFN currently appears the most promising combination. Several groups have now reported experience with this combination. Freund et al. treated 48 patients with IFN plus ara-C (20 mg/m² 5 days per week) and obtained 50% complete hematological remission and 4/48 PCR (71). Guilhot et al., in an interim report of a randomized study (30), compared IFN alone (104 patients) versus IFN plus ara-C (10 mg/m²/d for 10 days each month)

(103 patients). A higher CCR (15% v. 23%) was observed in the IFN plus ara-C group, but the difference did not reach significance. Long-term follow-up of this study is awaited to see if a significant survival advantage is achieved with the combination.

Kantarjian et al. (33) treated 60 patients with advanced CML (40 chronic phase >1 year from diagnosis and 20 accelerated-phase patients) using IFN plus ara-C 15 mg/m^2/d for 2 weeks every 4 weeks until remission. Chronic-phase patients receiving the combination had better complete hematological remission compared with IFN alone (55% v. 28%) and longer 3-year survival (75% v. 48%). In accelerated-phase patients response was not improved, and survival differences were accounted for by different patient characteristics; however, suppression of clonal evolution was observed in five patients.

Kantarjian et al. have also treated early chronic-phase patients with IFN plus ara-C (34). Earlier studies using ara-C 15 mg/m^2 daily for 7 days/month resulted in frequent IFN dose reductions, and so a later cohort of 101 patients were treated with ara-C 10 mg (total dose) daily continuously along with daily IFN 5×10^6 U/m^2. The lower dose of ara-C was well tolerated and allowed an actual delivered IFN dose of 3.6×10^6 U/m^2 daily. Very good responses were obtained with 40% of patients achieving major cytogenetic responses (Ph+ <35%).

Ferrajoli et al. treated 29 late chronic and accelerated-phase patients with IFN plus ara-C 15 mg/m^2 daily for 14 days/month (72). Two CCR and two minor cytogenetic responses occurred. Thaler et al. used a combination of IFN plus ara-C 10 mg/m^2 daily for 10 days/month in 84 untreated CML patients in chronic phase (35). Complete hematological responses were seen in 54%, cytogenetic responses in 44%, and major cytogenetic responses in 13%.

The combination of IFN plus ara-C was tolerable in these studies, but additional toxicity is observed consisting of nausea, diarrhea, fatigue, myalgia, and cytopenia (anemia, neutropenia, and thrombocytopenia). Additionally, in the Australian study, painful mouth ulceration was a feature in some patients possibly because a higher ara-C dose and longer duration (21 days) were used compared with the other studies.

There is a marked range of ara-C dose schedules used in these trials, ranging from 10 to 20 mg/m^2/day and duration of administration ranging from 10 days/month to 21 days every 42 days to continuous daily dosing. The Australian study reported here used the highest overall doses of ara-C per month, but whether this intensity is better remains unknown. Although the results of IFN plus Ara-C combinations are encouraging, it is unlikely that >50% of patients will achieve major benefit if cytogenetic responses are the ultimate goal.

The survival of patients with chronic-phase CML prior to the IFN era was 36–65 months, but recent studies using IFN now achieve median survival ranging from 61 to 89 months (73,74). However, it is very important to account for the proportion of risk groups in each study as well as differences in treatment policy. The Australian studies using IFN plus ara-C and high-dose IFN have survival of 76% at 6 years in the first study and 68% at 3 years in the later study. The later trial has poorer survival; however, there were twice as many high-risk patients in the later trial (9/32 [28%] v. 4/30 [13%]).

An interesting feature of the survival curves (Figs. 1 and 3) is the rapid decline between the first and second year which corresponds to the commonest time to undergo bone marrow transplantation and reflects transplant-related mortality. Patients were not censored from follow-up at the time of BMT since the reason for BMT was often failure of IFN therapy and so the mortality of BMT is associated with failure of IFN. The optimal timing of BMT continues to be controversial (74). Although BMT is the most common reason for mortality in this group of patients (11/19 deaths), many of the BMT patients would have died from disease progression within a short period of time if not transplanted.

Future investigation is likely to develop a multifaceted therapeutic and sequential approach to early chronic-phase patients. It is becoming increasingly evident that effective therapies in CML must be employed early and perhaps even as a matter of urgency. The likelihood of having normal residual stem cells and minimal drug-resistant leukemic clones is greatest at diagnosis. Such an approach could mean patients undergoing high-dose therapy followed by peripheral blood stem cell harvesting of Philadelphia-negative stem cells soon after diagnosis and then receiving IFN ± ara-C. A specific time limit might be set (e.g., 12 months), after which nonresponding patients would proceed to autografting and possibly adjuvant therapy with IFN or other agents postautograft. In fact, a study has already been initiated by the Australian CML study group using such a strategy (51).

The management options for CML remain quite varied, and no single therapy can yet be regarded as ideal. The use of IFN has provided a therapeutic foundation to which additive or synergistic therapies can be added. Considerable scope for exploring novel combinations and optimal doses of the current therapies remains.

REFERENCES

1. Kantarjian H, Deisseroth A, Kurzrock R, et al. Chronic myelogenous leukemia, a concise update. Blood 1993; 82:691–703.
2. Italian Cooperative Study Group on Chronic Myeloid Leukemia. Interferon alfa-2a as compared with conventional chemotherapy for the treatment of chronic myeloid leukemia. N Engl J Med 1994; 330:820–825.
3. Allan NC, Richards SM, Shepherd PC. UK Medical Research Council randomised multicentre trial of interferon-alpha for chronic myeloid leukaemia: improved survival irrespective of cytogenetic response. Lancet 1995; 345:1392–1397.

4. Borden EC. Interferons: pleiotropic cellular modulators. Clin Immunol Immunopathol 1992; 62:S18–S24.
5. Gresser I. Antitumour effects of interferons: past, present and future. Br J Haematol 1991; 79(suppl 1):1–5.
6. Clemens M. Interferons and oncogenes. Nature 1985; 313:531–532.
7. Keating A, Guinn BA, Laraya P, et al. α-Interferon downregulates transcription of bcr-abl in colonies arising from Ph(+) early hematopoietic progenitors in patients with chronic myeloid leukemia. Blood 1995; 86(suppl 1):527a. Abstract.
8. Bhatia R, McCarthy JB, Verfaillie CM. Interferon-α restores normal β1 integrin mediated growth inhibitory signalling in chronic myelogenous leukemia. Blood 1995; 86(suppl 1):600a. Abstract.
9. Upadhyaya G, Deisseroth AB, Emerson SG. CML progenitor cells are deficient in cell surface LFA-3: modulation by alpha-interferon in vitro and in vivo. Blood 1988; 72(suppl 1):836a.
10. Dowding C, Guo AP, Osterholz J et al. Interferon-α overrides the deficient adhesion of chronic myeloid leukemia primitive progenitor cells to bone marrow stromal cells. Blood 1991; 78:499–505.
11. Arthur CK, Ma DD. Combined interferon alfa-2a and cytosine arabinoside as first-line treatment for chronic myeloid leukemia. Acta Haematol 1993; 89(suppl 1): 15–21.
12. Kantarjian HM, Smith TL, O'Brien S, et al. Prolonged survival in chronic myelogenous leukemia after cytogenetic response to interferon-alpha therapy. Ann Intern Med 1995; 122:254–261.
13. Kantarjian H, Talpaz M, Keating M, et al. Therapy of Philadelphia chromosome (Ph)-positive chronic myelogenous leukemia (CML) with initial intensive chemotherapy (DOAP) followed by maintenance with human leukocyte alpha interferon. Blood 1986; 68:224a.
14. Talpaz M, Kurzrock R, Kantarjian H, et al. A phase II study of alternating alpha-2a-interferon and gamma interferon therapy in patients with chronic myelogenous leukemia. Cancer 1991; 68:2125–2130.
15. Kantarjian HM, Talpaz M, LeMaistre CF, et al. Intensive combination chemotherapy and autologous bone marrow transplantation leads to the reappearance of Philadelphia chromosome-negative cells in chronic myelogenous leukemia. Cancer 1991; 67:2959–2965.
16. Carella AM, Podesta M, Frassoni F, et al. Collection of 'normal' blood repopulating cells during early hemopoietic recovery after intensive conventional chemotherapy in chronic myelogenous leukemia. Bone Marrow Transplant 1993; 12:267–271.
17. Guilhot F. Interferon alfa and low-dose cytosine-arabinoside for the treatment of patients with chronic myelogenous leukemia in chronic phase. French CML Study Group. Semin Hematol 1993; 30(3 suppl 3):24–25.
18. Kantarjian HM, Keating MJ, Estey EH, et al. Treatment of advanced stages of Philadelphia chromosome-positive chronic myelogenous leukemia with interferon-alpha and low-dose cytarabine. J Clin Oncol 1992; 10:772–778.
19. Arthur CK, Ma DDF, Iland H, et al. A study of the effect of high dose interferon alpha-2a (HD-IFN) in early chronic phase chronic myeloid leukaemia (CML) patients with poor prognosis (Sokal ≥1.2) and of escalating dose in good prognostic patients (Sokal <1.2) after failing IFN + ara-C treatment. Thirty-fourth Annual Sci-

entific Meeting of the Haematology Society of Australia, Adelaide, Oct 13–16, 1996.
20. Elliott SL, Taylor KM, Taylor DL, et al. Cytogenetic response to α-interferon is predicted in early chronic phase chronic myeloid leukemia by M-bcr breakpoint location. Leukemia 1995; 9:946–950.
21. Williams BA, Taylor KM, Rodwell RL, et al. Adverse events and sudden blast crisis in patients with early chronic phase chronic myeloid leukemia (CML-ECP) achieving complete (CCR) and major cytogenetic responses (MCR) with interferon alpha (IFN). Thirty-third Annual Scientific Meeting of the Haematology Society of Australia, Brisbane, Oct 15–18, 1995:103.
22. Arthur CK, Hughes T, Taylor K. A pilot study of the addition of all-*trans* retinoic acid (ATRA) to interferon alpha 2a (IFN) for treatment of chronic myeloid leukaemia after failure of (1) IFN in chronic or accelerated phase, or (2) relapse post autologous bone marrow transplant. Thirty-fourth Annual Scientific Meeting of the Haematology Society of Australia, Oct 13–16, 1996.
23. Von Hoff D. In vitro data supporting interferon plus cytotoxic agent combinations. Semin Oncol 1991; 18(suppl 7):58–61.
24. Welander CE, Morgan T, Homesley HD, et al. Combined recombinant human interferon alpha2 and cytotoxic agents studied in a clonogenic assay. Int J Cancer 1985; 35:721–729.
25. Sokal JE, Gockerman JP, Bigner SH. Evidence for a selective anti-leukemic effect of cytosine arabinoside in chronic granulocytic leukemia. Leukemia Res 1988; 1: 453–458.
26. Sokal J, Bigner S. Low dose cytosine arabinoside in early and advanced chronic granulocytic leukemia. Blood 1986; 66(suppl 1):233a.
27. Robertson MJ, Tantravahi R, Griffin JD, et al. Hematologic remission and cytogenetic improvement after treatment of stable-phase chronic myelogenous leukemia with continuous infusion of low-dose cytarabine. Am J Hematol 1993; 43:95–102.
28. Imanishi J, Tanaka A. Experimental research from clinical applications of interferon. Jpn J Cancer Chemother 1984; 11:53–59.
29. Spiers ASD, Lorch CA, Harrison BA. Chronic granulocytic leukemia (CGL) in chronic phase with two Ph+ cell lines and suppression of one line by hydroxyurea. Blood 1986; 68(suppl 1):233a.
30. Guilhot F, Guerci A, Fiere D, et al. The treatment of chronic myelogenous leukemia by interferon and cytosine-arabinoside: rational and design of the French trials. Bone Marrow Transplant 1996; 17(suppl 3):S29–S31.
31. Guilhot F, Dreyfus B, Brizard A, et al. Cytogenetic remissions in chronic myelogenous leukemia using interferon alpha-2a and hydroxyurea with or without low-dose cytosine arabinoside. Leuk Lymph 1991; 4:49–55.
32. Silver RT, Benn P, Szatrowski TP, et al. Infusional cytosine arabinoside (ara-C) and recombinant interferon-a (rIFN-a) for the treatment of chronic myeloid leukemia (CML). Proc ASCO 1990; 9:209.
33. Kantarjian HM, Keating MJ, Estey EH, et al. Treatment of advanced stages of Philadelphia chromosome-positive chronic myelogenous leukemia with interferon-α and low dose cytarabine. J Clin Oncol 1992; 10:772–778.

34. Kantarjian H, O'Brien S, Beran M, et al. Interferon alpha (IFN-α) and low dose cytosine arabinoside (ara-C) therapy in Philadelphia chromosome (Ph)-positive chronic myelogenous leukemia (CML). Blood 1995; 86(suppl 1):529a.
35. Thaler J, Hilbe W. Comparative analysis of two consecutive phase II studies with IFN-α and IFN-α + ara-C in untreated chronic-phase CML patients. Bone Marrow Transplant 1996; 17(suppl 3):S25–S28.
36. Talpaz M, Kantarjian HM, McCredie K, et al. Hematologic remission and cytogenetic improvement induced by recombinant human IFN alpha A in chronic myelogenous leukemia. N Engl J Med 1986; 314:1065–1069.
37. Yin JL, Williams BG, Arthur CK, et al. Interferon response in chronic myeloid leukaemia correlates with ABL/BCR expression: a preliminary study. Br J Haematol 1995; 89:539–545.
38. Melo JV, Gordon DE, Tuszynski A, et al. Expression of the ABL-BCR fusion gene in Philadelphia-positive acute lymphoblastic leukemia. Blood 1993; 81:2488–2491.
39. Freund M, Von Wussow P, Diedrich H, et al. Recombinant human interferon (IFN) alpha-2b in chronic myelogenous leukaemia: dose dependency of response and frequency of neutralizing antibodies. Br J Haematol 1989; 72:350–356.
40. Morra E, Alimena G, Lazzarino M, et al. Evolving modalities of treatment with interferon alfa-2b for Ph1-positive chronic myelogenous leukaemia. Eur J Cancer 1991; 27(suppl 4):S14–S17.
41. Gastl G, Aulitzky Q, Tilg H, et al. Dose related effectiveness of alpha interferon in chronic myelogenous leukemia. Blut 1987; 54:251–252.
42. Taylor KMcD, Williams B, Elliot SL, et al. α-Interferon (α-IFN) dose escalation to suppress clonal evolution in chronic myelogenous leukemia. Thirtieth Annual Scientific Meeting of the Haematology Society of Australia, Melbourne, Oct 13–16, 1992:130.
43. Schofield JR, Robinson WA, Murphy JR, et al. Low doses of interferon-alpha are as effective as higher doses in inducing remissions and prolonging survival in chronic myeloid leukemia. Ann Intern Med 1994; 121:736–744.
44. Verma DS, Spitzer G, Gutterman JU. Human leukocyte interferon preparation blocks granulopoietic differentiation. Blood 1979; 54:1423–1427.
45. Neumann HA, Fauser AA. Effect of interferon on pluripotent hemopoietic progenitors (CFU-GEMM) derived from human bone marrow. Exp Hematol 1982; 10:587–590.
46. Witt PL, Storer BE, Bryan GT, et al. Pharmacodynamics of biological response in vivo after single and multiple doses of interferon-beta. J Immunother 1993; 13:191–200.
47. Allan NC, Richards S, Shepherd P. United Kingdom Medical Research Council randomized trial of interferon alpha in chronic-phase chronic myelogenous leukemia. European Hematologic Association Meeting, 1994:683. Abstract.
48. Inoue T, Tojo A, Tsuchimoto D, et al. Possible correlation between fusion pattern of BCR/ABL mRNA and clinical response to alpha-interferon in chronic myelogenous leukemia. Leukemia 1992; 6:948–951.
49. Fioretos T, Nilsson PG, Aman P, et al. Clinical impact of breakpoint position within M-bcr in chronic myeloid leukemia. Leukemia 1993; 7:1225–1231.

50. Lee M, Kantarjian H, Talpaz M, et al. Association of the responsiveness to interferon (IFN) therapy with BCR/ABL splicing patterns in Philadelphia chromosome (Ph)-positive chronic myelogenous leukemia (CML). Blood 1992; 80(suppl 1): 210a.
51. Hughes TP, Grigg A, Szer J, et al. Cyclophosphamide and rHuG-CSF to mobilise peripheral blood progenitors in early chronic phase chronic myeloid leukaemia. Thirty-third Annual Scientific Meeting of the Haematology Society of Australia, Brisbane, Oct 15–18, 1995:103.
52. Warrell RP Jr, Frankel SR, Miller WH Jr, et al. Differentiation therapy of acute promyelocytic leukemia with tretinoin (all-*trans*-retinoic acid). N Engl J Med 1991; 324:1385–1393.
53. Huang ME, Ye YC, Chen SR, et al. Use of all-*trans* retinoic acid in the treatment of acute promyelocytic leukemia. Blood 1988; 72:567–572.
54. Preisler HD, Raza A, Baccarani M. Proliferative advantage rather than classical drug resistance as the cause of treatment failure in chronic myelogenous leukemia. Leuk Lymph 1993; 11(suppl 1):303–306.
55. Strife A, Clarkson B. Biology of chronic myelogenous leukemia: is discordant maturation the primary defect? Semin Hematol 1988; 25:1–19.
56. Bedi A, Zehnbauer BA, Barber JP, et al. Inhibition of apoptosis of BCR-ABL in chronic myeloid leukemia. Blood 1994; 83:2038–2044.
57. Frey JR, Peck R, Bollag W. Antiproliferative activity of retinoids, interferon alpha and their combination in five human transformed cell lines. Cancer Lett 1991; 57: 223–227.
58. Bollag W, Holdener E. Retinoids in cancer prevention and therapy. Review. Ann Oncol 1992; 3:513–526.
59. Breitman TR, Keene BR, Hemmi H. Retinoic acid-induced differentiation of fresh human leukemia cells and the human myelomonocytic leukemia cell lines, HL-60, U-937 and THP-1. Cancer Surv 1983; 2:263–291.
60. Sidell N. Retinoic-acid induced growth inhibition and morphologic differentiation of human neuroblastoma cells in vitro. J Natl Cancer Inst 1982; 68:589–596.
61. Meyskens FL Jr, Kopecky KJ, Appelbaum FR, et al. Effects of vitamin A on survival in patients with chronic myelogenous leukemia: a SWOG randomized trial. Leuk Res 1995; 19:605–612.
62. Moore DM, Kalvakolanu DV, Lippman SM, et al. Retinoic acid and interferon in human cancer: mechanistic and clinical studies. Semin Hematol 1994; 31(4 suppl 5):31–37.
63. Bollag W. Retinoids and interferon: a new promising combination? Br J Haematol 1991; 79(suppl 1):87–91.
64. Zheng A, Savolainen ER, Koistinen P. All-*trans* retinoic acid combined with interferon-alpha effectively inhibits granulocyte-macrophage colony formation in chronic myeloid leukemia. Blood 1994; 84(suppl 1):153a.
65. Preisler HD, Raza A, Gezer S, et al. Inhibition of regrowth resistance and early cytogenetic response in the myelogenous leukemia. Blood 1995; 86(suppl 1):2107.
66. Preisler HD, Kotelnikov V, Hegde U, et al. A strategy overcoming regrowth resistance in chronic myelogenous leukemia (SORRCML). Blood 1993; 82(suppl 1): 556a.

67. McGlave PB, DeFabritiis P, Deisseroth A, et al. Autologous transplant therapy for chronic myelogenous leukemia prolongs survival: results from eight transplant centres. Lancet 1994; 343:1486–1488.
68. Adamson PC, Boylan JF, Balis FM, et al. Time course of induction of metabolism of all-*trans* retinoic acid and the up-regulation of cellular retinoic acid-binding protein. Cancer Res 1993; 53:472–476.
69. Adamson PC, Bailey J, Pluda J, et al. Pharmacokinetics of all-*trans*-retinoic acid administered on an intermittent schedule. J Clin Oncol 1995; 13:1238–1241.
70. Lazzarino M, Corso A, Regazzi M, et al. Modulation of all-*trans* retinoid acid pharmacokinetics in acute promyelocytic leukaemia by prolonged interferon-α therapy. Br J Haematol 1995; 90:928–930.
71. Freund M, Hild F, Grote-Metke A, et al. Combination of chemotherapy and interferon alfa-2b in the treatment of chronic myelogenous leukemia. Semin Hematol 1993; 30(suppl 3):11–13.
72. Ferrajoli A, Liberati AM, Caricchi P, et al. Interferon-α plus low-dose cytosine arabinoside in advanced phase chronic myelogenous leukaemia patients. Eur J Haematol 1995; 55:184–188.
73. Kumar L, Gulati SC. Alpha-interferon in chronic myelogenous leukaemia. Lancet 1995; 346:984–986.
74. Giralt S, Kantarjian H, Talpaz M. The natural history of chronic myelogenous leukemia in the interferon era. Semin Hematol 1995; 32:152–158.

APPENDIX: ACKNOWLEDGMENTS

Investigators and institutions participating in Australian CML-interferon studies. We wish to thank the doctors who participated in these studies or referred patients:

Interferon Plus Ara-C Study

D.D.F. Ma, J.P. Isbister, Royal North Shore Hospital, Sydney; M. Stevens, Royal Alexandra Hospital for Children, Camperdown; F. Firkin, St. Vincent's Hospital, Melbourne: M. Seldon, Royal Newcastle Hospital; A. Morley, Flinders Medical Centre, Adelaide; P. Harrison, Mater Misericordiae Hospital, Newcastle; C. Juttner, B. To, Institute of Medical & Veterinary Science, Adelaide; H. Iland, Kanematsu Institute, Royal Prince Alfred Hospital, Sydney; R. Ravich, S. Flecknoe-Brown.

Interferon Dose Escalation Study

D.D.F. Ma, J.P. Isbister, Royal North Shore Hospital, Sydney; A. Enno, S. Deveridge, Mater Misercordiae Hospital, Newcastle; J. Gallo, Lidcombe Hospital, Sydney; M. Hertzberg, Westmead Hospital, Sydney; F. Firkin, St. Vincent's

Hospital, Melbourne; M. Stevens, P. Shaw, L. Dalla-Pozza, Princess Alexandra Hospital for Children, Sydney; G. Young and H. Iland, Royal Prince Alfred Hospital, Sydney; A. Concannon, St. Vincent's Hospital, Sydney.

Interferon Plus Hydroxyurea

S.L. Elliot, K.M. Taylor, D.L. Taylor, R.L. Rodwell, M.M. Shuttlewood, S.J. Wright, B.F. Williams, Mater Misercordiae Hospital, Brisbane; P. Timms, Queensland University of Technology, Brisbane; P. Eliadis, I.H. Bunce, T.J. Frost, T.E. Olsen, Wesley Clinic, Brisbane; F. Firkin, St. Vincent's Hospital, Melbourne.

Interferon Plus ATRA

T. Hughes, Royal Adelaide Hospital, Adelaide; K.M. Taylor, Mater Misercordiae Hospital, Brisbane.

The studies of interferon plus Ara-C, interferon dose escalation and interferon plus ATRA were supported by grants from Roche Products, Dee Why, NSW, Australia.

The study of interferon plus hydroxyurea was supported by the J.P. Kelly foundation, Mater Misericordiae Hospital, Brisbane; Leukemia Foundation of Queensland; and Roche Products, Dee Why, NSW Australia.

I thank Leone Pemberton, Frances Power, and Elizabeth Melki for assistance with data management and preparation of the manuscript.

10
Allografting for Chronic Myelogenous Leukemia

David G. Savage
College of Physicians & Surgeons, Columbia University, New York, New York

John Michael Goldman
Imperial College School of Medicine, Hammersmith Hospital, London, England

INTRODUCTION

Allogeneic stem cell transplantation (alloSCT) remains the only curative therapy for chronic myelogenous leukemia (CML). There have been several advances in this field in the past decade. The bone marrow of HLA-identical siblings is no longer the only potential source of donor stem cells. Early data suggest that blood-derived stem cells are an effective substitute for marrow. AlloSCT can be performed using progenitor cells from other family members, volunteer unrelated donors (VUD), and umbilical cord blood. Evidence of early relapse can be detected by assays for the fusion gene, BCR-ABL, using the polymerase chain reaction. Most patients who relapse following alloSCT can be treated effectively by transfusion of lymphocytes from their original donor.

Despite these advances, alloSCT continues to suffer several limitations, including restricted availability, high cost, and substantial morbidity and mortality. The major challenges are to increase its applicability, to reduce graft-versus-host disease (GVHD), and to augment the graft-versus-leukemia (GVL) effect.

SOURCES OF ALLOGENEIC STEM CELLS

HLA Typing

The risks of alloSCT are lowest in patients who receive transplants from an HLA-identical sibling (1–4). Genes for the HLA system are inherited in Mendelian fashion. Thus, a patient and potential sibling donor only have a 1 in 4 chance of being HLA-identical. One can calculate the likelihood of a given patient having an HLA-matched sibling using the formula $1 - (0.75)^n$ in which n equals the total number of siblings. In North America and Europe, because family size is usually relatively small, most patients lack a histocompatible sibling (5–11).

To establish HLA identity between siblings, serological typing of the A, B, and DR loci (9,12,13) is usually adequate. More sophisticated methods are required for unrelated individuals (9,14–18). Several new techniques have been introduced, including one-dimensional isoelectric focusing to examine class I regions (19) and restriction fragment length polymorphisms (20) and sequence-specific oligonucleotide probes (12,21–23) for class II regions. Serology has been inadequate to demonstrate donor-recipient disparity for the C region of HLA class I. When examined by high-resolution methods the C locus appears to be a significant determinant of graft failure and GVHD (9,24–26). Molecular techniques have also made it possible to examine the DP and DQ regions of class II (9,15,16). High-resolution typing should provide a more accurate means to predict graft failure and GVHD in recipients of unrelated or mismatched donor transplants (15,17).

Functional assays should theoretically be able to predict the incidence and severity of GVHD and should therefore be of major value in excluding an unsatisfactory sibling donor and identifying the optimal donor when there is a choice. In practice, the mixed lymphocyte culture is useful only in confirming genetic identity at HLA loci and has no value in predicting GVHD or identifying alternative donors (9,27–30), as discussed below. A variety of assays have been developed that measure the frequency of alloreactive cytotoxic and helper T-cell precursors in the blood of the prospective donor. In some series a high frequency of cytotoxic T-cell precursors that react against recipient alloantigens correlates with an increased incidence of GVHD posttransplant (31–33), but in general the value of such assays is not yet established.

HLA-Identical Sibling Donors

Some patients will have more than one HLA-matched sibling. Donors are selected according to their general health, availability, and ability to give consent. Male or nulliparous female donors are generally preferred because of a lesser risk of GVHD (34,35). Younger donors are generally preferable to older donors

Allografting

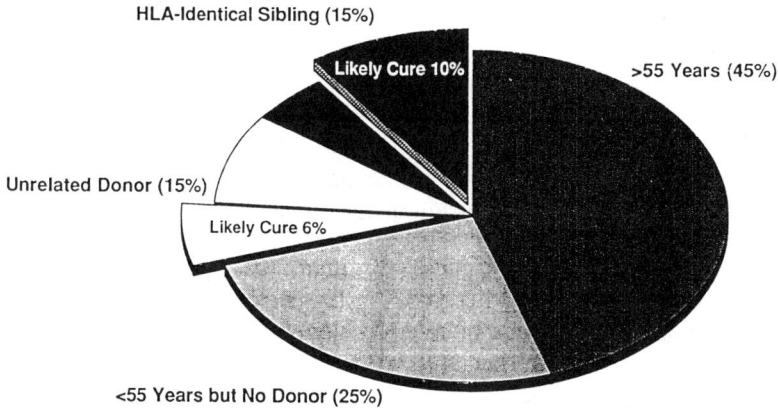

Figure 1 An estimate of the availability of donor and likelihood of cure by alloSCT for a notional 100 patients with newly diagnosed CML (Western Europe or North America). It is assumed that the median age is 50 years and the average number of siblings just over two. When the average family size is larger, the probability of finding a sibling donor is increased.

for the same reason. If both the recipient and donor lack serological evidence of cytomegalovirus (CMV) infection, the risk of CMV disease is negligible (36). If the patient is CMV-positive, seronegativity in the donor is probably not important (37). The donor should be free of infection with HIV and hepatitis viruses B and C. ABO and Rh compatibility is desirable but not mandatory.

Alternative Donors

For patients in whom alloSCT is indicated but who lack an HLA-identical sibling, there are three alternative sources: another family member, a volunteer unrelated donor, or umbilical cord blood (Fig. 1, Table 1).

Table 1 Potential Donors for Allogeneic Stem Cell Transplantation

Identical twin
HLA-identical sibling
HLA-identical or mismatched:
   other family member
   volunteer unrelated donor
   umbilical cord blood

Related Donors Other Than Genetically HLA-Identical Siblings

Family members who are not genetically HLA-identical with the patient have occasionally been used as donors with acceptable results (25,38–40). Such donors are usually classified as "phenotypically" HLA-identical because they share with the patient the six major antigens of the HLA system. In practice, if the "matched" donor is a parent or child of the patient, he or she must be genetically identical for one HLA haplotype and phenotypically identical for the other. Other family members may or may not share one HLA haplotype at the genetic level. The probability of finding such a donor in the patient's extended family may be greater than in an unrelated donor register, depending on the family's size, ethnic background, and frequency of intrafamilial marriage (41). Related family members mismatched for one or occasionally two HLA antigens have also served as donors (2–4,38,39,42–49).

Volunteer Unrelated Donors

In patients lacking a histocompatible family member, the search for a suitable unrelated donor may be extremely difficult because of the large number of possible HLA antigen combinations (9,13). On a theoretical basis, the number of possible HLA phenotypes is greater than the world population. Large national and international donor registries have been established to maximize the chance of finding an HLA match. Identification of a histocompatible individual is most likely when the search is carried out in potential donors who share a similar genetic background. For people of European ancestry it is estimated that a registry of 200,000 volunteers of European descent would allow a 40–50% chance of finding an HLA-matched donor (7,50,51). This chance is much lower for non-Caucasians, in part because the panels comprise mainly Caucasian volunteers (10).

Cord Blood Donors

Umbilical cord blood (UCB) transplantation is another form of alloSCT (52–60). When current guidelines are followed, this procedure poses little or no risk to the donor. Moreover, a suitable UCB graft is often available more quickly than a registry donor. Even when one or two HLA-antigen mismatched UCB is used, rates of graft failure and GVHD have been acceptable. The fact that GVHD is not a major problem may be due to the relative naïveté of immunocytes in UCB (61–63). The youth of UCB recipients may also be contributory, as children are generally less prone to severe GVHD than adults.

Because of the small number of hematopoietic stem cells in UCB collections, these transplants have been performed primarily in children and small adults (52,54–60). To date, only five UCB transplants have been described in detail in patients with CML (Table 2, Fig. 2). Four patients were children and one was a young adult; four had advanced phase disease. One patient died of interstitial pneumonia without evidence of engraftment (58); the others have fared well. Although UCB transplantation is not feasible for most patients with CML, the constraints of patient size and cell dose may be overcome if techniques to expand progenitor cell numbers ex vivo (64) can be developed.

STEM CELL COLLECTIONS

Marrow Stem Cell Harvest

Bone marrow is harvested in an operating room under general anesthesia (51). The marrow is removed by multiple aspirations from both posterior iliac crests until a sufficient number of cells has been obtained. Occasionally the anterior iliac crests and sternum must also be aspirated. The number of marrow cells is usually 1 to 3×10^8 nucleated cells/kg of the recipient's body weight, depending on the diagnosis, the type of transplant, and whether the marrow will be modified ex vivo. Donors usually complain of fatigue and pain for several days following the procedure. However, marrow harvest is generally well tolerated (50,65).

The harvested marrow may undergo T-cell depletion to minimize the risk of GVHD, although this may increase the risk of graft failure and disease relapse, as discussed below. When there is ABO incompatibility between donor and recipient, it may be advisable to remove erythrocytes or plasma from the harvested marrow.

Blood Stem Cell Harvest

Blood stem cell harvesting (BSCH) is a more convenient and less invasive approach to obtaining progenitor cells for alloSCT (64–75). BSCH is performed after treatment of the donor with hematopoietic growth factors (e.g., recombinant human granulocyte colony-stimulating factor) over a period of 5–6 days. Progenitor cells are collected by leukapheresis using cell-separator technology.

In contrast to marrow harvesting, endotracheal intubation and general anesthesia are not required for BSCH. However, some donors may have poor venous access and require insertion of a central catheter. One concern is that the short-term administration of pharmacological doses of a growth factor might conceivably perturb the normal donor's myelopoiesis sufficiently to cause later myelodysplasia and leukemia (68,78). Because of this concern, BSCHs have not yet been widely employed for unrelated donors.

As T-cell numbers are higher (by about 1 log) in blood-derived than marrow grafts (66,71,79), GVHD might be more significant than seen with conven-

Table 2 Clinical Details of Five Patients with CML Undergoing Umbilical Cord Blood Transplantation

Reference	Age (yrs)	Weight (kg)	Disease phase	Conditioning	Donor	HLA Ag mismatch (n)	Nucleated cell dose (×10^7/kg)	Engraftment	Survival (mos)
52	3	14	1st CP	Cy TBI	sibling	0	8.7	yes	>16
55	3	—	1st BC	Ara-C Bu Cy TBI	sibling	2	11.7	yes	>14
56	15	50	2nd CP	Cy TBI	sibling	3	4.8	yes	>18
58	13	40.4	2nd BC	Melph TBI	unrelated	3	1.6	no	1
59	26	—	2nd CP	Cy TBI	unrelated	1	1.0	yes	>8

BC = blast crisis; CP = chronic phase; Ara-C = arabinosyl cytosine; Bu = busulfan; Cy = cyclophosphamide; Melph = melphalan; TBI = total body irradiation.

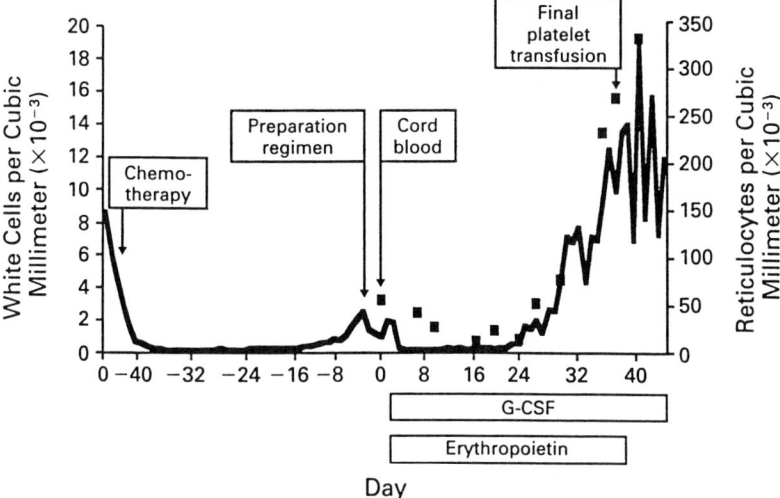

Figure 2 Umbilical cord blood transplantation in a 26-year-old woman with CML. Arabinosyl cytosine had been given for myeloblastic transformation, resulting in a second chronic phase. Conditioning consisted of antilymphocyte globulin, cyclophosphamide, and total body irradiation. From Ref. 59.

tional marrow transplantation. For the same reason, one would also anticipate the BSCT would be associated with greater GVL. Neither effect has been noted thus far. The primary observation is that allogeneic BSCT accelerates engraftment (80–83).

Overall, it is unclear whether allogeneic blood or marrow SCT is superior. This question is currently the subject of randomized studies in Seattle and Europe.

CONDITIONING

Prior to infusion of marrow or blood progenitor cells, the patient is "conditioned" by the administration of myeloablative doses of chemotherapy plus radiotherapy or chemotherapy alone. The aim is twofold; to destroy immunoreactive cells in the host, thus minimizing the chance of graft rejection; and to destroy residual leukemic cells. Initial attempts to transplant patients with CML using high dose regimens were directed mainly at those with advanced disease (84–87). More recently it has become apparent that the GVL effect may be of

Table 3 Some Conditioning Regimens Used for Allogeneic Transplantation for Chronic Myelogenous Leukemia

Regimen	Chemotherapy (mg/kg)	Usual TBI dose (Gy)	References
CyTBI	Cy 120	10–14.4	93,94
EtopoTBI	Etopo 60	13.2	92
BuCyTBI	Bu 7, Cy 50	12.0	91,95
BuCy$_4$	Bu 16, Cy 200	—	88,89
BuCy$_2$	Bu 16, Cy 120	—	90,93,94
BuMelph	Bu 16, Melph 140	—	96
ThiotepaCy	Thiotepa 15, Cy 150	—	73

Bu = busulfan; Cy = cyclophosphamide; Etopo = etoposide; Melph = melphalan; TBI = total body irradiation.

equal (or greater) importance in eradicating the leukemia. Nevertheless, high-dose regimens (Table 3) continue to be used for patients in chronic phase, who comprise the majority of individuals receiving allografts for CML.

Standard Regimens

Chemotherapy Plus Irradiation

The combination of cyclophosphamide and total body irradiation (CyTBI) (Table 3) is the most widely used. Cyclophosphamide is usually administered over 2 days (60 mg/kg/day) by continuous infusion. Either mesna (97) or continuous bladder irrigation (98) is used to reduce the risk of hemorrhagic cystitis. In Seattle TBI has been given either in a single dose or in six daily 200-cGy fractions or seven daily 225-cGy fractions (99,100). At Memorial-Sloan Kettering Cancer Center, cyclophosphamide has been combined with "hyperfractionated" TBI given as 120-cGy fractions three times daily to a total dose of 1320 or 1440 cGy (101). The Hammersmith Hospital (London) group employs 200-cGy fractions given twice daily for five or six doses (102). To achieve greater immunosuppression, TBI doses are generally higher for patients receiving transplants from unrelated or mismatched donors.

It has been suggested that fractionated treatment may be as myeloablative and immunosuppressive as a single dose of TBI (103–106). This issue has not been formally addressed in patients undergoing alloSCT for CML. A single, small randomized trial comparing single fraction TBI (10 Gy) versus fractionated TBI (12 Gy in six sessions) for patients with acute nonlymphocytic leukemia showed equivalent toxicity. Survival was marginally better with the fractionated regimen (107).

Allografting

There is no clear association between the incidence of interstitial pneumonitis and lung dose of irradiation in the range 5.6–13.0 Gy (108,109). Nevertheless, pulmonary damage is a potential toxicity of TBI. The primary objection to the use of lung shielding above a given dose is that leukemic cells in the ribs might escape destruction. This argument is less compelling when one recognizes the potency of the GVL effect. Current techniques would usually ensure some degree of shielding, so that the total lung exposure would be approximately 8–9 Gy.

Additional antileukemic activity may be achieved by intensification of the chemoradiotherapy (91,100,110). However, this is usually at the cost of greater toxicity. In the Seattle study (100) cited above, the lower dose of TBI (1200 cGy) was associated with a 36% actuarial risk of relapse at 4 years; in contrast, no relapse was seen in the patients given 1575 cGy. However, survival was not improved for the patients receiving the higher dose because of increased mortality from causes other than relapse (100). Increased doses of TBI are associated with greater GVHD (34,46,111) and veno-occlusive disease (112). Additional chemotherapy, such as busulfan (102,113,114), dimethylbusulfan (99), and anthracyclines (102,115), has provided no clear benefit.

Chemotherapy Alone

Because of its technical requirements, expense, and toxicity, various groups have used cytoreductive regimens which omit TBI (Table 3). The most popular is $BuCy_2$, which consists of busulfan (4 mg/kg/day for 4 days) followed by cyclophosphamide (60 mg/kg/day for 2 days) (90,92–94,110,116–122). A prior version of this combination, $BuCy_4$, employed a higher dose of cyclophosphamide (200 mg/kg) but was associated with excessive toxicity (88,89).

One difficulty with busulfan-based conditioning is the drug's variable pharmacokinetics (110,111,123,124). Hepatic veno-occlusive disease may be related to high plasma busulfan levels (112,125). The Seattle group has suggested that effective immunosuppression and myeloablation and less toxicity may be achieved with BuCy by adjusting the oral busulfan dose according to the busulfan plasma level (95). Newer parenteral preparations may also overcome the problem of variable bioavailability (124).

Chemoradiotherapy Versus Chemotherapy Alone

Two prospective randomized trials have compared CyTBI and $BuCy_2$ as conditioning therapy for HLA-identical sibling BMT in patients with CML in chronic phase: a single-center study reported from Seattle (93), and a multi-institutional trial reported from France (94). Event-free survival and overall survival were equivalent in patients receiving $BuCy_2$ and CyTBI in both reports. In the Seattle study, the incidence of GVHD, renal dysfunction, and infection was greater in the patients receiving CyTBI. The French investigators did not detect such differences. Relative to TBI, it is hoped that chemotherapy alone will be easier to give on an outpatient basis and will be associated with fewer complications such as cataract formation, growth retardation, and second malignancies (126). However, this remains to be shown.

Overall, both CyTBI and $BuCy_2$ are acceptable conditioning regimens for patients undergoing HLA-identical sibling alloSCT for CML in chronic phase. For advanced-phase disease (90,127), however, $BuCy_2$ may be associated with an unacceptable increase in transplant-related mortality (127).

For VUD and HLA-mismatched transplantation, more intensive immunosuppression is necessary to prevent rejection than is required for HLA-identical sibling alloSCT. As irradiation appears to provide more effective immunosuppression (128), CyTBI has been used in preference to chemotherapy alone. Recent reports have suggested that $BuCy_2$ may be an adequate alternative to TBI-based regimens in patients receiving VUD transplants (119,121,122,129). In other studies, however, excessive graft failure has been seen after conditioning with $BuCy_2$ (118,120). Whether high-dose chemotherapy alone is equivalent to TBI-based conditioning for VUD and mismatched donor transplants should be examined in prospective fashion.

Splenectomy and Splenic Irradiation

The role of splenectomy has not been addressed in a randomized trial. It was originally hoped that splenectomy would be an effective means to reduce the number of leukemic cells (130,131), but retrospective studies by the EBMT and Seattle groups have revealed no improvement in relapse rates or survival (132–136). Removal of the spleen may accelerate recovery of blood counts and reduce transfusion requirements in CML patients with marked splenomegaly (136–144). However, acute GVHD and infection also appear to be increased (138,139,141,142).

Compared to splenectomy, splenic irradiation has the advantage that surgery is not required. The EBMT group have recently reported that splenic irradiation (10 Gy) is associated with less relapse in a subset of patients transplanted in chronic phase with basophil counts >3% who receive non-T-cell-depleted grafts; however, there was no benefit for other patients (135).

Novel Regimens

The primary limitation of current cytoreductive regimens is their extrahematopoietic toxicity. As increased irradiation results in less leukemic relapse (100), radiation therapy which specifically targets lymphohematopoietic organs is being developed (145). These new modalities include ^{131}I-labeled monoclonal anti-

Allografting

bodies directed against CD33 (146,147) and CD45 (148); ^{166}Ho, a β emitter with high affinity for bone (149,150); and radioactive iron (^{52}Fe), which is taken up avidly by the erythropoietic marrow (151,152).

In view of the potent GVL effect of alloSCT for CML, less intensive conditioning might be feasible, particularly for chronic-phase disease. The Hammersmith group has achieved adequate immunosuppression and myeloablation using busulfan alone (16 mg/kg) before second transplant in patients relapsing after previous BMT (153). Investigators in Perugia have shown that high doses of the nucleoside analog fludarabine have immunosuppressive activity equivalent to cyclophosphamide in a mouse model of alloSCT (154). The M.D. Anderson group have reported intriguing preliminary results using a nonablative fludarabine-based regimen before alloSCT and DLT in patients with advanced acute nonlymphocytic leukemia and myelodysplasia (155).

COMPLICATIONS

Major transplant-related complications include GVHD, graft failure, VOD, interstitial pneumonia, and infection, as reviewed elsewhere (51,156–158). For the purposes of this chapter, we will focus on GVHD.

Clinical Features of GVHD

GVHD (156–158) occurring in the first 100 days following alloSCT has conventionally been termed the "acute" form of the disease. This disorder arises because immunologically competent cells in the graft recognize and attack antigens in normal host tissue. The skin, gut, and liver are the organs most commonly affected. Severity of acute GVHD varies markedly; some patients develop a localized maculopapular rash, whereas others have life-threatening bullous desquamation, diarrhea, and/or hepatic failure.

Of those patients surviving the first months of alloSCT, a minority will go on to develop chronic GVHD, which has features in common with other immune disorders, such as scleroderma. Chronic GVHD may be disfiguring and debilitating and may involve multiple organs (e.g., eyes, mouth, and lungs) in addition to skin, gut, and liver. Occasional patients die if left untreated.

Treatment of GVHD

To prevent GVHD, combined cyclosporine and methotrexate therapy is preferred (159–166). The optimal timing and dosage of these drugs have not been established (166). Compared to HLA-identical sibling transplantation, the use of VUD alloSCT is associated with a higher frequency of chronic GVHD

(164,167). Moreover, the incidence of acute GHVD is also probably increased after VUD transplants (167–169).

Despite cyclosporine and methotrexate prophylaxis, some degree of GVHD arises in most patients; this will usually respond to treatment with corticosteroids. Perhaps 10–15% of patients will develop severe acute GVHD that remains refractory to steroid therapy. Such patients often fail to respond to other measures (e.g., antithymocyte globulin, Campath) and die of organ damage or infection related to suppressed immunity.

The risk of GVHD is markedly reduced if the graft is depleted of T cells (46,167,170–173). However, removal of T cells also increases the risk of graft rejection and leukemic relapse. That T-cell depletion predisposes to rejection suggests that the T cells have an important role in facilitating engraftment. The inverse relationship between GVHD and relapse suggests that GVHD is accompanied by a GVL effect mediated by T cells (174). At most centers *in vitro* T cell depletion is reserved for patients receiving grafts from unrelated or mismatched donors.

RESULTS OF alloSCT

Chronic Phase

CML can be cured by alloSCT carried out while the patient remains in chronic phase (4,99,102,175–177). Most survivors of BMT have normal hematopoiesis for follow-up periods that now extend beyond 10 years. Such patients have no evidence of residual leukemia, i.e., no detectable Ph chromosome on cytogenetic analysis or leukemia-specific BCR-ABL transcripts by the polymerase chain reaction (170,178,179).

AlloSCT Using HLA-Identical Sibling Donors

For the past 15 years the International Bone Marrow Transplant Registry has gathered data on patients undergoing BMT for CML. For 1699 patients transplanted in chronic phase between 1987 and 1994 with bone marrow from HLA-identical siblings, the 3-year probability of leukemia-free survival is 57% (180) (Fig. 3). However, this figure is partially based on patients transplanted with donor marrow depleted *ex vivo* of T cells to reduce the risk of GVHD, an approach that may delay or impair donor hematopoietic stem cell engraftment and increase the risk of leukemic relapse (170,173,175,176), as mentioned above. In an IBMTR analysis performed in 1992, the 5-year survival and leukemia-free survival were 58% and 54%, respectively, for patients whose transplants were not T-cell-depleted (181). Most hematological relapses occurred within 3 years of the transplant; the overall probability of relapse at 5 years was

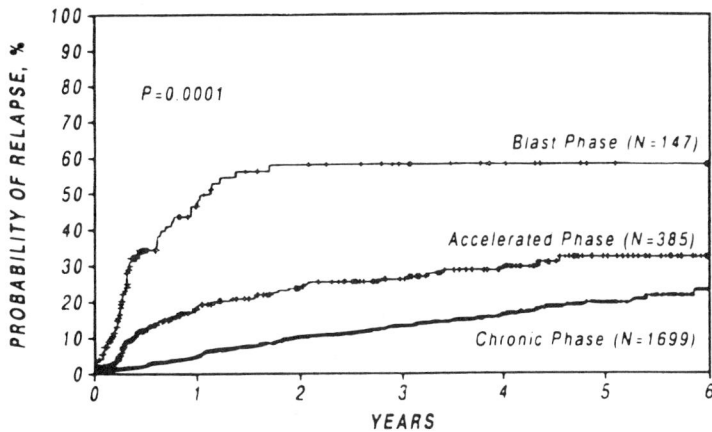

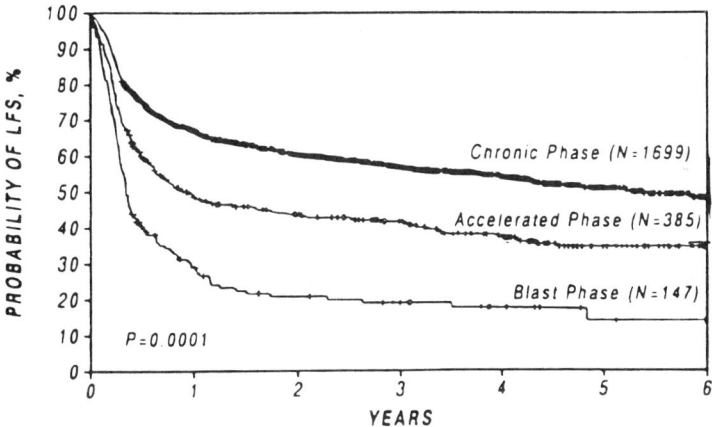

Figure 3 Probability of relapse (top) and leukemia free survival (LFS, bottom) after HLA-identical sibling bone marrow transplantation for CML in IBMTR series, 1987–1994. From Ref. 180.

19%. The relapse figure was 13% if recipients of T-cell-depleted marrow were excluded.

AlloSCT Using Volunteer Unrelated Donors

The incidence of successful engraftment is lower and GVHD and early mortality higher in recipients of marrow from HLA-identical volunteers than after BMT

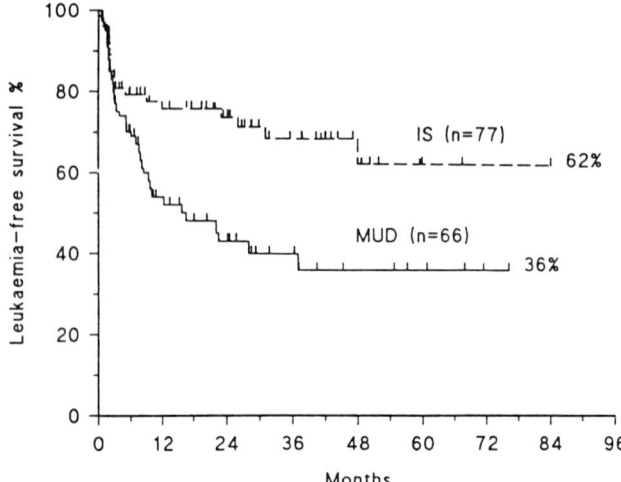

Figure 4 Actuarial leukemia-free survival for patients with CML in first chronic phase transplanted at the Hammersmith Hospital in London between 1988 and 1993. Results of identical sibling (IS, $n = 77$) donor transplants compared with "matched" unrelated donor (MUD, $n = 66$) transplants.

with marrow from HLA-matched siblings (4,167,172,182–185). This is likely to be related to imperfect matching for known HLA antigens or to unrecognized disparities between minor histocompatibility antigens. Recipients of HLA 1-antigen-mismatched marrow had a poorer outcome than those receiving HLA-matched marrow in two large multicenter series (4,167,182), although this difference was not observed in a single-institution study reported from Seattle (184). Acute and chronic GVHD are less frequent in recipients of marrow depleted of T cells *ex vivo*, but at the price of an increase in graft failure (3). Patients receiving unrelated donor grafts are also more likely to acquire serious viral or fungal infections in the first 6 months following alloSCT (164).

In 255 patients receiving VUD transplants who were analyzed by the IBMTR in 1992 (181), the overall survival and leukemia-free survival at 2 years were 38% and 35%, respectively. These results are inferior to what has been achieved with alloSCT using HLA-identical sibling donors (Figs. 3, 4). However, excellent results have been noted in a subset of younger patients transplanted with donors matched by high-resolution HLA typing (33) (Fig. 5).

Because of the greater risks of transplantation with unrelated donors, some centers reserve this approach for patients whose leukemia is resistant to more conservative therapy (e.g., hydroxyurea or IFN-α). Further assessment of the

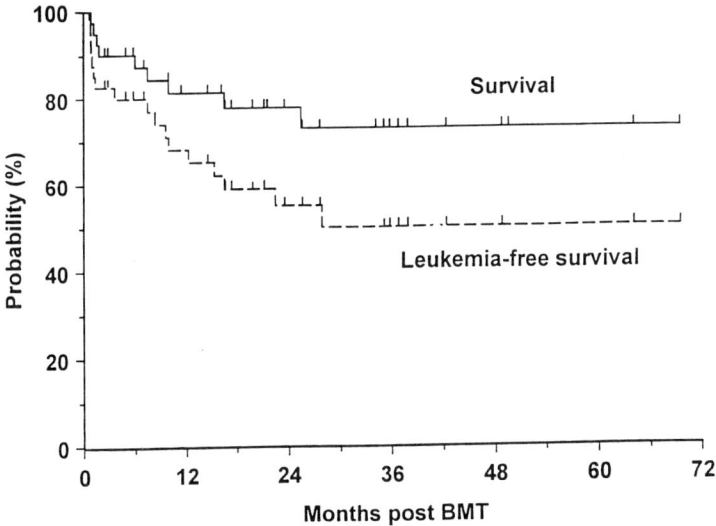

Figure 5 Probability of survival and leukemia-free survival for 40 Hammersmith Hospital patients in chronic phase at BMT, under 40 years of age, and matched with an unrelated donor by isoelectric focusing. From Ref. 33.

risk and benefit of unrelated donor BMT is required, particularly in older patients, and in relation to other potential treatments, such as IFN-α and autografting.

AlloSCT Using Family Members Other Than Genetically HLA-Identical Siblings

More than 500 patients lacking HLA-compatible siblings have been transplanted with marrow from family members other than genetically HLA-identical siblings (4,46,48,49,167,172,183,184,186). More intensive conditioning and immunosuppression are given to reduce the risk of graft rejection and GVHD (46,48), but mortality remains high. T-cell depletion of the graft results in less GVHD, but graft failure is more common and leukemia-free survival is not clearly improved (39,46).

AlloSCT for Advanced Disease

Patients with advanced disease have a poor prognosis with conventional treatment. AlloSCT is able to produce prolonged leukemia-free survival in a substantial minority of these patients, although the results are inferior to those achieved by allografting in chronic phase (4,46,84,86,90,92,99,102,126,167,170,182,186–191). The risk of GVHD (34,191), infection, and relapse is higher. As noted for chronic-phase disease, relapse is less common in patients who develop GVHD (192). The IBMTR actuarial figures for leukemia-free survival at 3 years following BMT with HLA-identical sibling donors performed in chronic and accelerated phase are 57% and 41%, respectively (180) (Fig. 3). In the Seattle series, as discussed by Clift (see Chap. 11), leukemia-free survival is comparable for patients transplanted in chronic and accelerated phase. Differing definitions of advanced-phase disease (191) may account for the superior outcome of Seattle patients transplanted in accelerated phase relative to those reported in the IBMTR series.

For patients transplanted in blastic phase, actuarial leukemia-free survival at 3 years is 18% in the IBMTR series (180) (Fig. 3). Patients allografted in frank blast crisis have an extremely dismal outlook, with a survival of between 0% and 6% (163,169). Rather than proceeding directly to alloSCT, many centers would first administer intensive "acute leukemia-type" therapy; better results may be possible following alloSCT in those patients who achieve a durable second chronic phase (163,169,193).

Prognosis

As discussed elsewhere in this volume (see Chap. 11), the prognosis of patients with CML undergoing alloSCT is determined by several factors, including disease phase (Fig. 3)(35,46,102,113,180,182,194), degree of HLA mismatch (Fig. 4) (1–4), and patient age (99,167,180,195). Patients <20 years of age have lower transplant-related mortality and higher leukemia-free survival than older patients. Outcome is somewhat poorer in patients >40 years of age (163), but there is no difference in survival between those 41–50 years versus those 51–60 years of age (see Chap. 11). Prognosis with BMT is better if the procedure is carried out in the first 1–2 years after diagnosis (35,99,180,195,196) (Fig. 6). Increased transplant-related mortality appears to be the primary reason for the unfavorable results of later transplantation (197). Prior busulfan therapy is an independent adverse risk factor (Fig. 6) (117,180,195), presumably due to the greater cumulative toxicity of this drug. It is unclear whether treatment with IFN-α for 6–18 months jeopardizes the result of a subsequent transplant (180,198,199).

GVL

The myeloablative conditioning regimen is undoubtedly essential to the cure of CML by transplantation. However, it has become evident that an immunologi-

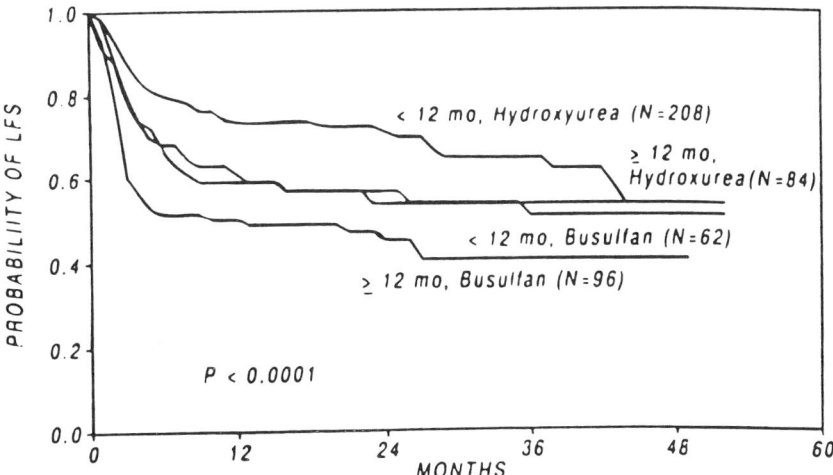

Figure 6 Probability of leukemia-free survival after HLA-identical sibling BMT for CML in first chronic phase according to interval between diagnosis and transplant and type of pre-BMT treatment. From Ref. 180.

cally mediated GVL effect is also important (174,197,200–204). The role of GVL is supported by the general observation that relapse occurs most often in patients who do not develop GVHD (35,174,200,201,205). Patients who receive syngeneic marrow have a higher incidence of relapse than recipients of marrow from HLA-identical siblings (180,201,206) (Fig. 7); the latter group has, in turn, an increased risk of relapse compared to patients receiving transplants from matched unrelated donors (35). GVHD is not seen in identical twin recipients and is less common with alloSCT from HLA-identical siblings than from unrelated donors. In HLA-identical sibling transplantation, when donor marrow is depleted of T lymphocytes, the incidence of GVHD falls and the frequency of leukemic relapse markedly rises. For VUD transplants, relapse is less common following T-cell depletion, presumably because the greater donor-recipient disparity compensates for the loss of GVL effect associated with removal of T cells (207).

In the event of leukemic relapse following transplantation, remission has been reinduced by the infusion of donor lymphocytes (208) (see below) or by abrupt discontinuation of immunosuppression (209), providing further evidence for the importance of GVL. T cells might mediate GVL by several mechanisms (202–204,210,211), including a natural killer cell response to leukemic cells (173,212–215), a T-cell response against tissue-specific antigens (202,216,217),

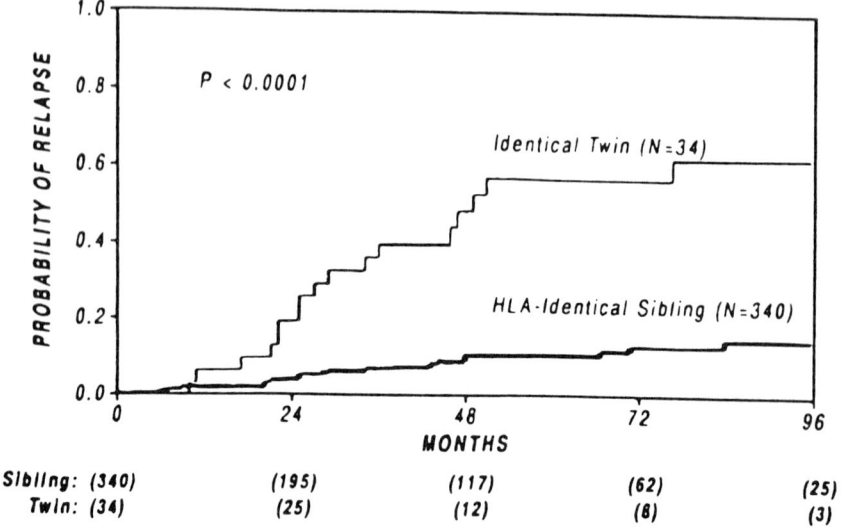

Figure 7 Probability of relapse after syngeneic and HLA-identical sibling BMT for CML in first chronic phase. From Ref. 180.

or release of cytokines (e.g., interleukin-2 or IFN-α or γ), which selectively suppress leukemic cell growth (218,219). In one study the combination of cyclosporine and selective depletion of donor CD8+ T-cells resulted in a reduction in acute GVHD without an increase in leukemic relapse (220,221), suggesting that GVHD and GVL are mediated by different T-cell subsets. The IBMTR has reported that syngeneic transplants are associated with increased relapse following BMT for acute and chronic myeloid leukemias but not acute lymphoblastic leukemia (206), suggesting that there may be an allogeneic GVL effect independent of GVHD (203). The mechanism for leukemic relapse is not established but may involve clonal evolution of residual leukemic cells, allowing immune escape from GVL (203,222).

MINIMAL RESIDUAL DISEASE

Patients can be monitored closely after transplant by serial cytogenetic studies and measurement of BCR-ABL transcripts using the reverse transcription-polymerase chain reaction (RT-PCR)(223–245).

Conventional Cytogenetics

Occasional patients may be found to have partially Ph-positive hematopoiesis months or years before hematological manifestations of relapse (242,246–249). Partially Ph-positive hematopoiesis has occasionally become entirely Ph-negative, a sequence of events that has been termed "transient cytogenetic relapse" (242,247). However, this phenomenon is generally associated with a high risk of subsequent progression to overt hematological relapse (242).

Polymerase Chain Reaction (PCR)

As blood and marrow samples give almost identical results for RT-PCR measurements of BCR-ABL transcripts (178,179,239,250), blood alone can be conveniently used (250). The assay can be rendered semiquantitative by using an artificial competing molecule that coamplifies and competes with the material collected from the patient (230,231,235)(Fig. 8). The proportion of Ph-positive metaphases in the bone marrow correlates with the number of BCR-ABL transcripts in blood. Ph-positive patients are invariably PCR-positive for BCR-ABL (237). One concern is that patients in apparent remission might harbor a pool of leukemic cells which fail to express BCR-ABL RNA; however, RT-PCR BCR-ABL transcript measurements and amplification of BCR-ABL in genomic DNA are usually concordant (245).

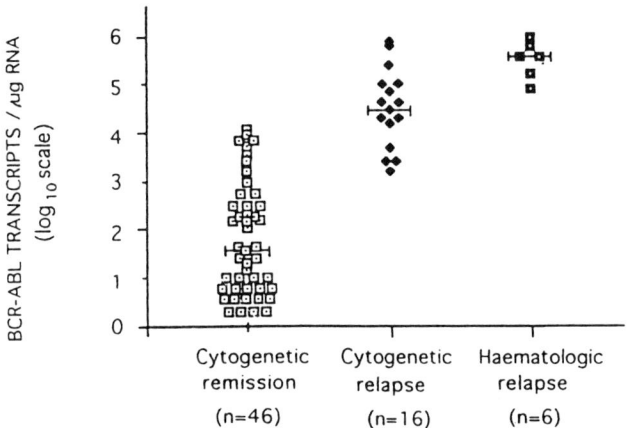

Figure 8 Number of BCR-ABL transcripts in patients in relapse after alloBMT related to cytogenetic and hematologic status. The majority of patients studied in cytogenetic remission were also negative for BCR-ABL transcripts and are therefore excluded from the figure. Data from the Hammersmith Hosptial, London, England.

It may be valuable to monitor patients with frequent PCR studies for some while after alloSCT, although results in the first 9 months posttransplant may be difficult to interpret. Increasing numbers of BCR-ABL transcripts after alloSCT predict for cytogenetic and subsequently hematological relapse in most cases (230–232,235). The majority of patients will be PCR-positive at least once in the first year after BMT, and almost half will have a positive result at 12 months (178,179,223,224,226). In some cases the PCR assay is positive for 3–9 months and then becomes negative (230,233,234), a phenomenon likely to be due to variable GVL activity. Other patients are persistently PCR-negative when studied repeatedly after alloSCT. Patients in both of these groups may become long-term disease-free survivors, but those who are persistently or intermittently PCR-positive >1 year after transplant are more likely to relapse than those who are persistently negative. Among 10-year survivors, most are PCR-negative but occasional patients are positive in blood or marrow without other evidence of relapse (251).

In patients who will eventually relapse the sequence of events is relatively consistent, although the speed of progression may be quite variable. Thus it is usually possible to identify a phase of *molecular relapse*, which proceeds subsequently to *cytogenetic relapse* and then to *hematological relapse*. Molecular relapse is defined as the observation of persisting high levels or rising levels of BCR-ABL transcripts >6 months posttransplant in the absence of a Ph chromosome in the marrow. As transcript levels rise further, an initially low number of Ph-positive metaphases can be identified, tantamount to cytogenetic relapse. Hematological relapse usually occurs when the proportion of Ph-positive marrow metaphases has reached 100%. This sequence presumably recapitulates the original evolution of disease before diagnosis. Occasional examples of a transient molecular relapse paralleling transient cytogenetic relapse have been seen.

In view of the probability that donor lymphocyte transfusion (DLT) is safer and more effective if initiated for a patient in molecular or cytogenetic relapse before the onset of hematological relapse, it may be advisable to monitor individual patients with PCR studies repeated at an interval of 1 or 2 months for the first 2 years posttransplant and thereafter at less frequent intervals.

Metaphase Fluorescence In Situ Hybridization (FISH)

Metaphase FISH allows direct visualization of the Ph translocation with high accuracy, while avoiding the risk of contamination associated with PCR. In contrast to interphase FISH, the technique examines dividing cells, which would theoretically be those most likely to have a role in leukemic relapse. The preparations are comparable to those used in standard cytogenetic analysis. However, more than 1000 metaphases can usually be examined in 3–6 hours by metaphase FISH, in contrast to 20 G-banded metaphases by the conventional technique.

Allografting

Using metaphase FISH in a small cohort of patients who had undergone alloSCT, El-Rifai and colleagues (241) have demonstrated that the absence of the Ph chromosome is predictive of remission and that increasing numbers of leukemic cells predict relapse.

The role of metaphase FISH relative to quantitative PCR has not been defined. The sensitivity of PCR may be as high as $1:10^4-10^5$ in the detection of Ph+ cells (247), in contrast to $1:10^2-10^3$ for metaphase FISH (241,253). One possibility is that using the two assays in combination might provide a powerful tool for detection of minimal residual disease (241).

MANAGEMENT OF RELAPSE

Hematological relapse after alloBMT occurs in 10–20% of recipients of unmanipulated donor marrow. The corresponding figure for patients treated with donor marrow depleted ex vivo of T cells is 60–80%. Relapse usually occurs within 3 years of BMT and evolves slowly over time (179). Occasional patients manifest blastic-phase disease as the first sign of relapse (99,153,248,254,255). Leukemic relapse has rarely been found in donor cells (255–257).

Relapse has been reported to occur as late as 7 years after transplant. At present there is no guarantee that even a 10-year disease-free survivor is cured, but this is likely in most cases (251). For treatment of relapse, one might administer conventional chemotherapy (254) or interferon-α (IFN-α), perform a second alloSCT, or infuse donor lymphocytes.

Interferon-α

When administered alone, IFN-α has clearly benefited a small group of patients with relapsed CML following alloSCT (249,258,259). Because of the risks of DLT, as discussed below, some clinicians would offer a trial of IFN-α as primary therapy to relapsing patients (249,258,259). Others would administer IFN-α in combination with DLT (208,260). The optimal approach has not been established. Whether routine prophylactic IFN-α therapy following alloSCT would reduce relapse has not been tested (261).

Second AlloSCT

Occasional relapsing patients have been treated successfully with a second BMT using the original donor (153,249,262,263). A second allograft is more likely to be successful if the interval between the two procedures exceeds 2 years (249,262). Because second transplants are associated with high mortality (249,263), less intensive conditioning may be appropriate (153).

Donor Lymphocyte Transfusion

Relapse following alloSCT can be treated by transfusion of leukocytes collected from the original donor without the use of cytotoxic drugs (212,264–281). Transfusion of donor-derived lymphocytes induces complete remission in 60–80% of patients who relapse into chronic phase and in some patients with more advanced disease. Most patients achieving complete cytogenetic remission revert from PCR-positive to PCR-negative. Responses generally occur within 1 to 9 months and are then usually durable.

DLT is most successful when performed in the first 2 years following alloSCT for patients manifesting molecular or cytogenetic (and not hematological) evidence of relapse (203,270,276,279). Remissions are also more common in patients who received T-cell-depleted transplants (258) and in those with limited GVHD prior to DLT. Following lymphocyte infusion, the development of acute and chronic GVHD is associated with a favorable response (203,279). However, in occasional patients the GVHD is severe and fatal.

The incidence and severity of GVHD correlate with lymphocyte dose (273,278). For patients with HLA-identical sibling donors who have relapsed in chronic phase, a dose escalation study suggested that 1×10^7 T cells per kg is the minimum dose required to induce remission without an unacceptable risk of GVHD (273). Higher numbers of T cells must be infused for accelerated-phase relapse (267). It is possible that lower lymphocyte doses may be effective for patients with mismatched or unrelated donors. However, the risk of GVHD doses not seem to be increased in patients receiving lymphocytes from unrelated donors (275).

In approximately 10–20% of patients, marrow aplasia occurs (260, 279,282). This complication is more likely in patients with overt hematological relapse and limited donor hematopoiesis prior to DLT (280). The pancytopenia usually improves with transfusion of progenitor cells from the original donor (208,276).

Because of the high success rate for DLT, it should probably be attempted before submitting a patient to a second transplant procedure. However, the precise timing of DLT is a matter of debate. At the Hammersmith Hospital, DLT is performed prior to hematological relapse in patients with increasing BCR-ABL transcripts in blood or Ph-positive metaphases in marrow (271,281). The optimal cell dose is not established (278,283). It is also not clear whether a patient who receives DLT for treatment of relapse should be given GVHD prophylaxis. Discontinuation of cyclosporine immunosuppression has been reported to reinduce complete remission even without DLT (209).

Novel Approaches

The efficacy of DLT is further evidence for a GVL effect, as mentioned above, but the nature of the effector cells is not known (202,203,210). The separation of GVL from GVHD is a fundamental challenge in transplantation. One approach is to perform the initial alloSCT using a T-cell-depleted graft, thus reducing the risk of severe acute GVHD in the immediate posttransplant period. Following engraftment and recovery from the early toxicity of the conditioning, DLT (or "lymphocyte add-back") is performed to confer the GVL effect (203,284,285). In CML patients who relapse following alloSCT, Giralt and colleagues (221) have reported that DLT selectively depleted of CD8+ cells were effective in treating the relapse with a low risk of GVHD. A group of Italian investigators (286) have treated leukemic relapse by infusing donor lymphocytes which had been transduced ex vivo with the *Herpes simplex* thymidine kinase gene; patients who developed unacceptable GVHD were treated with ganciclovir to eliminate the offending lymphocyte population. To augment GVL, the Hadassah group has infused interleukin-2 in conjunction with DLT (277). One of the most intriguing possibilities would be to generate cytotoxic T lymphocytes which are alloreactive against leukemia-specific antigens in vitro, and then to administer these targeted cells to patients as immunotherapy (217,287–289).

LIMITATIONS OF AlloSCT

As discussed above, alloSCT has a number of limitations as treatment of CML. Appropriate donors can be found for only a minority of patients. Only about 15% of all patients with CML in chronic phase can be allografted using sibling donors (Fig. 1). Nonsibling family members and unrelated volunteers are found to be acceptable donors for perhaps another 15%. GVHD affects 40–60% of "good-risk" patients and is fatal in perhaps 10% overall. GVHD is more severe in patients with advanced disease, in older patients, and in those who receive grafts from donors other than HLA-identical siblings.

AN INTEGRATED APPROACH

The primary objective in the newly diagnosed patient with CML is to prevent or delay transformation to blastic phase. Guidelines for management of a patient <60 years of age are provided in Figure 9 and in Chapter 11. These approaches are in general agreement.

If an HLA-identical sibling is available, alloSCT should be performed as early as feasible. For patients 40 years of age or older, one might postpone the transplant to allow a trial of IFN-α. If the patient achieves a cytogenetic response, alloSCT could be postponed until there is evidence of IFN-α resistance. Debatable points are the use of blood-derived rather than marrow cells, the

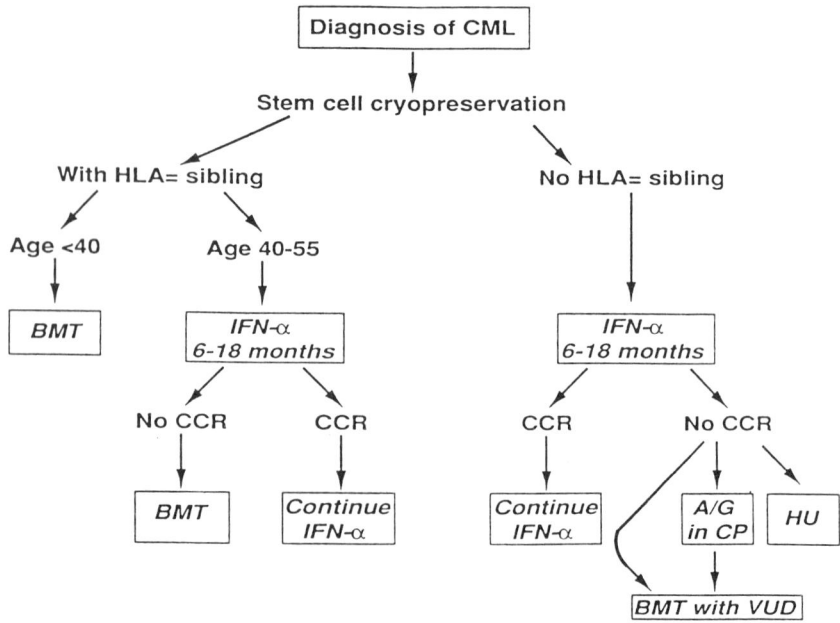

Figure 9 A possible approach to the management of CML in patients under 60 years of age. (CCR = continuous cytogenetic response; VUD = volunteer unrelated donor; BMT = bone marrow transplantation; IFN = interferon.)

upper age limit for alloSCT, the age at which an initial trial of IFN-α is appropriate, and the duration of IFN-α therapy if a cytogenetic response is not achieved within 6 months.

If a patient has no HLA-identical sibling, an initial trial of IFN-α would seem reasonable. If a durable cytogenetic response is obtained, IFN-α should probably be continued indefinitely. For patients who cannot tolerate IFN-α or who fail to achieve cytogenetic conversion after treatment for 12–18 months, consideration should be given to a different strategy, such as hydroxyurea therapy. If an appropriate alternative donor has been identified in the interim, this option should be considered. Patients reluctant to undergo the formidable risks involved in alloSCT may be candidates for autografting. Points that are still a matter of debate include the duration of therapy with IFN-α, whether to proceed to allografting rather than autografting, what degree of HLA incompatibility is acceptable, and the details of conditioning and GVHD prophylaxis at transplant.

REFERENCES

1. Clift RA, Hansen JA, Thomas ED, et al. Marrow transplantation from donors other than HLA-identical siblings. Transplantation 1979; 28:235–242.
2. Beatty PG, Nash RA, Mickelson EM, et al. Marrow transplantation from related donors other than HLA-identical siblings. N Engl J Med 1985; 313:765–771.
3. Anasetti C, Amos D, Beatty PG, et al. Effect of HLA compatibility on engraftment of bone marrow transplants in patients with leukemia or lymphoma. N Engl J Med 1989; 320:197–204.
4. Szydlo RM, Goldman JM, Klein JP, et al. Results of allogeneic bone marrow transplantation for leukemia using donors other than HLA-identical siblings. J Clin Oncol 1997; 15:1767–1777.
5. Westoff CF. Fertility in the United States. Science 1986; 234:544–549.
6. Vowels MR, Honeyman M. Ziegler J, et al. Searches for matched and closely matched related and unrelated marrow donors undertaken in a pediatric unit. J Pediatr Child Health 1992; 28:379–382.
7. Beatty PG, Dahlberg S, Mickelson EM, et al. Probability of finding HLA-matched unrelated marrow donors. Transplantation 1988: 45:714.
8. Anasetti C, Howe C, Petersdorf EW, Martin PJ, Hansen JA. Marrow transplants from HLA matched unrelated donors: an NMDP update and the Seattle experience. Bone Marrow Transplant 1994; 13:693–695.
9. Charron DJ. HLA matching in unrelated donor bone marrow transplantation. Curr Opinion Hematol 1996; 3:416–422.
10. Freytes CO, Beatty PG. Representation of Hispanics in the National Marrow Donor Program. Bone Marrow Transplant 1996; 17:323–327.
11. Mori M, Graves M, Milford EL, Beatty PG. Computer program to predict likelihood of finding an HLA-matched donor: methodology, validation, and application. Biol Blood Marrow Transplant 1996; 2:134–144.
12. Terasaki PI, McLelland JD. Microdroplet assay of human serum cytotoxins. Nature 1964; 204:998–1000.
13. Poynton C. Matching techniques and HLA typing. In: Treleaven J, Barrett J, eds. Bone Marrow Transplantation in Practice. Edinburgh; Churchill Livingstone, 1992: 187–206.
14. Tiercy J-M, Roosnek E, Speiser D, et al. Replacement of HLA class II serology by the HLA-DR microtitre plate oligotyping assay: a one-year experience in unrelated bone marrow donor selection. Br J Haematol 1993; 85:417–418.
15. Santamaria P, Reinsmoen NL, Lindstrom AL, et al. Frequent HLA class I and DP sequence mismatches in serologically (HLA-A, HLA-B, HLA-DR) and molecularly (HLA-DRB1, HLA-DQA1, HLA-DQB1) HLA-identical unrelated bone marrow transplant pairs. Blood 1994; 83:280–287.
16. Nademanee A, Schmidt GM, Parker P, et al. The outcome of matched unrelated donor bone marrow transplantation in patients with hematologic malignancies using molecular typing for donor selection and graft-versus-host disease prophylaxis regimen of cyclosporine, methotrexate, and prednisone. Blood 1995; 86:1228–1234.

17. Speiser DE, Tiercy J-M, Rufer N, et al. High resolution HLA matching associated with decreased mortality after unrelated bone marrow transplantation. Blood 1996; 87:4455–4462.
18. Devergie A, Apperley JF, Labopin M, et al. European results of matched unrelated donor bone marrow transplantation for chronic myeloid leukemia. Impact of HLA class II matching. Bone Marrow Transplant 1997; 20:11–20.
19. Neefjes JJ, Breur-Vriesendrop BS, van Seventer GA, Iványi P, Ploegh HL. An improved biochemical method for the analysis of HLA-class I antigens. Definition of new HLA-class I subtypes. Human Immunol 1986; 16:169–181.
20. Noreen HJ, Davidson ML, McCullough J, Bach FH, Segall M. HLA class II typing by restriction fragment length polymorphism (RFLP) in unrelated bone marrow transplant patients. Transplant Proc 1989; 21:2968–2970.
21. Tiercy J-M, Morel C, Freidel AC, et al. Selection of unrelated donors for bone marrow transplantation is improved by HLA class II genotyping with oligonucleotide hybridization. Proc Natl Acad Sci 1991; 88:7121–7125.
22. Petersdorf EW, Longton GM, Anasetti C, et al. The significance of HLA-DRB1 matching on clinical outcome after HLA-A, B, DR identical unrelated donor marrow transplantation. Blood 1995; 86:1606–1613.
23. Williams F, Mawhinney H, Middleton D. Application of an HLA-B PCR-SSOP typing method to a bone marrow donor registry. Bone Marrow Transplant 1997; 19:205–208.
24. Petersdorf EW, Longton GM, Anasetti C, et al. Association of HLA-C disparity with graft failure after marrow transplantation from unrelated donors. Blood 1997; 89:1818–1823.
25. Petersdorf EW, Stanley JF, Martin PJ, Hansen JA. Molecular diversity of the HLA-C locus in unrelated marrow transplantation. Tissue Antigens 1994; 44: 93–99.
26. Nagler A, Brautbar C, Slavin S, Bishara A. Bone marrow transplantation using unrelated and family donors: the impact of HLA-C disparity. Bone Marrow Transplant 1996; 18:891–897.
27. DeGast GC, Mickelson EM, Beatty PG, et al. Mixed leukocyte culture reactivity and graft-versus-host disease in HLA-identical marrow transplantation for leukemia. Bone Marrow Transplant 1992; 9:87–90.
28. Lim SH, Patton WM, Jobson S. et al. Mixed lymphocyte reactions do not predict severity of graft-versus-host disease (GvHD) in HLA-DR compatible sibling bone marrow transplants. Clin Pathol 1988; 41:1155–1157.
29. Mickelson EM, Bartsch GE, Hansen JA, Dupont B. The MLC assay as a test for HLA-D region compatibility between patients and unrelated donors: results of a National Marrow Donor Program involving multiple centers. Tissue Antigens 1993; 42:465–472.
30. Mickelson EM, Guthrie LA, Etzioni R, Anasetti C, Martin PJ, Hansen JA. Role of the mixed lymphocyte culture (MLC) reaction in marrow donor selection: matching for transplants from related haploidentical donors. Tissue Antigens 1994; 44:83–92.
31. Roosnek E, Hoogendjik S, Zawadynski S, et al. The frequency of pre-transplant cytotoxic lymphocyte precursors with anti-host specificity predicts survival of pa-

tients transplanted with bone marrow from donors other than HLA-identical siblings. Transplantation 1993; 56:691–696.
32. Spencer A, Brookes PA, Kaminski E, et al. Cytotoxic T lymphocyte precursor frequency analyses in bone marrow transplantation with volunteer unrelated donors. Value in donor selection. Transplantation 1995; 59:1302–1308.
33. Spencer A, Szydlo RM, Brookes PA, et al. Bone marrow transplantation for chronic myeloid leukemia with volunteer unrelated donors using ex vivo or 'in vivo' T-cell depletion: major prognostic impact of HLA class I identity between donor and recipient. Blood 1995; 86:3590–3597.
34. Nash RA, Pepe MS, Storb R, et al. Acute graft-versus-host disease: analysis of risk factors after allogeneic marrow transplantation and prophylaxis with cyclosporine and methotrexate. Blood 1992; 80:1838–1845.
35. Enright H, Davies SM, DeFor T, et al. Relapse after non-T-cell-depleted allogeneic bone marrow transplantation for chronic myelogenous leukemia: early transplantation, use of an unrelated donor, and chronic graft-versus-host disease are protective. Blood 1996; 88:714–720.
36. Meyers JD, Flournoy N, Thomas ED, et al. Non-bacterial pneumonia after allogeneic bone marrow transplantation: a review of ten years experience. Rev Infect Dis 1982; 4:1119–1132.
37. Meyers JD. Prevention and treatment of cytomegalovirus infection after marrow transplantation. Bone Marrow Transplant 1988; 3:95–104.
38. Anasetti C, Beatty PG, Storb R, et al. Effect of HLA incompatibility on graft-versus-host disease, relapse, and survival after marrow transplantation for patients with leukemia or lymphoma. Hum Immunol 1990; 29: 79–91.
39. Ash RC, Horowitz MM, Gale RP, et al. Bone marrow transplantation from related donors other than HLA-identical siblings: effect of T-cell depletion. Bone Marrow Transplant 1991; 7:443–452.
40. Hansen, JA, Anasetti C, Petersdorf EW, Choo SY, Mickelson EM, Martin PJ. The status of clinical marrow transplantation and current issues in donor matching. In: Tsuju K, Aizawa M, Sasazuki T, eds. HLA 1991—Proceedings of the Eleventh International Histocompatibility Workshop and Conference. Oxford; Oxford Science Publications, 1992; 13.
41. Schipper RF, D'Amaro J. Outshoorn M. The probability of finding a suitable related donor for bone marrow transplantation in extended families. Blood 1996; 87:800–804.
42. Hows JM, Yin JL, Marsh J, et al. Histocompatible unrelated volunteer donors compared with HLA nonidentical family donors in marrow transplantation for aplastic anemia and leukemia. Blood 1986; 68:1322–1328.
43. Hansen JA, Petersdorf EW, Choo SY, Martin PJ, Anasetti C. Marrow transplantation from HLA partially matched relatives and unrelated donors. Bone Marrow Transplant 1995; 15(suppl 1):S128–S139.
44. Fujimori Y, Kanamaru A, Hashimoto N, et al. Second transplantation with CD34+ bone marrow cells selected from a two-loci HLA-mismatched sibling for a patient with chronic myeloid leukaemia. Br J Haematol 1996; 94:123–125.
45. Ottinger H, Beelen D, Sayer H, Schaefer UW, Grosse-Wilde H. Bone marrow transplantation from partially matched HLA-matched related donors in adults with

leukaemia: the experience at the University Hospital of Essen, Germany. Br J Haematol 1996; 92:913–921.
46. Henslee-Downey PJ, Abhyankar SH, Parrish RS, et al. Use of partially mismatched related donors extends access to allogeneic marrow transplant. Blood 1997; 89:3864–3872.
47. Munn RK, Henslee-Downey PJ, Romond EH, et al. Treatment of leukemia with partially matched related bone marrow transplantation. Bone Marrow Transplant 1997; 19:421–427.
48. Speiser DE, Hermans J, van Biezen A, et al. Haploidentical family member transplants for patients with chronic myeloid leukaemia: a report of the Chronic Leukaemia Working Party of the European Group for Blood and Marrow Transplantation. Bone Marrow Transplant 1997; 19:1197–1204.
49. Soiffer RJ, Mauch P, Fairclough D, et al. CD6+ T cell depleted allogeneic bone marrow transplantation from genotypically HLA non-identical related donors. Biol Blood Marrow Transplant 1997; 3:11–17.
50. Gahrton G. Bone marrow transplantation with unrelated volunteer donors. Eur J Cancer 1991; 27:1537–1539.
51. Bociek RG, Stewart DA, Armitage JO. Bone marrow transplantation—current concepts. J Invest Med 1995; 43:127–135.
52. Bogdaníc V, Nemet D, Kastelan A, et al. Umbilical cord blood transplantation in a patient with Philadelphia chromosome-positive chronic myeloid leukemia. Transplantation 1993; 56:477–479.
53. Gale RP. Cord-blood-cell transplantation—a real *Sleeper*. N Engl J Med 1995; 332:392–394.
54. Wagner JE, Kernan NA, Steinbuch M, Broxmeyer HE, Gluckman E. Allogeneic sibling umbilical-cord-blood transplantation in children with malignant and non-malignant disease. Lancet 1995; 346:214–219.
55. Abecasis MM, Machado AM, Boavida G, et al. Haploidentical cord blood transplantation contaminated with maternal T cells in a patient with advanced leukaemia. Bone Marrow Transplant 1996; 17:891–895.
56. Fernández MN, Regidor C, Díez JL, et al. HLA haploidentical cord blood cell transplant in a 15-year-old, 50 kg weight patient: successful treatment for chronic myeloid leukemia after myeloid blastic transformation. Bone Marrow Transplant 1996; 17:1175–1178.
57. Gluckman E. The therapeutic potential of fetal and neonatal hematopoietic stem cells. N Engl J Med 1996; 335:1839–1840.
58. Kurtzberg J, Laughlin M, Graham ML, et al. Placental blood as a source of hematopoietic stem cells for transplantation into unrelated recipients. N Engl J Med 1996; 335:157–166.
59. Laporte J-P, Gorin N-C, Rubinstein P, et al. Cord-blood transplantation from an unrelated donor in an adult with chronic myelogenous leukemia. N Engl J Med 1996; 335:167–170.
60. Wagner JE, Rosenthal J, Sweetman R, et al. Successful transplantation of HLA-matched and HLA-mismatched umbilical cord blood from unrelated donors: analysis of engraftment and acute graft-versus-host disease. Blood 1996; 88:795–802.

61. Harris DT, Schumacher MJ, Locascio J, et al. Phenotypic and functional immaturity of human umbilical cord blood T lymphocytes. Proc Natl Acad Sci USA 1992; 89:10006–10010.
62. Roncarolo MG, Bigler M, Cuiti E, Martino S, Tovo P-A. Immune responses by cord blood cells. Blood Cells 1994; 20:573–586.
63. Garban F, Ericson M, Roucard C, et al. Detection of empty HLA class II molecules on cord blood B cells. Blood 1996; 87:3970–3976.
64. DiGiusto DL, Lee R, Moon J, et al. Hematopoietic potential of cryopreserved and ex vivo manipulated umbilical cord blood progenitor cells evaluated in vitro and in vivo. Blood 1996; 87:1261–1271.
65. Stroncek DF, Holland PV, Bartsch G, et al. Experiences of the first 493 unrelated marrow donors in the National Marrow Donor Program. Blood 1993; 81:1940–1946.
66. Dreger P, Haferlach T, Eckstein V, et al. Harvesting G-CSF-mobilised peripheral blood progenitor cells for allogeneic transplantation. Safety, kinetics of mobilisation and composition of the graft. Br J Haematol 1994; 87:609–613.
67. Bensinger WI. Transplantation of allogeneic peripheral blood stem cells mobilized by recombinant granulocyte colony stimulating factor. Blood 1995; 85:1655.
68. Goldman J. Peripheral blood stem cells for allografting. Blood 1995; 85:1413–1415.
69. Körbling M, Przepiorka D, Huh YO, et al. Allogeneic blood stem cell transplantation for refractory leukemia and lymphoma: potential advantage of blood over marrow allografts. Blood 1995; 85:1659–1665.
70. Lane RA, Law P, Maruyama M, et al. Harvesting and enrichment of hematopoietic progenitor cells mobilized into the peripheral blood of normal donors by granulocyte-macrophage colony-stimulating factor (GM-CSF) or G-CSF: potential role in allogeneic marrow transplantation. Blood 1995; 85:275–282.
71. Russell JA, Luider J, Weaver M, et al. Collection of progenitor cells for allogeneic transplantation from peripheral blood of normal donors. Bone Marrow Transplant 1995; 15:111–115.
72. Schmitz N, Dreger P, Suttorp M, et al. Primary transplantation of allogeneic peripheral blood progenitor cells mobilized by filgrastim (granulocyte colony-stimulating factor). Blood 1995; 85:1666–1672.
73. Bacigalupo A, Van Lint MT, Valbonesi M, et al. Thiotepa cyclophosphamide followed by granulocyte colony-stimulating factor mobilized allogeneic peripheral blood cells in adults with advanced leukemia. Blood 1996; 88:353–357.
74. Tanaka R, Matsudaira T, Aizawa J, et al. Characterization of peripheral blood progenitor cells (PBPC) mobilized by filgastrim (rHuG-CSF) in normal volunteers: dose-effect relationship for filgrastim with the character of mobilized PBPC. Br J Haematol 1996; 92:795–803.
75. Miflin G, Charley C, Stainer C, Anderson S, Hunter A, Russell NH. Stem cell mobilization in normal donors for allogeneic transplantation: analysis of safety and factors affecting efficacy. Br J Haematol 1996; 95:345–348.
76. Russell JA, Brown C, Bowen T, et al. Allogeneic blood cell transplants for haematological malignancy: preliminary comparison of outcomes with bone marrow transplantation. Bone Marrow Transplant 1996; 17:703–708.

77. Waller CF, Bertz H, Wenger MK, et al. Mobilization of peripheral blood progenitor cells for allogeneic transplantation: efficacy and toxicity of a high-dose rhG-CSF regimen. Bone Marrow Transplant 1996; 18:279–283.
78. Hasenclever D, Sextro M. Safety of alloPBSCT donors: biometrical considerations on monitoring long term risks. Bone Marrow Transplant 1996; 17(suppl 2):S28–S30).
79. Weaver CH, Longin K, Buckner CD, Bensinger W. Lymphocyte content in peripheral blood mononuclear cells collected after the administration of recombinant human granulocyte colony stimulating factor. Bone Marrow Transplant 1994; 13:411–415.
80. Bensinger WI, Buckner CD, Demirer T, Storb R, Appelbaum FA. Transplantation of allogeneic peripheral blood stem cells. Bone Marrow Transplant 1996; 17(suppl 2):S56–S57.
81. Schmitz N, Bacigalupo A, Labopin M, et al. Transplantation of allogeneic peripheral blood progenitor cells—the EBMT experience. Bone Marrow Transplant 1996; 17(suppl 2):S40–S46.
82. Miflin G, Russell NH, Hutchinson RM, et al. Allogeneic peripheral blood stem cell transplantation for haematological malignancies—an analysis of kinetics of engraftment and GVHD risk. Bone Marrow Transplant 1997; 19:9–13.
83. Przepiorka D, Anderlini P, Ippoliti C, et al. Allogeneic blood stem cell transplantation in advanced hematologic cancers. Bone Marrow Transplant 1997; 19:455–460.
84. Doney K, Buckner CD, Sale GE, Ramberg R, Boyd C, Thomas ED. Treatment of chronic granulocytic leukemia by chemotherapy, total body irradiation and allogeneic bone marrow transplantation. Exp Hematol 1978; 6:738–747.
85. Fefer A, Cheever MA, Thomas ED, et al. Disappearance of Ph1-positive cells in four patients with chronic granulocytic leukemia after chemotherapy, irradiation and marrow transplantation from an identical twin. N Engl J Med 1979; 300:333–337.
86. Doney KC, Buckner CD, Thomas ED, et al. Allogeneic bone marrow transplantation for chronic granulocytic leukemia. Exp Hematol 1981; 9:966–971.
87. Fefer A, Cheever MA, Greenberg PD, et al. Treatment of chronic granulocytic leukemia with chemoradiotherapy and transplantation of marrow from identical twins. N Engl J Med 1982; 306:63–68.
88. Tutschka PJ, Santos GW, Elfenbein GJ. Marrow transplantation in acute leukemia following busulfan and cyclophosphamide. Blut 1980; 25:375–380.
89. Santos GW, Tutschka PJ, Brookmeyer R, et al. Marrow transplantation for acute non-lymphocytic leukemia after treatment with busulfan and cyclophosphamide. N Engl J Med 1983; 309:1347–1353.
90. Copelan EA, Grever MR, Kapoor N, Tutschka PJ. Marrow transplantation following busulfan and cyclophosphamide for chronic myelogenous leukaemia in accelerated or blastic phase. Br J Haematol 1989; 71:487–491.
91. Petersen FB, Buckner CD, Appelbaum FR, et al. Busulfan, cyclophosphamide and fractionated total body irradiation as a preparatory regimen for marrow transplantation in patients with advanced hematological malignancies: a phase I study. Bone Marrow Transplant 1989; 4:617–623.

92. Blume KG, Kopecky KJ, Henslee-Downey JP, et al. A prospective randomized comparison of total body irradiation—etoposide versus busulfan-cyclophosphamide as preparatory regimens for bone marrow transplantation in patients with leukemia who were not in first remission: a Southwest Oncology Group study. Blood 1993; 81:2187–2193.
93. Clift RA, Buckner CD, Thomas ED, et al. Marrow transplantation for chronic myeloid leukemia: a randomized study comparing cyclophosphamide and total body irradiation with busulfan and cyclophosphamide. Blood 1994; 84:2036–2043.
94. Devergie A, Blaise D, Attal M, et al. Allogeneic bone marrow transplantation for chronic myeloid leukemia in first chronic phase: a randomized trial of busulfan-cytoxan versus cytoxan-total body irradiation as preparative regimen: a report from the French Society of Bone Marrow Graft (SFGM). Blood 1995; 85:2263–2268.
95. Demirer T, Buckner CD, Appelbaum FR, et al. Busulfan, cyclophosphamide and fractionated total body irradiation for allogeneic marrow transplantation in advanced acute and chronic myelogenous leukemia: phase I dose escalation of busulfan based on targeted plasma levels. Bone Marrow Transplant 1996; 17:341–346.
96. Vey N, De Prijck B, Faucher C, et al. A pilot study of busulfan and melphalan as preparatory regimen prior to allogeneic bone marrow transplantation in refractory or relapsed hematological malignancies. Bone Marrow Transplant 1996; 18:495–499.
97. Hows JM, Mehta A, Ward L, et al. Comparison of mesna with forced diuresis to prevent cyclophosphamide induced haemorrhagic cystitis in marrow transplantation: a prospective randomised study. Br J Cancer 1984; 50:753–756.
98. Storb R, Thomas ED, Weiden PL, et al. Aplastic anemia treated by allogeneic bone marrow transplantation. A report on 49 new cases from Seattle. Blood 1976; 48:817–823.
99. Thomas ED, Clift RA, Fefer A, et al. Marrow transplantation for the treatment of chronic myelogenous leukemia. Ann Intern Med 1986; 104:155–163.
100. Clift RA, Buckner CD, Appelbaum FR, et al. Allogeneic marrow transplantation in patients with chronic myeloid leukemia in the chronic phase: a randomized trial of two irradiation regimens. Blood 1991; 77:1660–1665.
101. Cunningham I, Castro-Malaspina H, Flomenberg N, et al. Improved results of bone marrow transplantation (BMT) for chronic myelogenous leukemia using marrow depleted of T cells by soybean lectin agglutination and E-rosette depletion. In: Gale RP, Champlin RE, eds. Progress in Bone Marrow Transplantation. New York: Alan R. Liss, 1987:359–363.
102. Goldman JM, Apperley JF, Jones L, et al. Bone marrow transplantation for patients with chronic myeloid leukemia. N Engl J Med 1986; 314:202–207.
103. Peters LJ, Withers R, Cundiff JH, Dicke KA. Radiobiological considerations in the use of total body irradiation for bone marrow transplantation. Radiology 1979; 131:243–247.
104. Cosset JM, Baume D, Pico JL, et al. Single dose versus hyperfractionated total body irradiation before allogeneic bone marrow transplantation: a non-randomized

comparative study of 54 patients at the Institut Gustave-Roussy. Radiat Oncol 1989; 15:151–160.
105. Altschuler C, Resbeut M, Maraninchi D, et al. Fractionated total body irradiation and allogeneic bone marrow transplantation for standard risk leukaemia. Radiat Oncol 1989; 16:289–295.
106. Barrett-Lee P. In: Treleaven J, Barrett J, eds. Bone Marrow Transplantation in Practice. Edinburgh: Churchill Livingstone, 1992; 187–206.
107. Deeg HJ, Sullivan KM, Buckner CD, et al. Marrow transplantation for acute non-lymphoblastic leukemia in first remission: toxicity and long term follow-up of patients conditioned with single or fractionated total body irradiation. Bone Marrow Transplant 1986; 1:151–157.
108. Sloane JP, Depledge M, Powles RL, Morgenstern GR, Trickey BS, Dady PJ. Histopathology of the lung afer total body irradiation. J Clin Pathol 1983; 36: 546–554.
109. Weiner RS, Bortin MM, Gale RP, et al. Interstitial pneumonitis after bone marrow transplantation. Assessment of risk factors. Ann Intern Med 1986; 104:168–175.
110. Copelan EA, Deeg HJ. Conditioning for allogeneic marrow transplantation in patients with lymphohematopoietic malignancies without the use of total body irradiation. Blood 1992; 80:1648–1658.
111. Deeg HJ, Spitzer TR, Cottler-Fox M, Cahill R, Pickle LW. Conditioning-related toxicity and acute graft-versus-host disease in patients given methotrexate/cyclosporine prophylaxis. Bone Marrow Transplant 1991; 7:193–198.
112. Bearman SI. The syndrome of hepatic veno-occlusive disease after marrow transplantation. Blood 1995; 85:3005–3020.
113. Speck B, Bortin MM, Champlin R. Allogeneic bone marrow transplantation for chronic myelogenous leukemia. Lancet 1984; 1:665–668.
114. Lynch MH, Petersen FB, Appelbaum FR, et al. Phase II study of busulfan, cyclophosphamide and fractionated total body irradiation as a preparatory regimen for allogeneic bone marrow transplantation in patients with advanced myeloid malignancies. Bone Marrow Transplant 1995; 15:59–64.
115. Schattenberg A, Preijers F, Mensink E, et al. Survival in first or second remission after lymphocyte-depleted transplantation for Philadelphia chromosome-positive CML in first chronic phase. Bone Marrow Transplant 1997; 19:1205–1212.
116. Tutschka PJ, Copelan EA, Klein JP. Bone marrow transplantation for leukemia following a new busulfan and cyclophosphamide regimen. Blood 1987; 70:1382–1388.
117. Biggs JC, Szer J, Crilley P, et al. Treatment of chronic myeloid leukemia with allogeneic bone marrow transplantation after preparation with BuCy2. Blood 1992; 80:1352–1357.
118. Mehta J, Powles R, Mitchell P, et al. Graft failure after bone marrow transplantation from unrelated donors using busulfan and cyclophosphamide for conditioning. Bone Marrow Transplant 1994; 13:583–587.
119. deMagalhaes-Silverman M, Bloom EJ, Donnenberg A, et al. Toxicity of busulfan and cyclophosphamide (BU/CY2) in patients with hematologic malignancies. Bone Marrow Transplant 1996; 17:329–333.

120. Sahebi F, Copelan E, Crilley P, et al. Unrelated allogeneic bone marrow transplantation using high-dose busulfan and cyclophosphamide (BU-CY) for the preparative regimen. Bone Marrow Transplant 1996; 17:685–689.
121. Klein JL, Avalos BR, Belt P, et al. Bone marrow engraftment following unrelated donor transplantation utilizing busulfan and cyclophosphamide preparatory chemotherapy. Bone Marrow Transplant 1996; 17:479–483.
122. Bertz H, Potthoff K, Mertelsmann R, Finke J. Busulfan/cyclophosphamide in volunteer unrelated donor (VUD) BMT: excellent feasibility and low incidence of treatment-related toxicity. Bone Marrow Transplant 1997; 19:1169–1173.
123. Vassal G, Deroussent A, Challine D, et al. Is 600 mg/m^2 the appropriate dosage of busulfan in children undergoing bone marrow transplantation? Blood 1992; 79: 2475–2479.
124. Ehninger G, Schuler U, Renner U, et al. Use of a water-soluble busulfan formulation—pharmacokinetic studies in a canine model. Blood 1995; 85:3247–3249.
125. Grochow LB, Jones RJ, Brundrett RB, et al. Pharmacokinetics of busulfan: correlation with veno-occlusive disease in patients undergoing bone marrow transplantation. Cancer Chemother Pharmacol 1989; 25:55–61.
126. Clift RA, Storb R. Marrow transplantation for CML: the Seattle experience. Bone Marrow Transplant 1996; 17(suppl 3):S1–S3.
127. Ringdén O, Ruutu T, Remberger M, et al. A randomized trial comparing busulfan with total body irradiation as conditioning in allogeneic marrow transplant recipients with leukemia: a report from the Nordic Bone Marrow Transplantation Group. Blood 1994; 83:2723–2730.
128. Appelbaum FR. The influence of total dose, fractionation, dose rate and distribution of total body irradiation on bone marrow transplantation. Semin Oncol 1993; 20(suppl 4):3–10.
129. Topolsky D, Crilley, Styler, MJ, Bulova S, Brodsky I, Marks DI. Unrelated donor bone marrow transplantation without T cell depletion using a chemotherapy only conditioning regimen. Low incidence of failed engraftment and severe acute GVHD. Bone Marrow Transplant 1996; 17:549–554.
130. Clift RA, Buckner CD, Thomas ED, et al. Treatment of chronic granulocytic leukaemia in chronic phase by allogeneic marrow transplantation. Lancet 1982; 2: 621–622.
131. Goldman JM, Baughan ASJ, McCarthy DM, et al. Marrow transplantation for patients in chronic phase of chronic granulocytic leukaemia. Lancet 1982; 2:623–625.
132. Gratwohl A, Gluckman E, Goldman J, Zwaan F. Effect of splenectomy before bone marrow transplantation on survival in chronic granulocytic leukaemia. Lancet 1985; 2:1290–1291.
133. Gratwohl A, Hermans J, v. Biezen A, et al. No advantage for patients who receive splenic irradiation before bone marrow transplantation for chronic myeloid leukemia: results of a prospective randomized study. Bone Marrow Transplant 1992; 10:147–152.
134. Gratwohl A, Hermans J, v. Biezen A, et al. Splenic irradiation before bone marrow transplantation for chronic myeloid leukemia: update of a prospective randomized study. Leuk Lymph 1994; 7(suppl 1):227–231.

135. Gratwohl A, Hermans J, von Biezen A, et al. Splenic irradiation before bone marrow transplantation. Br J Haematol 1996; 95:494–500.
136. Kalhs P, Schwarziger I, Anderson G, et al. A retrospective analysis of the long-term effect of splenectomy on late infections, graft-versus-host disease, relapse, and survival after allogeneic marrow transplantation for chronic myelogenous leukemia. Blood 1995; 86:2028–2032.
137. Banaji M, Bearman SI, Buckner CD, et al. The effect of splenectomy on engraftment and platelet transfusion requirements in patients with chronic myelogenous leukemia undergoing marrow transplantation. Am J Hematol 1986; 22:275–283.
138. Tollemar J, Ringdén O, Boström L, Nilsson B, Sundberg B. Variables predicting deep fungal infections in bone marrow transplant recipients. Bone Marrow Transplant 1989; 4:635–641.
139. Boström L, Ringdén O, Jacobsen N. Zwaan F, Nilsson B. A European multicenter study of chronic graft-versus-host disease: the role of cytomegalovirus serology in recipients and donors, acute graft-versus-host disease and splenectomy. Transplantation 1990; 49:1100–1105.
140. Helenglass G, Treleaven J, Parikh P, Aboud H, Smith C, Powles RL. Delayed engraftment associated with splenomegaly in patients undergoing bone marrow transplantation for chronic myeloid leukaemia. Bone Marrow Transplant 1990; 5:247–251.
141. Michallet M, Corront B, Bosson JL, et al. Role of splenectomy in incidence and severity of acute graft-versus-host disease: a multicenter study of 157 patients. Bone Marrow Transplant 1991; 8:13–17.
142. Ringdén O, Nilsson B. Death by graft-versus-host disease is associated with HLA-mismatch, high recipient age, low marrow cell dose and splenectomy. Transplantation 1993; 40:39–43.
143. Martino R, Altes A, Muniz-Diaz E, et al. Reduced transfusion requirements in a splenectomized patient undergoing bone marrow transplantation. Acta Haematol 1994; 92:167–168.
144. von Bueltzingslowewen A, Bordignoni P, Dorveaux Y, et al. Splenectomy may reverse pancytopenia occurring after allogeneic bone marrow transplantation. Bone Marrow Transplant 1994; 14:339–340.
145. Corcoran MC, Press OW, Matthews DC, Appelbaum FR, Bernstein ID. The role of radioimmunotherapy in bone marrow transplantation. Curr Opin Hematol 1996; 3:438–445.
146. Schwartz MA, Lovett DR, Redner A, et al. Dose-escalation trial of M195 labeled with iodine 131 for cytoreduction and marrow ablation in relapsed or refractory myeloid leukemias. J Clin Oncol 1993; 11:294–303.
147. Caron PC, Schwartz MA, Co MS et al. Murine and humanized constructs of monoclonal antibody M195 (anti-CD33) for the therapy of acute myelogenous leukemia. Cancer 1994; 73(suppl 3):1049–1056.
148. Matthews DC, Appelbaum FR, Eary JF, et al. Development of a marrow transplant regimen for acute leukemia using targeted hematopoietic irradiation delivered by ^{131}I-labeled anti-CD45 antibody, combined with cyclophosphamide and total body irradiation. Blood 1995; 85:1122–1131.

149. Appelbaum FR, Brown PA, Sandmaier BM, et al. Specific marrow ablation before marrow transplantation using an aminophosphonic acid conjugate ^{166}Ho-EDTMP. Blood 1992; 80:1608–1613.
150. Parks NJ, Kawakami TG, Avila MJ, et al. Bone marrow transplantation in dogs after radio-ablation with a new Ho-166 amino phosphonic acid bone-seeking agent (DOTMP). Blood 1993; 82:318–325.
151. Ferrant A, Cogneau M, Leners N, et al. ^{52}Fe for additional marrow ablation before bone marrow transplantation. Blood 1993; 81:3435–3439.
152. Jacquy C, Ferrant A, Leners N, Cogneau M, Jamar F, Michaux JL. Additional myeloablation with ^{52}Fe before bone marrow transplantation. Bone Marrow Transplant 1997; 19:191–196.
153. Cullis JO, Schwarer AP, Hughes TP, et al. Second transplants for patients with chronic myeloid leukaemia in relapse after original transplant with T-depleted donor marrow: feasibility of busulphan alone for re-conditioning. Br J Haematol 1992; 80:33–39.
154. Terenzi A, Aversa F, Perruccio, et al. Efficacy of fludarabine as immunosuppressor for bone marrow transplantation conditioning. Blood 1996; 88(suppl 1):2373a.
155. Giralt S, Estey E, Albitar M, et al. Engraftment of allogeneic hematopoietic progenitor cells with purine analog-containing chemotherapy: harnessing graft-versus-leukemia without myeloablative therapy. Blood 1997; 89:4531–4536.
156. Treleaven J, Barrett J. Bone Marrow Transplantation in Practice. Edinburgh: Churchill Livingstone, 1992.
157. Armitage J. Bone marrow transplantation. N Engl J Med 1994; 330:827–838.
158. Ferrara JLM, Deeg HJ, Burakoff SJ. Graft-Versus-Host Disease. 2nd ed. New York; Marcel Dekker, 1997.
159. Ramsay NKC, Kersey JH, Robinson LL, et al. A randomized study of the prevention of acute graft-versus-host disease. N Engl J Med 1982; 306:392–397.
160. Storb R, Deeg HJ, Pepe M, et al. Methotrexate and cyclosporine compared with cyclosporine alone for prophylaxis for acute graft versus host disease after marrow transplantation for leukemia. N Engl J Med 1986; 314:729–735.
161. Storb R, Deeg HJ, Pepe M, et al. Methotrexate and cyclosporine versus cyclosporine alone for prophylaxis of graft-versus-host disease in patients given HLA-identical marrow grafts for leukemia: long-term follow-up of a controlled trial. Blood 1989; 73:1729–1734.
162. Ringdén O, Klaesson S, Sundberg B, Ljungman P, Lonnqvist B, Persson U. Decreased incidence of graft-versus-host disease and improved survival with methotrexate combined with cyclosporin compared with monotherapy in recipients of bone marrow from donors other than HLA identical siblings. Bone Marrow Transplant 1992; 9:19–25.
163. Marks DI, Hughes TP, Szydlo RM, et al. HLA-identical sibling donor bone marrow transplantation for chronic myeloid leukaemia in first chronic phase: influence of GVHD prophylaxis on outcome. Br J Haematol 1992; 81:383–390.
164. Marks DI, Cullis JO, Ward KN, et al. Allogeneic bone marrow transplantation for chronic myeloid leukemia using sibling and volunteer unrelated donors: a comparison of complications in the first two years. Ann Intern Med 1993; 119:207–214.

165. Deeg HJ, Lin D, Leisenring W, et al. Cyclosporine or cyclosporine plus methylprednisolone for prophylaxis of graft-versus-host disease: a prospective, randomized trial. Blood 1997; 89:3880–3887.
166. Gratwohl A, Hermans J, Apperley J, et al. Acute graft-versus-host disease: grade and outcome in patients with chronic myelogenous leukemia. Blood 1995; 86:813–818.
167. McGlave P, Bartsch G, Anasetti C, et al. Unrelated donor marrow transplantation therapy for chronic myelogenous leukemia: initial experience of the National Marrow Donor Program. Blood 1993; 81:543–550.
168. Hows J, Bradley BA, Gore S, et al. Prospective evaluation of unrelated donor bone marrow transplantation. Bone Marrow Transplant 1993; 12:371–380.
169. Hansen JA, Gooley TA, Martin PJ, Appelbaum FR, Chauncey TR, Clift RA, Petersdorf EW, Radich J, Sanders JE, Storb RF, Sullivan KM, Anasetti C. Bone marrow transplantation from unrelated donors for patients with chronic myeloid leukemia. N Engl J Med 1998; 338:962–968.
170. Apperley JF, Mauro FR, Goldman JM, et al. Bone marrow transplantation for chronic myeloid leukaemia in first chronic phase: importance of a graft-versus-leukaemia effect. Br J Haematol 1988; 69:239–245.
171. Devergie A, Reiffers J, Vernant JP, et al. Long-term follow-up after bone marrow transplantation for chronic myelogenous leukemia: factors associated with relapse. Bone Marrow Transplant 1990; 5:379–386.
172. McGlave P. Bone marrow transplants in chronic myelogenous leukemia: an overview of determinants of survival. Sem Hematol 1990; 27(suppl 4):23–30.
173. Marmont AM, Horowitz MM, Gale RP, et al. T-cell depletion of HLA-identical transplants in leukemia. Blood 1991; 78:2120–2130.
174. Weiden P, Flournoy N, Thomas E, et al. Antileukemic effects of graft-versus-host disease in human recipients of allogeneic marrow grafts. N Engl J Med 1979; 300:1068–1073.
175. Thomas ED, Clift RA. Indications for marrow transplantation in chronic myelogenous leukemia. Blood 1989; 73:861–864.
176. Goldman JM, Gale RP, Horowitz MM, et al. Bone marrow transplantation for chronic myelogenous leukemia in chronic phase: increased risk of relapse associated with T-cell depletion. Ann Intern Med 1988; 108:806–814.
177. Italian Cooperative Study Group on Chronic Myeloid Leukaemia. Evaluating survival after allogeneic bone marrow transplant for chronic myeloid leukaemia in chronic phase: a comparison of transplant versus no-transplant in a cohort of 258 patients first seen in Italy between 1984 and 1986. Br J Haematol 1993; 85:292–299.
178. Morgan GJ, Hughes T, Janssen JWG, et al. Polymerase chain reaction for detection of residual leukaemia. Lancet 1989; 1:928–929.
179. Hughes TP, Morgan GJ, Martiat P, Goldman JM. Detection of residual leukemia after bone marrow transplant for chronic myeloid leukemia: role of the polymerase chain reaction in predicting relapse. Blood 1991; 77:874–878.
180. Horowitz MM, Rowlings PA, Passweg JR. Allogeneic bone marrow transplantation for CML: a report from the International Bone Marrow Transplant Registry. Bone Marrow Transplant 1996; 17(suppl 3):S5–S6.

181. Savage DG, Goldman JM. Approaches to the treatment of chronic myelogenous leukemia. Int J Hematol 1994; 60:1–21.
182. Beatty PG, Ash R, Hows JM, McGlave PB. The use of unrelated bone marrow donors in the treatment of patients with chronic myelogenous leukemia: experience of four marrow transplant centers. Bone Marrow Transplant 1989; 4:287–290.
183. Gajewski J, Cecka M, Champlin R. Bone marrow transplantation utilizing HLA-matched unrelated marrow donors. Blood Rev 1990; 4:132–138.
184. Beatty PG, Hansen JA, Longton GM et al. Marrow transplantation from HLA-matched unrelated donors for treatment of hematological malignancies. Transplantation 1991; 51:443–447.
185. Mackinnon S, Hows JM, Goldman JM, et al. Bone marrow transplantation for chronic myeloid leukemia: the use of histocompatible unrelated volunteer donors. Exp Hematol 1989; 18:421–425.
186. Champlin R, Ho W, Arenson E, Gale RP. Allogeneic bone marrow transplantation for chronic myelogenous leukemia in chronic or accelerated phase. Blood 1982; 60:1038–1041.
187. McGlave PB, Arthur DC, Weisdorf D, et al. Allogeneic bone marrow transplantation as treatment for accelerating chronic myelogenous leukemia. Blood 1984; 63: 219–222.
188. Martin PJ, Clift RA, Fisher LD, et al. HLA-identical marrow transplantation during accelerated-phase chronic myelogenous leukemia: analysis of survival and remission duration. Blood 1988; 72:1978–1984.
189. Clift RA, Buckner CD, Thomas ED, et al. Marrow transplantation for patients in accelerated phase of chronic myeloid leukemia. Blood 1994; 84:4368–4373.
190. Clift RA. Marrow transplantation for chronic myeloid leukemia. Cancer Treat Rep 1995; 76:1–42.
191. Savage DG, Szydlo RM, Chase A, Apperley JF, Goldman JM. Bone marrow transplantation for chronic myeloid leukaemia: the effects of differing criteria for defining chronic phase on probabilities of survival and relapse. Br J Haematol 1997; 99:30–35.
192. Copelan EA, Penza SL, Elder PJ, et al. Influence of graft-versus-host disease on outcome following allogeneic transplantation with radiation-free preparative therapy in patients with advanced leukemia. Bone Marrow Transplant 1996; 18:907–911.
193. Lipton JH, Messner HA, Curtis JE, Atkins HL, Minden MD. Intensive remission induction therapy for chronic myeloid leukemia in blast phase with a goal of post-remission bone marrow transplant—a pilot study. Eur J Haematol 1996; 57:42–5.
194. Gratwohl A, Hermans J. Allogeneic bone marrow transplantation for chronic myeloid leukemia. Bone Marrow Transplant 1996; 17(suppl 3):S7–S9.
195. Goldman JM, Szydlo R, Horowitz MM, et al. Choice of pretransplant treatment and timing of transplants for chronic myelogenous leukemia in chronic phase. Blood 1993; 82:2235–2238.
196. Enright H, Daniels K, Arthur DC, et al. Related donor marrow transplant for chronic myeloid leukemia: patient characteristics predictive of outcome. Bone Marrow Transplant 1996; 17:537–542.
197. Champlin R. Allogeneic, syngeneic and autologous bone marrow transplantation for chronic myelogenous leukemia. Leukemia 1993; 7:1084–1086.

198. Giralt SA, Kantarjian HM, Talpaz M, et al. Effect of prior interferon alfa therapy on the outcome of allogeneic bone marrow transplantation for chronic myelogenous leukemia. J Clin Oncol 1993; 11:1055–1061.
199. Beelen DW, Graeven U, Elmaagacli AH, et al. Prolonged administration of interferon-α in patients with chronic-phase Philadelphia chromosome-positive chronic myelogenous leukemia before allogeneic bone marrow transplantation may adversely affect transplant outcome. Blood 1995; 85: 2981–2990.
200. Weiden PL, Sullivan KM, Thomas ED, et al. Antileukemic effect of chronic graft-versus-host disease in human recipients of allogeneic marrow grafts. N Engl J Med 1981; 304:1529–1531.
201. Horowitz MM, Gale RP, Sondel PM, et al. Graft-versus-leukemia reactions after bone marrow transplantation. Blood 1990; 75:555–562.
202. Barrett AJ, Malkovska V. Graft-versus-leukaemia: understanding and using the alloimmune response to treat haematological malignancies. Br J Haematol 1996; 93:754–761.
203. Mavroudis D, Barrett J. The graft-versus-leukemia effect. Curr Opin Hematol 1996; 3:423–429.
204. Truitt RL, Johnson BD. Principles of graft-versus-leukemia reactivity. Biol Blood Marrow Transplant 1995; 1:61–68.
205. Sullivan KM, Weiden PL, Storb R, et al. Influence of acute and chronic graft-versus-host disease on relapse and survival after bone marrow transplantation from HLA-identical siblings as treatment of acute and chronic leukemia. Blood 1989; 73:1720–1728.
206. Gale RP, Horowitz M, Ash R, et al. Identical-twin bone marrow transplants for leukemia. Ann Intern Med 1994; 120:646–652.
207. Hessner MJ, Endean DJ, Caster JT, et al. Use of unrelated marrow grafts compensates for reduced graft-versus-leukemia reactivity after T-cell-depleted allogeneic marrow transplantation for chronic myelogenous leukemia. Blood 1995; 86:3987–3996.
208. Kolb HJ, Mittermüller J, Clemm C, et al. Donor leukocyte transfusions for treatment of recurrent chronic myelogenous leukemia in marrow transplant patients. Blood 1990; 76:2462–2465.
209. Collins RH Jr, Rogers ZR, Bennett M, Kumar V, Nikein A, Fay JW. Hematologic relapse of chronic myelogenous leukemia following allogeneic bone marrow transplantation: apparent graft-versus-leukemia effect following abrupt discontinuation of immunosuppression. Bone Marrow Transplant 1992; 10:391–395.
210. Butturini A, Gale RP. Graft versus leukemia in humans. In: Buckner CD, Clift RA, eds. Technical and Biological Components of Marrow Transplantation. Boston: Kluwer, 1995; 299–314.
211. Fowler DH, Breglio J, Nagel G, Hirose C, Gress RE. Allospecific CD4+, Th1/Th2 and CD8+, Tc1/Tc2 populations in murine GVL: type I cells generate GVL and type II cells abrogate GVL. Biol Blood Marrow Transplant 1996; 2:118–125.
212. Hauch M, Gazzola MV, Small T, et al. Anti-leukemia potential of interleukin-2 activated natural killer cells after bone marrow transplantation for chronic myelogenous leukemia. Blood 1990; 75:2250–2262.

213. Antin JH. Graft-versus-leukemia: no longer an epiphenomenon. Blood 1993; 82: 2273–2277.
214. Glass B, Uharek L, Zeis M, Loeffler H, Mueller-Ruchholtz W, Gassmann W. Graft-versus-leukaemia activity can be predicted by natural cytotoxicity against leukaemia cells. Br J Haematol 1996; 93:412–420.
215. Wong EK, Eaves C, Klingemann H-G. Comparison of natural killer activity of human bone marrow and blood cells in cultures containing IL-2, IL-7 and IL-12. Bone Marrow Transplant 1996; 18:63–71.
216. Sosman JA, Oettel KR, Smith SD, Hank JA, Fisch P, Sondel PM. Specific recognition of human leukemic cells by allogeneic T-cells. II. Evidence for HLA-D restricted determinants on leukemic cells that are crossreactive with determinants present on unrelated nonleukemic cells. Blood 1990; 75:2005–2016.
217. Molldrem J, Dermime S, Parker K, et al. Targeted T-cell therapy for human leukemia: cytotoxic T lymphocytes specific for a peptide derived from proteinase 3 preferentially lyse human myeloid leukemia cells. Blood 1996; 88:2450–2457.
218. Bunjes D, Theobald M, Hertenstein B, et al. Successful therapy with donor buffy coat transfusions in patients with relapsed chronic myeloid leukemia after bone marrow transplantation is associated with high frequencies of host-reactive interleukin 2-secreting T helper cells. Bone Marrow Transplant 1995; 15:713–719.
219. Jiang Y-Z, Barrett AJ. Cellular and cytokine-mediated effects of CD4-positive lymphocyte lines generated in vitro against chronic myelogenous leukemia. Exp Hematol 1995; 23:1167–1172.
220. Champlin R, Ho W, Gajewski J, et al. Selective depletion of CD8+ T-lymphocytes for prevention of graft-versus-host disease after allogeneic bone marrow transplantation. Blood 1990; 76:418–423.
221. Giralt S, Hester J, Huh Y, et al. CD8-depleted donor lymphocyte infusion as treatment for relapsed chronic myelogenous leukemia after allogeneic bone marrow transplantation. Blood 1995; 86: 4337–4343.
222. Dermime S, Mavroudis D, Jiang Y-Z, Hensel N, Molldrem J, Barrett AJ. Immune escape from a graft-versus-leukemia effect may play a role in the relapse of myeloid leukemias following allogeneic bone marrow transplantation. Bone Marrow Transplant 1997; 19:989–999.
223. Lange W, Snyder DS, Castro R, Rossi JJ, Blume KG. Detection by enzymatic amplification of *bcr/abl* mRNA in peripheral blood and bone marrow cells of patients with chronic myelogenous leukemia. Blood 1989; 73:1735–1741.
224. Roth MS, Antin JH, Bingham EL, Ginsberg D. Detection of Philadelphia chromosome-positive cells by the polymerase chain reaction following bone marrow transplant for chronic myelogenous leukemia. Blood 1989; 74:882–885.
225. Delage R, Soiffer RJ, Dear K, Ritz J. Clinical significance of *bcr-abl* gene rearrangement detected by polymerase chain reaction after allogeneic bone marrow transplantation in chronic myelogenous leukemia. Blood 1991; 78:2759–2767.
226. Negrin RS, Blume KG. The use of the polymerase chain reaction for the detection of minimal residual malignant disease. Blood 1991; 78:255–258.
227. Lee M, Khouri I, Champlin R, et al. Detection of minimal residual disease by polymerase chain reaction of bcr/abl transcripts in chronic myelogenous leukae-

mia following allogeneic bone marrow transplantation. Br J Haematol 1992; 82: 708–714.

228. Roth M, Antin JH, Ash R, et al. Prognostic significance of Philadelphia chromosome-positive cells detected by the polymerase chain reaction after allogeneic bone marrow transplant for chronic myelogenous leukemia. Blood 1992; 79:276–282.

229. Thompson JD, Brodsky I, Yunis JJ. Molecular quantification of residual disease in chronic myelogenous leukemia after bone marrow transplantation. Blood 1992; 79:1629–1635.

230. Cross NCP, Feng L, Chase A, Bungey J, Hughes TP, Goldman JM. Competitive polymerase chain reaction to estimate the number of BCR-ABL transcripts in chronic myeloid leukemia patients after bone marrow transplantation. Blood 1993; 82:1929–1936.

231. Cross NCP, Hughes TP, Lin F, et al. Minimal residual disease after allogeneic bone marrow transplantation for chronic myeloid leukaemia in first chronic phase: correlations with acute graft-versus-host disease. Br J Haematol 1993; 84:67–74.

232. Lion T, Henn T, Gaiger A, Kalhs P, Gadner H. Early detection of relapse after bone marrow transplantation in patients with chronic myelogenous leukaemia. Lancet 1993; 341:275–276.

233. Miyamura K, Tahara T, Tanimoto M, et al. Long persistent bcr-abl positive transcript detected by polymerase chain reaction after marrow transplant for chronic myelogenous leukemia without clinical relapse: a study of 64 patients. Blood 1993; 81:1089–1093.

234. Xu MW, Piao XH, Addy L, Jamal N, Minden MD, Messner HA. Minimal residual disease in bone marrow transplant recipients with chronic myeloid leukemia. Bone Marrow Transplant 1994; 14:299–306.

235. Cross NCP. Quantitative PCR techniques and applications. Br J Haematol 1995; 89:693–697.

236. Frassoni F, Martinelli G, Saglio G, et al. bcr/abl chimeric transcript in patients in remission after marrow transplantation for chronic myeloid leukemia: higher frequency of detection and slower clearance in patients grafted in advanced disease as compared to patients grafted in chronic phase. Bone Marrow Transplant 1995; 16:595–601.

237. Lin F, Chase A, Bungey J, Goldman JM, Cross NC. Correlation between the proportion of Philadelphia chromosome positive metaphase cells and levels of BCR-ABL mRNA in chronic myeloid leukemia. Genes Chromosomes Cancer 1995; 13:110–114.

238. Preudhomme C, Wattel E, Lai JL, et al. Good predictive value of combined cytogenetic and molecular follow up in chronic myelogenous leukemia after non T-cell depleted allogeneic bone marrow transplantation: a report on 38 consecutive cases. Leuk Lymph 1995; 18:265–271.

239. Radich JP, Gehly G, Gooley T, et al. Polymerase chain reaction detection of the *BCR-ABL* fusion transcript after allogeneic marrow transplantation for chronic myeloid leukemia: results and implications in 346 patients. Blood 1995; 85:2632–2638.

240. Costello RT, Kirk J, Gabert J. Value of PCR analysis for long term survivors after allogeneic bone marrow transplant for chronic myelogenous leukemia: a comparative study. Leuk Lymph 1996; 20:239–243.
241. El-Rifai W, Ruutu T, Vettenranta K, Temtamy S, Knuutila S. Minimal residual disease after allogeneic bone marrow transplantation for chronic myeloid leukaemia: a metaphase-FISH study. Br J Haematol 1996; 92:365–369.
242. Lin F, Kirkland MA, van Rhee F, et al. Molecular analysis of transient cytogenetic relapse after allogeneic bone marrow transplantation for chronic myeloid leukemia. Bone Marrow Transplant 1996; 18:1147–1152.
243. Lin F, van Rhee F, Goldman JM, Cross NCP. Kinetics of increasing BCR-ABL transcript numbers in chronic myeloid leukemia patients who relapse after bone marrow transplantation. Blood 1996; 87:4473–4478.
244. Santini V, Zoccolante A, Bosi A, et al. Detection of bcr/abl transcripts by RT-PCR and their colorimetric evaluation in chronic myeloid leukemia patients receiving allogeneic bone marrow transplantation. Haematologica 1996; 81:201–207.
245. Zhang JG, Lin F, Chase A, Goldman JM, Cross NCP. Comparison of genomic DNA and cDNA for detection of residual disease after treatment of chronic myeloid leukemia with allogeneic bone marrow transplantation. Blood 1996; 87: 2588–2593.
246. Apperley JF, Rassool F, Parreira A, et al. Philadelphia-positive metaphases in the marrow after bone marrow transplantation for chronic granulocytic leukemia. Am J Hematol 1986; 22:199–204.
247. Arthur CK, Apperley JF, Guo AP, Rassool F, Gao LM, Goldman JM. Cytogenetic events after bone marrow transplantation for chronic myeloid leukemia in chronic phase. Blood 1988; 71:1179–1186.
248. Zaccaria A, Rosti G, Sessarego M, et al. Relapse after allogeneic bone marrow transplantation for Philadelphia chromosome positive chronic myeloid leukemia: cytogenetic analysis of 24 patients. Bone Marrow Transplant 1988; 3:413–423.
249. Arcese W, Gratwohl A, Niederwiser D, et al. Outcome for patients who relapse after allogeneic bone marrow transplantation for chronic myeloid leukemia. Blood 1993; 82:3211–3219.
250. Lin F, Goldman JM, Cross NCP. A comparison of the sensitivity of blood and bone marrow for the detection of minimal residual disease in chronic myeloid leukaemia. Br J Haematol 1994; 86:683–685.
251. Van Rhee F, Lin F, Cross NC, et al. Detection of residual leukaemia more than 10 years after allogeneic bone marrow transplantation. Bone Marrow Transplant 1994; 14:609–612.
252. Frenoy N, Chabli A, Sol O, et al. Application of a new nested PCR to the detection of minimal residual disease bcr/abl transcripts. Leukemia 1994; 8:1411–1414.
253. Zhao L. Kantarjian H, Van Oort J, Cork A, Trujillo J, Liang J. Detection of residual proliferating leukemic cells by fluorescence in situ hybridization in CML patients in complete remission after interferon treatment. Leukemia 1993; 7:L168–171.
254. Nevill TJ, Barnett MJ, Robinson KS, Greer W, Phillips GL. Return to durable haematopoiesis after blast phase relapse of chronic myeloid leukaemia following bone marrow transplantation. Br J Hematol 1992; 80:256–258.

255. Marmont A, Frassoni F, Bacigalupo A, et al. Recurrence of Ph^1-positive leukemia in donor cells after marrow transplantation for chronic granulocytic leukemia. N Engl J Med 1984; 310:903–906.
256. McCann SR, Lawler M, Humphries P, et al. Recurrence of Philadelphia chromosome-positive leukemia in donor cells after marrow transplantation for chronic granulocytic leukemia: confirmation by microsatellite analysis. Blood 1992; 79: 2803–2805.
257. McCann SR, Lawler M, Bacigalupo A. Recurrence of Philadelphia chromosome-positive leukemia in donor cells after marrow transplantation for chronic granulocytic leukemia. Leuk Lymph 1993; 10:419–425.
258. Higano CS, Raskind WH, Singer JW. Use of interferon alfa-2a to treat hematologic relapse of chronic myelogenous leukemia after bone marrow transplantation. Acta Haematol 1993; 89(suppl 1):8–14.
259. Pigneux A, Devergie A, Pochitaloff M, et al. Recombinant alpha-interferon as treatment for chronic myelogenous leukemia in relapse after allogeneic bone marrow transplantation: a report of the Société Française de Greffe de Moelle. Bone Marrow Transplant 1995; 15:819–824.
260. Porter DL, Roth MS, McGarigle C, Ferrara JLM, Antin JH. Induction of graft-versus-host disease in immunotherapy for relapsed chronic myeloid leukemia. N Engl J Med 1994; 300:100–106.
261. Klingemann H-G, Grigg AP, Wilkie-Boyd K, et al. Treatment with recombinant interferon-α early after bone marrow transplantation in patients at high risk for relapse. Blood 1991; 78:3306–3311.
262. Mrsic M, Horowitz MM, Atkinson K, et al. Second HLA-identical sibling transplants for leukemia recurrence. Bone Marrow Transplant 1992; 9:269–275.
263. Barrett AJ, Locatelli F, Treleaven JG, Gratwohl A, Szydlo RM, Zwaan FE. Second transplants for leukaemic relapse after bone marrow transplantation: high early mortality but favourable effect of chronic GVHD on continued remission. Br J Haematol 1991; 79:567–574.
264. Slavin S, Or R, Naparstek W, et al. Cellular-mediated immunotherapy of leukemia in conjunction with autologous and allogeneic bone marrow transplantation in experimental animals and man. Blood 1988; 72(suppl 1):407a.
265. Cullis JO, Jiang YZ, Schwarer AP, Hughes TP, Barrett AJ, Goldman JM. Donor leukocyte infusions for chronic myeloid leukemia after allogeneic bone marrow transplantation. Blood 1992; 79:1379–1381.
266. Bär BM, Schattenberg A, Mensink EJBM, et al. Donor leukocyte infusions for chronic myeloid leukemia relapsed after allogeneic bone marrow transplantation. J Clin Oncol 1993; 11:513–519.
267. Drobyski WR, Keever CA, Roth MS, et al. Salvage immunotherapy using donor leukocyte infusions as treatment for relapsed chronic myelogenous leukemia after allogeneic bone marrow transplantation: efficacy and toxicity of a defined T-cell dose. Blood 1993; 82:2310–2318.
268. Hertenstein B, Wiesneth M, Novotny J, et al. Interferon-α and donor buffy coat transfusions for treatment of relapsed chronic myeloid leukemia after allogeneic bone marrow transplantation. Transplantation 1993; 56:1114–1118.
269. Jiang YZ, Cullis J, Kanfer E, et al. T cell and NK cell mediated graft-versus-

leukemia reactivity following donor buffy coat transfusion to treat relapse after marrow transplantation for chronic myeloid leukemia. Bone Marrow Transplant 1993; 11:133–138.
270. Boiron JM, Cony-Makhoul P, Mahon FX, Pigneux A, Puntous M, Reiffers J. Treatment of hematological malignancies relapsing after allogeneic bone marrow transplantation. Blood Rev 1994; 8:234–240.
271. Van Rhee F, Feng L, Cullis JO, et al. Relapse of chronic myeloid leukemia after allogeneic bone marrow transplant: the case for giving donor leukocyte transfusions before the onset of hematologic relapse. Blood 1994; 83:3377–3383.
272. Kolb HJ, Schattenberg A, Goldman JM, et al. Graft-versus-leukemia effect of donor lymphocyte transfusions in marrow grafted patients. European Group for Blood and Marrow Transplantation Working Party Chronic Leukemia. Blood 1995; 86:2041–2050.
273. Mackinnon S, Papadopoulos EB, Carabasi MH, Reich L, Collins NH, O'Reilly RJ. Adoptive immunotherapy using donor leukocytes following bone marrow transplantation for chronic myeloid leukemia: is T cell dose important in determining biological response? Bone Marrow Transplant 1995; 15:591–594.
274. Mackinnon S, Papadopoulos EB, Carabasi MH, et al. Adoptive immunotherapy evaluating escalating doses of donor leukocytes for relapse of chronic myeloid leukemia after bone marrow transplantation: separation of graft-versus-leukemia responses from graft-versus-host disease. Blood 1995; 86:1261–1268.
275. Slavin S, Naparstek E, Nagler A, Ackerstein A, Kapelushnik J, Or R. Allogeneic cell therapy for relapsed leukemia after bone marrow transplantation with donor peripheral blood lymphocytes. Exp Hematol 1995; 23: 1553–1562.
276. Van Rhee F, Kolb H. Donor leukocyte transfusions for leukemic relapse. Curr Opin Hematol 1995; 2:423–430.
277. Slavin S, Naparstek E, Nagler A, et al. Allogeneic cell therapy with donor peripheral blood cells and recombinant human interleukin-2 to treat leukemia relapse after allogeneic bone marrow transplantation. Blood 1996; 87:2195–2204.
278. Bacigalupo A, Soracco M, Vassallo F, et al. Donor lymphocyte infusions (DLI) in patients with chronic myeloid leukemia following allogeneic bone marrow transplantation. Bone Marrow Transplant 1997; 19:927–932.
279. Collins RH Jr, Shpilberg O, Drobyski WR, et al. Donor leukocyte infusions in 140 patients with relapsed malignancy after allogeneic bone marrow transplantation. J Clin Oncol 1997; 15:433–444.
280. Keil F, Haas OA, Fritsch G, et al. Donor leukocyte infusion for leukemic relapse after allogeneic marrow transplantation: lack of residual donor hematopoiesis predicts aplasia. Blood 1997; 89:3113–3117.
281. Van Rhee F, Savage D, Blackwell J, et al. Adoptive immunotherapy for relapse of chronic myeloid leukemia after allogeneic bone marrow transplant: equal efficacy of lymphocytes from sibling and matched unrelated donors. Bone Marrow Transplant 1997; 20:553–560.
282. Garicochea B, van Rhee F, Spencer A, et al. Aplasia after donor lymphocyte infusion (DLI) for CML in relapse after sex-mismatched BMT: recovery of donor-type haemopoiesis predicted by non-isotopic in situ hybridisation. Br J Haematol 1994; 88:400–402.

283. Collins R, Wolff S, List A, et al. Prospective multicenter trial of donor buffy coat infusion for relapsed hematologic malignancy post-allogeneic bone marrow transplantation. Blood 1994; 84(suppl 1):333a.
284. Naparstek E, Or R, Nagler A, et al. T-cell-depleted allogeneic bone marrow transplantation for acute leukemia using Campath-1 antibodies and post-transplant administration of donor's peripheral blood lymphocytes for prevention of relapse. Br J Haematol 1995; 89:506–515.
285. Barrett AJ, Mavroudis D, Molldrem J, et al. Optimizing the dose and timing of lymphocyte add-back in T-cell depleted BMT between HLA-identical siblings. Blood 1996; 88:1830a.
286. Bonini C, Ferrari G, Verzeletti S, et al. HSV-TK gene transfer into donor lymphocytes for control of allogeneic graft-versus-leukemia. Science 1997; 276:1719–1724.
287. Faber L, van Luxemburg-Heijs S. Veenhof W, et al. Generation of CD4+ cytotoxic T-lymphocyte clones from a patient with severe graft-versus-host disease after allogeneic bone marrow transplantation implications for graft-versus-leukemia reactivity. Blood 1995; 86:2821–2828.
288. Faber LM, van Luxemburg-Heijs SAP, Rijnbeek M, Willemze R, Falkenburg JHF. Minor histocompatibility antigen-specific leukemia-reactive cytotoxic T cell clones can be generated in vitro without in vivo priming using chronic myeloid leukemia cells as stimulators in the presence of α-interferon. Biol Blood Marrow Transplant 1996; 2:31–36.
289. Choudhury A, Gajewski JL, Liang JC, et al. Use of leukemic dendritic cells for the generation of antileukemic cellular cytotoxicity against Philadelphia chromosome-positive chronic myelogenous leukemia. Blood 1997; 89:1133–1142.

11
Treatment Algorithm in CML: Bone Marrow Transplantation as Frontline Therapy

Reginald A. Clift
Fred Hutchinson Cancer Research Center, Seattle, Washington

INTRODUCTION

Three treatment modalities are available for patients with newly diagnosed chronic myeloid leukemia (CML): chemotherapy in doses that do not require marrow rescue; daily subcutaneous interferon (IFN); and intensive cytoreduction by chemotherapy or radiotherapy requiring the restoration of hematopoiesis by the infusion of allogeneic (or syngeneic) stem cells (BMT).

The use of chemotherapy in doses intended to control the hematological manifestations and symptoms of CML in chronic phase (CP) has usually been referred to as conventional therapy. However, the widespread acceptance of BMT and IFN as nonexperimental therapy means that these therapies must also be considered conventional and, given the results, treatments other than these are best described as palliative.

All three therapeutic approaches are well described elsewhere in this book. The purpose of this chapter is to advance the proposition that when newly diagnosed patients have suitable donors they should be treated by BMT as soon as possible. Since most patients have the diagnosis of CML established while they are in CP, this chapter deals mainly with that phase. The data are derived from experience with BMT in Seattle, but similar results have been reported from several large transplant centers. Unless otherwise indicated, all data refer to transplants from genotypically HLA-identical siblings.

"SURVIVAL" IS VERY IMPORTANT

In 1979 Fefer et al. (1) reported experience in transplanting four patients in CP from identical twin donors after treatment with a busulfan derivative (dimethylbusulfan, DMB), cyclophosphamide (CY), and a single exposure of 920 cGy of total body irradiation (TBI). The leukemic clone was successfully eliminated in all patients (1). These studies were extended, and in 1982, a report described the total experience through 1979 of transplants for CML from identical twins (22 patients, 12 of them in CP) (2). Figure 1 presents the probabilities of survival and relapse for the 12 patients transplanted in CP, updated as of July 1996. These patients were treated with a regimen consisting of DMB, CY, and TBI. There is evidence that syngeneic transplants are associated with a markedly increased risk of relapse compared with allogeneic transplants using the same conditioning regimen. However, it is clear from Figure 1 that syngeneic transplantation after an effective conditioning regimen has a high probability of curing patients with CML in CP, and that an allogeneic effect is not essential for cure.

Encouraged by the demonstration that prolonged disease-free survival could be obtained in patients transplanted in CP from identical twins, the first marrow transplants from HLA-identical siblings for patients with CML in CP took place in Seattle in 1979, and the first 10 such transplants were reported in 1982 (3). At the time of publication, four of these patients had died, all within 100 days of transplant (three from interstitial pneumonia [IP] and one from acute graft-versus-host disease [GVHD]), and only one patient had relapsed (4.3

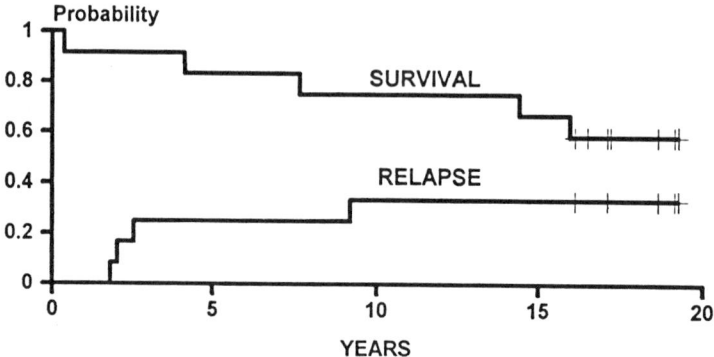

Figure 1 Kaplan-Meier probability of survival and the cumulative incidence of persistent cytogenetic relapse for 12 patients with CML in CP transplanted from syngeneic donors through 1979 after a regimen of CY, dimethylbusulfan, and TBI and first reported in 1982 (2). Survival and events were updated as of July 1996.

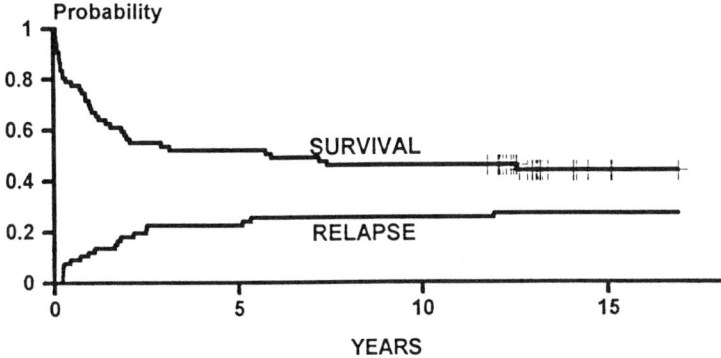

Figure 2 Kaplan-Meier probability of survival and the cumulative incidence of persistent cytogenetic relapse for 67 patients with CML in CP transplanted in Seattle from HLA-identical siblings through 1983 and first reported in 1986 (6). Survival and events updated as of July 1996.

years after transplant). These results and those of others (4,5) led to an increasing use of transplantation for patients with CML and, in 1986, the Seattle team published its complete experience through 1983 which involved 167 patients with CML transplanted from HLA-identical siblings (6). This report revealed the opportunities and problems provided by this form of therapy which have since been amply confirmed by many investigators. Sixty-seven of these patients were transplanted while in CP; the probabilities of survival and relapse for these updated through July 1996 are presented in Figure 2. The latest relapse was at 12 years after transplantation occurring as a cerebral chloroma in a patient with normal marrow cytogenetics. These patients were treated with regimens and support that have been superseded by improved protocols, but the figure shows that prolonged disease-free survival frequently can be expected after transplantation while in CP. It also shows that the risk of relapse persists for many years after allogeneic transplantation.

"RELAPSE" IS DIFFICULT TO DEFINE

There are several difficulties in defining relapse and leukemia-free survival which are unique to the setting of transplantation for the treatment of CML. We can recognize four levels of relapse; in order of detection sensitivity these are molecular, cytogenetic, hematological, and clinical relapse. As is often the case, there is an inverse relationship between sensitivity and solidity. The markers of both molecular and cytogenetic relapse sometimes disappear spontaneously without therapeutic intervention. This phenomenon is more common when the relapses are detected soon after transplant, and occurs more frequently in patients with molecular than in those with cytogenetic relapses. Patients who have experienced such transient relapses are more likely to have a subsequent persistent relapse. Spontaneous remissions have not been reported in patients with hematological or clinical relapse. Only clinical relapse is associated with symptoms that encourage patients to seek medical assistance. The detection of other forms of relapse is therefore subject to monitoring design and performance although, of course, hematological relapse is by far the easiest to detect. Statistics on molecular or cytogenetic relapse are particularly unreliable in the absence of a strategy and discipline which produces frequent sampling.

"LEUKEMIA-FREE SURVIVAL" CAN BE MISLEADING

Relapse after transplantation for CML differs from that after transplantation for other types of leukemia in that it is less likely to result in early death. Indeed, the pace of disease progression is frequently very slow after posttransplant relapse, particularly for patients with minimal cytogenetic relapse (7,8). Some patients will have stable relapsed disease over many years with no increase in the proportion of Ph-positive metaphases, and they may not even require early treatment intervention. This phenomenon has also been recognized after autologous transplantation (9). The prolonged survival of relapsed patients is further enhanced by the relative effectiveness of therapies for dealing with this situation. Methods of treatment other than second transplant are available, and it has been shown that a longer delay between the first and second transplant improves the chance of a successful outcome.

Two methods that have been used widely for the treatment of posttransplant relapse are treatment with IFN alone or with the infusion of lymphocytes from the marrow donor. Treatment with IFN alone is effective in producing both clinical and cytogenetic remission in patients who have relapsed after transplantation, and complete remissions are more frequent when this treatment is initiated in the early stages of relapse (7,10,11). Because of this, most patients are treated while in cytogenetic relapse and statistics on hematological or clinical relapse after transplantation are of limited value in settings where such a policy is followed.

The same considerations apply to the use of IFN in this setting as to its use in the management of patients with CML who have not had marrow transplants; that is, success requires high doses of IFN, the treatment is toxic and expensive, and it is not known how often successful treatment can be discontinued without relapse. Kolb et al. produced hematological and cytogenetic remission by treatment with IFN accompanied by the infusion of donor buffy coat cells in three patients who relapsed after transplantation (12); he discusses this approach elsewhere in this volume. This form of treatment has a high success rate for patients in early relapse with most patients achieving hematological remission, many achieving cytogenetic remission, and some becoming negative to PCR testing for BCR-ABL (12–14). Most patients have reactivation of acute GVHD, which has sometimes been fatal. Another serious complication of this treatment is the development of marrow aplasia, presumably in patients whose hematopoiesis became entirely of host origin when they lost the myeloid component of their grafts in the same process that produced relapse. Lymphocyte transfusions without IFN have also been demonstrated to be effective in producing remission (15).

As mentioned above, successful second transplants have been reported. For second transplants, chemotherapy only is used when the first transplant was with a TBI-containing regimen; TBI-containing regimens are used when the first transplant regimen consisted of chemotherapy only. In cases where immune tolerance of donor tissues persists, the regimen need not be constrained by the need to overcome graft rejection. In Seattle through 1990, 12 patients who relapsed after transplants from identical twins received second transplants. Two of these patients relapsed a second time and died, and four remain alive and disease-free between 6 and 15 years after the first and between 4 and 14 years after the second transplant. A short interval between the first and second transplants appears to be associated with a high incidence of regimen-related toxicity and mortality, and current practice in Seattle is to aim at an interval of at least 1 year. This is usually feasible because of the other treatment approaches available and because of the usually slow rate of disease progression.

Cullis et al. (16) reported 16 patients who received second transplants from their primary donors for relapse after transplantation with T-depleted marrow from HLA-identical siblings. Eight patients were alive disease-free a median of 424 days after the second transplant (range 158–1789 days). Five of these patients had been conditioned for second transplant with a regimen of BU only. In Seattle 30 patients who had received transplants from HLA-identical siblings received second transplants through 1989. Twenty of these patients relapsed after the second transplant and died, and four patients remain alive and disease-free between 8 and 15 years after the first and 7 and 11 years after the second transplant. Fifteen of these patients were in CP when they received the first transplant, and one of these died from rejection, seven died after a second relapse, three died from VOD, and one from *Aspergillus* infection. Two of these patients survive disease-free, 7 and 10 years after the second and 8 and 12 years after the first transplants. Clearly, second transplants for patients transplanted for CML who relapse are possible but are much less likely to be successful than first transplants.

For all the reasons described above, statistics on leukemia-free survival are of limited value in assessing the role and timing of marrow transplantation for the treatment of CML, and statistics on relapse should be accompanied by statements of the monitoring and follow-up practices employed. It is entirely possible that two studies with identical leukemia-free survival could be subject to major differences of interpretation because the measured event was usually death in one study and relapse in the other. This complexity is very important in a setting where death is not an early consequence of relapse. Moreover, statistics on overall survival are particularly important in discussing intervention in a disease where the median age at diagnosis is high and survival from diagnosis without major therapeutic intervention is measured in years and where the prevailing (and mistaken) impression is that marrow transplant is necessarily accompanied by substantial early regimen-related mortality.

EFFECT OF PHASE

The best results in treating CML by marrow transplantation are achieved by treating patients early in the course of their disease. Figure 3 presents the Seattle survival experience with patients categorized according to phase of disease at the time of transplantation.

The group of patients in CP constitutes our entire experience from August 1983 through June 1995 in treating patients with one of the two most recently used regimens. One of these regimens (CY-TBI) consisted of cyclophosphamide (CY) 60 mg/kg on each of 2 successive days followed by 12.0 Gy of total body irradiation (TBI) in six daily fractions; the other regimen was busulfan (BU) 16

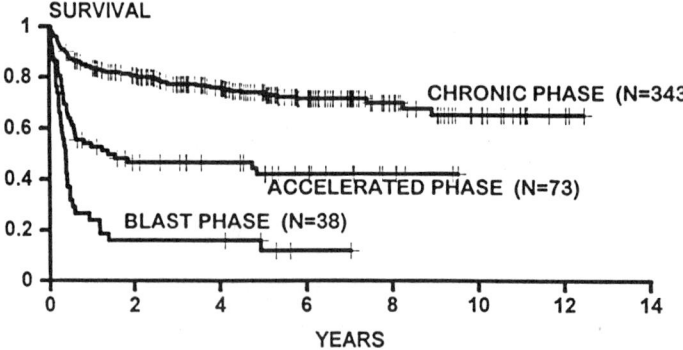

Figure 3 Kaplan-Meier probabilities of survival for patients transplanted from HLA-identical family members in CP (since 1983), in AP or BP (since 1985). The survival was calculated as of February 1996.

mg/kg administered over 4 days, followed by 60 mg/kg CY on each of 2 successive days (17). This regimen (BU-CY) has low toxicity and is effective in facilitating allogeneic engraftment. In 1994 we reported a randomized study comparing this regimen with the CY-TBI regimen in patients receiving marrow transplants from HLA-identical related donors for the treatment of CML in CP (18). All patients received a combination of methotrexate and cyclosporine as prophylaxis against acute graft-versus-host disease (GVHD). There was no significant difference between the CY-TBI and the BU-CY groups in the 3-year probabilities of survival (0.80 for both) or relapse (0.13 for both), in event-free survival (CY-TBI 0.68, BU-CY 0.71), or in speed of engraftment or incidence of veno-occlusive disease of the liver. The 4-year probabilities of survival and event-free survival for patients transplanted within 1 year of diagnosis were 0.86 and 0.72, respectively, for each group. Significantly more patients in the CY-TBI group experienced major creatinine elevations. There was significantly more acute GVHD in the CY-TBI group. Fever days, positive blood cultures, hospitalizations, and inpatient hospital days were significantly more common in the CY-TBI group than in the BU-CY group. Since completion of that study, all patients older than 14 years transplanted in Seattle while in CP from HLA-identical siblings have been treated with the BU-CY regimen, and, as of the end of 1995, 343 CML CP patients had been treated with either the BU-CY of the CY-TBI regimen.

The groups of patients transplanted in accelerated (AP) or blast (BP) phase contains all such patients transplanted with unmodified marrow and a variety of regimens from January 1985 through June 1995. It is clear that survival after transplantation in CP is superior to that in more advanced stages of the disease. Figure 4 presents the cumulative incidences of persistent relapse for these patients, and Figure 5 presents the probabilities of survival, leukemia-free survival, and persistent relapse for the patients transplanted in CP. There is no difference between the relapse rate for patients transplanted in CP or AP, but the relapse incidence is much higher in patients transplanted in BP. Comparison of Figures 3 and 4 shows that the nonrelapse mortality is higher in the AP patients than in those transplanted in CP. This may be a consequence of the more intensive regimens employed for patients in AP; current practice in Seattle is to use the same regimens for patients in AP and CP. A report of the Seattle experience of marrow transplantation during AP was published in 1994 (19).

EFFECT OF DELAY

The most obvious and easily understood adverse consequence of delaying transplantation for patients newly diagnosed in CP with acceptable marrow donors is a change in phase from CP to AP or BP. Using long-established algorithms it

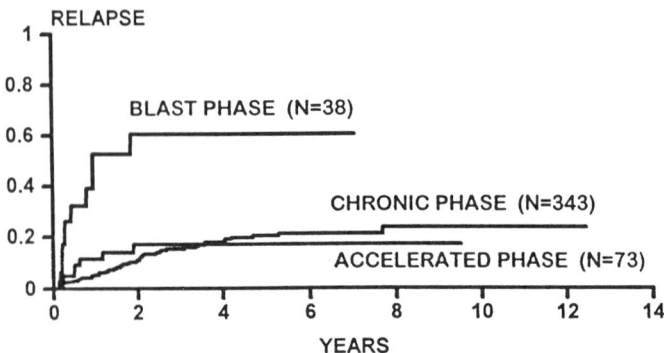

Figure 4 Cumulative incidences of persistent cytogenetic relapse for patients transplanted from HLA-identical family members in CP (since 1983), in AP or BP (since 1985). The survival was calculated as of January 1996.

is possible to identify three prognostically useful categories of newly diagnosed patients (20,21). The best-risk group (about 20% of patients) had a median survival of between 5 and 6 years, which implies a median duration of CP lasting about 5 years with a transformation rate into AP or about 5% during the first year. There is evidence that more recent therapeutic approaches with the use of HU (22) and of IFN (23) can delay the development of transformation. Nevertheless, patients may still go to bed in CP and wake up the next morning in BP. For the patient with a matched sibling donor, this is a tragic development with a prognostic shift from a group with an 80% expectation of survival at 5 years after BMT to <10%. At the moment, nothing except early transplantation can completely remove this possibility.

There is another, more serious, adverse effect of delay. The interval between diagnosis and transplant influences the outcome of BMT for patients transplanted in CP and for patients transplanted in AP. This observation, which was first recognized early in the Seattle experience (3) and has now been confirmed in many studies (24), is crucial to the design of treatment strategies. Delay is also associated with an increased risk of relapse, but multivariable analysis demonstrates that these two associations are independent. This is to be expected since posttransplant relapse does not have an early influence on survival, and it suggests that the advantage of early transplantation will become even greater as the impact of an increased relapse rate upon survival develops.

We do not know why patients who remain in chronic phase without obvious physical, hematological, or cytogenetic change have an increasing risk of dying of the complications of BMT. No single cause of death accounts for the difference. The diagnosis of CML in CP is frequently made fortuitously, and it seems likely that the deterioration in survival prospects is associated with making the diagnosis rather than with the inception of disease, which implicates physician intervention as a possible cause. BU was the standard treatment for CML until recently, when most physicians began to use HU instead.

Consequently, in earlier studies, patients with a long interval between diagnosis and transplantation were much more likely to have been treated with BU than with HU. This has made it difficult to examine separately the effect of delayed transplantation and the effect of pretreatment with BU. However, the IBMTR study (24) shows that palliative treatment with BU has an independent adverse effect on the outcome of subsequent BMT and that delay was detrimental even in patients who did not receive BU. It may well be that treatment with HU is also detrimental, which could only be recognized if there were a comparative series of patients who had received no treatment before transplant. A population of patients with newly diagnosed CML may not have a uniform susceptibility to the influence of delay on posttransplant survival. We have transplanted eight patients in CP 8 or more years after diagnosis; with a follow-up between 2 and 10 years, four of these patients have died (on days 90, 147, and 175 and at 4.5 years), and there are four survivors (three of them in uninterrupted remission) between 2.5 and 12.5 years after transplant. Thus, the effect of delay may be different in different groups of patients. The adverse effect of delaying marrow transplantation has also been demonstrated for patients transplanted in AP.

Figure 6 presents the survival of patients transplanted in Seattle in CP categorized by the interval between diagnosis and transplant. It can be seen that

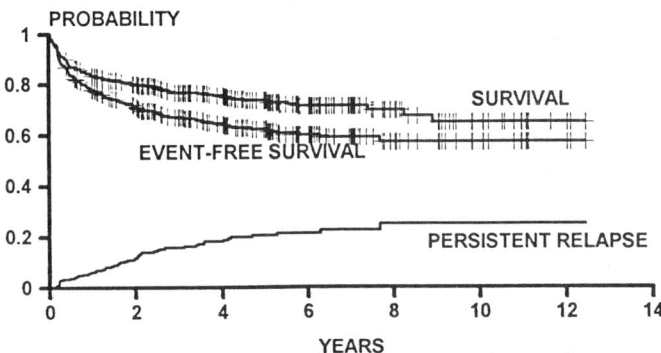

Figure 5 Kaplan-Meier probabilities of survival and of relapse-free survival and the cumulative incidence of relapse for all patients transplanted in CP from HLA-identical family members since 1983. The statistics were calculated in January 1996.

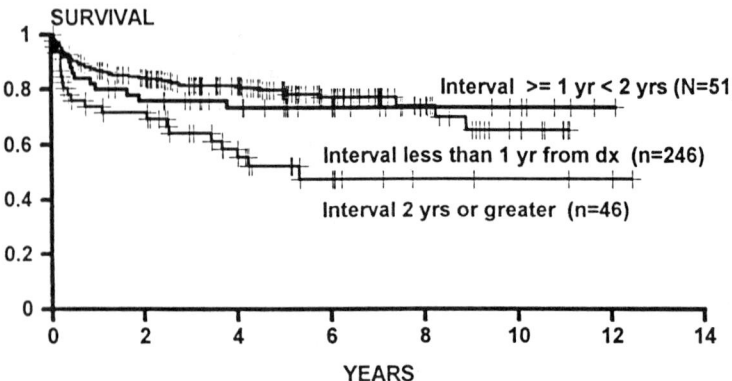

Figure 6 Kaplan-Meier probabilities of survival for patients transplanted from HLA-identical family members for CML in CP, categorized on the basis of the interval between diagnosis and transplant. The statistics were calculated in January 1996.

the survival of patients transplanted within 2 years of diagnosis is markedly superior to that of patients transplanted later, and this difference is statistically significant ($p = 0.001$).

EFFECT OF AGE

Age is an adverse risk factor for survival after marrow transplant. The median age at diagnosis of CML is 67 years (25), and most centers will not transplant patients older than 55. Successfully transplanting older patients could dramatically increase the number of patients cured of CML. In a study of the influence of age on the outcome of transplantation for the treatment of CML in CP (26), only 10 patients were <20 years of age and none of these died. Using patients aged 20–30 years as the reference group, the relative risks of dying for patients aged 30–40, 40–50, and 50–60 years were 1.24 ($p = 0.57$, C.L. 0.59–2.57), 2.30 ($p = 0.02$, C.L. 1.13–4.71), and 2.54 ($p = 0.01$, C.L. 1.18–5.48), respectively. Thus, age 30–40 years was not associated with a significantly increased risk of dying, but patients 40 through 50 and 50 through 60 years had a significantly increased risk of dying compared with patients <40 years. However, patients aged 50–60 did not have an increased risk of dying compared to patients aged 40–50 years. Of the five patients aged 60 years, two died (one on day 45 of idiopathic pneumonia syndrome (27) and one on day 472 of varicella hepatitis). There were no relapses, and the survivors are currently 901, 960, and 1106 days after transplant.

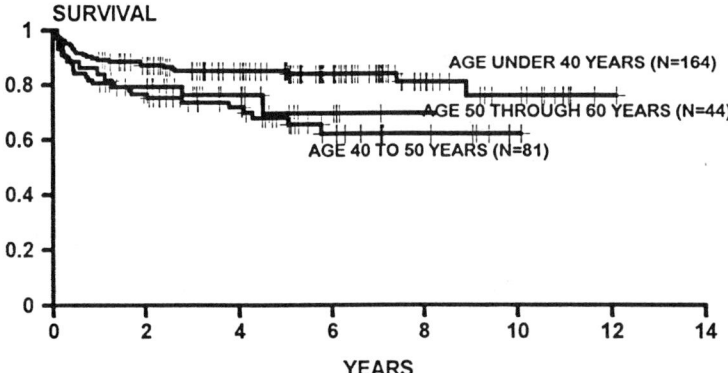

Figure 7 Kaplan-Meier probabilities of survival for patients transplanted <2 years after diagnosis from HLA-identical family member for CML in CP, categorized on the basis of age at the time of transplant. The statistics were calculated in February 1996.

Figure 7 describes the Kaplan-Meier probabilities of survival for patients transplanted for CML in CP within 2 years of diagnosis, categorized as <40 years, 40–50 years, and 50–60 years of age at the time of transplant.

UNRELATED DONORS

Less than 30% of newly diagnosed patients will have HLA-matched relatives, and 50% of these will be unacceptable because of age. Thus the benefits of marrow transplantation from a matched related donor can only be offered to about 15% of newly diagnosed patients.

We and others have been studying the use of volunteer unrelated donors, an approach made possible by the establishment of the National Marrow Donor Program. This has received substantial government support and has been the model for National Donor Registries in several other countries. The resulting network of donor registries provides access to the names and basic tissue types of more than 1 million volunteers around the world.

CML is a disease which, because of its relatively slow progression, is well suited to the search for a suitable unrelated donor. A recent report (28) described results for 312 patients with CML aged 55 years or less, transplanted from unrelated donors. Two hundred thirty-six had donors with whom they were extremely well matched for tissue antigens, and 194 of these patients were in CP when transplanted. The 3-year survival for patients in CP transplanted from well-matched donors within 1 year of diagnosis was 75%. This study demonstrated that the results of unrelated donor transplants for CML can approach those of HLA-identical sibling transplants, and the authors emphasized the importance of optimizing donor selection and HLA matching early in the course of the disease.

It is clear that these strict criteria for identifying HLA-matched unrelated donors have paid off in producing results not noticeably different from those with related donors. However, there is a downside to this strategy—it reduces the availability of donors. We do not know for sure, but we believe that using our present criteria we can locate well-matched unrelated donors for approximately 40% of patients with newly diagnosed CML, and about half of these patients will be of an acceptable age. Thus, we should be able to transplant about 35% of patients with newly diagnosed CML from HLA-matched donors, either related or unrelated, and about 70% of these should be cured.

STRATEGY FOR USING BMT TO TREAT CML

The results reported above are derived from the Seattle experience. The proposed strategy is obviously applicable only when applied at a center with similar experience. Patients aged 55 years or less who have HLA-identical family members available to act as marrow donors should be offered marrow transplantation as soon as possible after diagnosis. For such patients, there is nothing to be gained and much to be lost by delay.

The Seattle protocols now accept patients aged 65 years or less, and our growing experience justifies recommending early transplantation to patients through the age of 60 years. The situation in counseling older patients is complicated by the fact that delay has the additional risk of moving them into an age group in which the development of "unacceptable" disabilities is more common. Even if age per se is not a contraindication to transplantation, a larger proportion of older patients will not be acceptable because of health problems.

Patients aged 55 years or less who do not have acceptable related donors should be treated with IFN, and a search should be initiated for a suitable unrelated donor. If a well-matched donor is found, the transplant should be performed as soon as logistically feasible unless complete cytogenetic remission has been achieved.

REFERENCES

1. Fefer A, Cheever MA, Thomas ED, et al. Disappearance of Ph^1-positive cells in four patients with chronic granulocytic leukemia after chemotherapy, irradiation and marrow transplantation from an identical twin. N Engl J Med 1979; 300:333.
2. Fefer A, Cheever MA, Greenberg PD, et al. Treatment of chronic granulocytic

leukemia with chemoradiotherapy and transplantation of marrow from identical twins. N Engl J Med 1982; 306:63.
3. Clift RA, Buckner CD, Thomas ED, et al. The treatment of chronic granulocytic leukaemia in chronic phase by allogeneic marrow transplantation. Lancet 1982; ii: 621.
4. Goldman JM, Baughan ASJ, McCarthy DM, et al. Marrow transplantation for patients in the chronic phase of chronic granulocytic leukaemia. Lancet 1982; ii:623.
5. McGlave PB, Arthur DC, Kim TH, Ramsay NKC, Hurd DD, Kersey J. Successful allogeneic bone marrow transplantation for patients in the accelerated phase of chronic granulocytic leukaemia. Lancet 1982; 2:625.
6. Thomas ED, Clift RA, Fefer A, et al. Marrow transplantation for the treatment of chronic myelogenous leukemia. Ann Intern Med 1986; 104:155.
7. Arcese W, Goldman JM, D'Arcangelo E, et al. Outcome for patients who relapse after allogeneic bone marrow transplantation for chronic myeloid leukemia. Blood 1993; 82:3211.
8. Buckner CD, Clift RA. Timing of allogeneic marrow transplants for patients with chronic myeloid leukemia. In: Champlin RE, Gale RP, eds. Advances and Controversies in Bone Marrow Transplantation. Keystone Symposia, 1994. New York: Alan R. Liss, 1994.
9. McGlave PB, DeFabritiis P, Deisseroth A, et al. Autologous marrow transplant therapy for chronic myelogenous leukemia prolongs survival: results from eight transplant groups. Lancet 1994; 343:1486.
10. Higano CS, Raskind W, Singer JW. Use of alpha interferon for the treatment of relapse of chronic myelogenous leukemia in chronic phase after allogeneic bone marrow transplantation. Blood 1992; 80:1437.
11. Higano C, Raskind W, Flowers M. Alpha interferon (IFN) results in high complete cytogenetic response rate in patients with cytogenetic-only relapse of chronic myelogenous leukemia (CML) after marrow transplantation (BMT). Blood 1993; 82(10 suppl 1):169a. Abstract.
12. Kolb HJ, Mittermüller J, Clemm C, et al. Donor leukocyte transfusions for treatment of recurrent chronic myelogenous leukemia in marrow transplant patients. Blood 1990; 76:2462.
13. Zuo L, Keever CA, Roth MS, et al. Salvage immunotherapy using donor leukocyte infusions as treatment for relapsed chronic myelogenous leukemia after allogeneic bone marrow transplantation: efficacy and toxicity of a defined T-cell dose. Blood 1993; 82:2310.
14. Porter DL, Roth MS, McGarigle C, Ferrara JLM, Antin JH. Induction of graft-versus-host disease as immunotherapy for relapsed chronic myeloid leukemia. N Engl J Med 1994; 330:100.
15. Cullis JO, Jiang YZ, Schwarer AP, Hughes TP, Barrett AJ, Goldman JM. Donor leukocyte infusions for chronic myeloid leukemia in relapse after allogeneic bone marrow transplantation. Blood 1992; 79:1379.
16. Cullis JO, Schwarer AP, Hughes TP, et al. Second transplants for patients with chronic myeloid leukaemia in relapse after original transplant with T-depleted marrow: feasibility of using busulphan alone for reconditioning. Br J Haematol 1992; 80:33.
17. Tutschka PJ, Copelan EA, Kapoor N. Replacing total body irradiation with busul-

fan as conditioning of patients with leukemia for allogeneic marrow transplantation. Transplant Proc 1989; 21:2952.
18. Clift RA, Buckner CD, Thomas ED, et al. Marrow transplantation for chronic myeloid leukemia: a randomized study comparing cyclophosphamide and total body irradiation with busulfan and cyclophosphamide. Blood 1994; 84:2036.
19. Clift RA, Buckner CD, Thomas ED, et al. Marrow transplantation for patients in accelerated phase of chronic myeloid leukemia. Blood 1994; 84:4368.
20. Tura S, Baccarani M, Corbelli G. Staging of chronic myeloid leukaemia. Br J Haematol 1981; 47:105.
21. Sokal JE, Baccarani M, Tura S, et al. Prognostic discrimination among younger patients with chronic granulocytic leukemia: relevance to bone marrow transplantation. Blood 1985; 66:1352.
22. Hehlmann R, Heimpel H, Hasford J, et al. Randomized comparison of busulfan and hydroxyurea in chronic myelogenous leukemia: prolongation of survival by hydroxyurea. Blood 1993; 82:398.
23. Italian Cooperative Study Group on Chronic Myeloid Leukemia. Interferon alfa-2a as compared with conventional chemotherapy for the treatment of chronic myeloid leukemia. N Engl J Med 1994; 330:820.
24. Goldman JM, Szydlo R, Horowitz MM, et al. Choice of pretransplant treatment and timing of transplants for chronic myelogenous leukemia in chronic phase. Blood 1993; 82:2235.
25. Anonymous. SEER Cancer Statistics Review: 1973–1990. Bethesda, MD: NCI, 1993.
26. Clift RA, Buckner CD, Appelbaum FR, et al. The influence of patient age on the outcome of transplantation during chronic phase (CP) of chronic myeloid leukemia (CML). Blood 1995; 86:617. Abstract.
27. Kantrow SP, Hackman RC, Boeckh M, Myerson D, Crawford SW. Idiopathic pneumonia syndrome after bone marrow transplantation. ALA/ATS International Conference 1994. Abstract.
28. Hansen JA, Gooley T, Clift R, Petersdorf EW, Martin PJ, Anasetti C. Unrelated donor marrow transplants for patients with chronic myeloid leukemia. Blood 1995; 86:123a. Abstract.

12
Autologous Stem Cell Transplantation for Chronic Myeloid Leukemia

Josy Reiffers, F.X. Mahon, J.M. Boiron, H. Chahine, C. Faberes,
T. Cousin, P. Cony-Makhoul, A. Pigneux, P. Agape, A. Broustet,
and G. Marit
*Université Victor Segalen, Bordeaux 2,
Bordeaux, France*

INTRODUCTION

Chronic myelogenous leukemia (CML) is a clonal myeloproliferative disorder due to an acquired cytogenetic abnormality in a pluripotential stem cell (1). The Philadelphia chromosome (Ph), which is the hallmark of the disease, is the result of a reciprocal translocation involving chromosomes 9 and 22 and juxtaposing the ABL proto-oncogene on chromosome 9 with the BCR gene normally located on chromosome 22 (2).

Allogeneic stem cell transplantation (AlloSCT) remains the only curative treatment for CML, but most CML patients (up to 70%) are either too old for such a transplant (>50 years of age) or lack a suitable HLA-identical (sibling or unrelated) donor (3). Recombinant alpha-interferon (IFN), first introduced by the Houston group in the late 1980s, is capable of inducing hematological and cytogenetic remissions, but the percentage of IFN-responding patients does not exceed 25–40% (4,5). Thus, for patients who either cannot undergo AlloSCT or do not respond to IFN, other treatments have to be proposed. Autologous stem cell transplantation (ASCT), which is one of these alternative treatments, is reviewed in this chapter.

ASCT FOR CML IN TRANSFORMATION

Autologous stem cell transplantation was first attempted for patients with CML in transformation in order to restore a second chronic phase with a similar duration to the first one. It was pioneered by Buckner et al. (6) who used bone marrow harvested during chronic phase to rescue hematopoiesis after a supralethal myeloablative conditioning regimen including total body irradiation (TBI). Subsequently, Goldman et al. reported that blood cells collected at diagnosis could efficiently be used to reconstitute hematopoiesis (7).

The results of ASCT for CML in transformation have been extensively reviewed (8–11) and can be summarized as follows: hematopoietic recovery is quicker after blood cell than bone marrow transplantation; following ASCT, some patients exhibit a "cytogenetic conversion" due to the reemergence of Ph-negative cells and seem to have a prolongation of survival; unsurprisingly, the survival of patients transplanted in the accelerated phase is longer than that of those transplanted in blast crisis; patients who have received a "double" transplant have a longer survival than those undergoing a single transplant; a second chronic phase is obtained in most cases but its duration is usually short, as most patients develop a recurrent blast crisis within 6–9 months due to the clone implicated in the first transformation. Thus, in most patients, restoring a prolonged second chronic phase has not proved possible, so ASCT has progressively been abandoned for patients with CML in transformation.

ASCT IN CHRONIC PHASE

Autotransplants in chronic phase are now increasingly used. Since preliminary results suggest that ASCT could prolong survival (or increase IFN sensitivity) and that some transplants can be performed using Ph-negative (and sometimes BCR-ABL-negative) cells.

Does ASCT Prolong Survival?

As no prospective study has compared ASCT with IFN, it is still unknown whether ASCT could prolong survival in CML, and if so in what category of patients. Many unicentric and multicentric studies have now been published; their main results are summarized in Table 1. They are very difficult to compare as there is a wide heterogeneity in the characteristics of patients (inclusion criteria) and transplants (conditioning regimens, source of stem cells, treatment administered after ASCT). Despite this heterogeneity, the results look similar. Meloni et al. reported 34 patients who were transplanted in chronic phase after a conditioning regimen consisting of melphalan (60 mg/m^2) and busulfan (4 mg/kg/day, 4 days). All patients engrafted, and only one patient died early from interstitial pneumonitis (12). At the time of analysis, 31 of the 34 patients were alive in chronic phase, but the follow-up from transplant was short (around 1

Table 1 Summary of Results of ASCT for CML in Chronic Phase

Number of patients	Source of stem cells[a]	Cytogenetic conversion[b]	Outcome[c]	Reference
34	Unmanipulated BSC	18/32 patients	31/34 A/W (median follow-up of 12 months)	12
21	Unmanipulated BSC	11/17 patients	5-year survival of 56%	13
23	Unmanipulated BSC	14/23 patients	3-year survival of 23%	14
22	Unmanipulated BSC or marrow = 10 Mobilized BSC = 9 Purged marrow = 3	5/22 patients	Median survival of 34 months	15
5	Mafosfamide-treated marrow	5/5 patients	2/5 A/W	34
16	Cultured marrow	7/11 patients	12/16 A/W (median follow-up of)	35
6	IFN-gamma-treated marrow	5/6 patients	5/6 A/W	36
23	Mobilized BSC	7/16 patients treated in early chronic phase achieved a complete response	5-year survival of 64%	41

[a]BSC: Blood stem cells.
[b]More than 50% Ph-negative cells in most cases.
[c]A/W: Alive and well (in chronic phase).

year). The authors also reported that 18 of the 32 evaluated patients had a reduction of Ph-positive metaphases >50% following transplantation.

In London (Hammersmith Hospital), 21 patients were treated with high-dose chemotherapy (busulfan, 4 mg/kg/day × 4 combined with cyclophosphamide or melphalan) ($n = 18$) or cyclophosphamide and TBI followed by the reinfusion of unmanipulated blood stem cells. The 5-year survival from transplantation was 56%. Eleven of the 17 patients studied during the first year post-transplantation had a cytogenetic conversion and seemed to have a prolonged survival (13).

In France, 23 patients with bad prognosis CML (initial Sokal index >1.2; $n = 16$, or no response to IFN; $n = 7$) were transplanted with blood stem cells collected at diagnosis, after a conditioning regimen consisting of busulfan (4 mg/kg/day × 4) and melphalan (140 mg/m^2) (14). Their 3-year transformation-free survival was 66.8 ± 23%, which is similar to that of the London and Rome series.

Khouri et al. have summarized the experience of the M.D. Anderson Cancer Center at Houston (15). They have transplanted 22 patients who either had shown resistance to IFN or were unable to tolerate IFN treatment. Eighteen patients achieved a complete hematological response, and five a partial or complete cytogenetic response. The median survival of these 22 patients was 34 months (from transplantation).

Obviously, the results of the retrospective analysis of multicentric studies correspond to those of unicentric studies. In the report by McGlave et al. (16), 142 patients transplanted during chronic phase in eight major transplant centers were analyzed; their 4-year survival was around 60% and was influenced by the age of patients at the time of transplantation. The source of stem cells (blood versus marrow) and the use of ex vivo cell treatment did not influence survival. In the retrospective analysis of the European Blood and Marrow Transplantation Registry (EBMTR), we have now analyzed 174 patients who underwent autologous blood (66%) or marrow (34%) stem cell transplantation during chronic phase after different conditioning regimens. Most of these patients were treated with IFN-α after transplantation. The actuarial percentage of patients surviving at 5 years was 68.4 ± 11% and was significantly higher for younger patients and, more importantly, for those who achieved hematological or cytogenetic responses following ASCT. Interestingly, in this series of patients, we found that survival was not influenced by the source of stem cells (marrow versus peripheral blood; purged versus unpurged stem cells) and that ASCT was able to restore IFN sensitivity in some patients who had exhibited IFN resistance prior to ASCT.

In summary, ASCT performed during chronic phase has an acceptable toxicity (as the transplant-related mortality does not exceed 5%) and produces a 5-year survival from transplantation around 50–70%. This result compares favorably with those of AlloSCT, but unlike AlloSCT, most patients surviving after ASCT have persistent disease. Thus, ASCT is not a curative treatment in CML but could prolong survival. This needs to be confirmed prospectively. If ASCT is able to prolong survival, it is interesting to discern what category of patients with CML in chronic phase could benefit from ASCT. As seen above (4,5), some patients respond to IFN and those who achieve a major (≥65% Ph-negative cells) or complete cytogenetic response have a 85–90% chance of surviving at 5 years. For these patients, it cannot be excluded that ASCT might prolong survival, but this would be very difficult to demonstrate. As most of these IFN-responding patients do not have a high Sokal index, it can be imagined that ASCT could be indicated for patients with high-risk CML.

In France we have performed "straight ASCT" in 20 CML patients with a Sokal index >1.2. These patients were given busulfan and melphalan, then were reinfused with blood stem cells. Fifteen of them received IFN after ASCT, and three achieved a major cytogenetic response. Fifteen of the 20 patients are still alive 1–61 months after transplant. Some authors have also suggested that ASCT could benefit patients who have exhibited resistance to IFN. In the series of Khouri et al. (15), ASCT did not seem to prolong survival in these IFN-resistant patients, whereas in the EBMT retrospective analysis, some patients were restored to IFN sensitivity after ASCT (18). Thus, the possible restoration of IFN sensitivity after ASCT needs to be further evaluated.

The indication of ASCT is also debated in patients who have an HLA-identical sibling or unrelated donor. As the early transplant-related mortality of AlloSCT is relatively high (about 30%), it has been suggested to reserve AlloSCT for patients who did not respond to IFN and/or ASCT, at least for those >35–40 years of age or those having either a mismatch family donor or an unrelated donor.

What Source of Stem Cells?

ASCT can be performed with either unpurged bone marrow or blood stem cells. As the concentration of blood progenitor cells is very high in CML at diagnosis, one single leukapheresis usually contains more than 10×10^4 CFU-CM/kg (7). When transplanted, these cells engraft very quickly (about 15 days), which is more rapidly than observed after autologous bone marrow transplantation (19). It has now been reported that both peripheral blood and bone marrow in early chronic phase contain some Ph-negative progenitors (20–22). These normal progenitors are able to engraft and are probably responsible for the cytogenetic conversions which are regularly seen after ASCT (9,11,23). Thus, as peripheral blood seems to be equivalent to bone marrow for observing cytogenetic conversion and to contain more progenitors (leading to quicker engraftment) than bone marrow, most autologous transplants are now performed with blood stem cells.

Whatever the source of stem cells (blood or marrow), the main question concerns purging. It is must unlikely that ASCT would cure CML if Ph-positive multipotent stem cells are reinfused to the patients. Moreover, Deisseroth et al. (24), using gene marking techniques, have reported that transplanted leukemic progenitor cells could contribute to relapse after ASCT. Thus many attempts have been made to eradicate Ph-positive leukemic cells from the graft.

Ex vivo purging techniques include the use of hyperthermia (25), cyclophosphamide derivatives (hydroxycyclophosphamide and mafosfamide-AZTA Z) (26), long-term cultures (27), interferons or interleukin-2 (28,29), and, more recently, ribozymes (30), antisense oliognucleotides (31), or tyrosine kinase inhibitors (32). Other methods have also been reported (33). Some of their in vitro results are encouraging as incubation of CML marrow cells with these latter agents could lead to a decrease in the number of Ph-positive colonies (as compared to unmanipulated cells). The clinical results are more disappointing (or difficult to interpret). Carlo-Stella et al. have reported 10 patients who were transplanted with marrow treated ex vivo with mafosfamide (34). After a median follow-up of 16 months, only three patients are alive without disease transformation (two among the five patients transplanted in first chronic phase). Barnett et al. have reported 16 patients transplanted in first chronic phase with cultured marrow (35). Twelve of these patients are alive without transformation 12–68 months after ASCT. However, hematological recovery was delayed (about 30 days), and three patients died from transplant-related complications; moreover, the transplanted patients were selected on the basis of a laboratory assessment of their marrow to test its capacity to initiate normal long-term culture-initiating cells after 10 days of culture. This assay excluded about one-third of the patients.

McGlave et al. reported six patients transplanted in first chronic phase with marrow treated ex vivo with interferon gamma (36). One patient died early, and the other five were alive at the time of publication with some minor cytogenetic responses; however, the follow-up from transplant was very short (12 months). The other techniques of purging, such as those using c-myb or BCR-ABL antisense oligonucleotides, have not been extensively tested clinically. They did not seem to impair hematological reconstitution in one patient reported by De Fabritiis et al. (21), but this needs to be confirmed in a larger number of patients.

Therefore, although interesting, these clinical protocols using purged stem cells need to be further explored, as their possible advantage (prolongation of survival over unpurged ASCT) is not yet demonstrated. They also have some drawbacks such as a delayed engraftment, and do not seem to induce cytogenetic responses more frequently than after unpurged ASCT (12,14,23). Besides these latter purging methods, it has also been proposed to select Ph-negative, BCR-ABL-negative progenitors from the CD34-positive fraction. These normal progenitors probably belong to subfractions of CD34 + CD38-Lin-negative or CD34 + CD33-Lin-negative subpopulations, or even CD34 + Thy-positive cells (20). They could be expanded using different culture techniques. In our laboratory, we have treated CML blood cells with 5-fluorouracil (5-Fu) to gain access to primitive progenitors, then grown these 5-Fu-resistant cells with different combinations of cytokines. Cytogenetic and molecular evaluation of the cells grown showed that, at least in some cases, Ph-negative, BCR-ABL-negative cells were preferentially expanded (37).

In vivo purging is another strategy to decrease the number (or percentage) of leukemic stem cells from the graft. In 1985, we treated some CML patients with intensive nonmyeloblative chemotherapy. During recovery from chemotherapy-induced marrow aplasia, we collected bone marrow from four of these patients and used it for transplantation. The transplanted marrow contained 25, 46, 100, and 100% Ph-positive cells, respectively. After transplant a long-lasting complete cytogenetic response was observed in the patient transplanted with 75% Ph-negative cells (38). Such a strategy, which had been used in 1981 by Körbling et al. (39), was reintroduced by Carella et al. when growth factors became available. They treated 49 patients with a combination of idarubicin (5 mg/m^2/day, 3–5 days), cytosine arabinoside (800 mg/m^2/day, 3–5 days), and etoposide (150 mg/m^2/day, 3 days) (ICE protocol) followed by G-CSF.

Leukaphereses performed as soon as the white blood cell count reached 0.8×10^9/L contained >50% Ph-negative metaphases in patients treated during the first year from diagnosis (40). The percentage of Ph-negative cells in leukaphereses was significantly lower in patients treated during late chronic phase or transformation than in those treated in early chronic phase. The authors reported the results of 23 patients in chronic phase who underwent autologous transplantation of such mobilized cells and were subsequently treated by IFN-α or interleukin-2 (41). As seen above, these patients were selected among 49 patients treated in chronic phase with the ICE protocol.

Although most patients achieved a cytogenetic response (seven of the 15 patients transplanted in early chronic phase achieved a complete cytogenetic response), the overall survival did not seem to be longer than that observed after unpurged stem cell transplantation, as the estimated proportion of patients alive at 5 years was 64%. Other authors used a combination of hydroxyurea and G-CSF to mobilize Ph-negative cells and found that this approach was comparable in efficacy to that of the ICE protocol and probably less toxic (42). Simonsson et al. enrolled 160 patients with CML. They planned to treat these patients with three courses of intensive chemotherapy, high-dose IFN-α, and hydroxyurea and to collect bone marrow when Ph-negativity was achieved (43). Ph-negativity was obtained in 5–35% cases after each course of chemotherapy. Thirty patients were autotransplanted with Ph-negative cells, and 25 were alive at the time of report. However, with 31 months median follow-up, the 6-year actuarial survival from diagnosis of the initial population of 130 patients was 68%, which is similar to that observed after unpurged ASCT.

Ph-negative blood cells can be mobilized with growth factors alone without necessarily using chemotherapy in addition. We have recently treated 23 patients with G-CSF (lenograstim 150 mg/m^2/day) (44). They were in either major or complete cytogenetic response under IFN treatment when G-CSF was initiated. Leukaphereses performed after 5–12 days of lenograstim contained no Ph-positive metaphases in 57% of cases. Interestingly, Ph-negative leukaphereses were obtained in some patients who were not in complete response after

IFN-α. Similar results have also been reported by Carreras et al. (45), suggesting that, at least in some patients, G-CSF could preferentially stimulate Ph-negative cells. The results of ASCT using Ph-negative progenitors collected in these latter conditions cannot be evaluated yet, as the number of patients transplanted is too low and the follow-up from transplantation too short.

Finally, another method of in vivo purging could be serial transplantation. Based upon the experience of Daley et al. on transplantation of BCR-ABL-infected stem cells in mice, most stem cells competing for hematopoietic reconstitution after an initial transplant could be normal (46). So the transplantation of these cells collected after a first transplant could lead to a significant prolongation of Ph-negativity when used for a second transplant (47).

CONCLUSION

As for AlloSCT, the results of ASCT for CML in blast crisis are very poor. When performed during chronic phase, ASCT gives results which suggest that it could prolong survival, but this needs to be demonstrated with a prospective randomized study. Up to now, the different methods of purging, although producing interesting in vitro results, have failed to prolong survival significantly.

REFERENCES

1. Fialkow PJ, Jacobson RJ, Papayannopoulo T. Chronic myelocytic leukemia: clonal origin in a stem cell common to granulocyte, platelet and monocyte/macrophage. Am J Med 1977; 63:125–130.
2. De Klein A, Geurts van Kessel A, Grosveld G, et al. A cellular oncogene is translocated to the Philadelphia chromosome in chronic myelocytic leukaemia. Nature 1982; 300:765–770.
3. Goldman JM, Apperley JF, Jones LM, et al. Bone marrow transplantation for patients with chronic myeloid leukemia. N Engl J Med 1986; 314:202–207.
4. Kantarjian HM, Smith TL, O'Brien S, Beran M, Pierce S, Talpaz M. Prolonged survival in chronic myelogenous leukemia following cytogenetic response to alpha interferon therapy. Ann Intern Med 1995; 122:254–261.
5. Italian Cooperative Study Group on Chronic Myeloid Leukemia. Interferon alpha-2a as compared with conventional chemotherapy for the treatment of chronic myeloid leukemia. N Engl J Med 1994; 330:820–825.
6. Buckner CD, Stewart P, Clift RA, et al. Treatment of blastic transformation of chronic granulocytic leukemia by chemotherapy, total body irradiation and infusion of cryopreserved autologous marrow. Exp Hematol 1978; 6:96–109.
7. Goldman JM, Th'ng KH, Park DS, Spiers ASD, Lowenthal RM, Ruutu T. Collection, cryopreservation and subsequent viability of haemopoietic stem cells intended for treatment of chronic granulocytic leukemia in blast-cell transformation. Br J Haematol 1978; 40:185–195.

8. Butturini A, Keating A, Goldman J, Gale RP. Autotransplants in chronic myelogenous leukaemia: strategies and results. Lancet 1990; 335:1255–1258.
9. Reiffers J, Mahon FX, Boiron JM, et al. Autografitng in chronic myeloid leukemia: an overview. Leukemia 1996; 10:385–388.
10. Reiffers J, Trouette R, Marit G, et al. Autologous blood stem cell transplantation for chronic granulocytic leukemia in transformation: a report of 47 cases. Br J Haematol 1991; 77:339–345.
11. Haines Me, Goldman, JM, Worsley AM, et al. Chemotherapy and autografting for chronic granulocytic leukemia in transformation: probable prolongation of survival in some patients. Br J Haematol 1984; 58:711–721.
12. Meloni G, De Fabritiis P, Alimena F, et al. Autologous bone marrow transplantation or peripheral blood stem cell transplantation for patients which chronic myelogenous leukemia in chronic phase. Bone Marrow Transplant 1990; 4(suppl 4): 92–94.
13. Hoyle C, Gray R, Goldman J. Autografting for patients with CML in chronic phase: an update. Br J Haematol 1994; 86:76–81.
14. Reiffers J, Cahn JY, Montastruc M, et al. Peripheral blood stem cell transplantation followed by recombinant alpha interferon for chronic myelogenous leukemia in chronic phase: preliminary results. Stem Cells 1993; 11:23–24.
15. Khouri IF, Kantarjian H, Talpaz M, et al. Results with high-dose chemotherapy and unpurged autologous stem cell transplantation in 73 patients with chronic myelogenous leukemia: the MD Anderson experience. Bone Marrow Transplant 1996; 17:775–779.
16. McGlave PB, De Fabritiis P, Deisseroth J, et al. Autologous transplants for chronic myelogenous leukemia: results from eight transplant groups. The Lancet 1994; 343: 1486–1488.
17. Reiffers J, Goldman J, Meloni G, Cahn JY, Gratwohl A on behalf of the Chronic Leukemia Working Party of the EBMT. Autologous stem cell transplantation in chronic myelogenous leukemia: a retrospective analysis of the European Group for Bone Marrow Transplantation. Bone Marrow Transplant 1994; 14:407–410.
18. Boiron JM, Cahn JY, Carlo-Stella C, et al. Autologous Stem Cell Transplantation (ASCT) for patients with chronic myeloid leukemia (CML) in first chronic phase (CP1) not responding to alpha-interferon (IFN). Blood 1996; 88(suppl 1):126a.
19. Rieffers J. Autologous transplantation in chronic myelogenous leukemia. Blood Transf Immunohaemat 1985; 28:509–520.
20. Kirk JA, Reems JA, Roecklein BA, et al. Benign marrow progenitors are enriched in CD34+/HLA-DR^{lo} population but not in the CD34+/38^{lo} population in chronic myeloid leukemia: an analysis using interphase fluorescence in situ hybridization. Blood 1995; 86:737–743.
21. Petzer AL, Eaves CJ, Lansdorp PM, Ponchio MJ, Barentt MJ, Eaves AC. Characterization of primitive subpopulation of normal leukemic cells in the blood of patients with newly diagnosed as well as established chronic myeloid leukemia. Blood 1996; 88:2162–2171.
22. Coulombel L, Kalousek DK, Eaves CJ, Gupta CM, Eaves AC. Long-term marrow culture reveals chromosomally normal hematopoietic progenitor cells in patients with Philadelphia chromosome positive chronic myelogenous leukemia. N Engl J Med 1983; 308:1493–1498.

23. Brito-Babapulle F, Bowcock SJ, Marcus RE, et al. Autografting for patients with chronic myeloid leukemia in chronic phase: peripheral blood stem cells may have a finite capacity for maintaining haematopoiesis. Br J Haematol 1989; 73:76–81.
24. Diesseroth AB, Zu Z, Claxton D, et al. Genetic marking shows that Ph+ cells present in autologous transplant of chronic myelogenous leukemia (CML) contribute to relapse after autologous bone marrow in CML. Blood 1994; 83:3068–3076.
25. Osman Y, Moriyama Y, Shibata A. Enhanced elimination of Ph+ chromosome cells in vitro by combined hyperthermia and other drugs (AZT, IFN-α, TNF, and quercetin): its application to autologous bone marrow transplantation for CML. Exp Hematol 1995; 23:444–452.
26. Carlo-Stella C, Mangoni L, Piovani G, et al. In vitro purging in chronic myelogenous leukemia: effect of mafosfamide and recombinant granulocyte-macrophage colony-stimulating factor. Bone Marrow Transplant 1991; 8:265–271.
27. Barnett MJ, Eaves J, Phillips GL, et al. Successful autografting in chronic myeloid leukemia after maintenance of marrow cultures. Bone Marrow Transplant 1989; 4:345–351.
28. Becker M, Fabrega S, Belloc F, Rice A, Barbu V, Reiffers J. Interferon gamma is effective for BM purging in a patient with CML. Bone Marrow Transplant 1993; 12:155–158.
29. Gambacorti-Passerini C, Rivoltini L, Fizzotti M, et al. Selective purging by human interleukin-2 activated lymphocytes of bone marrow contaminated with a lymphoma line or autologous leukaemic cells. Br J Haematol 1991; 78:197–205.
30. James H, Mills K, Gibson I. Investigating and improving the specificity of ribozymes directed against the bcr-abl translocation . Leukemia 1996; 10:1054–1064.
31. De Fabritiis P, Amadori S, Petti MC, et al. In vitro purging with BCR-ABL antisense oligonucleotides does not prevent haematologic reconstitution after autologous bone marrow transplantation. Leukemia 1995; 9:662–668.
32. Druker BJ, Tamura S, Buchdunger E, et al. Effects of a selective inhibitor of the Abl tyrosine kinase on the growth of Bcr-Abl positive cells. Nature Med 1996; 2:561–565.
33. O'Brien SG, Goldman JM. Current approaches to hematopoietic stem-cell purging in chronic myeloid leukemia. J Clin Oncol 1995; 13:541–546.
34. Carlo-Stella C, Mangoni L, Almici C, et al. Autologous transplant for chronic myelogenous leukemia using marrow treated ex vivo with mafosfamide. Bone Marrow Transplant 1994; 14:425–432.
35. Barnett MJ, Eaves CJ, Phillips GL, et al. Autografting with cultured marrow in chronic myeloid leukemia: results of a pilot study. Blood 1994; 84:724–732.
36. McGlave PB, Arther D, Miller WJ, Lasky L, Kersey J. Autologous transplantation for CML using marrow treated ex vivo with recombinant human interferon gamma. Bone Marrow Transplant 1990; 6:115–120.
37. Jazwiec B, Mahon FX, Pigneux A, Pigeonnier V, Reiffers J. 5-Fluorouracil resistant CD34+ cell population from peripheral blood of CML patients contains Bcr-Abl negative progenitor cells. Exp Hematol 1995; 23:1509–1514.
38. Reiffers J, Maraninchi D, Marit G, et al. Autologous transplantation of Ph-positive cell depleted marrow in chronic granulocytic leukemia. In: Dicke K, Spitzer G,

Jagannath S, eds. Autologous Bone Marrow Transplantation. Houston: University of Texas M.D. Anderson Hospital and Tumor Institute, 1987:199–203.
39. Körbling M, Burke P, Braine H, Elfenbein G, Santos G, Kaiser H. Successful engraftment of blood derived normal hemopoietic stem cells in chronic myelogenous leukemia. Exp Hematol 1981; 9:684–690.
40. Carella AM, Podesta M, Frassoni F, et al. Collection of normal blood repopulating cells during early hematopoietic recovery after intensive conventional chemotherapy in chronic myelogenous leukemia. Bone Marrow Transplant 1993; 12:267–271.
41. Carella AM, Chimirri F, Podesta M, et al. High-dose chemo-radiotherapy followed by autologous Philadelphia chromosome-negative blood progenitor cell transplantation in patients with chronic myelogenous leukemia. Bone Marrow Transplant 1996; 17:201–205.
42. Johnson J, Owen RG, Child JA, et al. Mobilization of Philadelphia-negative peripheral blood mononuclear cells in chronic myeloid leukaemia using hydroxyurea and G-CSF (filgrastim). Br J Haematol 1996; 93:863–868.
43. Simonsson B, Oberg G, Björeman M, et al. Intensive treatment in order to minimize the Ph-positive clone in CML. Bone Marrow Transplant 1996; 17(suppl 3): S63–S64.
44. Reiffers J, Taylor K, Gluckman E, Gorin N, Carella A, Destée D. Ph-negative blood progenitors cells can be successfully collected with lenograstim in patients with chronic myeloid leukemia good responders to alpha-interferon. Bone Marrow Transplant 1996; 17(suppl 1).
45. Carreras E, Sierra J, Rovira M, et al. Successful autografting in chronic myelogenous leukemia using Philadelphia negative blood progenitor cell mobilized with rHuG-GCF alone in a patient responding to alpha-interferon. Br J Haematol 1997.
46. Daley GQ, Van Etten RA, Baltimore D. Induction of chronic myelogenous leukemia in mice by the $P210^{bcr/abl}$ gene of the Philadelphia chromosome. Science 1990; 247:824–830.
47. Daley GQ, Goldman JM. Autologous transplant for CML revisited. Exp Hematol 1993; 21:734–737.

13
Philadelphia Chromosome-Negative Chronic Myelogenous Leukemia

Jorge E. Cortes
M.D. Anderson Cancer Center, Houston, Texas

John F. Seymour
Royal Melbourne Hospital, Parkville, Australia

INTRODUCTION

The Philadelphia chromosome (Ph) results from a balanced translocation between the long arms of chromosomes 9 and 22, t(9;22)(q34;q11). Since its first description in 1960 by Nowell and Hungerford (1), it has been considered the hallmark of chronic myelogenous leukemia (CML) (2,3) as it is found in the majority of patients with this disease. However, a small percentage of patients with clinical features suggestive of CML do not have the Ph chromosome. The true frequency of this phenomenon is unclear, in part because of the different diagnostic criteria used to select the cases studied in different series. Earlier series reported as many as 29% of patients with CML to lack evidence of the Ph chromosome by standard cytogenetic methods (4), but it has become clear that some patients previously considered as Ph-negative CML should be reclassified on morphological criteria as having one of the myelodysplastic syndromes (MDS) (5). Consequently, more recent series suggest that Ph-negative cases comprise only 5–10% of all patients with CML (6,7). Significant controversy on the nature of this disease persists, with a wide range of interpretations to this phenomenon, ranging from those who have considered it as a "nonentity" (8) to those who consider it to be indistinguishable from Ph-positive CML (9). As more information on the molecular mechanisms of Ph-negative CML has become available, the biology of the disease is now better understood.

MOLECULAR CHARACTERIZATION

From the initial clinical descriptions of patients with Ph-negative CML, it was clear that this diagnostic label embraced a heterogeneous group of patients (4). Although most early series reported a generally poor prognosis for this group of patients (4,10,11), some studies identified a bimodal survival pattern, with some patients having a short survival while others followed a similar course as patients with Ph-positive CML (4), consistent with the presence of populations of patients with two distinct disease processes.

Masked, Variant, and Complex Translocations

In 1983 it was identified that the c-abl ongogene is translocated from its normal location in the long arm of chromosome 9 to the long arm of chromosome 22 within what was then called the bcr region (12,13), providing the molecular explanation for the Ph-chromosome. A first attempt to understand the mechanisms underlying some cases of Ph-negative CML was the study of complex and variant chromosomal translocations (14). Several investigators have reported that up to 3–10% of patients with CML show a variation of the Ph-chromosome by standard cytogenetic analysis (15,16), and more sensitive techniques such as fluorescence in situ hybridization (FISH) may identify some additional cases that escape detection by standard cytogenetic analysis (17). Variant translocations involve chromosome 22 [t(V;22)] or chromosome 9 [t(V;9)], and complex translocations involve usually a three- or four-way translocation affecting chromosomes 9 and 22 and at least one other chromosome (14).

Hagemeijer et al. (19) first reported two CML patients with complex translocations t(9;12;22)(q34;q13;q11) and t(4;9;22)(p16;q34;q11) in whom, by in situ hybridization, a translocation of the c-abl similar to that of Ph-positive CML was identified. Later this group and others reported similar mechanisms on patients with variant translocations involving chromosome 22, t(V;22) (20,21). Based on these results, and considering that the initial description of the Ph chromosome identified it as a minute chromosome 22 (1), patients in whom chromosome 22 was involved in simple or complex translocations were considered to represent a manifestation of the same molecular event as the Ph chromosome. It was proposed that even single variant translocation involving chromosome 22, t(V;22), in fact represents complex translocations in which some part of 9q34 was involved (20). These patients were subsequently considered to have "Ph-positive disease."

Conversely, variant translocations involving only chromosome 9, t(V;9), were still considered to represent a separate disease entity. However, it soon became evident that the molecular events characteristic of the Ph chromosome could be identified in most of these patients. Bartram et al. (21) first reported on a patient with a clinical diagnosis of CML with a t(9;12)(q34;q21) without detectable Ph chromosome. By using in situ hybridization and Southern blotting techniques, they documented a rearrangement within the bcr region and a joint translocation of bcr and c-abl to the derivative chromosome 12 (21). Numerous other reports of similar cases followed, establishing the presence of molecular events characteristic of Ph-positive disease in patients with most variant or complex translocations, leading to the current view that these patients should be considered as having "Ph-positive" CML (22–24).

Ph-Negative, bcr-Positive CML

In 1986 Morris et al. reported five CML patients with a normal karyotype in which they investigated the presence of a BCR/ABL junction (25) by Southern blot. Two of the patients harbored rearrangements of the bcr region similar to that seen in Ph-positive cases, whereas three others had no evidence of rearrangement (25). Several groups subsequently reported small series of patients with Ph-negative CML with rearrangement of bcr (26–29). Therefore, some patients with Ph-negative CML have molecular features indistinguishable from those of patients with Ph-positive CML, with rearrangement in the bcr region, juxtaposition of c-abl, and expression of the aberrant 8.5-kb mRNA and its product, the 210-kD bcr-abl protein.

Two distinct mechanisms have been proposed to explain the lack of detectable karyotypic abnormalities despite the obvious molecular events. One postulated model suggests that an interstitial insertion of c-abl into bcr occurs. According to this mechanism, there is a two-break deletion of chromosome 9q34 which is then inserted between the two ends of a single break at chromosome 22q11 (25,29–33). The length of the 9q34 inserted into chromosome 22 is variable (33), but the common feature in all cases described is the lack of detection of 3' fragments of bcr in chromosome 9. The second proposed mechanism is the occurrence of a standard translocation t(9;22)(q34;q11) followed by a second translocation that reverses the original translocation, reconstituting chromosome 22 while leaving a fragment of 9q34 including c-abl in place (34–37). In this schema, the second break in both chromosomes 9 and 22 occurs distal to the initial translocation t(9;22)(q34;q11), thus leaving 3' fragment of bcr in chromosome 9 that can be identified by in situ hybridization (35) or FISH (36). It is likely that both mechanisms occur, although it is possible that the single-event mechanism is more frequent (30). Interestingly, a few Ph-negative CML patients have been reported in which bcr is rearranged, but the mechanism appears to be the translocation of bcr from chromosome 22 to chromosome 9 (38–41). The BCR-ABL fusion gene can therefore be localized by FISH to chromosome 9 (38–41). There has been at least one CML patient reported with Ph-negative, bcr rearrangement-positive disease in whom a novel 7.3-kb bcr mRNA was detected, with no evidence of the 8.5-kb bcr/abl transcript (42).

bcr-Negative CML

Overall, in approximately 30–50% of patients with Ph-negative CML, bcr rearrangement can be detected and the common bcr-abl transcripts (b3a2 or b2a2) identified. However, there remains a small but significant number of patients in whom bcr rearrangement cannot be identified by standard molecular techniques. As discussed below, this represents a group of patients with heterogeneous clinical characteristics, and the molecular mechanisms driving the pathological processes are likely to be similarly heterogeneous.

However, recent evidence suggests that a portion of patients considered to have Ph-negative bcr rearrangement-negative have a variant bcr/abl junction. Early studies recognized the variability in the breakpoints in patients with Ph-positive and Ph-negative CML (27,28,43). Several authors have identified patients with Ph-positive and Ph-negative disease in which a small 3'-bcr probe did not identify rearrangement of bcr whereas a larger probe encompassing 5' sequences uncovered the rearrangement. This phenomenon has been described in both Ph-positive (27) and Ph-negative (28,43) disease. In these patients, the 3' sequences corresponding to those hybridized by the shorter probe are deleted and the breakpoint occurs at a more 5' location. More frequent application of methods using the larger universal probe in most recent studies has led to the identification of an increasing number of patients with Ph-positive CML in which the bcr rearrangement could be located either 3' or 5' of the bcr region (44–48). The area affected during rearrangement of bcr in these patients is highly variable, but this variability shows that regions other than the M-bcr can be affected in Ph-positive CML. Similar variability in the breakpoint in c-abl gene has been described; both van der Plas et al. (49) and Iwata et al. (50) have reported Ph-positive CML patients with a breakpoint that excludes exon a2, resulting in a b2a3 (49) or a b3a3 (5) fusion transcript.

A number of breakpoint cluster regions outside M-bcr that are reproducibly involved in translocations have been well characterized. A small but increasing number of patients have been described in whom the breakpoint occurs in the first intron of the m-bcr gene (rather than the M-bcr region), thus creating an e1a2 junction between the first exon of the bcr gene and exon 2 of c-abl (51–56; Cortes J, unpublished). The resulting protein product is of a similar size to the p190BCR/ABL expressed in most cases of Ph-positive acute lymphoblastic leukemia. Six patients with such a breakpoint have been reported (51–56), and we have observed three additional unpublished cases. All patients had the Ph chromosome, but no bcr rearrangement could be detected by using the conventional probes for CML (51–56; Cortes J, unpublished).

In other patients the breakpoint occurs in a region 3' to M-bcr, between exons e19 and e20 (also known as c3 and c4) resulting in an e19a2 (or c3a2) junction which translates into a slightly larger protein; p230BCR/ABL (57–59). The name µ-bcr has been proposed for this region (59). All patients reported with these breakpoints express the Ph chromosome. However, Hochhaus et al. recently reported a patient with Ph-negative CML in which a novel BCR-ABL fusion gene was detected (60). The BCR-ABL resulted from a breakpoint 5' from M-bcr resulting in a junction between exon e6 of the bcr gene and exon a2 of c-abl. This translated into a protein slightly larger than the p185BCR/ABL (60). Although only one patient has been reported with this rearrangement, it illustrates the fact that the absence of the Ph chromosome and rearrangement in the M-bcr region (which is currently investigated in most patients) in a patient with CML is not sufficient to exclude bcr rearrangement. As reviewed by Hochhaus et al. (60), the structure of the bcr and c-abl genes provides for a large number of potential in frame BCR-ABL fusions with variability in the bcr and c-abl breakpoint regions. Therefore, patients must be thoroughly investigated for rearrangements of the bcr and abl genes before they are classified as Ph-negative, bcr rearrangement-negative. The use of pulsed-field gel electrophoresis may be useful in detecting some of these patients (61). Recently, a PCR technique in which cDNA is amplified using four oligonucleotide primers has been developed and found useful in detecting unusual bcr breakpoints (60,62). Western blot for the BCR-ABL chimeric protein (63) might be another useful tool in detecting rearrangement of bcr. It is possible that with more extensive investigation, most patients will demonstrate rearrangement of the bcr gene.

However, it remains probable that regardless of the completeness of investigation, some patients do not have any bcr rearrangement and that their disease process is related to other mechanisms within the bcr or abl genes, or unrelated to them. It is established that in the murine system, point mutations within the ABL gene, independent of any involvement by bcr, can result in functional activation and leukemogenesis. Therefore, Melo et al. (67) looked for evidence of such point mutations involving c-abl in 25 patients with Ph-negative, bcr rearrangement-negative CML using restriction fragment length polymorphism and single-strand conformational polymorphism (67). No such point mutations were found. Cogswell et al. reported a high incidence of ras mutations in patients with Ph-negative, bcr rearrangement-negative CML (64). Five of the nine patients investigated with these characteristics had evidence of ras mutations, compared to none of the 39 patients with Ph-positive CML in chronic phase, and one of 18 with Ph-positive CML in blastic phase (64). These results are concordant with the 57–69% incidence of point mutations in ras found in patients with CMML (65,66). Other studies, however, have not confirmed this high frequency of ras mutations in Ph-negative, bcr rearrangement-negative CML (66). It is obvious that there is much still to be learned from patients with

Ph-negative, apparently bcr rearrangement-negative disease, and the understanding of the molecular mechanisms will clarify some of the clinical variability and controversies that we will now analyze.

CLINICAL CHARACTERISTICS

It is difficult to describe the clinical features and outcome of patients with Ph-negative CML. Not only is there marked heterogeneity within this disease category, but in many reported series, some patients should be reclassified as having other hematological diagnoses, most frequently CMML or other MDS. However, since the earliest reports of patients with Ph-negative CML, some distinctive features are consistently identified. These patients tend to be older, have lower white blood cell (WBC) and platelet counts, and frequently lack basophilia (4,10,11). Their response to chemotherapy was found to be poor, and their survival shorter than patients with Ph-positive CML (4,10,11). However, on clinical grounds two groups of patients could be identified: some had these atypical clinical features and short survival whereas the clinical characteristics and outcome in others resembled those of patients with Ph-positive CML, consistent with the inclusion of both bcr-positive and bcr-negative categories, respectively (4).

In their initial description of the presence of molecular evidence of the BCR-ABL fusion in CML patients with normal karyotype, Morris et al. provide molecular correlation to this heterogeneity (25). In this report, two of the five patients investigated had bcr rearrangement. These two patients had clinical characteristics undistinguishable from Ph-positive CML disease. In contrast, the three patients without rearrangement were older, responded poorly to treatment, and had a short survival (25). Since then, several investigators have confirmed the identical clinical characteristics of patients with Ph-positive CML and those with Ph-negative, bcr rearrangement-positive disease (7,27,28,68–70). Wiedemann et al. (28) investigated 28 patients who had been diagnosed with Ph-negative CML for bcr rearrangement. After consideration of the clinical characteristics at diagnosis, 10 of the 17 patients were considered to be clinically indistinguishable from CML, whereas the others could be reclassified into other diseases. All 10 with typical CML features, but none of the other seven, had bcr rearrangement (28).

Similarly, Shtalrid et al. (27) described seven patients with Ph-negative, bcr rearrangement-positive disease, all of whom had clinical features identical to those of Ph-positive CML. Two other groups have compared the clinical characteristics of Ph-negative, bcr rearrangement-positive patients to those of Ph-positive patients seen at their institutions during the same study period (7,69,70). The two groups found nearly identical clinical features (7,69,70). The only dissenting report is that of Dreazen et al. (29), who described 10 patients with Ph-negative, bcr rearrangement-positive CML and noticed heterogeneity in their clinical features. Four of the patients in this group had clinical features that these investigators consider uncharacteristic of classical Ph-positive CML, including lack of splenomegaly despite a high WBC, low platelet count, no eosinophilia and/or basophilia, and poor response to treatment (29). Therefore, the authors questioned the notion that the bcr/abl fusion gene determines the clinical features of the disease. However, these authors failed to recognize the heterogeneity that exists even within patients with Ph-positive disease. All the atypical characteristics shown by the four patients with uncharacteristic CML can be seen in patients with CML, and some of these features are recognized adverse prognostic features in CML (71,72). In fact, the four patients with atypical disease despite the presence of bcr rearrangement could be considered to be in accelerated phase (71), accounting for their adverse outcomes. Further, when patients in early chronic phase are compared, the clinical characteristics, including the frequency of poor prognostic features, are similar for patients with Ph-positive and Ph-negative, bcr rearrangement-positive disease (7). Therefore, it is now accepted that patients with bcr rearrangement, whether Ph-positive or Ph-negative, have the same disease.

The reports on the clinical characteristics of patients with Ph-negative, bcr rearrangement-negative CML have been variable. Some have reported patients with clinical features at diagnosis indistinguishable from those of patients with Ph-positive disease (9,73). Others, however, have found significant differences when comparing these patients to those with bcr rearrangement-positive disease (whether Ph-positive or Ph-negative) (7,68–70). Patients with bcr rearrangement-negative disease have been found at diagnosis to be older, to have lower white blood cell and platelet counts, to be more frequently anemic, to have higher monocyte counts both in peripheral blood and bone marrow, less basophilia, a lower percentage of immature myeloid precursors in peripheral blood, and a higher percentage of erythroblasts in the bone marrow (7,69,70).

In analyzing these apparently conflicting results, two factors should be considered. First, despite the statistical significance of the differences between the two groups in some of the clinical characteristics in some of the comparative studies (7,69,70), there is considerable overlap in the clinical characteristics of these groups of patients (68). Second, it is possible that some of the patients considered as Ph-negative, bcr rearrangement-negative in some studies can be reclassified into other diseases. In some series, a revision of the original clinical features of patients considered to have Ph-negative CML have led to reclassification of these patients into other diseases, including true CMML and unclassified myeloproliferative disorders (5,8,28). This has led some investigators to consider Ph-negative CML as a nonentity (8).

However, as mentioned above, there is a group of patients with clinical features indistinguishable from those of Ph-positive disease (9,73). When analyzing these differences, Shepherd et al. identified an intermediate group of patients with features distinct from those of CMML and of Ph-positive CML (74), and proposed the name atypical CML (aCML) (74). This is an ill-defined group which is not yet universally accepted and whose clinical and molecular characteristics as well as its outcome are not completely understood (see below); however, it highlights the heterogeneity of this group of patients.

Finally, the variable molecular mechanisms responsible for rearrangements in the bcr gene may result in different phenotypes (59,75). Most of the reported CML patients with the e1a2 BCR/ABL junction expressing the p190BCR/ABL product have presented with monocytosis (51–56). Also, these patients are somewhat older (five evaluable patients reported, ages 44, 52, 65, 77, 81) and have lower WBC, but have basophilia and a high percentage of circulating immature granulocytes (51–56). In contrast, patients with a c3a2 junction may have a predominance of mature granulocytes in the peripheral blood (57,59). As these alternative BCR/ABL junctions are identified, more inclusive molecular analysis will have to be a part of the diagnostic approach of patients with CML. This will clarify whether the clinical heterogeneity can be explained by molecular mechanisms.

The majority of patients with Ph-negative bcr-negative CML have been reported to have normal karyotypes. As mentioned earlier, many of the earlier reported cases considered to be Ph-negative disease had translocations involving chromosome 9q34 (76). These are now considered to have variant or complex Ph-chromosomes. A variety of other cytogenetic abnormalities have been described in patients with Ph-negative CML. Although none is particularly predominant, abnormalities in chromosome 8, in particular trisomy 8, have been reported in several patients (9,69,73,76). Most other cytogenetic abnormalities reported are nonspecific.

DIFFERENTIAL DIAGNOSIS

As discussed in the preceding section, there are some conditions that can be confused with Ph-negative, bcr rearrangement-negative CML that should be considered in the differential diagnosis. Shepherd et al. proposed the existence of a distinct entity called atypical CML (aCML) (74). This condition can be differentiated from classical CML, called by these authors CGL, by the presence of dysplastic features, and absence or low percentage of basophils. Other distinctive features include a somewhat lower WBC count and higher monocyte count. Patients with aCML are more likely to have thrombocytopenia ($<150 \times 10^9$/L). However, compared to patients with CMML, patients with aCML have a higher percentage of circulating immature precursors and a smaller proportion of erythroid cells in the bone marrow. Diagnostic criteria for aCML, CGL, and CMML have been proposed by the French-American-British (FAB) Cooperative Leukemia Group (77,78). These criteria, however, should be considered only guidelines and should not be used in the classification of individual patients. As mentioned above, there is significant overlap in the clinical characteristics of all of these disease groups.

Although aCML has been proposed as an intermediate disease between CML (or CGL) and CMML, the dysplastic features are an important characteristic of this disease, and it has been proposed that this disease might represent a link with the myelodysplastic syndromes (79). Oscier recently described 10 patients with clinical features of aCML at one point during their disease course, all of whom had initially presented with disease features more characteristic of a myelodysplastic syndrome (79). The molecular mechanisms underlying aCML have not been studied in depth, but it is clear that at least some patients with bcr rearrangement-positive CML may have features of aCML. Ganesan et al. described bcr rearrangements in two patients with CML with dysplastic features, increased monocytes, and low basophil count which would meet the criteria for aCML (80). Also, some of the CML patients with the p190BCR/ABL junction that have been reported in the literature could be classified as aCML (55). However, Wiedemann et al. (28) found no evidence of increased abl kinase activity using a protein tyrosine kinase assay in three patients with aCML. Other molecular abnormalities may also be present.

A high frequency of ras mutations has been reported in patients with Ph-negative, bcr rearrangement-negative CML (64), and some of this patients could meet the criteria for a CML. It would be interesting to determine whether these patients have molecular abnormalities intermediate between CGL and CMML, e.g., some form, possibly a variant, of BCR/ABL, and high incidence of ras mutations.

Another disease that must be considered in the differential diagnosis of Ph-negative, bcr rearrangement-negative CML is chronic neutrophilic leukemia (CNL). This is a rare myeloproliferative disorder first described in 1920 (81), and is characterized by a persistent and unexplained leukocytosis consisting predominantly of mature granulocytes. These patients are usually older, have a moderately elevated WBC count usually $<100 \times 10^9$/L, with rare circulating immature forms, mild anemia, normal to mildly decreased platelet count, moderate splenomegaly, normal to elevated leukocyte alkaline phosphatase, and myeloid hyperplasia in the bone marrow (82–84). CNL is a clonal disorder (85,86) and is associated with dysfunction of the neutrophils involved (87,88). In some cases it has been found to be associated with polycythemia vera (89–91), monoclonal gammopathy of undetermined significance (92,93), and multiple myeloma (94,95), but the neutrophilic expansion is clonal (89–91,94). Transformation into a blastic phase has been reported (96,97) and occurs more frequently in cases with dysplastic features, consistent with the natural history of other MDS (98,99). The few reported cases suggest that patients with CNL do not have the Ph chromosome or any bcr rearrangement (100). It is reasonable to consider proof of the absence of bcr rearrangement a requirement for the diagnosis of CNL (83,84,101).

However, Pane et al. (59) reported five patients with CNL and the Ph-chromosome. Interestingly, they identified in these patients a distinctive BCR/ABL junction, c3a2, giving rise to a fusion protein of predicted 230 kD. They propose that the condition associated with this rearrangement should be called neutrophilic-chronic myeloid leukemia (CML-N), while the term CNL should be used for patients who meet the criteria for the disease but do not have this molecular marker (59). A favorable response to interferon therapy has been reported in some patients with CNL (101).

TREATMENT AND PROGNOSIS

The initial descriptions of patients with Ph-negative CML reported a poor response to therapy and short survival compared to patients with Ph-positive disease (4,10,11), although a subgroup with an outcome similar to Ph-positive patients could be identified (4). As with the clinical characteristics at diagnosis, Morris et al. (25) provided the first evidence of correlation between the molecular findings and the outcome of the disease. The two initial patients in whom bcr rearrangement was identified were in chronic phase at 4 and 6 years from diagnosis, whereas the three patients without rearrangement responded poorly to treatment, had progressive thrombocytopenia, and all died before 10 months from diagnosis (25). This duality of outcome according to molecular findings has been confirmed by several investigators (7,68–70). Patients with Ph-negative, bcr rearrangement-positive disease have an outcome similar to Ph-positive CML (7,22,27,28,69,70,80).

This is best appreciated when patients in similar stage of their disease are compared. In the M.D. Anderson experience investigating only patients with early chronic phase CML, 17 patients with Ph-negative, bcr-positive disease were compared to 508 Ph-positive patients who presented during the same period of time. Fourteen Ph-negative, bcr-positive patients were treated with alpha interferon and 12 had a complete hematological remission. The other three patients were treated with hydroxyurea and two had resistant disease. With a median follow-up of 51 months, the median survival for the 17 patients was 68 months, which compares to a median survival of 73 months for the Ph-positive group (7). These patients should be considered for treatment options in the same manner as patients with Ph-positive disease, including alpha interferon and bone marrow transplantation.

Patients with Ph-negative, bcr-negative disease have a significantly worse outcome. The median survival of 35 patients with early chronic phase presenting to M.D. Anderson was 25 months (7). This was significantly worse than both Ph-positive and Ph-negative, bcr-positive disease, but better than the median survival of 9 months for patients with CMML in the same study (7). Martiat et al. (69) also reported an inferior survival for Ph-negative, bcr-negative patients (median 36 months) compared to those with Ph-negative, bcr-positive disease (median 58 months). They found no difference with the median survival of 30 months observed for patients with CMML (69). However, the characteristics of disease progression differ in some studies. Kurzrock et al. noted the absence of transformation to blast phase in any of the 11 patients investigated as would be expected in Ph-positive CML (73). These Ph-negative, bcr-negative patients had clinical characteristics indistinguishable from CML at diagnosis, but with disease progression developed marked organomegaly, extramedullary manifestations, and bone marrow failure but only rarely myelofibrosis (73). These features are similar to those of progressive CMML.

In contrast, other studies have described a natural history similar to that of patients with Ph-positive CML. Four of seven patients reported by Costello et al. (102) and three of six by Dobrovic et al. (68) evolved into a blastic phase. These differences are probably related in part to the inclusion in some series of patients who could be classified into other disorders with features distinctive from CML. It is likely, however, that some heterogeneity in the outcome of patients exists. The possibility that related but distinctive molecular events are associated with different outcomes as well as different clinical characteristics at presentation should be considered. For example, the one Ph-negative patient described by Hochhaus et al. (60) with an e6a2 BCR/ABL fusion gene had a transformation characterized by extramedullary infiltration with no increased blasts in the peripheral blood or bone marrow, similar to the progression in the cases reported by Kurzrock et al. (73), although with no organomegaly or bone marrow failure.

There is little information on the therapy for patients with Ph-negative, bcr-negative disease. Most patients reported in the literature have been treated with hydroxyurea or busulfan, but there is some information on treatment with alpha interferon. Kantarjian et al. initially reported a poor response to interferon, with only one of the six patients treated (17%) having a hematological response (70). In contrast, Costello et al. report that response to interferon cases was favorable in most cases, but most patients received also other chemotherapeutic agents (102). Interestingly, Kurzrock et al. reported only two complete hematological responses among six patients treated with interferon (33%) (73). However, these were the only two complete hematological responses among the 11 Ph-negative, bcr-negative CML patients in their series. Therefore, although the response rate to interferon is significantly lower than in Ph-positive or Ph-negative, bcr-positive CML, it might still be the alternative of choice for these patients. However, there is still much to be learned about the treatment for these patients. The trials that include such patients should have strict inclusion criteria that exclude other confounding diseases, and perform a more inclusive molecular analysis to investigate bcr rearrangements in the bcr gene but outside the M-bcr region.

REFERENCES

1. Nowell PC, Hungerford DA. A minute chromosome in human chronic granulocytic leukemia. Science 1960; 132:1497.
2. Melo JV. The molecular biology of chronic myeloid leukemia. Leukemia 1996; 10:751–756.
3. Kurzrock R, Gutterman JU, Talpaz M. The molecular genetics of Philadelphia chromosome positive leukemias. N Engl J Med 1988; 319:990–998.
4. Ezdinli EZ, Sokal JE, Crosswhite L. Philadelphia-chromosome-positive and negative chronic myelocytic leukemia. Ann Intern Med 1970; 72:175–182.
5. Pugh WC, Pearson M, Vardiman JW, Rowley JD. Philadelphia chromosome-negative chronic myelogenous leukemia: a morphologic reassessment. Br J Haematol 1985; 60:457–467.
6. Kantarjian HM, Keating MJ, Walters RS, et al. Clinical and prognostic features of Philadelphia chromosome-negative chronic myelogenous leukemia. Cancer 1986; 58:2023–2030.
7. Cortes JE, Talpaz M, Beran M, et al. Philadelphia chromosome-negative chronic myelogenous leukemia with rearrangement of the breakpoint cluster region. Cancer 1995; 75:464–470.
8. Travis LB, Pierre RV, DeWald GW. Ph1-negative chronic granulocytic leukemia: a nonentity. Am J Clin Pathol 1986; 85:186–193.
9. Selleri L, Emili G, Luppi M, et al. Chronic myelogenous leukemia with typical clinical and morphological features can be Philadelphia chromosome negative and bcr negative. Hematol Pathol 1990; 4:67–77.
10. Canellos GP, Whang-Peng J, DeVita VT. Chronic granulocytic leukemia without the Philadelphia chromosome. Am J Clin Pathol 1976; 65:467–470.
11. Whang-Peng J, Canellos GP, Carbone PP, Tijo JH. Clinical implications of cytogenetic variants in chronic myelocytic leukemia (CML). Blood 1968; 32:755–766.
12. Heisterkamp N, Stephenson JR, Groffen J, et al. Localization of the c-abl oncogene adjacent to a translocation break point in chronic myelocytic leukemia. Nature 1983; 306:239–242.
13. Groffen J, Stephenson JR, Heisterkamp N, de Klein A, Bartram CR, Grosveld G. Philadelphia chromosomal breakpoints are clustered within a limited region, bcr, on chromosome 22. Cell 1984; 36:93–99.
14. Huret JL. Complex translocations, simple variant translocations and Ph-negative cases in chronic myelogenous leukemia. Hum Genet 1990; 85:565–568.
15. de Braekeleer M. Variant Philadelphia translocations in chronic myeloid leukemia. Cytogenet Cell Genet 1987; 44:215–222.

16. Ishihara T, Minamihisamatsu M. The Philadelphia chromosome. Consideration based on studies of variant translocation. Cancer Genet Cytogenet 1988; 32: 75–92.
17. Seong DC, Liu P, Sicialiano J, et al. Detection of variant Ph-positive chronic myelogenous leukemia involving 1, 9, and 22 by fluorescence in situ hybridization. Cancer Genet Cytogenet 1993; 65:100–103.
18. Bartram CR, de Klein A, Hagemeijer A, et al. Translocation of c-abl oncogene correlates with the presence of a Philadelphia chromosome in chronic myelocytic leukemia. Nature 1983; 306:277–280.
19. Hagemeijer A, Bartram CR, Smit EME, van Agthoven AJ, Bootsma D. Is the chromosomal region 9q34 always involved in variants of the Ph1 translocation? Cancer Genet Cytogenet 1984; 13:1–6.
20. Hagemeijer A, de Klein A, Godde-Salz E, et al. Translocation of c-abl to masked Ph in chronic myeloid leukemia. Cancer Genet Cytogenet 1985; 18:95–104.
21. Bartram CR, Kleihauer E, de Klein A, et al. c-abl and bcr are rearranged in a Ph1-negative CML patient. EMBO J 1985; 4:683–686.
22. Kurzrock R, Blick MB, Talpaz M, et al. Rearrangement in the breakpoint cluster region and the clinical course in Philadelphia-negative chronic myelogenous leukemia. Ann Intern Med 1986; 105:673–679.
23. Zaccaria A, Testoni N, Tassinari A, et al. Cytogenetic and molecular studies in patients with chronic myeloid leukemia and variant Philadelphia translocations. Cancer Genet Cytogenet 1989; 42:191–201.
24. Morris CM, Rosman I, Archer SA, Cochrane JM, Fitzgerald PH. A cytogenetic and molecular analysis of five variant Philadelphia translocations in chronic myeloid leukemia. Cancer Genet Cytogenet 1988; 35:179–197.
25. Morris CM, Reeve AE, Fitzgerald PH, Hollings PE, Beard MEJ, Heaton DC. Genomic diversity correlates with clinical variation in Ph-negative chronic myeloid leukemia. Nature 1986; 320:281–283.
26. Van der Plas DC, Hermans ABC, Soekarman D, et al. Cytogenetic and molecular analysis in Philadelphia negative CML. Blood 1989; 73:1038–1044.
27. Shtalrid M, Talpaz M, Blick M, et al. Philadelphia-negative chronic myelogenous leukemia with breakpoint cluster region rearrangement: molecular analysis, clinical characteristics, and response to therapy. J Clin Oncol 1988; 6:1569–1575.
28. Wiedemann LM, Kahri KK, Shivji MKK, et al. The correlation of breakpoint cluster region rearrangement and p210ph1/abl expression with morphological analysis of Ph-negative chronic myeloid leukemia and other myeloproliferative disease. Blood 1988; 71:349–355.
29. Dreazen O, Rassool F, Sparkes RS, Klisak I, Goldman JM, Gale RP. Do oncogenes determine clinical features in chronic myeloid leukemia? Lancet 1987; i: 1402–1405.
30. Nishigaki H, Misawa S, Inazawa J, Abe T. Absence in Ph-negative, M-BCR rearrangement-positive chronic myelogenous leukemia of linkage between 5′ ABL and 3′ M-BCR sequences in Philadelphia translocation. Leukemia 1992; 6:385–392.
31. Dreazen O, Klisak I, Rassool F, Goldman JM, Sparkes RS, Gale RP. The bcr

gene is joined to c-abl in Ph1 chromosome negative chronic myelogenous leukemia. Oncogene Res 1988; 2:167–175.
32. Zaccari A, Testoni N, Tassinari A, et al. Molecular and cytogenetic studies of a patient with Philadelphia-negative, BCR-positive chronic myeloid leukemia and t(12;12)(q13;p12). Genes Chrom Cancer 1990; 1:284–288.
33. Rassool F, Martiat P, Taj A, Klisak I, Goldman J. Interstitial insertion of varying amounts of ABL-containing genetic material into chromosome 22 in Ph-negative CML. Leukemia 1990; 4:273–277.
34. Morris CM, Heisterkamp N, Kennedy MA, Fitzgerald PH, Groffen J. Ph-negative chronic myeloid leukemia: molecular analysis of ABL insertion into M-BCR on chromosome 22. Blood 1990; 76:1812–1818.
35. Inazawa J, Nishigaki H, Takahira H, et al. Rejoining between 9q+ and Philadelphia chromosomes results in normal-looking chromosomes 9 and 22 in Ph1-negative chronic myelocytic leukemia. Hum Genet 1989; 83:115–118.
36. Calabrese G, Stuppia L, Franchi PG, et al. Complex translocations of the Ph chromosome and Ph negative CML arise from similar mechanisms, as evidenced by FISH analysis. Cancer Genet Cytogenet 1994; 78:153–159.
37. Morris C, Kennedy M, Heisterkamp N, et al. A complex chromosome rearrangement forms the BCR-ABL fusion gene in leukemic cells with a normal karyotype. Genes Chromosomes Cancer 1991; 3:263–271.
38. Nacheva E, Holloway T, Brown K, Bloxham D, Green AR. Philadelphia-negative chronic myeloid leukemia: detection by FISH of BCR-ABL fusion gene localized either to chromosome 9 or chromosome 22. Br J Haematol 1993; 87: 409–412.
39. Brunel V, Sainty D, Costello R, et al. Translocation of BCR to chromosome 9 in a Philadelphia-negative chronic myeloid leukemia. Cancer Genet Cytogenet 1995; 85:82–84.
40. Hagemeijer A, Buijs A, Smit E, et al. Translocation of BCR to chromosome 9: a new cytogenetic variant detected by FISH in two Ph-negative, BCR-positive patients with chronic myeloid leukemia. Genes Chromosomes Cancer 1993; 8:237–245.
41. Richards EM, Bloxham DM, Nacheva E, Marcus RE, Green AR. BCR rearrangement in apparent essential thrombocythaemia. Br J Haematol 1993; 85:625–626.
42. Bartram CR. bcr Rearrangement without juxtaposition of c-abl in chronic myelocytic leukemia. J Exp Med 1985; 162:2175–2179.
43. Popenoe DW, Schaefer-Rego K, Mears JG, Bank A, Leibowitz D. Frequent and extensive deletion during the 9,22 translocation in CML. Blood 1986; 68:1123–1128.
44. Bartram CR, Bross-Bach U, Schmidt H, Waller HD. Philadelphia-positive chronic myelogenous leukemia with breakpoint 5′ of the breakpoint cluster region but with the bcr gene. Blut 1987; 55:505–511.
45. Negrini M, Tallarico A, Pazzi I, Castagnoli A, Cuneo A, Castoldi GL. A new chromosomal breakpoint in Ph positive, bcr negative chronic myelogenous leukemia. Cancer Genet Cytogenet 1992; 61:11–13.
46. Leibowitz D, Schaefer-Rego K, Popenoe DW, Mears JG, Bank A. Variable breakpoints on the Philadelphia chromosome in chronic myelogenous leukemia. Blood 1985; 66:243–245.

47. Saglio G, Guerrasio A, Tassinari A, et al. Variability of the molecular defects corresponding to the presence of a Philadelphia chromosome in human hematologic malignancies. Blood 1988; 72:1203–1208.
48. Selleri L, Narni F, Emilia G, et al. Philadelphia-positive chronic myeloid leukemia with a chromosome 22 breakpoint outside the breakpoint cluster region. Blood 1987; 70:1659–1664.
49. Van der Plas DC, Soekarman D, van Gent AM, Grosveld G, Hagemeijer A. bcr-abl mRNA lacking abl exon a2 detected by polymerase chain reaction in a chronic myelogenous leukemia patient. Leukemia 1991; 5:457–461.
50. Iwata S, Mizutani S, Nakazawa S, Yata J. Heterogeneity of the breakpoint in the ABL gene in cases with BCR/ABL transcript lacking ABL exon a2. Leukemia 1994; 8:1696–1702.
51. Sawyers CL, Timson L, Kawasaki ES, Clark SS, Witte ON, Champlin R. Molecular relapse in chronic myelogenous leukemia patients after bone marrow transplantation detected by polymerase chain reaction. Proc Natl Acad Sci USA 1990; 87:563–567.
52. Zaccaria A, Tassinari A, Testoni N, Lauria F, Tura S, Algeri R. Alternative BCR/ABL transcripts in chronic myeloid leukemia. Blood 1990; 76:1663–1668.
53. Nakamura Y, Hirosawa S, Aoki N. Consistent involvement of the 3' half part of the first BCR intron in adult Philadelphia-positive leukemia without M-bcr rearrangement. Br J Haematol 1993; 83:53–57.
54. Selleri L, von Lindern M, Hermans A, Meijer D, Torelli G, Grosveld G. Chronic myeloid leukemia may be associated with several bcr-abl transcripts including the acute lymphoid leukemia-type 7kb transcript. Blood 1990; 75:1146–1153.
55. Melo JV, Myint H, Galton DAG, Goldman JM. p190BCR/ABL chronic myeloid leukemia: the missing link with chronic myelomonocytic leukemia? Leukemia 1994; 8:208–211.
56. Guo JQ, Hirsch-Ginsberg CF, Xian YM, et al. Acute lymphoid leukemia molecular phenotype in a patient with benign-phase chronic myelogenous leukemia. Hematol Pathol 1993; 7:91–106.
57. Saglio G, Guerrasio A, Rosso C, et al. New type of BCR/ABL junction in Philadelphia chromosome-positive chronic myelogenous leukemia. Blood 1990; 76:1819–1824.
58. Wada H, Mizutani S, Nishimura J, et al. Establishment and molecular characterization of a novel leukemic cell line with Philadelphia chromosome expressing p230 BCR/ABL fusion protein. Cancer Res 1995; 55:3192–3196.
59. Pane F, Frigeri F, Sindona M, et al. Neutrophilic-chronic myeloid leukemia: a distinct disease with a specific molecular marker (BCR/ABL with C3/A2 junction). Blood 1996; 88:2410–2414.
60. Hochhaus A, Reiter A, Skladny H, et al. A novel BCR-ABL fusion gene (e6a2) in a patient with Philadelphia chromosome-negative chronic myelogenous leukemia. Blood 1996; 88:2236–2240.
61. Min GL, Martiat P, Pu GA, Goldman J. Use of pulsed field gel electrophoresis to characterize BCR gene involvement in CML patients lacking M-BCR rearrangement. Leukemia 1990; 4:650–656.
62. Cross NCP, Melo JV, Feng L, Goldman JM. An optimized multiplex polymerase

chain reaction (PCR) for detection of BCR-ABL fusion mRNAs in hematological disorders. Leukemia 1994; 8:186–189.
63. Guo JQ, Lian JY, Xian YM, et al. BCR-ABL protein expression in peripheral blood cells of chronic myelogenous leukemia patients undergoing therapy. Blood 1994; 83:3629.
64. Cogswell PC, Morgan R, Dunn M, et al. Mutations of the ras protooncogenes in chronic myelogenous leukemia: a high frequency of ras mutations in bcr/abl rearrangement-negative chronic myelogenous leukemia. Blood 1989; 74:2629–2633.
65. Padua RA, Carter G, Hughes E, et al. RAS mutations in myelodysplasia detected by amplification, oligonucleotide hybridization, and transformation. Leukemia 1988; 2:503–510.
66. Hirsch-Ginsberg C, LeMaistre AC, Kantarjian H, et al. RAS mutations are rare events in Philadelphia chromosome-negative/bcr gene rearrangement-negative chronic myelogenous leukemia, but are prevalent in chronic myelomonocytic leukemia. Blood 1990; 76:1214–1219.
67. Melo JV, Goldman JM. Specific point mutations that activate v-abl are not found in Philadelphia-negative chronic myeloid leukemia, Philadelphia-negative acute lymphoblastic leukemia or blast transformation of chronic myeloid leukemia. Leukemia 1992; 6:786–790.
68. Dobrovic A, Morley AA, Seshadri R, Januszewicz EH. Molecular diagnosis of Philadelphia negative CML using the polymerase chain reaction and DNA analysis: clinical features and course of M-bcr negative and M-bcr positive CML. Leukemia 1991; 5:187–190.
69. Martiat P, Michaux JL, Rodhain J, et al. Philadelphia-negative (Ph−) chronic myeloid leukemia (CML): comparison with Ph+ CML and chronic myelomonocytic leukemia. Blood 1991; 78:205–211.
70. Kantarjian HM, Shtalrid M, Kurzrock R, et al. Significance and correlations of molecular analysis results in patients with Philadelphia chromosome-negative chronic myelogenous leukemia and chronic myelomonocytic leukemia. Am J Med 1988; 85:639–644.
71. Kantarjian HM, Keating MJ, Smith TL, Talpaz M, McCredie KB. Proposal for a simple synthesis prognostic staging system in chronic myelogenous leukemia. Am J Med 1990; 88:1–8.
72. Sokal JE, Cox EB, Baccarani M, et al. Prognostic discrimination in good-risk chronic granulocytic leukemia. Blood 1984; 63:789–799.
73. Kurzrock R, Kantarjian HM, Shtalrid M, Gutterman JU, Talpaz M. Philadelphia chromosome-negative chronic myelogenous leukemia without breakpoint cluster region rearrangement: a chronic myeloid leukemia with a distinct clinical course. Blood 1990; 75:445–452.
74. Shepherd PCA, Ganesan TS, Galton DAG. Haematological classification of the chronic myeloid leukemias. Balliere's Clin Hematol 1987; 1:887–906.
75. Melo JV. The diversity of BCR-ABL fusion proteins and their relationship to leukemia phenotype. Blood 1996; 88:2375–2384.
76. van der Plas DC, Grosveld G, Hagemeijer A. Review of clinical, cytogenetic,

and molecular aspects of Ph-negative CML. Cancer Genet Cytogenet 1991; 52: 143–156.
77. Galton DAG. Haematological differences between chronic granulocytic leukemia, atypical chronic myeloid leukaemia and chronic myelomonocytic leukaemia. Leuk Lymph 1992; 7:343–350.
78. Bennett JM, Catovsky D, Daniel MT, et al. The chronic myeloid leukaemias: guidelines for distinguishing chronic granulocytic, atypical chronic myeloid, and chronic myelomonocytic leukaemia. Proposal from the French-American-British Cooperative Leukaemia Group. Br J Hematol 1994; 87:746–754.
79. Oscier DG. Atypical chronic myeloid leukaemia, a distinct clinical entity related to the myelodysplastic syndrome? Br J Hematol 1996; 92:582–586.
80. Ganesan TS, Rassool F, Guo A-P, et al. Rearrangement of the bcr gene in Philadelphia chromosome-negative chronic myeloid leukemia. Blood 1986; 68:957–960.
81. Tuohy EA. A case of splenomegaly with polymorphonuclear neutrophil hyperleukocytosis. Am J Med Sci 1920; 160:18–25.
82. Rubin H. Chronic neutrophilic leukemia. Ann Intern Med 1966; 65:93–100.
83. You W, Weisbrot IM. Chronic neutrophilic leukemia. Report of two cases and review of the literature. Am J Clin Pathol 1979; 233–242.
84. Zittoun R, Rea D, Hoang-Ngoc L, Ramond S. Chronic neutrophilic leukemia. A study of four cases. Ann Hematol 1994; 68:55–60.
85. Kwong YL, Cheng G. Clonal nature of chronic neutrophilic leukemia. Blood 1993; 82:1035–1036.
86. Lugassy G. Clonality of chronic neutrophilic leukemia. Blood 1994; 83:619.
87. Kaplan SS, Berkow RL, Joyce RA, Basford RE, Barton JC. Neutrophil function in chronic neutrophilic leukemia: defective respiratory burst in response to phorbol esters. Acta Haematol 1992; 87:16–21.
88. Dotten DA, Pruzanski W, Wong D. Functional characterization of the cells in chronic neutrophilic leukemia. Am J Hematol 1982; 12:157–165.
89. Lugassy G, Farhi R. Chronic neutrophilic leukemia associated with polycythemia vera. Am J Hematol 1989; 31:300–301.
90. Iurlo A, Foa P, Maido AT, Luksch R, Capsoni F, Polli EE. Polycythemia vera terminating in chronic neutrophilic leukemia. Am J Hematol 1990; 35:139–140.
91. Foa P, Iurlo A, Saglio G, Guerrasio A, Capsoni F, Maiolo AT. Chronic neutrophilic leukemia associated with polycythemia vera: pathogenetic implications and therapeutic approach. Br J Hematol 1991; 78:286–288.
92. Florensa L, Woessner S, Vicente P, Roig Marti A, Sole F, Perez A. Chronic neutrophilic leukemia associated with monoclonal gammopathy of undetermined signficance. A multimethod study. Ann Hematol 1993; 676:129–131.
93. Ito T, Kojima H, Otani K, et al. Chronic neutrophilic leukemia associated with monoclonal gammopathy of undetermined significance. Acta Haematol 1996; 95: 140–143.
94. Standen GR, Steers FJ, Jones L. Clonality of chronic neutrophilic leukemia associated with myeloma: analysis using the X-linked probe M27 beta. J Clin Pathol 1993; 46:297–298.

95. Cehrlei C, Undar B, Akkoc N, Onvural B, Altungoz O. Coexistence of chronic neutrophilic leukemia with light chain myeloma. Acta Haematol 1994; 91:32–34.
96. Bareford D, Jacobs P. Chronic neutrophilic leukemia. Am J Clin Pathol 1980; 73: 837.
97. Shindo T, Sakai C, Shibata A. Neutrophilic leukemia and blastic crisis. Ann Intern Med 1977; 87:66–67.
98. Zoumbos CN, Symeonidis A, Kourakli-Symeonidis A. Chronic neutrophilic leukemia with dysplastic features: a new variant of the myelodysplastic syndromes. Acta Haematol 1989; 82:156–160.
99. Cervantes F, Rozman M, Vives-Corrons JL, Rozman C. Chronic neutrophilic leukemia with dysplastic features. Acta Haematol 1990; 84:109.
100. Storek J. Chronic neutrophilic leukemia: case report documenting the absence of bcr-abl rearrangement. Am J Hematol 1992; 41:304.
101. Meyer S, Feremans W, Cantiniaux B, Capel P, Huygen K, Dicato M. Successful alpha-2b-interferon therapy for chronic neutrophilic leukemia. Am J Hematol 1993; 43:307–309.
102. Costello R, Lafage M, Toiron Y, et al. Philadelphia chromosome-negative chronic myeloid leukemias; a report of 14 new cases. Br J Haematol 1995; 90:346–352.

14
Monitoring Changes in the Breakpoint Cluster Region During Therapy for CML: M.D. Anderson Cancer Center Experience

Claire F. Verschraegen
M.D. Anderson Cancer Center, Houston, Texas

INTRODUCTION

Interferon-based therapy prolongs the overall survival of patients with chronic myelogenous leukemia (CML) by extending the length of time their disease remains in the chronic phase (1–4). The overall median survival range in patients treated with interferon is 60–89 months. Patients who had a major cytogenetic response also have a significantly longer survival than those who did not. Based on the responses observed after interferon therapy, the chronic phase has been divided into early (<12 months since diagnosis), and late (>12 months since diagnosis) phases. The course of CML varies in individual patients. Some patients remain in the chronic phase for >10 years, whereas in others the disease enters the blastic phase within 2 years from diagnosis (5).

Ongoing studies are looking at the combination of interferon with chemotherapeutic agents such as cytosine arabinoside (6), homoharringtonine (7), and hydroxyurea (8). Patients treated with allogeneic bone marrow transplantation for CML in chronic phase have an overall disease free survival of 40–70% at 5 years, with a relapse rate of <20% (9,10). However, as a therapeutic approach, allogeneic bone marrow transplantation is limited by the necessity of an HLA-identical donor, the age of the recipient (the younger, the better the results), the timing of the transplantation during the course of the disease (the earlier, the better the results), and the risks inherent to allogeneic transplantation (20–25% mortality in the first 5 years). When all these factors are considered, only 15–25% of patients are candidates for transplantation. The choice of therapy depends on the risk acceptance by the patient and the probability of survival (11,12).

The course of CML is commonly monitored by karyotypic analysis of bone marrow samples, to look for the presence of the Philadelphia chromosome (Ph) (13). Response criteria to therapy are defined as followed: a complete hematological response requires normalization of the peripheral blood counts and differential (white blood cell count <10 × $10^3/\mu L$; platelet count <450 × $10^3/\mu L$; and no immature peripheral blasts, promyelocytes, or myelocytes) and disappearance of all signs and symptoms of the disease, including palpable splenomegaly (14). Patients in whom a complete hematological response is shown are further categorized by their best cytogenetic response (lowest percentage of Ph-positive metaphases): a complete response denotes the disappearance of all Ph-positive metaphases (0%), the observations of 1–34% Ph-positive metaphases is a partial response and of 35% to 90% Ph-positive metaphases a minor response (15). A major cytogenetic response includes complete and partial cytogenetic remissions—i.e., <35% Ph-positive metaphases.

DETECTION METHODS FOR THE GENETIC ANOMALY

Today, various tests are available to evaluate the presence of the Ph chromosome translocation. Until now, the cytogenetic analysis of bone marrow samples was the gold standard with which to determine response to therapy (13). However, this technique is not very sensitive. So newer techniques have been developed to refine the evaluation of the disease. Most of these techniques can be used to detect any residual disease after treatment. Some quantitative techniques are currently evaluated for measurement of residual disease, and correlations are made to prognosis and survival.

Cytogenetic analysis requires bone marrow aspirates which are either used immediately or submitted to a short-term culture with fetal calf serum to promote cell division. Cells are harvested, and following standard procedures, chromosomal preparations are mounted on slides. If possible, 25–100 metaphases are analyzed after Giemsa banding to detect the typical t(9;22) translocation (16). Practically, 20–25 metaphases are analyzed. This number results in a high standard error in categorizing the cytogenetic response, in evaluating the accuracy of response between two time points, and in assessing the amount of minimal residual disease. The ratio of Ph-positive cells to the total number of metaphases analyzed is used to define the cytogenetic response (see above). The disadvantages of this time-consuming method include: (1) the requirement of serial bone marrow aspirations; (2) the low sensitivity; (3) the need for a sufficient number of mitotic cells in metaphase: up to 20% of treated patients have

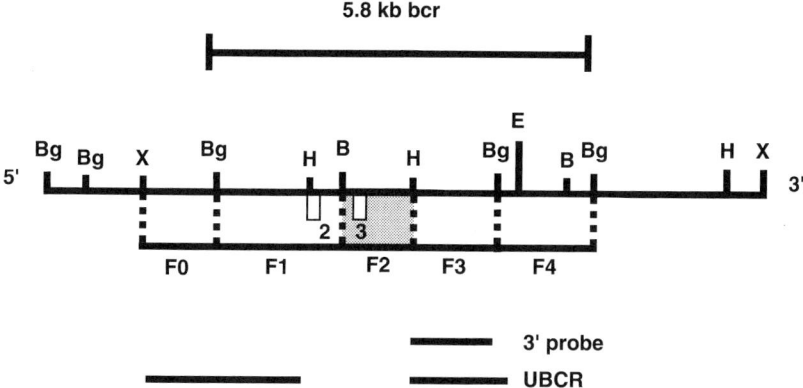

Figure 1 The breakpoint cluster region of chromosome 22. Bg, Bgl II; B, BamHI; H, HindIII; E, EcoRI; X, XbaI; 2 and 3, location of exons 2 and 3, respectively; gray area, area not mapped by the technique we used. F0, F1, F2, F3, and F4, fragments of the breakpoint cluster region arbitrarily designated according to the site of restriction enzyme activity. From Ref. 31.

insufficient metaphases; and (4) the need for typical translocations; any translocation below the level of karyotypic detection will be missed.

Southern blotting for quantification of the breakpoint cluster region (BCR) rearrangement has been used to study bone marrow or blood samples (17). White blood cells are isolated by Ficoll gradient centrifugation or lysis of red blood cells. DNA is extracted by standard methods and digested with a panel of restriction enzymes (Fig. 1). The digested DNA fragments are isolated by electrophoresis on an agarose gel. Separated fragments are transferred onto a cellulose membrane. Specific probes (Fig. 1) are used to detect the different segments of digested DNA. A germline band and one or more bands of the BCR showing rearrangement are obtained. The germline represents the normal chromosome; the rearranged bands, the translocated chromosomal DNA. Southern blot analysis has been useful in diagnosing patients with Ph-negative CML and BCR rearrangement, and patients with acute lymphocytic leukemia and p210 Ph-positive disease not identified by cytogenetic studies. Southern blotting is now accepted in clinical practice (18).

The intensity of the bands can be quantified by isotopic counters after hybridization (19,20). In molecular studies, the percentage of rearranged BCR band is calculated as the ratio of the signal from the band of the rearranged BCR to the signal from the same and the normal (unrearranged) BCR gene. A theoretical 2:1 ratio exists between the cytogenetic and the molecular results. For example, a cell population that is 100% Ph-positive would be expected to have a BCR rearrangement value of 50% [the abnormal t(9;22) chromosome/ the same abnormal t(9;22) chromosome plus the normal chromosome], and a 50% Ph-positive cell population would have an expected BCR rearrangement of 25% (one-quarter of the DNA carries the 9-22 translocation). This method has been used at M.D. Anderson Cancer Center to evaluate whether the quantity of abnormal DNA is a prognostic determinant of survival (21).

Polymerase chain reaction (PCR) has been used to detect the presence of BCR/ABL mRNA in bone marrow, blood, or marrow imprint samples (22). For PCR analysis, RNA is extracted from the sample by standard methods and submitted to reverse transcriptase amplification. Two oligonucleotide primers mapped on both sides of the translocation are used to amplify the translocated area (23). Often, a nested amplification is necessary to detect the translocation (24). The amplified RNA transcripts are then separated by gel electrophoresis and compared with known controls. Various quantitative PCR methods are being developed. The PCR technique is highly sensitive and can detect one abnormal cell out of 100,000 cells. However, the significance of the persistence of a very low percentage of Ph chromosomes is not well established (25–27). Some patients have been known to be Ph-positive by PCR analysis but have remained free of clinical disease for many years and may be considered cured (28). Longitudinal surveys will help to define the role of PCR in evaluating minimal residual disease.

Other tests are being evaluated for their ability to detect the Ph chromosome. Most of these are in the early stages of development but have a significant potential to improve the monitoring of CML therapy.

Fluorescence in situ hybridization (FISH) is a quantitative method for estimating the presence of the BCR/ABL translocation. This technique can be applied to blood or bone marrow samples and yields a result that is independent from the cycling status of the cells. Two probes of different colors are usually used to map the chromosomes of interest (29,30).

Western blot analysis allows the detection of the p210 or the p190 proteins, the protein products of BCR/ABL translocations (31). It is an experimental tool that has been used to gain insights in the physiopathology of CML. A study by Guo et al. has shown that the protein level can be measured quantitatively in circulating white blood cells. The expression of BCR/ABL protein products parallels the course of the disease, as measured by cytogenetic studies. This technique may be effective for monitoring both p210 and p190 diseases (32).

QUANTIFICATION OF THE BCR REARRANGEMENT

The intensity of the rearranged bands revealed by Southern blotting can be quantified by densitometric analysis (19,20). Thus we hypothesized that the quantifi-

Table 1 Comparison of Cytogenetic vs. Molecular Analyses of 465 Samples

Percent BCR quantification	Percent Ph-positive metaphases No. of samples (percent total, percent column)			
	0	1–34	35–95	>95
0	75 (16,83)	11 (2,23)	0	0
1 to <17.5	9 (2,10)	32 (7,65)	44 (10,50)	29 (6,12)
17.5–47.5	6 (1,7)	5 (1,10)	41 (9,47)	181 (39,76)
>47.5	0	1 (0,2)	3 (1,3)	28 (6,12)
Total	90	49	88	238

Abbreviations: BCR, breakpoint cluster region; Ph, Philadelphia chromosome.

cation of the BCR rearrangement can be used to monitor the efficacy of therapy and to establish a survival prognosis in patients with CML. We also compared results obtained on blood samples with those obtained on bone marrow samples (21).

The BCR rearrangement was quantified in 300 patients who were treated for Ph-positive CML with an interferon-based therapy. Eighty-nine patients were in the early chronic phase, 132 in late chronic phase, 54 in accelerated phase, and 25 in blastic phase. Four hundred sixty-five bone marrow samples were examined using cytogenetic and molecular (BCR quantification after Southern blotting) analyses. The details of these techniques have been explained elsewhere (33). A correlation was made between 72 of these bone marrow samples and blood samples obtained at the same time as the bone marrow aspiration and submitted to densitometric quantification after Southern blotting.

A BCR rearrangement was detected in 388 of 474 tested samples and was quantified in 465 samples. Complete cytogenetic remission was observed in 99 samples of which 75 (75%) were negative for a BCR rearrangement and 24 had a BCR rearrangement. In nine of these samples the BCR rearrangement was not quantified. In the remaining 15 samples, the median BCR quantification was 12.4% (range, 2.1–38.5%). No BCR rearrangements were detected in 11 (3%) of the 375 samples with Ph-positive metaphases. The percentage of Ph-positive metaphases in these 11 samples ranged from 4% to 24% (median 5%). BCR quantification and cytogenetic analysis were performed on 465 samples (Table 1). Of 90 samples with no detectable Ph-positive metaphases, 75 (83%) had no BCR rearrangement. Of 49 samples in partial cytogenetic remission, 32 (65%) showed partial and 11 (23%) showed complete molecular remission, for a total response rate of 88%. Of 88 samples in minor cytogenetic response, 44 (50%) were classified as partial molecular remission. Of the 238 samples with no response (>95% Ph-positive metaphases), 29 (12%) had a BCR value of <17.5%.

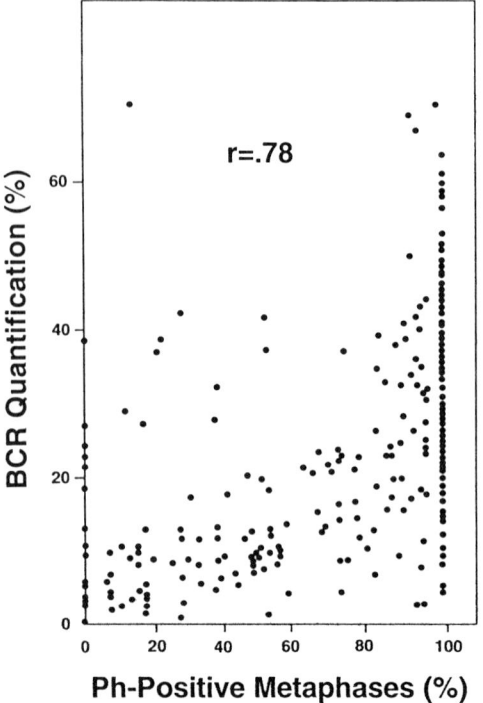

Figure 2 Correlation between BCR quantification and cytogenetics in 465 samples.

A good correlation was found between the percentages of Ph-positive metaphases and the BCR quantification (Fig. 2; $r = 0.78$; $p < 0.001$). The distribution of patients by CML phase and the corresponding BCR quantification are shown in Table 2.

Figures 3 and 4 show the survival of patients by their best cytogenetic and molecular responses, respectively. A significant difference is seen between the occurrence of a complete or a partial response, and a minor or no remission ($p \leq 0.001$) by both cytogenetic and molecular studies. To understand which technique would yield a better prognosis when results were discordant, we evaluated the survival of patients who had achieved a specific cytogenetic remission according to the BCR quantification (< or >17.5% BCR quantification). Figure 5 shows the survival of patients whose disease did not respond to therapy according to cytogenetic criteria (>95% Ph-positive metaphases). A trend for better survival is seen for patients with a partial molecular response ($p \leq 0.05$).

BCR quantification was performed on 72 of 79 blood samples tested by molecular studies. A bone marrow sample was obtained at the same time as the

Table 2 Patient Distribution by CML Phases

CML phase	No. of patients	Median percent BCR quantification (range)
Newly diagnosed	28	30 (3.7–68.8)
Early chronic	61	30 (0–85)
Late chronic	132	28 (0–71.1)
Accelerated	54	32 (0–66.7)
Blastic	25	32 (14.7–51.6)

Abbreviations: CML, chronic myelogenous leukemia; BCR, breakpoint cluster region.

blood sample and submitted to molecular and cytogenetic studies (Table 3). Molecular studies were negative in 35 samples each of blood and bone marrow, and positive in 42 samples each. The two remaining samples were discordant by molecular analysis. However, molecular results of the blood samples corresponded to the karyotypic analyses. An excellent correlation was obtained between BCR quantification values of blood and bone marrow samples (Pearson correlation coefficient $r = 0.94$) (Fig. 6).

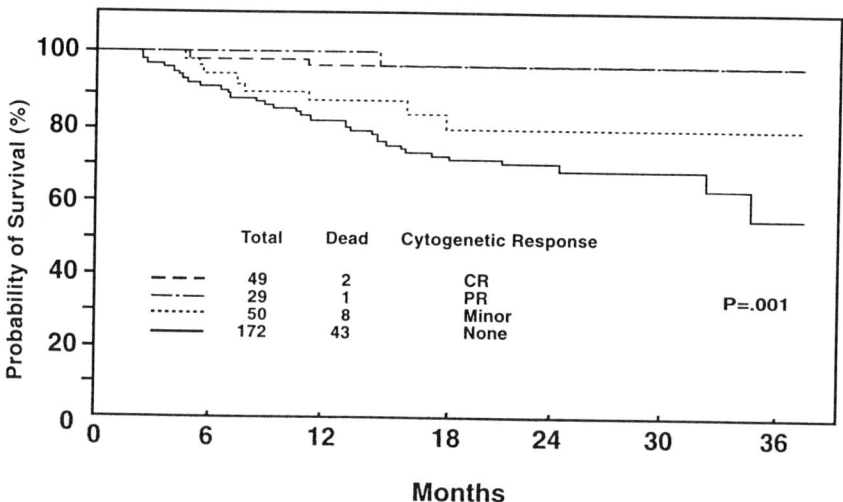

Figure 3 Survival analysis by cytogenetic response in patients with Philadelphia-positive chronic myelogenous leukemia. Survival is calculated from the time of the best cytogenetic response.

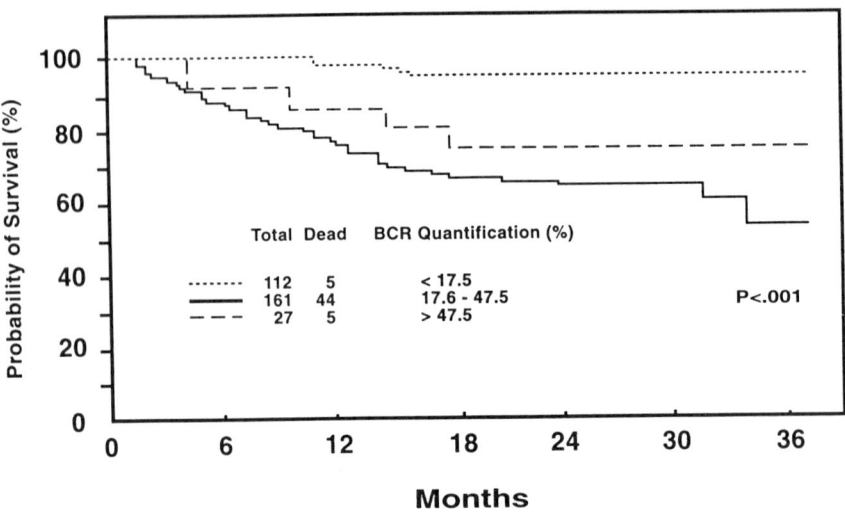

Figure 4 Survival analysis according to the BCR quantification in patients with Philadelphia-positive chronic myelogenous leukemia. Survival is calculated from the time of the best cytogenetic response.

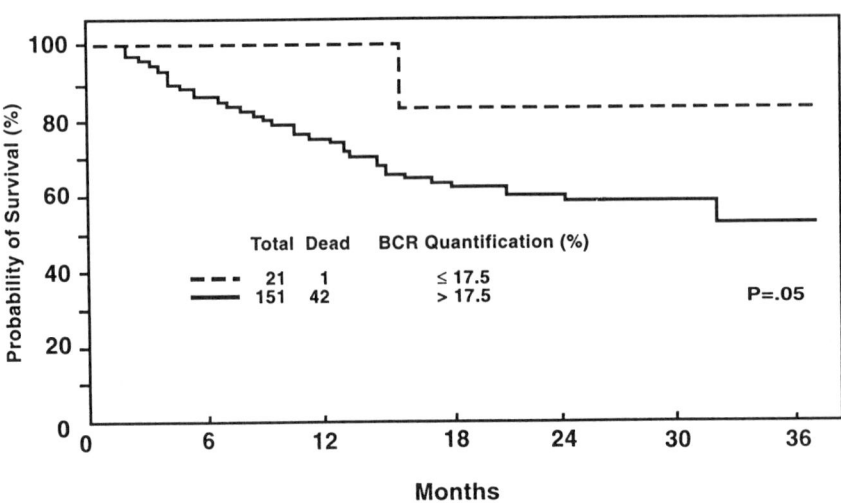

Figure 5 Survival analysis according to the BCR quantification in patients with Philadelphia-positive chronic myelogenous leukemia who did not have a cytogenetic response despite therapy. Survival is calculated from the time of the best cytogenetic response.

Table 3 Percentage of BCR Quantification on Bone Marrow and Blood Samples Drawn on the Same Day

No. of samples	Ph %	Median BCR % (range)	
		Bone marrow samples	Blood samples
35	0	0	0
1	0	positive	negative
1	5	0	6.31
6	0	positive	positive
3	0	3.11 (2.79–3.31)	5.01 (0.91–6.31)
4	1–34	6.08 (3.16–9.93)	15.72 (4.03–25.75)
16	35–95	16.21 (3.16–39.49)	10.17 (2.49–43.23)
8	>95	24.01 (18.34–55.05)	20.72 (14.97–66.32)
5	no results	14.97 (4.71–17.1)	12.38 (10.65–16.33)

Abbreviations: BCR, breakpoint cluster region; Ph, Philadelphia chromosome.

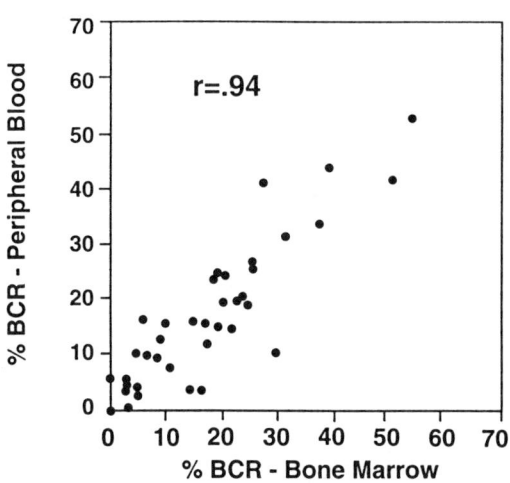

Figure 6 Comparison of BCR quantification done on bone marrow samples versus blood samples.

DISCUSSION

A good correlation was found between cytogenetic and molecular studies on a large number of bone marrow samples obtained from patients diagnosed with Ph-positive CML (Fig. 2). The BCR quantification may overestimate the degree of response as defined by karyotypic quantification (34), because 23% of samples showed a partial cytogenetic response but had a complete molecular response, 50% of samples with a minor cytogenetic response were classified as partial molecular response, and 12% of samples with no cytogenetic response had a partial molecular response (Table 1). The same observation was made by the CALGB group (34). What is the biological significance of this discordance? Twenty-one patients with a partial molecular response despite the absence of cytogenetic response had a better survival than patients with no molecular response (Fig. 5). This observation may be explained by the proliferative advantage of the Ph-positive clone, which results in a higher detection of Ph-positive metaphases in dividing (cytogenetic studies) vs. clonal and total cell populations (molecular studies).

Alternatively, because the analysis of BCR rearrangement is done on a mixed pool of myeloid and nonmyeloid cells, and some of the latter (T-cell lymphocytes) may not have BCR rearrangements, the BCR quantification may yield a relatively lower value than if done on the myeloid subset only. BCR quantification done on the myeloid subset may yield a better correlation with cytogenetic studies. If this is the case, no survival advantage should be seen between patients whose disease shows a molecular response that differs from the cytogenetic response.

The comparison between bone marrow samples and peripheral blood samples shows that results are interchangeable, a finding also reported by Stock et al. (34) (Fig. 6). Peripheral blood samples could replace bone marrow samples in DNA analyses if the equal or superior prognostic value in discordant cases to cytogenetic studies is confirmed (34). Furthermore, the technical cost of cytogenetic analysis is two or three times higher than the cost of molecular analysis performed on peripheral blood.

BCR quantification was found to be predictive for the survival of patients treated for Ph-positive CML. With a median follow-up of 78 weeks from the time of sample measurement, patients with high BCR values had a significantly shorter survival than those with low BCR values (Fig. 4). Despite the small number of patients in each subgroup and the short follow-up, we were able to identify a survival trend for patients whose disease showed a low BCR value but no cytogenetic response (Table 4). A low BCR value (≤17.5%) might indicate a more favorable prognosis in patients with no cytogenetic response (Fig. 5).

Our data show that 24% of 99 cases of cytogenetic remission (no Ph chromosome detected) had a detectable BCR rearrangement and 13% of 86

Table 4 Survival from the Date of the Best Cytogenetic Response by BCR Quantification

Ph %	BCR %	No. of patients	Probability of survival at 2 years (%)
0	0	41	98
	1 to <17.5	4	100
	≥17.5	4	75
1–34	<17.5	25	95
	≥17.5	4	100
35–95	<17.5	21	84
	≥17.5	29	75
>95	<17.5	21*	85
	≥17.5	151	67

Abbreviations: BCR, breakpoint cluster region; Ph, Philadelphia chromosome.
*Significance ($p = 0.05$) was shown between cytogenetic and molecular results for these 21 patients.

cases of molecular remission had a Ph chromosome. In patients whose disease is in complete remission by either test, the concordance rate is 68% (75 of 110). In 10% (11 of 110) of the cases we studied, the diagnosis of residual CML was missed by molecular studies as opposed to 22% (24 of 110) that were missed by cytogenetic studies. Thus, we advocate the use of BCR quantification to detect residual disease in patients who demonstrate a complete cytogenetic response.

In summary, cytogenetic studies and BCR quantification have shown relatively good concordance for monitoring patients on therapy for Ph-positive CML. As a single variable, BCR quantification was found to be a significant prognostic determinant and might be superior to cytogenetic analysis for survival prognosis in discordant samples. BCR quantification on blood samples yields results equivalent to those from bone marrow samples, and should be substituted for bone marrow studies when clinically indicated (34). BCR quantification overestimated the response in up to 50% of the cases in patients whose disease showed minor or no cytogenetic response. The clinical significance of this observation needs to be evaluated on a larger group of patients over a longer period of time.

Molecular studies by Southern blotting and BCR quantification will need to be compared with other techniques such as PCR (35), fluorescence in situ hybridization (36), and Western blotting (32) to evaluate the merits of each technique in providing prognostic determinants of clinical response and survival.

REFERENCES

1. Talpaz M, Kantarjian HM, McCredie K, Trujillo JM, Keating MJ, Gutterman JU. Hematologic remission and cytogenetic improvement induced by recombinant human interferon alpha in chronic myelogenous leukemia. N Engl J Med 1986; 314: 1065–1068.
2. Italian Study Group on Chronic Myeloid Leukemia. Interferon-alfa-2a as compared with conventional chemotherapy for the treatment of chronic myeloid leukemia. N Engl J Med 1994; 330:820–825.
3. Hehlmann R, Heimpel H, Hasford J, et al. Randomized comparison of interferon-alpha with busulfan and hydroxyurea in chronic myelogenous leukemia. Blood 1994; 84:4064–4068.
4. Allan NC, Richards SM, Sheperd PCA. UK Medical Research Council randomised, multicentre trial of interferon-α1 for chronic myeloid leukaemia: improved survival irrespective of cytogenetic response. Lancet 1995; 345:1392–1396.
5. Kantarjian HM, Deisseroth AB, Kurzrock R, Estrov Z, Talpaz M. Chronic myelogenous leukemia: a concise update. Blood 1993; 82:691–703.
6. Kantarjian HM, Keating MJ, Estey EH, et al. Treatment of advanced stages of Philadelphia chromosome-positive chronic myelogenous leukemia with interferon-α and low-dose cytarabine. J Clin Oncol 1992; 10:772–778.
7. O'Brien S, Kantarjian HM, Feldman E, et al. Homoharringtonine produces high hematologic and cytogenetic response rates in Philadelphia-chromosome positive chronic myelogenous leukemia. Blood 1992; 80:358a.
8. Guilhot F, Abgrall JF, Harrousseau JL, et al. A multicenter randomised study of alfa 2b interferon and hydroxyurea with or without cytosine-arabinoside in previously untreated patients with Ph+ chronic myelocytic leukemia: preliminary cytogenetic results. Leuk Lymph 1993; 11:181–183.
9. Gratwohl A, Hermans J, Niederwieser D, et al. Bone marrow transplantation for chronic myeloid leukemia: long term results. Bone Marrow Transplant 1993; 12:509–516.
10. Speck B, Bortin MM, Champlin R, et al. Allogeneic bone marrow transplantation for chronic myelogenous leukemia. Lancet 1984; 1:665–668.
11. Wagner JE, Zahurak M, Piantadosi S, et al. Bone marrow transplantation of chronic myelogenous leukemia in chronic phase: evaluation of risks and benefits. J Clin Oncol 1992; 10:779–789.
12. Goldman JM, Szydlo R, Horowitz MM, et al. Choice of pretransplant treatment and timing of transplants for chronic myelogenous leukemia in chronic phase. Blood 1993; 82:2235–2238.
13. Rowley JD. A new consistant chromosomal abnormality in chronic myelogenous leukemia identified by quinacrine fluorescence and Giemsa staining. Nature 1973; 243:290–293.
14. Kurzrock R, Gutterman JU, Talpaz M. The molecular genetics of Philadelphia chromosome-positive leukemias. N Engl J Med 1988; 319:990–998.
15. Kantarjian HM, Smith TL, O'Brien S, Beran M, Pierce S, Talpaz M. Prolonged survival in chronic myelogenous leukemia after cytogenetic response to interferon-α therapy. Ann Intern Med 1995; 122:254–257.
16. ISCN. An international system for human cytogenetic nomenclatures. Harnden DG,

Klinger HP, eds. Basel, Switzerland: Karger, 1985 (published in collaboration with Cancer Genet Cytogenet).
17. Southern EM. Detection of specific sequences among DNA fragments separated by gel electrophoresis. J Mol Biol 1975; 98:503–517.
18. Westbrook CA. The role of molecular techniques in the clinical management of leukemia. Cancer 1992; 70(S6):1695–1700.
19. Grossman A, Silver R, Szatrowski T, Gutfriend A, Verma R, Benn P. Densitometric analysis of Southern blot autoradiographs and its application to monitoring patients with chronic myeloid leukemia. Leukemia 1991; 5:540–545.
20. Ayscue L, Ross D, Ozer H, Rao K, Gulley M, Dent G. bcr/abl recombinant DNA analysis versus karyotype in the diagnosis and therapeutic monitoring of chronic myeloid leukemia. Am J Clin Pathol 1990; 94:404–408.
21. Verschraegen C, Talpaz M, Hirsch-Ginsberg C, et al. Quantification of the breakpoint cluster region rearrangement for clinical monitoring in Philadelphia chromosome-positive chronic myeloid leukemia. Blood 1995; 85:2705–2710.
22. Crisan D, Farkas DH. Bone marrow biopsy imprint preparations: use for molecular diagnostics in leukemias. Ann Clin Lab Sci 1993; 23:407–422.
23. Lee MS, Kantarjian HM, Talpaz M, et al. Detection of minimal residual disease by polymerase chain reaction in Philadelphia chromosome positive chronic myelogenous leukemia following interferon therapy. Blood 1992; 79:1920–1923.
24. Cross NCP, Hughes TP, Lin F, et al. Minimal residual disease after allogeneic bone marrow transplantation for chronic myeloid leukaemia in first chronic phase: correlations with acute graft-versus-host disease and relapse. Br J Haematol 1993; 84:67–74.
25. Hochhaus A, Lin F, Reiter A, et al. Variable numbers of BCR-ABL transcripts persist in CML patients who achieve complete cytogenetic remission with interferon-α. Br J Haematol 1995; 91:126–131.
26. Lee M, Khouri I, Champlin R, et al. Detection of minimal residual disease by polymerase chain reaction in Philadelphia chromosome positive chronic myelogenous leukemia following allogeneic bone marrow transplantation. Br J Haematol 1992; 82:708–714.
27. Italian Cooperative Study Group on Chronic Myeloid Leukemia. Chronic myeloid leukemia, BCR-ABL transcript, response to alpha-interferon and survival. Leukemia 1995; 9:1648–1652.
28. van Rhee F, Lin F, Cross NC, et al. Detection of residual leukaemia more than 10 years after allogeneic bone marrow transplantation for chronic myelogenous leukaemia. Bone Marrow Transplant 1994; 14:609–612.
29. Seong DC, Song MY, Henske EP, et al. Analysis of interphase cells for the Philadelphia translocation using painting probe made by inter-Alu-polymerase chain reaction from a radiation hybrid. Blood 1994; 83:2268–2273.
30. Bentz M, Cabot G, Moos M, et al. Detection of chimeric BCR-ABL genes on bone marrow samples and blood smears in chronic myeloid and acute lymphoblastic leukemia by in situ hybridization. Blood 1994; 83:1922–1928.
31. Guo JQ, Wang JY, Arlinghaus RB. Detection of BCR-ABL proteins in blood cells of benign phase chronic myelogenous leukemia patients. Cancer Res 1991; 51:3048–3051.
32. Guo JQ, Lian JY, Xian YM, et al. BCR-ABL protein expression in peripheral blood

cells of chronic myelogenous leukemia patients undergoing therapy. Blood 1994; 83:3629–3637.
33. Haber LM, Childs CC, Hirsch-Ginsberg C, et al. Strategy for breakpoint cluster region analysis in chronic myelocytic leukemia in a routine clinical laboratory. Am J Clin Pathol 1990; 94:762–767.
34. Stock W, Westbrook C, Peterson B, et al. Molecular monitoring of bcr/abl fusion gene in chronic myelogenous leukemia: peripheral blood analysis is comparable to a bone marrow examination. Blood 1993; 82(10S1):331a.
35. Lin F, Chase A, Bungey J, Goldman JM, Cross NCP. Correlation between the proportion of Philadelphia chromosome positive metaphases and levels of BCR-ABL mRNA in chronic myeloid leukaemia. Genes Chromos Cancer 1995; 13:110–114.
36. el-Rifai W, Ruutu T, Vettenranta K, Temtamy S, Knuutila S. Minimal residual disease after allogeneic bone marrow transplantation for chronic myeloid leukaemia: a metaphase-FISH study. Br J Haematol 1996; 92:365–369.

15
Monitoring the Course of Chronic Myelogenous Leukemia by Fluorescence In Situ Hybridization

Chu-Myong Seong
Ewha Woman's University, Seoul, Korea, and M. D. Anderson Cancer Center, Houston, Texas

Hagop M. Kantarjian, Moshe Talpaz, Richard Champlin, and Michael Siciliano
M. D. Anderson Cancer Center, Houston, Texas

INTRODUCTION

In situ hybridization is based on the base pairing of the DNA probe to complementary sequences in cells of the sample. Fluorescence detection has been the most popular technique for a variety of reasons including its high sensitivity, signal resolution, and, most of all, the potential to simultaneously detect multiple target regions (1,2). The different types of DNA probes useful for clinical applications can be categorized according to the complexity of the respective target sequences. Most genomic DNA fragments cloned in plasmid-, phage-, cosmid-, P1-, or yeast artificial chromosome (YAC) vectors, detect unique loci in the genome. To reach efficiencies needed for diagnostic applications, probes comprising at least 20–50 kB (i.e., cosmid size probes) are required. Larger chromosomal regions and even whole chromosomes can be "painted" by using probe pools derived from for examples, flow-sorted or microdissected chromosomes, or from somatic hybrid cell lines containing only one human chromosome or segments thereof (3–5). In this review, recent advances in the analysis of CML made by fluorescence in situ hybridization (FISH) studies and future prospects will be discussed.

VALUE OF METAPHASE-FLUORESCENCE IN SITU HYBRIDIZATION (M-FISH) TO DETECT VARIANT Ph TRANSLOCATION

Variations of the typical Ph (VPh) translocation occur in 3% of CML cases (6,7); VPh-CML is often difficult to detect by standard cytogenetic procedures, and the incidence of VPh may be higher than suspected. Chromosome-specific probes using dual *Alu* primers to direct polymerase chain reaction (PCR) amplification of human DNA from hybrid cells containing regions of the human genome (i.e., chromosomes 1, 9, and 22) in rodents were generated. Because FISH probes made in this manner do not recognize centromeric sequences (8), such probes could be used to delineate complex VPh chromosomes rapidly and unambiguously. This is especially true in translocations involving multiple chromosomes (i.e., variant Ph-positive CML involving chromosome 1, 9, and 22), for which FISH with inter-*Alu* PCR probes should allow accurate and fast analysis of chromosome abnormalities (9). It is important that the method identifies these events in the less than ideal metaphases that often occur in clinical samples and in which the abnormalities are difficult to resolve by standard cytogenetic procedures.

ANALYSIS OF INTERPHASE CELLS FOR THE PHILADELPHIA TRANSLOCATION BY FISH

Identification of the Ph chromosome in interphase nuclei had been first attempted using a combination of cosmid probes (10). Digitized images were collected with a cooled charged coupled device (CCD) camera and displayed after computer enhancement. A combination of the two colors indicated the presence of the Ph chromosome. The small size of the region detected by these probes raises questions as to their reliability for large-scale clinical use. Inter-*Alu*-PCR product from the YAC showed that 64% of the interphase nuclei from the bone marrow (BM) of a CML patient contained more than two signals, whereas 96% of normal diploid cells had two signals or less, as expected (11). Because these signals appeared as dots in the interphase nuclei, there was a possibility of false negatives (missing some true targets because of incomplete hybridization) or false positives (counting artificial spots). However, in a sufficiently large sample size, it was suggested that the presence of cancer cells in a population could be detected.

We examined the usefulness of a larger size probe derived by inter-All-polymerase chain reaction of DNA from an interspecific somatic cell hybrid containing approximately 5 MB of human DNA covering the ABL gene region on human chromosome 9q34 to give a clear, yet resolvable signal for detection of three domains of hybridization in CML interphases and two domains in normal cells (Fig. 1). We also evaluated the effectiveness of combining that probe with a BCR probe in two-color procedures for high-efficiency quantitation of

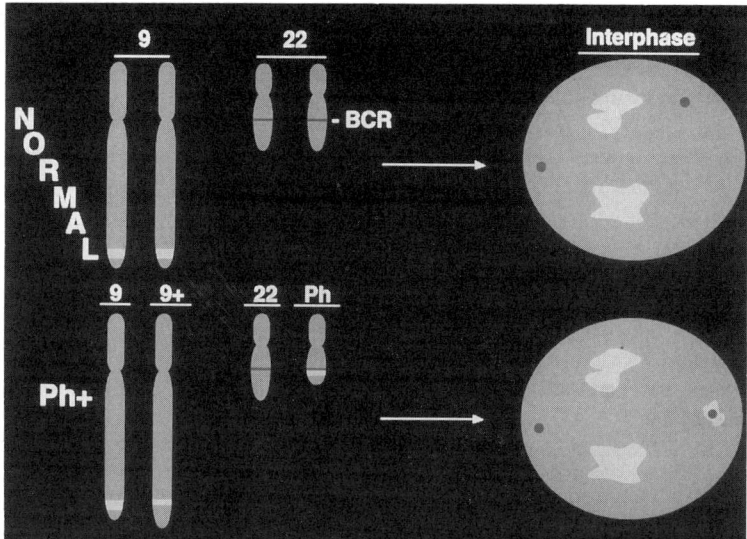

Figure 1 Cartoon showing the region of human chromosome 9 identified by the E6B probe and chromosome 22 identified by the BCR probe and the appearance of the probe in metaphase (left) and interphase cells of (right) before (top) and after (bottom) development of the Ph chromosome.

the frequency of Ph-positive cells. Such quantitation enables the detection of Ph-positive cells in heterogeneous cell populations with obvious application to research and management of the disease (12).

An experiment was performed with a subset of samples from the previous series—five normals and five CML patients. All interphase cells (not just polys) were counted (three domains: 79.2%; two domains: 20.6%). However, interphase FISH with E6B does have its limitations. At present, it appears that the signal generated by the large probe, although very efficient for resolving the domains in polys, is often diffuse in other cell types that may include more immature cycling cells. In addition, about 5% of the cells from normals and 9% of the cells from CML patients were judged unscorable.

HYPERMETAPHASE FLUORESCENCE IN SITU HYBRIDIZATION (HMF)

Quantitative Monitoring of Ph-Positive Cells During IFN-α Treatment

While extremely reliable when a good harvest of metaphases is obtained from a marrow culture, more than 20–25 metaphases are rarely recovered from pa-

Table 1 A Practical Monitoring Approach to Patients on Therapy

1. Cytogenetic studies at diagnosis to detect Ph-positive disease and clonal evolution, then yearly to monitor clonal evolution.
2. On therapy:
   a. PB I-FISH studies as long as Ph-positive disease is expected to be more than 5–10%
   b. Shift to HMF (BM) when Ph-positive cells are <5% to monitor MRD
3. Value of HMF in monitoring CML course, and in assessing MRD with IFN-α therapy or post BMT:
   a. Monitor minor interval changes of % Ph-positive cells (as low as 5% changes)
   b. May consider stopping IFN-α therapy if 0 out of 1000 Ph-positive metaphases by HMF
   c. Optimize therapy (additional agents; DLI) for significant but minor changes in disease status

tients on therapy. Consequently, in patients with CML receiving treatment, monitoring the effect of therapy by cytogenetic studies (CG) is limited with respect to detection minimal residual disease (MRD) and identifying significant changes in Ph-positive cell frequency. Analyzing greater numbers of metaphases per sample would provide higher resolution and greater efficiency in addressing these issues.

Long-term exposure (24 hours) of bone marrow cultures to colcemid (0.1 µg/mL) maximized the frequency of metaphase collection. Such preparations were subjected to FISH using a probe that overlapped the region of the translocation at chromosome 9q34. This detected the Ph translocation in the resultant large number of overly contracted chromosome spreads. The procedure was validated and verified by studying 70 double-blind marrow samples from patients in different stages of Ph-positive CML, and from patients with Ph-negative hematological malignancies (controls). This hypermetaphase FISH (HMF) method clearly identified Ph-positive metaphases and allowed the analysis of 500 metaphases per sample in <1 hour after FISH (13). In this analysis, 24% of patients were reclassified into a cytogenetic response category that was more appropriate than the one assigned by CG (Table 1). It was also successful in providing response data in patients with insufficient metaphases for regular CG studies. Of significance was the ability of HMF to detect MRD in three of 19 patients in complete cytogenetic response by routine CG, thus providing insight into their true response status, which may influence treatment decisions (dose schedule, additional agents, need to continue therapy). Furthermore, in patients shown to be 0% Ph-positive by HMF on 500 cells, an argument could be made to reduce or stop IFN-α therapy, while continuing close monitoring by HMF. Studies on 500 cells have very narrow confidence intervals (±2%) and minor changes (<4%) observed at periodic intervals (e.g., every 3–6 months) can be reliable measurements of the efficiency of a particular therapy and disease evolution.

The maximum frequency of cancer cells present at the indicated confidence levels (at 99%, 95%) were: 0.11, 0.007 when 0 cancer cells were seen in 400 metaphases; and 0.009, 0.006 when 0 cells were seen in 500 metaphases. Thus, in the standard HMF analysis, when 500 cells are studied and no cancer cell hypermetaphases are identified, there is a 99% confidence that there are <1% cancer cells in the sample. With respect to the assessment of minimal residual disease during therapy, a complete cytogenetic response by CG may in fact be only a partial cytogenetic response by HMF, or it may be a complete response of high quality (0 Ph-positive cells in 500 cells analyzed). This should help in decisions regarding continuation of IFN-α therapy and/or addition of other agents (e.g., low-dose cytosine-arabinoside [ara-C]), dose schedule adjustment, or even discontinuation of therapy.

The major limitation of HMF is the inability of the procedure to detect cytogenetic clonal evolution, an indicator of worse prognosis (14), as it is focused on scoring the single cytogenetic event of interest (in this case, the Ph chromosome). There is also recent evidence that clonal evolution may not carry the same poor prognostic impact in such cases as when occurring with other features (15).

Early Detection of Relapse by HMF After Allogeneic Bone Marrow Transplantation (BMT)

Using probes that identify Ph-positive cells, HMF was compared with standard CG in the follow-up evaluations of 51 patients with CML following allogeneic BMT (21,22). Among them, 12 (23.5%) were negative for Ph by standard CG but were positive by HMF. Among these 12 patients, six (50%) experienced CML relapse after median 103 days (range 63–185 days), and the 5-year actuarial survival was 28%. None of the other 35 patients who were Ph-negative by CG and HMF have relapsed; their actuarial survival was 67% at 5 years (Fig. 2).

Early recognition of CML relapse post BMT is becoming increasingly important with the recent documentation that donor lymphocyte infusions (DLI) can reinduce complete remission via a graft-versus-leukemia effect in patients relapsing into chronic phase. This approach was most effective when applied early in the course of relapse. Kolb et al. (16) reported that among 84 patients, 14 (82%), 39 (78%), and one (12.5%) achieved complete remission after DLI for cytogenetic relapse, hematological relapse, and transformed phase relapse, respectively. Van Rhee et al. (17) reported a higher remission rate and a lower risk of marrow aplasia and other complications in patients transplanted early in cytogenetic relapse than in overt hematological relapse. Early intervention, when donor-derived hematopoietic cells are dominant, might prevent the complications associated with pancytopenia.

We conclude that in patients with CML after allogeneic BMT, HMF should be considered as a quantitative technique to detect and monitor the results of therapy for CML.

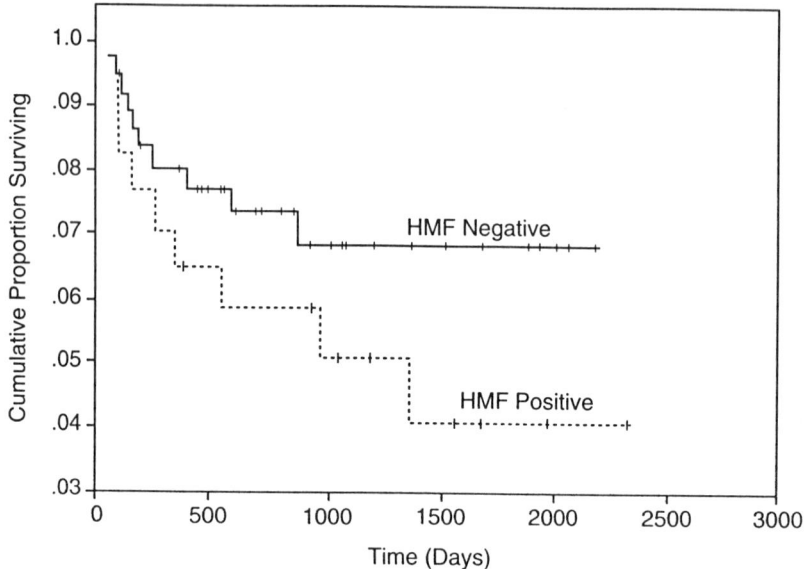

Figure 2 DFS based on Ph status by HMF.

Analysis of Ph-Negative BCR-Positive CML by HMF

Approximately 5–10% of patients with a morphologic diagnosis of CML are Ph-negative (18). They tend to be older (median age >65 years) and to have monocytosis, thrombocytopenia, a poor response to chemotherapy, and an overall shorter survival than Ph-positive CML patients. Thirty percent of them have rearrangement of BCR by Southern blot (Ph-negative BCR-positive) and are indistinguishable from patients with Ph-positive CML in relation to characteristics, response, and prognosis.

We recently analyzed six such patients by HMF. The detailed cytogenetic and molecular analyses are shown in Table 2. Two of the six patients showed an insertion of 9q34 into chromosome 22q11 with a frequency of 74.2% and 92%. In both cases, the insertion was easily identified by HMF. In addition, HMF detected a low frequency of Ph-positive cells at diagnosis in two patients (patients 2 and 5) and during hematological relapse in two other patients (patients 1 and 6). The pattern of UBCR was identical to the classical pattern in Ph-positive CML. The p210 results correlated well in two patients (patients 2 and 5) but were discordant in one (patient 2), in whom high p210 expression with of a low Ph-positive frequency might suggest the presence of a cryptic BCR-ABL junction. The HMF analysis was useful in identifying Ph-positive clones, in Ph-negative BCR-positive CML, and characterized the nature of the chromosome aberration, i.e., an insertion. It identified two distinct subsets of

Table 2 Summary of Standard Cytogenetic Studies, Southern and Western Blots, and HMF in the Study Group

Patients	Karyotype (CG)	BCR/ABL Rearrangement	P210$^{BCR-ABL}$ Expression	HMF(%)
1	46, XY[20]	positive	+	22/400(5.5%)-Chromosome 9 29/500(5.8%)-Chromosome 22
2	46, XY[23]	positive	++++	25/475(5.2%)-Chromosome 9 22/500(4.4%)-Chromosome 22
3	45,X,-Y[24] 46, XY [1]	positive	na	371/500(74.2%)-Chromosome 9 0/500(0%)-Chromosome 22
4	46,XY,del(19)(p13.2)[19] 46, XY [1]	positive	na	462/501(92%)-Chromosome 9 0/800(0%)-Chromosome 22
5	46, XX[20]	positive	+	17/400(4.2%)-Chromosome 9 18/500(3.6%)-Chromosome 22
6	46,XY[20]	positive	na	2/800(0.3%)-Chromosome 9 1/800(0.1%)-Chromosome 22

Ph-negative BCR-positive CML: one with an insertion of 9q34 into 22q11, the other with a low frequency of typical Ph chromosome translocations. The use of HMF with other complementary molecular studies (i.e., Southern and Western studies) in larger study groups may help further define the heterogeneity and prognosis in Ph-negative BCR-positive CML.

BLOOD VERSUS BONE MARROW STUDIES FOR PH MONITORING BY FISH

The technique for monitoring Ph frequency with HMF involves the invasive and painful procedure of bone marrow aspiration. One of our aims has been to develop a noninvasive, yet highly reliable, method to monitor the frequency of Ph-positive cells in CML patients undergoing therapy, By testing the use of interphase (I-FISH) on peripheral blood (PB), we chose to target polymorphonuclear leukocytes (polys), which have better resolution with I-FISH techniques. The I-FISH results (five normals and 26 CML) were compared with their respective bone marrow (BM) HMF results to verify the correlation between the frequency of Ph-positive cells obtained by the two methods. The BCR/ABL translocation probe (Vysis) was used to detect BCR/ABL gene fusion (Fig. 3), and this probe was highly effective in identifying Ph-positive cells in the majority of cells in PB polys. Our FISH probe containing only approximately 5 Mb of human DNA surrounding the ABL locus on human chromosome 9 probe was used to detect BCR/ABL gene fusions in BM metaphases. The percent Ph-positive by I-FISH was estimated using the method of Thall et al. (20). The correlation between the percent of Ph positivity by I-FISH on polys and percent of Ph positivity metaphases by BM HMF in 26 samples was excellent ($r = 0.983$, $p < 0.0001$) (Fig. 4).

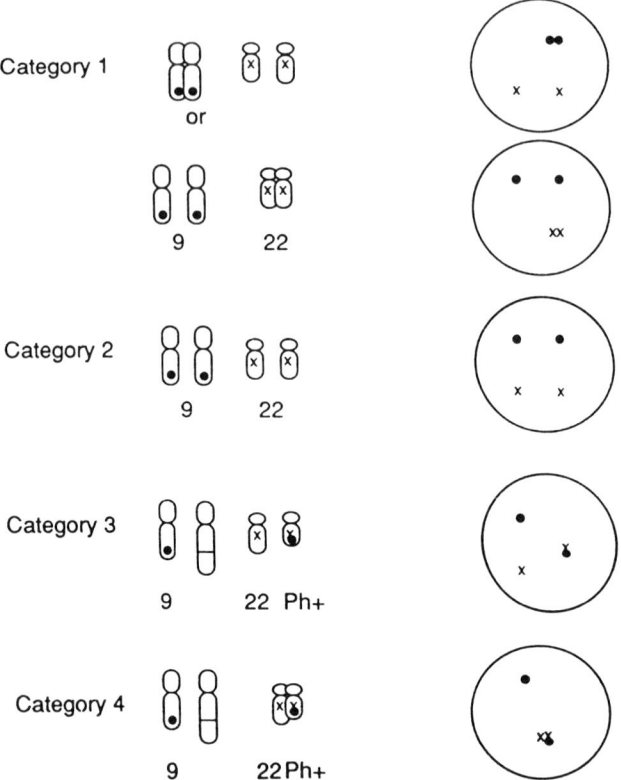

Figure 3 Cartoon of I-FISH showing normal and Ph+ cell by the ABL probe and the BCR probe: category 1, 2: normal and category 3, 4: Ph+.

Peripheral blood I-FISH was not suitable for CML patients with minimal residual disease (i.e., <5% Ph positivity), because of the false positivity potential. In such cases, other procedures like HMF are necessary. However, PB I-FISH is a practical and less invasive monitoring procedure allowing rational treatment decisions at particular periods during the course of therapy, when Ph-positive disease is reduced, but not eliminated, below the conventional cytogenetic levels.

CONCLUSION AND RECOMMENDATION

Peripheral blood I-FISH is most useful in assessing early treatment response of patients receiving IFN-α therapy or DLI. However, the background rate of 5% false positivity limits its use to assess minimal residual disease. More sensitive quantitative methods (HMF) should be performed for that purpose. HMF recog-

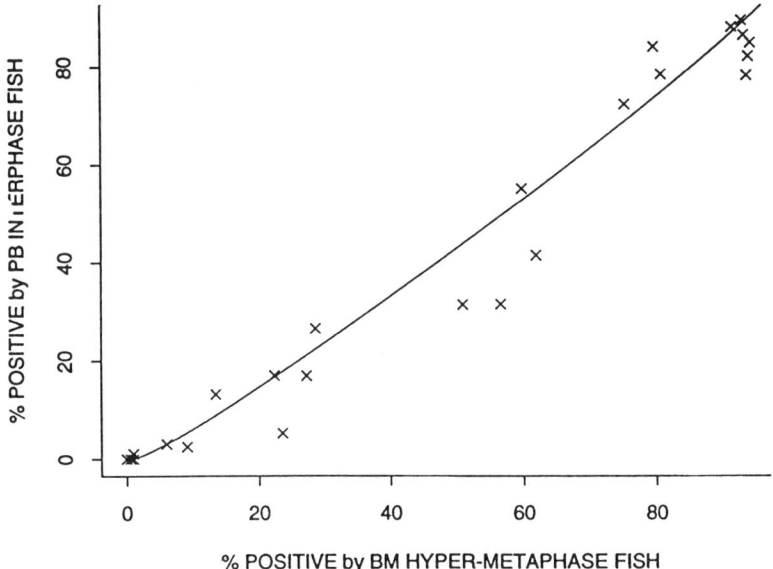

Figure 4 Scatter plot and fitted regression line where Y = percent Ph+ in PMNs by I-FISH and where X = percent Ph+ in BM cells by HMF.

nized Ph-positive cells in 16% of patients characterized as having a complete cytogenetic response after IFN-α therapy and identified statistically significant differences between the frequencies of Ph-positive cells in samples that differed by <4% during therapy. In addition, HMF was a useful quantitative technique to detect and monitor Ph-positive disease after allogeneic BMT or peripheral blood stem cell transplantation, since early detection of CML relapse post-BMT is increasingly important for DLI intervention.

REFERENCES

1. Raap AK, Dirks RW, Jiwa NM, Nderlof PM, van der Ploeg M. In situ hybridization with hapten-modified DNA probes. In: Racz P, Haase AT, Gluckman JC, eds. Modern Pathology of AIDS and Other Retroviral Infections. Basel: S. Karger, 1990: 17–28.
2. Lichter P. Cremer T. Chromosome analysis by non-isotopic in situ hybridization. In: Rooney DE, Czepulkowski BH, eds. Human Cytogenetics. New York: Oxford University Press, 1992:157–192.
3. Lichter P, Boyle AL, Cremer T, Ward DC. Analysis of genes and chromosomes by nonisotopic in situ hybridization. Genet Anal Tech Appl 1991;8:24–35.
4. Tkachuk DC, Pinkel D, Kuo W-L, Weier H-U, Gray JW. Clinical applications of fluorescence in situ hybridization. Genet Anal Tech Appl 1991; 18:67–74.

5. Joos S, Fink TM, Rätsch A, Lichter P. Mapping and chromosome analysis: the potential of fluorescence in situ hybridization. J Biotechnol 1994. In press.
6. Heim S. Mitelman F. Multistep cytogenetic scenario in CML. Adv Viral Oncol 1987; 7:53–76.
7. Potter AM, Watmore AE, Cooke P, Lilleyman JS, Sokol RJM. Significance of nonstandard Philadelphia chromosomes in CML. Br J Cancer 1981; 44:51–54.
8. Lie P, Siciliano J, Seong D, et al. Dual Alu PCR primers and conditions for isolation of human painting probes from hybrid cells. Cancer Genet Cytogenet. Submitted.
9. Seong D, Liu P, Siciliano J, et al. Detection of variant Ph1-positive CML involving chromosome #1,#9, and #22 by FISH. Cancer Genet Cytogenet 1993; 65:100.
10. Tkachuk DC, Westbrook CA, Andreeff M, et al. Detection of *bcr-abl* fusion in chronic myelogenous leukemia by in situ hybridization. Science 1990; 250:559.
11. Lengauer C. Riethman HC, Speicher MR, et at. Metaphase and interphase cytogenetics with Alu-PCR-amplified yeast artificial chromosome clones containing the BCR gene and the opotooncogenes c-*raf*-1, c-*fms*, and c-*erbB*-2. Cancer Res 1992: 52:2590.
12. Seong DC. Song MY, Henske E, et al. Analysis of interphase cells for the Philadelphia translocation using painting probe made by inter-alu PCR from a radiation hybrid. Blood 1994; 83:2268.
13. Seong D, Kantarjian H, R. J. Siciliano M. Hypermetaphase FISH for quantitative monitoring of Ph-positive cells in patients with CML during treatment. Blood 1995; 86:2343.
14. Kantarjian HM, Deisseroth A, Kurzrock R, Estrov Z, Talpaz M. Chronic myelogenous leukemia: a concise update. Blood 1993; 82:691.
15. Majlis A, Kantarjian H, Smith T, et al. What is the significance of cytogenetic clonal evolution (CE) in patients (PTS) with Philadelphia chromosome (Ph)-positive chromonic myelogenous leukemia (CML)? Blood 1994; 84(suppl 1):150a.
16. Kolb H. Schtternberg A, Goldman J, Hertenstein B, Hassan A. Graft-versus-leukemia effect of DLI in marrow grafted patients. Blood 1995; 86:2041–2050.
17. Van Rhee F, Lin F, Cullis J, et al. Relapse of chronic myeloid leukemia after allogeneic bone marrow transplant: the case for giving donor leukocyte transfusions before the onset of hematologic relapse. Blood 1994; 83:3377–3383.
18. Kantarjian HM, Smith TL, McCredie KB, et al. Chronic myelogenous leukemia: a multivariate analysis of the associations of patient characteristics and therapy with survival. Blood 1985; 66:1326.
19. Kantarjian HM, Walters S, McCredie KB, et al. Clinical and prognostic features of Philadelphia chromosome negative chronic myelogenous leukemia. Cancer 1986; 58:2023.
20. Thall P, Jacoby D, Zimmerman S. Estimating genomic category probabilities from fluorescent in situ hybridization counts and misclassification. Appl Statistics 1996. In press.
21. Seong CM, Giralt S, Kantarjian H, Siciliano M, Champlin R. Early detection of relapse by HMF after BMT for CML. J Clin Oncol (in press).
22. Seong CM, Giralt S, Kantarjian H, Siciliano M, Champlin R. Usefulness of detection of MRD by HMF after BMT for CML. Bone Marrow Transplant 1997; 19: 565–570.

16
Molecular Monitoring of CML During Interferon Treatment: Insights from the Cancer and Leukemia Group B Experience

Wendy Stock

Loyola University Medical Center, Maywood, Illinois

INTRODUCTION

Quantitation of Philadelphia chromosome-positive cells in bone marrow samples has become an important endpoint in the evaluation of treatment response in patients with chronic myeloid leukemia (CML) (1,2). Several randomized clinical trials have now shown a significant survival benefit for CML patients who have achieved a complete cytogenetic response with disappearance of the Philadelphia chromosome during treatment with alpha interferon (3–6). An alternative monitoring method for patients with CML involves molecular detection of rearrangements of the *bcr* gene using Southern blot analysis (7–9). The proportion of leukemic and normal cells in a CML patient sample may be quantitated based on the relative strengths of the Southern blot signals and may be used to monitor the disappearance of malignant cells during treatment. Southern blot quantitation represents an additional method for monitoring treatment response in this disease (10,11). This technique is useful for detection of leukemia cells when the malignant cells comprise 5–100% of the specimen in question and, therefore, is an appropriate method for monitoring response to treatment with alpha interferon.

Southern blot monitoring is also useful in CML cases where *bcr/abl* gene rearrangement is present in the absence of a cytogenetically detectable Philadelphia chromosome. Use of the polymerase chain reaction (PCR) to detect *bcr/abl* transcripts with reverse transcriptase technology (RT-PCR) has further enhanced the sensitivity of molecular monitoring of minimal residual disease in patients who have undergone intensive therapy for CML (12). Both Southern blot and RT-PCR analyses can be performed easily on blood, as well as bone marrow samples, thereby providing a theoretical advantage to the patient and treating physician over serial monitoring using quantitative cytogenetics of bone marrow samples. Until recently, however, no prospective studies comparing blood and marrow monitoring of CML in comparison to standard cytogenetic monitoring during treatment had been performed.

The focus of this chapter is to review our experience in the Cancer and Leukemia Group B (CALGB) with the clinical utility and efficacy of prospective, quantitative Southern blot monitoring for CML patients receiving interferon-based therapy. Briefly, the monitoring technique will be reviewed, and applications will be discussed and followed by review of both our and other groups' data in large clinical trials. Special emphasis will be placed on clinical insights gained from prospective monitoring trials in patients receiving interferon-based therapy for CML.

QUANTITATIVE SOUTHERN BLOT ANALYSIS OF THE *bcr/abl* FUSION GENE

Gene rearrangement of *bcr* and *abl* detected by recombinant DNA technology is the molecular counterpart of the translocation t(9;22)(q34;q11) identified on karyotypic analysis as a truncated chromosome 22 known as the Philadelphia chromosome. This translocation relocates the proto-oncogene *c-abl* from chromosome 9q34 to within the *bcr* (breakpoint cluster region) gene on chromosome 22q11 (7). The Philadelphia chromosome is found in >95% of patients with CML; however, there are cases of CML which are Philadelphia chromosome-negative because mitotic cells are required for cytogenetic analysis, and/or the genetic exchange is masked by additional chromosomal involvement, or is limited to the exchange of submicroscopic chromosomal segments. The *bcr/abl* fusion gene can be detected using Southern blot analysis in virtually all cases of Philadelphia chromosome-positive disease; in addition, from 30% to 50% of these Philadelphia chromosome-"negative" CML can be detected using this technique (8).

There are two major types of *bcr/abl* rearrangements based on differences in chromosomal breakpoint. In the vast majority of cases of CML, the breakpoint falls within a small, 5.8-kb segment which contains four exons, designated b1 to b4 (7,13). The breakpoint occurs either between exons b2 and b3, or b3 and b4 of the *bcr* gene. The resulting fusion gene is transcribed and translated into a 210-kD (p210) protein. These *bcr/abl* rearrangements can be detected on Southern blots. The breakpoint location in the *bcr* gene can be roughly estimated using two molecular probes from the major breakpoint cluster region (M-bcr) hybridized to Southern blots prepared with three enzymatic digests using specific restriction endonucleases. Using this method, it is also possible to calculate the percentage of leukemia cells in each sample. Our technique for preparing the Southern blots is described in brief below.

A buffy coat is prepared from heparinized bone marrow aspirate and blood specimens, red blood cells are lysed, and DNA is extracted using standard methods (14). In each case, approximately 10 µg of extracted DNA is enzymatically digested with *Bam*H1, *Hind*III, and *Bgl*II. The enzymatic digests are electrophoresed on standard agarose gels, and Southern blotting is performed by sequential hybridizations with two probes from the M-bcr of the *bcr* gene (one from exon 2 and the other from exon 4). This method will identify the majority of *bcr* breakpoints in patients with CML, and makes it possible to estimate whether the breakpoint is in the 5′ or 3′ region of the M-bcr. Southern blots prepared from CML patients with a breakpoint in the major breakpoint cluster region of the *bcr* gene will have two identifiable bands; one represents the normal germline *bcr* gene, and the other represents the abnormal, rearranged *bcr* gene.

Using densitometric techniques, it is possible to quantify directly the proportion of leukemia cells relative to normal cells in the sample (Fig. 1). The intensity of the rearranged *bcr* band can be compared to the intensity of the normal *bcr* band in each sample. In our studies, data were collected as the ratio of the rearranged *bcr* band to the normal *bcr* band using an algebraic correction to calculate the percentage of CML cells in each sample (15).

PROSPECTIVE COMPARISON OF BLOOD AND BONE MARROW SOUTHERN BLOT MONITORING

Previous reports described the ability to utilize peripheral blood as a means of detecting *bcr/abl* rearrangements on Southern blot. It became clear that a prospective comparison of blood and marrow monitoring was essential in order to validate the routine use of blood monitoring in patients receiving interferon therapy. The CALGB has recently published a prospective monitoring study, and a retrospective analysis comparing blood and marrow monitoring has been performed by the team at M.D. Anderson Cancer Center (15,16). Both groups found strong correlation between Southern blot results of matched blood and bone marrow samples. Similarly, we found an excellent correlation between blood and marrow results when sequential sampling timepoints during treatment were evaluated.

In the CALGB prospective study, blood and marrow samples from 64 adults with previously untreated CML were evaluated prior to initiation of treatment and at specified sequential follow-up timepoints during interferon-based treatment for CML on a CALGB protocol. Blood and marrow specimens were

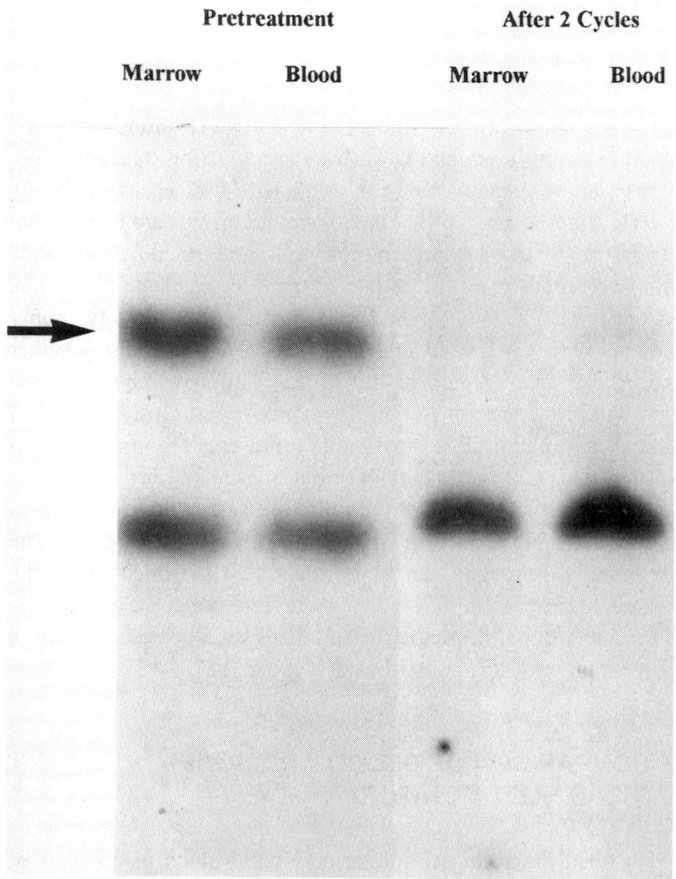

Figure 1 Quantitative Southern blot monitoring in blood and marrow specimens. The upper band (arrow) is the rearranged *bcr* allele; the lower band represents the germline *bcr* allele. Pretreatment quantitative densitometric analysis showed a *bcr* gene rearrangement in 100% of the cells. After two treatment cycles, the percentage of malignant cells had decreased to 14% (marrow) and 20% (blood), respectively.

highly correlated at both high and low levels of detectable malignant cells (Fig. 2). Importantly, in our study, in all cases where a complete molecular response was observed in blood samples (no detectable rearranged *bcr* gene on Southern blot), there was complete concordance with the matched marrow sample. The retrospective comparison of blood and marrow Southern blot monitoring per-

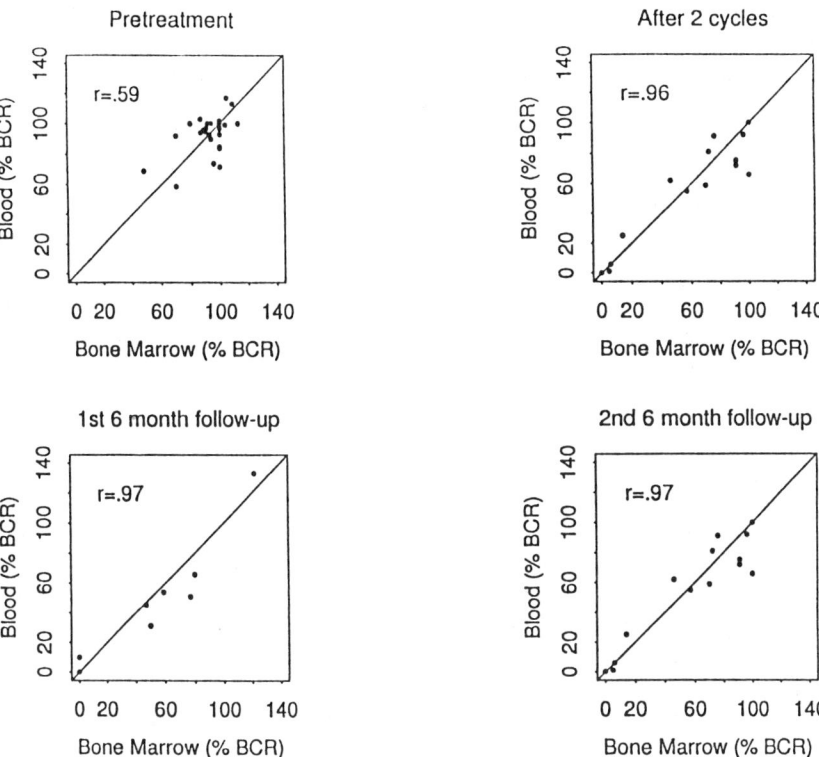

Figure 2 Comparison of bone marrow and blood *bcr* gene rearrangements in 83 matched cases. The percentage of malignant cells in the bone marrow are displayed on the X axis; in the blood, on the Y axis. The diagonal line is the line of identity; if blood and marrow specimens have an identical percentage of *bcr*-rearranged cells, the point falls on the line. The distance of a point from the line represents the difference between matched marrow and blood values. The point at position (100,100) in the pretreatment diagram represents a total of 19 cases (upper left) with identical marrow and blood values, and a total of two matched cases following two treatment cycles (upper right). The points at position (0,0) in the diagrams following two treatment cycles, at the first 6-month follow-up, and at the second 6-month follow-up represent four, six, and two matched cases, respectively. (Modified from Ref. 15.)

formed by Verschraegen et al. also showed the results between marrow and blood are interchangeable (16). Molecular monitoring using blood samples rather than bone marrow is a very important consideration for patient acceptability and cost, as it obviates the need for frequent bone marrow examinations.

COMPARISON OF SOUTHERN BLOT AND CYTOGENETIC MONITORING METHODS

A critical comparison of molecular monitoring using Southern blot *bcr* gene rearrangements with cytogenetic analysis is essential, since monitoring of the disappearance of the Philadelphia chromosome has been the standard monitoring method and has been shown to correlate strongly with delay of blastic transformation. Furthermore, disappearance of the Philadelphia chromosome appears to be an important surrogate marker of overall survival in several large series (1,3–6,17,18). We found that a strong correlation exists between Southern blot (blood or marrow) and standard marrow cytogenetic monitoring (Table 1). Analysis of sequential, matched samples showed no statistically significant difference between the mean or median values for the percentage of malignant cells detected with either method; similarly, Southern blot and cytogenetic monitoring were concordant when serial monitoring of individual patients was examined (15). Therefore, this study validates the use of quantitative Southern blot methods for monitoring patients receiving interferon-based treatment of CML.

Comparison of the two methods for evaluation of residual disease states may also provide some insight into the dynamics of remission induction in chronic-phase CML, and highlights some of the potential differences between

Table 1 Comparison of Quantitative Southern Blot Results from Blood Samples and Marrow Cytogenetic Results in Chronologically Matched Samples

Sample	N	Median % CML cells (range)		Intraclass correlation (95% CI)
		SB (blood)	Cytogenetics	
Pretreatment	49	100% (40–117)	100% (50–100)	0.29 (0.05, 0.49)
After 2 cycles	21	42% (0–100)	30% (0–100)	0.89 (0.78, 0.94)
6 months later	13	31% (0–133)	27% (0–100)	0.92 (0.78, 0.97)
12 months later	5	63% (43–100)	88% (56–97)	0.52 (0.00, 0.90)

Medians and ranges of the percentages of malignant cells detected and the intraclass correlation coefficient with 95% CI are shown for pretreatment samples, following two treatment cycles, and after two subsequent follow-up samples at 6-month intervals. (Modified from Ref. 15.)

Southern blot and cytogenetic monitoring. In our study, cytogenetic analysis tended to indicate a higher percentage of malignant cells than Southern blot monitoring when minimal disease states existed. We reviewed samples from 17 patients with <15% malignant cells by Southern blot or cytogenetic analysis (15). Interestingly, four discordant cases were found in which Southern blot analysis detected no evidence of a *bcr* gene rearrangement, yet demonstrated from 12% to 20% Philadelphia chromosome-positive metaphase cells by cytogenetic analysis. The converse was not found; specifically, we found no cases in which Southern blot was "positive" (*bcr* rearrangement detected) while the cytogenetics was "negative" (Philadelphia-negative).

Since the Southern blot technique described above measures the entire cell population of a given sample, whereas cytogenetic analysis examines only the dividing cells. These findings suggest that the Philadelphia-positive clone has a proliferative advantage and results in a higher detection rate in dividing cells (cytogenetic studies) than the total cell population (molecular studies), which contains both cells that have a *bcr* gene rearrangement (Philadelphia-positive) and those without *bcr* gene rearrangements (Philadelphia-negative). The M.D. Anderson, using similar methodology, has also reported discordant cases such as these and they also found cases where cytogenetic analysis detected no malignant cells while Southern blots had a *bcr* rearrangement (16). The clinical significance of the discrepant cases is unclear. At the present time, the four "discordant" patients who were complete responders by Southern blot on our study remain well and without evidence of progressive disease. One of these patients subsequently achieved a complete cytogenetic response (15).

Interestingly, Verschraegen et al. have reported that Southern blot responses in the absence of significant cytogenetic responses was predictive of long-term survival (16). Therefore, longitudinal follow-up of these, and additional, discordant cases for survival will be needed to understand more completely the clinical relevance of these findings. Until such data are available, however, our current recommendation is that a marrow cytogenetic evaluation should be performed in patients who become *bcr*-negative by Southern blot to avoid overestimating the degree of response and to obtain information about the possibility of clonal evolution of the disease.

The studies summarized above validate the use of quantitative Southern blotting of blood samples as a valuable monitoring tool in interferon-treated CML. Clearly, monitoring using blood samples has advantages in terms of patient acceptability, flexibility, and cost (in many laboratories, cytogenetic analysis is more than two times more costly than Southern blot quantification). In conclusion, quantitative Southern blotting may be used for diagnosis and monitoring. In cases where a complete response is noted by Southern blot, cytogenetic analysis should be done to confirm the Southern blot findings and contribute any additional clinical information about disease evolution.

MOLECULAR ANALYSIS AS A MEANS OF PREDICTING RESPONSE TO INTERFERON

Another practical question that molecular studies in CML have addressed is whether identification of the molecular breakpoint has clinical, prognostic value. As mentioned previously, in CML, the molecular breakpoint falls within a 5.8-kb segment containing exons b1–b4. Using Southern blotting techniques, the breakpoint may be localized either 5' or 3' to a central *Hind*III restriction site which conventionally separates a 5' and 3' area of the M-bcr (7,13). When the breakpoint is in the 3' area, exon b3 is always included in the fusion *bcr/abl* transcript. When the site is in the 5' area, exon b3 can be either maintained or removed; therefore, two different mRNAs are transcribed, called a2b3 and a2b2, respectively. These two transcripts differ by 75 bp and the protein that is coded by a2b3 has 25 amino acids more (7,13,19).

A number of studies, initially using specific restriction endonucleases and Southern blotting to identify 5' and 3' breakpoints, and more recently using a reverse-transcriptase PCR assay to identify the a2b2 or a2b3 transcripts, have addressed the question of whether breakpoint location has prognostic significance and is predictive of response to treatment and/or duration of chronic phase (20–27). The results of such studies have been mixed and are difficult to interpret for a variety of reasons, including differences in the definition of the breakpoint region (Southern blotting studies), use of different prognostic models for CML, and the fact that the vast majority of these studies were small retrospective analyses of patients who received a variety of different treatments including chemotherapy or interferon treatment. One of the largest studies published to date is a prospective analysis of breakpoint significance using an RT-PCR analysis of interferon treatment in 146 chronic-phase patients from the Italian Cooperative Study Group on CML (28). Sixty-two patients were identified with the a2b2 transcript and 84 had the a2b3 transcript. Patients were analyzed for cytogenetic response and for survival. There were no significant differences noted between the two groups for either cytogenetic response or overall 5-year survival rates. Similarly, they found that the rate of progression from chronic to accelerated and blastic phase was clearly independent of transcript type. Perhaps further progress in the definition of the molecular lesions and longer follow-up may eventually reveal differences; currently, the available data do not support a significant role for defining the M-bcr breakpoint in the management of CML.

Whereas the location of the breakpoint within the M-bcr has not been shown to be prognostically significant, a very limited amount of data suggests that Southern blot quantitation of the *bcr/abl* gene at the time of diagnosis may be useful for predicting response to interferon. We have observed an occasional, newly diagnosed patient who presents prior to any treatment with a lower percentage of malignant cells by quantitative Southern blot analysis (from 40% to

75% *bcr*-rearranged at the time of diagnosis rather than the usual 90–100%). In our study of 64 patients, three such cases were observed (15). Conversely, at the time of diagnosis in these cases, the Philadelphia chromosome was detected in 90–100% of the metaphases examined (minimum of 20 metaphases studied). Interestingly, all three of these patients subsequently became complete cytogenetic and molecular (Southern blot) responders to the interferon/cytarabine combination.

This is an intriguing observation and suggests that CML patients with a low percentage of *bcr*-rearranged cells at the time of diagnosis may identify a group who are more likely to respond to treatment with interferon, although the small number of patients observed precludes any definitive statement about the true prognostic significance. Additional quantitative monitoring studies of larger numbers of patients are needed to confirm these findings. Information from only one other study begins to address this specific question. In their study, Vershraegen et al. also found five of 28 patients with more than 90% Philadelphia-positive metaphases at diagnosis who had a low percentage of *bcr*-rearranged cells (16). However, these patients were not monitored specifically for response to interferon, and because overall survival was excellent in patients with both high and low BCR values, these investigators found no significant differences between the two groups.

MOLECULAR DETECTION OF MINIMAL RESIDUAL DISEASE IN INTERFERON-TREATED PATIENTS

A number of studies employing the polymerase chain reaction (PCR) to detect *bcr/abl* transcripts have addressed the issue of minimal residual disease status following complete cytogenetic and/or Southern blot responses to interferon-based therapy as primary treatment for CML. The majority of these studies used a two-step nested reverse-transcriptase based assay for detection of *bcr/abl* transcripts with a sensitivity of detection of approximately one *bcr/abl* positive cell against a background of 100,000 normal cells (15,29,30,31).

Overwhelmingly, the data from these studies demonstrate that *bcr/abl* transcripts persist even in patients who are long-term complete cytogenetic responders to interferon; however, the number of transcripts detected may be variable and of clinical significance. In one of the earlier studies of minimal residual disease following interferon therapy, Lee and colleagues studied 40 samples from 29 patients in complete cytogenetic remission for from <12 months to >60 months (30). They found that the abnormal transcript was present in all samples, even in those from patients with long-term cytogenetic remissions. In serial monitoring studies, Opalka et al. and our group have found an occasional patient who is found to be PCR-negative at one sampling timepoint, but later is found to be PCR-positive in subsequent samples while remaining negative by cytogenetic and Southern blot analysis (15,29). Therefore, although a negative PCR result may be found rarely, it is clear that a single negative result at one timepoint is not sufficient to define a patient as truly *bcr/abl*-negative; serial samples should be obtained. Similar to the strong correlation of blood and bone marrow PCR monitoring found following allogeneic bone marrow transplantation for CML, use of blood samples rather than marrow for detection of minimal residual disease following interferon treatment for CML is appropriate (32,33). Summarizing the data described above, it appears that there is little prognostic significance in the detection of *bcr/abl* transcripts from interferon-treated patients in complete cytogenetic and Southern blot responders since the vast majority remain positive, even in long-term remission.

Recent efforts have focused on the clinical relevance of quantifying the number of abnormal transcripts present during interferon treatment using a competitive PCR reaction. Using a competitive PCR assay, Gaiger et al. reported that rising numbers of *bcr/abl* transcripts correlate with disease progression in patients with chronic-phase CML (34). Similarly, quantitative, serial PCR monitoring of patients following allogeneic bone marrow transplantation for CML indicates that rising numbers of transcripts may be an early predictor of relapse (35). Using quantitative PCR to monitor patients treated with interferon, Hochhaus et al. found concordance between bone marrow cytogenetic quantification of the Philadelphia chromosome and *bcr/abl* transcript levels in blood or marrow samples (33). In their monitoring study, Lion et al. found that increasing numbers of transcripts correlated with progression of disease in interferon-treated patients and that the PCR findings preceded any cytogenetic or hematologic evidence of progression by a median of 6 months (36). In another study, Hochhaus et al. found that although all interferon patients in complete cytogenetic response have residual disease by quantitative PCR, the number of transcripts present at the time of complete cytogenetic response may predict which patients are likely to eventually relapse. They were able to define a level of transcript below which patients appear to remain in long-term clinical remission (37). In summary, these recent studies suggest that quantification of minimal residual disease using competitive PCR analysis of the *bcr/abl* transcript may be useful in predicting the durability of response in interferon-treated patients who are complete cytogenetic responders.

RECOMMENDATIONS FOR THE USE OF MOLECULAR STUDIES DURING INTERFERON TREATMENT

The studies described above demonstrate that quantitative Southern blotting and PCR techniques are valuable additions to cytogenetic monitoring during interferon treatment in patients with CML. Serial, quantitative Southern blotting may be done using blood samples, thereby increasing the ease and decreasing the cost, of monitoring of both Philadelphia chromosome-positive and -negative CML patients by decreasing the need for frequent bone marrow examinations. As mentioned, when patients have achieved a complete response by Southern blotting, it is reasonable to do a bone marrow examination for cytogenetic analysis in order to avoid overestimating the degree of response. In patients who have achieved a complete response by Southern blot, recent data suggest that competitive PCR analysis for quantification of residual *bcr/abl* transcripts in blood samples is useful for prediction of the quality and duration of interferon response. This type of "two-tiered" molecular approach provides a logical approach for assessment of response for individual CML patients receiving interferon therapy, as well as to analyze large clinical trials in CML. As competitive PCR techniques become standardized, long-term, large-scale monitoring studies will provide additional information about the clinical utility of this type of monitoring approach for patients receiving interferon-based therapy for CML.

ACKNOWLEDGMENTS

This work was supported, in part, by CA37027, and an American Cancer Society Career Development Award.

REFERENCES

1. Talpaz M, Kantarjian HM, McCredie K, et al. Interferon-alpha produces sustained cytogenetic responses in chronic myelogenous leukemia: Philadelphia chromosome positive patients. Ann Intern Med 1991; 113:532–538.
2. Ozer H, George SL, Schiffer CA, et al. Prolonged subcutaneous administration of recombinant alpha 2b interferon in patients with previously untreated Philadelphia chromosome-positive chronic-phase chronic myelogenous leukemia: effect of remission duration and survival: Cancer and Leukemia Group B Study 8583. Blood 1993; 82:2975.
3. Italian Cooperative Study Group on Chronic Myeloid Leukemia. Interferon alfa-2a as compared with conventional chemotherapy for the treatment of chronic myeloid leukemia. N Engl J Med 1994; 319:990.
4. Hehlmann R, German CML Study Group. Randomized comparison of interferon-alpha with busulfan and hydroxyurea in chronic myelogenous leukemia. Blood 1994; 84:4064.
5. Ohnishi K, Tomonaga M, Kamada N. et al. A randomized trial comparing interferon-alpha with busulfan for newly diagnosed chronic myelogenous leukemia in chronic phase. Blood 1995; 86:906.
6. Guilhot F, Chastang C, Guerci A, et al. Interferon alpha2b and cytarabine increase

survival and cytogenetic response in chronic myeloid leukemia. Results of a randomized trial. Blood 1996; 88(suppl 1):551. Abstract.
7. Groffen J. Stephenson JR, Heisterkamp N, et al. Philadelphia chromosomal breakpoints are clustered within a limited region, bcr, on chromosome 22. Cell 1984; 36:93.
8. Kurzrock R, Gutterman JU, Talpaz M. The molecular genetics of Philadelphia chromosome-positive leukemias. N Engl J Med 1988; 319:990.
9. Bartram CR, Kleihauer E, DeKlein A, et al. C-abl and bcr are rearranged in a Ph negative CML patient. EMBO J 1985; 4:683.
10. Grossman A, Silver RT, Szatrowski TP, et al. Densitometric analysis of Southern blot autoradiographs and its application to monitoring patients with chronic myelogenous leukemia. Leukemia 1991; 5:540.
11. Ayscue LH, Ross DW, Ozer H, et al. *BCR/ABL* recombinant DNA analysis versus karyotype in the diagnosis and therapeutic monitoring of chronic myeloid leukemia. Am J Clin Pathol 1990; 94:404.
12. Lee MS, Chang KS, Freireich EJ, et al. Detection of minimal residual bcr/abl transcripts by a modified polymerase chain reaction. Blood 1988; 72:893.
13. Heisterkamp N. Stam K, Groffen J, et al. Structural organization of the bcr gene and its role in the Ph' translocation. Nature 1985; 315:758.
14. Westbrook CA, Hooberman AL, Spino C, et al. Clinical significance of the *BCR/ABL* gene in adult acute lymphoblastic leukemia. A Cancer and Leukemia Group B study (8762). Blood 1992; 80:2983.
15. Stock W, Westbrook CA, Peterson B, et al. Value of molecular monitoring during the treatment of chronic myeloid leukemia: A Cancer and Leukemia Group B study. J Clin Oncol 1997; 15:26.
16. Verschraegen CF, Talpaz M, Hirsch-Ginsberg CF, et al. Quantification of the breakpoint cluster region rearrangement for clinical monitoring in Philadelphia chromosome-positive chronic myeloid leukemia. Blood 1995; 85:2705.
17. Kantarjian HM, Deisseroth A, Kurzrock, et al. Chronic myelogenous leukemia: a concise update. Blood 1993; 82:691.
18. Italian Cooperative Study Group on Chronic Myeloid Leukemia. Alpha interferon versus chemotherapy in chronic myeloid leukemia: updating the Italian study. Blood 1994; 84(suppl 1):153a. Abstract.
19. Shtivelman E, Lifshitz B, Gale RP, et al. Alternative splicing of RNAs transcribed from the human *abl* gene and from the *bcr/abl* fused gene. Cell 1986; 47:277.
20. Eisenberg A, Silver R, Arlin Z, et al. The location of breakpoints within the breakpoint cluster region (bcr) of chromosome 22 in chronic myeloid leukemia. Leukemia 1988: 2:642.
21. Shtalrid M, Talpaz M, Kurzrock R, et al. Analysis of breakpoints within the bcr gene and their correlation with the clinical course of Philadelphia-positive chronic myeloid leukemia. Blood 1988; 72:485.
22. Mills KI, MacKenzie E, Birnie GD. The site of the breakpoint within the bcr is a prognostic factor in Philadelphia-positive CML patients. Blood 1988:72:1237.
23. Mills KI, Benn P, Birnie GD. Does the breakpoint within the major breakpoint cluster region (M-bcr) influence the duration of chronic phase in chronic myeloid leukemia? An analytical comparison of current literature. Blood 1991;78:1155.

24. Ogawa H. Sugiyami H, Soma T, et al. No correlation between location of bcr breakpoint and clinical state in Ph-positive CML patients. Leukemia 1989:3:492.
25. Opalka B, Wandl UB, Stutenkemper R, et al. No correlation between the type of bcr-abl hybrid messenger RNA and platelet counts in chronic myelogenous leukemia. Blood 1992; 80:1854.
26. Elliott SL, Taylor KM, Taylor DL, et al. Cytogenetic response to alpha-interferon is predicted in early chronic phase chronic myeloid leukemia by M-bcr breakpoint location. Leukemia 1995; 9:946.
27. Shepherd P, Suffolk R, Halsey J, et al. Analysis of molecular breakpoint and m-RNA transcripts in a prospective randomized trial of interferon in chronic myeloid leukaemia: no correlation with clinical features, cytogenetic response, duration of chronic phase, or survival. Br J Haematol 1995; 89:546.
28. Italian Cooperative Study Group on Chronic Myeloid Leukemia. Chronic myeloid leukemia, BCR/ABL transcript, response to alpha-interferon and survival. Leukemia 1995; 9:1648.
29. Opalka B, Wandl UB, Becher R, et al. Minimal residual disease in patients with chronic myelogenous leukemia undergoing long-term treatment with recombinant interferon alpha-2b alone or in combination with interferon gamma. Blood 1991; 87:2188.
30. Lee M-S, Kantarjian H, Talpaz M, et al. Detection of minimal residual disease by polymerase chain reaction in Philadelphia chromosome-positive chronic myelogenous leukemia following interferon therapy. Blood 1992; 79:1920.
31. Martiat P. Detection of residual BCR/ABL transcripts in chronic myeloid leukaemia patients in complete remission using the polymerase chain reaction and nested primers. Br J Haematol 1990; 75:355.
32. Lin F, Goldman JM, Cross NCP. A comparison of the sensitivity of blood and bone marrow for the detection of minimal residual disease in chronic myeloid leukaemia. Br J Haematol 1994; 86:683.
33. Hochhaus A. Lin F, Reiter A, et al. Quantification of residual disease in chronic myelogenous leukemia patients on interferon-alpha therapy by competitive polymerase chain reaction. Blood 1996; 87:1549.
34. Gaiger A, Henn T. Horth E, et al. Increase of BCR-ABL chimeric mRNA in tumor cells of patients with chronic myeloid leukemia precedes disease progression. Blood 1995; 86:2731.
35. Cross NCP, Feng L, Chase A, et al. Competitive polymerase chain reaction to estimate the number of BCR-ABL transcripts in chronic myeloid leukemia patients after bone marrow transplantation. Blood 1993; 82:1929.
36. Lion T, Gaiger A, Henn T, et al. Use of quantitative polymerase chain reaction to monitor residual disease in chronic myelogenous leukemia during treatment with interferon. Leukemia 1995; 9:1353.
37. Hochhaus A, Reiter A, Skladny H, et al. Molecular heterogeneity in complete cytogenetic responders after interferon-alpha-therapy of chronic myelogenous leukemia: levels of minimal residual disease predict risk of relapse. Blood 1997; 88(suppl 1): 664a. Abstract.

17
Oligonucleotide Therapeutics for Chronic Myelogenous Leukemia

Alan M. Gewirtz
University of Pennsylvania, Philadelphia, Pennsylvania

INTRODUCTION

The notion that gene expression might be modified through use of exogenous nucleic acids derives from studies by Paterson and co-workers who first used reverse-complementary (antisense), single-stranded DNA to inhibit translation of a corresponding RNA in a cell-free system in 1977 (1). The following year Zamecnik and Stephenson showed that a short (13-mer) DNA oligonucleotide antisense to the Rous sarcoma virus could inhibit viral replication in culture (2). The latter investigators are widely credited on this basis for having first suggested the therapeutic utility of reverse-complementary nucleic acids. In the mid-1980s, Mizuno et al. (3) and Simons and Kleckner (4) demonstrated the existence of naturally occurring antisense RNAs in prokaryotes and showed that these molecules played a role in regulating expression of their corresponding genes. These observations were particularly important because the existence of naturally occurring antisense RNAs lent credibility to the belief that modification of gene expression by reverse-complementary sequences was more than a laboratory phenomenon, and kindled hope that oligonucleotides could be utilized in living cells to manipulate gene expression. The work of Izant and Weintraub (5,6) further buttressed belief in this potential by demonstrating that expression of antisense RNA in eukaryotic cells could also modulate expression of the complementary gene. These seminal papers, and the many that have since followed, have stimulated the development of technologies employing nucleic acids to manipulate gene expression.

Virtually all available gene disruption methods rely on some type of nu-

- ANTI-GENE
  - Homologous Recombination-Viral Vector
  - Triplex Formation- Oligodeoxynucleotide
  - Transcription Factor Decoy- Oligonucleotide
- ANTI-mRNA
  - Ribozyme
  - Oligodeoxynucleotide
  - RNA Binding Protein Decoy- Oligonucleotide

Figure 1 Strategies for disrupting gene expression.

cleotide sequence recognition for targeting specificity. They differ where and how they perturb the flow of genetic information. From an operational point of view, strategies for modulating gene expression may be thought of as either "antigene" or anti-mRNA (Fig. 1). Antigene strategies focus primarily on gene targeting by homologous recombination (7), by triple-helix-forming oligodeoxynucleotides (TFOs) (8), and by the use of oligonucleotide transcription factor decoy molecules (9,10). Homologous recombination remains the gold standard of all the disruption methodologies since it physically destroys the gene of interest. Nevertheless, from a clinical point of view, this approach is considerably constrained by the fact that it remains very inefficient, requires a selection process to detect cells in which the desired combination event has occurred, and, as of this writing, is restricted to a small number of cell types. TFOs hybridize in the major groove of DNA by Hoogsteen or reverse Hoogsteen bonding and can disturb gene function by preventing the binding of transcription factors, by inhibiting unwinding of the duplexed DNA strands, or by inducing mutations in the targeted gene (11–13). This approach to manipulating gene expression is also significantly constrained by the need for polypurine/polypyrimidine target sequences. In addition, problems of TFO delivery to the cell and to the correct intracellular location also need to be solved. The potential use of transcription factor decoy molecules is still in its infancy.

A larger body of work has focused on perturbing the use of mRNA. These are the so-called antisense strategies because of their reliance on the formation of reverse complementary (antisense) Watson-Crick base pairs between the targeting construct or vector, and the mRNA whose function is to be disrupted. It is, of course, the specificity of the Watson-Crick base pairing which allows a particular mRNA species to be selectively targeted. The antisense strategies rely on either introducing the reverse complementary nucleic acid sequence into the target cell or expressing the reverse complementary sequence in the target cell from a transfected viral or plasmid vector. Therefore, the reverse complement may be DNA or RNA. If hybridization between the target mRNA and the exogenous RNA nucleotide sequence occurs, a duplex is created which, in effect, forms a "jam" that prevents the ribosomal complex from reading along the message. If the ribosomal complex cannot read the message, the appropriate tRNA are not assembled and the encoded peptide is not made. If an exogenous DNA molecule is employed, hybridization allows for binding of RNase H, which destroys the RNA but leaves the DNA molecule intact to hybridize with yet another mRNA target. Either would appear to be a relatively foolproof mechanism for preventing mRNA utilization, but, as was true for triple-stranded DNA molecules, RNA-RNA or RNA-DNA duplexes can be unwound by a variety of repair/editing enzymes such as helicase and RNA unwindase (14). Peptide assembly is thereby unperturbed. Such effects were very convincingly demonstrated by Shakin et al. (15) using a globin mRNA model. Associated consequences of mRNA duplex formation may therefore play strong supporting roles in bringing about antisense effects.

The power of the antisense strategy has been demonstrated in experiments in which critical biological information has been gathered and subsequently confirmed using alternative or complementary experimental methods. The biologic function of a number of hematopoietic genes has been accurately predicted using antisense oligonucleotides, and clinically relevant data have flowed from such work (16–23). With this brief resume as background, I will discuss below the development of oligonucleotides as potential therapeutic agents for chronic myelogenous leukemia. Understandably, work from my own laboratory will be emphasized, but seminal contributions from other laboratories will hopefully not be ignored.

GENE TARGETS FOR OLIGONUCLEOTIDES IN CML

bcr/abl

If one considers the molecular pathogenesis of CML (Fig. 2), a number of potentially interesting gene targets present themselves. First and foremost is the bcr/abl mRNA itself. As has no doubt been discussed numerous times in this volume, bcr/abl mRNA is the product of a neogene created by a reciprocal translocation involving the c-abl gene on chromosome 9 and the bcr gene on chromosome 22 (recently reviewed in 24). This translocation results in the formation of the Philadelphia chromosome, and the neogene bcr/abl. There are three major bcr/abl variants depending on where the invariant portion of abl is fused with bcr. These are designated b1a2 (p185), b2a2, and b3a2 (both encode p210). A

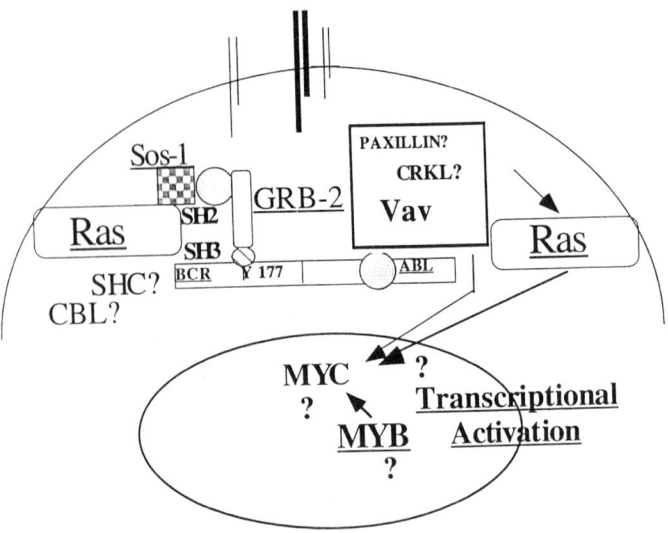

Figure 2 Transcriptional activation.

fourth variant e 19a2 (p230), which is associated with a chronic neutrophilia, has been recently described. Each of these genes may be considered tumor-specific, and they are likely both necessary and required for the CML transformation of hematopoietic cells. Because they are tumor-specific, and pathogenetically important, they are an obvious oligonucleotide target in this disease.

Szczylik and colleagues were among the first to suggest that oligonucleotides targeting bcr/abl might be of therapeutic utility (25). These workers found that when primary leukemic blast cells were exposed to synthetic 18-mer oligodeoxynucleotides complementary to b2a2 or b3a2 BCR-ABL junctions, leukemic cell colony formation in vitro was significantly suppressed. In contrast, granulocyte-macrophage colony formation from normal marrow progenitors was unaffected by the same oligonucleotides. Suppression of colony growth was found to be sequence-specific as well, in that mismatched oligonucleotides had no effect on colony formation and oligonucleotides targeting one breakpoint did not inhibit growth of cells expressing the other. Finally, when equal proportions of normal marrow progenitors and blast cells were mixed, exposed to the oligodeoxynucleotides, and assayed for residual colony formation, the majority of residual cells were normal. These findings suggested that BCR-ABL-targeted oligonucleotides represented a means for specifically killing CML cells. This work was followed by a number of reports from the same group, and others, which reported very similar findings (26–30).

Not all investigators have been able to reproduce the results described above (31–36). O'Brien and colleagues, for example, examined the effects of antisense oligonucleotides of various lengths, sequences, and chemistry on the proliferation of eight different cell lines—five derived from patients with chronic myelogenous leukemia (CML), and three from other sources (31). They found that phosphodiester oligonucleotides had little antiproliferative activity in their system, presumably because of degradation by nucleases present in fetal calf serum or rapid intracellular breakdown. Phosphorothioate oligonucleotides antisense, but not sense, to the B2A2 and B3A2 breakpoints significantly inhibited the proliferation of three CML cell lines (BV173, LAMA84, and KYO1). However, the antiproliferative effect appeared to be independent of the type of breakpoint expressed by each cell line, suggesting that the inhibition was sequence-dependent but not sequence-specific. Other investigators have reported that inhibition of CML cell growth with oligonucleotides is not sequence-dependent, suggesting that an aptameric effect is responsible (35).

Ribozymes have been applied against this target and appear to give rise to more specific, but still imperfect, cleavage of their target (37–39). An explanation for some of the controversy surrounding the ability of this breakpoint to be specifically cleaved may be found in recent work from the Sczakiel laboratory (40). These investigators have previously reported that rapid association of antisense sequence with its target is the most critical determinant of antisense efficacy (41). In the course of designing oligonucleotides and ribozymes directed to the bcr/abl breakpoint, kinetic probing combined with calculations of the local folding potential indicated that the bcr/abl fusion point sequences are not easily accessible for complementary nucleic acid hybridization (40). The study suggested that selective and efficient antisense sequences should be directed against the bcr portion neighboring the fusion point as well as the first eight nucleotides of the abl sequence. To effectively inhibit this target, then, relatively high doses of oligonucleotides may be required, and these in turn may produce nonspecific effects. In addition, if ribozymes with unfavorable kinetics are employed to target the sequence, inhibition is likely to be inefficient and therefore difficult to measure.

In spite of the controversy over whether bcr/abl mRNA can be effectively destroyed, several groups have proceeded to determine the potential therapeutic utility of antisense bcr/abl nucleic acids for inhibiting CML cell growth. The general strategy has been to transplant CML blast cells into SCID mice and then to examine the effects of oligonucleotides on leukemic cell growth and animal survival, an approach originally reported by our group in 1992 (42). For example, Skorski et al. (43) injected SCID mice with Ph+ CML blast crisis cell line (BV173) and monitored expression of bcr/abl transcripts in bone marrow, spleen, peripheral blood, liver, and lungs. Once disease was established in these mice, treatment with a 26-mer bcr/abl AS-ODN at a dose of 1 mg/day for 9 days decreased bcr-abl mRNA levels in mouse tissues and induced the disappearance of CD10+ and clonogenic leukemic cells. Further, antisense-treated mice survived 18–23 weeks, while control and sense-treated mice were dead 8–13 weeks after leukemic cell injection.

Nevertheless, since all animals eventually succumb to disease, attempts to improve on these results have naturally evolved. One strategy has been to target multiple, in theory cooperating, mRNA species. Since c-myc is thought to be a downstream target of bcr/abl signaling and to be required for bcr/abl induced transformation (44,45), targeting bcr/abl and c-myc simultaneously might be expected to have enhanced treatment efficacy, and this in fact has been reported (46,47). An alternative strategy has been to combine the use of oligonucleotides with traditional chemotherapy, in the context of either ex vivo bone marrow purging (48) or treating CML-bearing SCID mice directly with "low-dose" cyclophosphamide and bcr/abl targeted oligonucleotides (49). With regard to marrow purging, Skorski et al. reported that a 1:1 mix of Ph+ leukemic cells that had been exposed to a combination of low-dose mafosfamide and bcr-abl AS-ODN appeared to be effectively (~100%) purged of Ph+ cells by clonogenic assay. Indeed, bcr-abl transcripts were only found in untreated cells, in cells treated with mafosfamide or with AS-ODN alone, but not in those treated with combinational therapy. This strategy was extended to direct in vivo treatment where CML bearing SCID mice were treated intravenously with bcr/abl oligonucleotides and 25% of what would normally be a therapeutically effective dose of cyclophosphamide. This treatment strategy was reported to result in cure of 50% of the animals.

Alternative Gene Targets in CML

While bcr/abl is an obvious target for antigene therapeutics, a number of considerations suggest that it may not be as ideal a target as first considerations would suggest. It must be recalled that since anti-mRNA strategies based on the use of oligodeoxynucleotides are transient interventions, the target has to be expressed when oligonucleotides are physically present in the cell. In addition, it is straightforward that the strategy will only be effective if the target cell fails to tolerate transient downregulation of the targeted mRNA. There is reasonable evidence to suggest that bcr/abl mRNA is not expressed in CML stem cells, in spite of the fact that the translocation is present (50). Since CML is a stem cell disorder, it is reasonable to hypothesize that the candidate gene for perturbation must be expressed at the stem cell level in order to be effective. If this is not the case, a constant supply of CML progenitors will be derived from the untreated stem cell. In addition to this important consideration, it is not at all clear that transient perturbation of bcr/abl expression results in cell death (51,52). Finally, given the known redundancy of signaling pathways, one might also be concerned that bcr/abl-mediated activation of RAS might have alternative pathways in primary malignant cells. For all these reasons then, we chose to pursue nonobvious mRNA targets.

c-myb

Myb protein is encoded by the c-myb proto-oncogene, a member of a transcription factor family composed of at least two other highly homologous genes, designated A-myb and B-myb (53,54). Located on chromosome 6q in humans, c-myb's predominant transcript encodes a ~75-kDa nuclear binding protein (Myb) which recognizes the core consensus sequence 5'-PyAAC(G/Py)G-3'(55). The protein plays a major role in regulating G1/S transition in cycling hematopoietic cells, and likely functions as a transactivator of a number of important cellular genes such as the Kit receptor (16), CD4 (56), and CD34 (57).

Attempts to exploit the c-myb gene as an antisense ODN target in CML were an outgrowth of studies that sought to define the role of Myb protein in regulating normal human hematopoiesis (19). These studies revealed that exposing normal bone marrow mononuclear cells (MNC) to c-myb antisense ODN resulted in a decrease in cloning efficiency and progenitor cell proliferation. The effect was lineage-indifferent since c-myb antisense DNA inhibited granulocyte-macrophage colony forming units (CFU-GM), CFU-E (erythroid), and CFU-Meg (megakaryocyte). In contrast, c-myb ODN with the corresponding sense sequence had no consistent effect on hematopoietic colony formation when compared to growth in control cultures. Finally, inhibition of colony formation was also dose-related. Inhibition of the targeted mRNA was also demonstrated. Sequence-specific, dose-related biologic effects accompanied by a specific decrease or total elimination of the targeted mRNA were strong pieces of evidence to suggest that the effects we were observing were due to an "antisense" mechanism. As mentioned above, the mechanism responsible for inhibition of hematopoietic cell growth appeared to be an inducible block in G1/S transition (58). In other investigations, it was also determined that hematopoietic progenitor cells appeared to require Myb protein during specific stages of development—in particular, when they were actively cycling (59), as might be expected given the above functional description of Myb protein. Accordingly, Myb appeared to be critical for normal hematopoietic cell development, a finding that was largely confirmed using the technique of homologous recombination (60).

Myb protein is also required for leukemic hematopoiesis. Evidence to support this statement includes the fact that Myb is widely expressed in malignant cell lines, and inhibition of Myb with oligonucleotides inhibits malignant cell line growth (61). Growth of cells derived from primary patient material is also inhibited (62). However, to be useful as a therapeutic target, leukemic cells would have to be more dependent on Myb protein than their normal counterparts. To examine this critical issue we incubated phagocyte and T-cell-depleted normal human marrow mononuclear cells (MNC), human T-lymphocyte leukemia cell line blasts (CCRF-CEM), or 1 : 1 mixtures of these cells with sense or antisense oligodeoxynucleotides to codons 2–7 of human c-myb mRNA (62). As antisense oligonucleotide exposure was intensified, normal myeloid colonies continued to grow in the cultures while leukemic colonies were increasingly suppressed. The growth of AML blasts from 18 of 23 patients studied also exhibited significant (~75%) decrease in colony and cluster formation compared to untreated or sense oligomer-treated controls. When 1 : 1 mixing experiments were carried out with primary AML blasts and normal MNC, we were again able to preferentially eliminate AML blast colony formation while normal myeloid colonies continued to form. Accordingly, these experiments suggested that leukemic cell growth could be preferentially inhibited after exposure to c-myb antisense ODN. These findings and several other considerations were important motivating factors in developing the anti-myb oligonucleotide. In particular, we were concerned that given the apparent redundancy in many signaling cascades, transient perturbation in bcr/abl signaling might be compensated for by alternative pathways. Perhaps more realistically, we were also concerned that transient perturbation of bcr/abl signal transduction might not lead to cell death. Finally, we were concerned that bcr/abl might not be expressed in the most primitive CML hematopoietic cells. Data to support this concern are now in the literature.

We therefore began to systematically explore the potential therapeutic efficacy of a c-myb-targeted antisense oligonucleotide (42,63). Eight cases were initially evaluated, and in each case bcr-abl expression as detected by RT-PCR correlated with colony growth in cell culture. In cases inhibited by exposure to c-myb antisense ODNs (7/11), bcr-abl expression was also greatly decreased or nondetectable. These results suggested that bcr-abl-expressing CFU might be substantially or entirely eliminated from a population of blood or marrow mononuclear cells by exposure to the antisense oligodeoxynucleotides. To explore this possibility further, replating experiments were carried out on samples from two patients. We hypothesized that if CFU belonging to the malignant clone were present at the end of the original 12-day culture period, but not detectable because of failure to express bcr-abl, they might reexpress the message upon regrowth in fresh cultures. Accordingly, cells from these patients were exposed to ODN and then plated into methylcellulose cultures formulated to favor growth of either CFU-GM or CFU-GEMM. As was found with the original specimens, untreated control cells and cells exposed to sense ODN had RT-PCR detectable bcr-abl transcripts. Those exposed to the c-myb antisense ODN had none. One of the paired dishes from these cultures was the solubilized with fresh medium, and all cells contained therein were washed, disaggregated, and replated into fresh methylcellulose cultures *without* reexposing the cells to ODN. After 14 days, CFU-GM and CFU-GEMM colony cells were again probed for bcr-abl expression. Control and sense-treated cells had RT-PCR detectable mRNA, but none was found in the antisense-treated colonies. These results suggest that elimination of bcr-abl-expressing cells and CFU was highly efficient and perhaps permanent.

Why does downregulating Myb kill leukemic cells preferentially? Our initial studies on the function of the c-kit receptor in hematopoietic cells suggested that c-kit might be a Myb-regulated gene (16). Additional studies have since confirmed this (64–66). Since c-kit encodes a critical hematopoietic cell tyrosine kinase receptor (16), we have hypothesized that dysregulation of c-kit expression may be an important mechanism of action of Myb AS ODN. In support of this hypothesis it has been shown that when hematopoietic cells are deprived of c-kit R ligand (Steel Factor), they undergo apoptosis (67). It has also recently been shown that when $CD56^{bright}$ NK cells, which express c-kit, are deprived of their ligand (Steel Factor), they too undergo apoptosis, perhaps because bcl-2 is downregulated (68). Malignant myeloid hematopoietic cells, in particular CML cells, also express c-kit and respond to Steel Factor. Accordingly, we postulate that perturbation of Myb expression in malignant hematopoietic cells may force them to enter an apoptotic pathway by downregulating c-kit. Preliminary studies of K562 cells exposed to c-myb antisense ODN demonstrates that such cells do in fact undergo nuclear degenerative changes characteristic of apoptosis. Of necessity, we must also postulate that normal progenitor cells, at least at some level of development, are more tolerant of this transient disturbance. Since neither Steel nor White Spotting (W) mice (which lack the Kit receptor or its ligand, respectively) are aplastic, this is a tenable hypothesis.

The in vitro studies described above were carried out primarily with unmodified DNA. Such molecules are subject to endo- and exonuclease attack at the phosphodiester bonds and are therefore of little utility in vivo. Since we could not give this material to patients, we next evaluated phosphorothioate modified oligonucleotides. These DNA molecules are much more resistant to nuclease attack and are therefore more suited to in vivo administration. To test the efficacy of these compounds in a clinically relevant model, we established a human leukemia/SCID mouse model system (42). SCID mice were injected IV with K562 chronic myeloid leukemia cells after cyclophosphamide conditioning. K562 cells express c-myb, the antisense oligodeoxynucleotide target, and the tumor-specific bcr-abl oncogene which was utilized for tracking the human leukemia cells in the mouse host. After tumor cell injection, animals developed blasts in the peripheral blood within 4–6 weeks. After peripheral blood blast cells appeared, mean (±SD) survival of untreated mice (n = 20) was 6 ± 3 days. Dying animals had prominent central nervous system infiltration, marked infiltration of the ovary, and scattered abdominal granulocytic sarcomas. Infusion of either sense or scrambled sequence c-myb phosphorothioate ODN (24 bp; codons 2–9) for 3, 7, or 14 days had no statistically significant effect on sites of disease involvement or animal survival in comparison to control animals. In contrast, animals treated for 7 or 14 days with c-myb AS ODN survived 3.5 to 8 times longer ($p<0.001$) than the various control animals (n = 60). In addition, animals receiving c-myb AS DNA had either rare microscopic foci or no obviously detectable CNS disease, and a >50% reduction of ovarian involvement. A 3-day infusion of myb AS (100 μg/d) was without effect. Infusing mice (n = 12) with AS ODN (200 μg/day × 14 days) complementary to the c-kit proto-oncogene, which K562 cells do not express, also had no effect on disease burden or survival (n = 12). These results suggested that phosphorothioate modified c-myb antisense DNA might be efficacious for the treatment of human leukemia in vivo.

Receptors and Signaling Proteins

Other potential mRNA targets for treating CML might also be envisioned. These may be found among the surface receptors and signaling proteins constitutive to hematopoietic cells. For example, we have previously suggested that the Kit receptor might serve this purpose (16,21,42). As noted above, Kit appears to be a c-myb-regulated gene, and downregulation of Kit in hematopoietic cells is associated with induction of apoptosis, perhaps an important mechanistic component of anti-Myb's ability to kill malignant cells. Directly comparing the ability of anti-Myb and anti-Kit targeted oligonucleotides to inhibit the growth of leukemic cells suggests this possibility and at the same time supports the potential of Kit-targeted oligonucleotides in the treatment of CML and other leukemias (Table 1).

A newer target, which may prove to be of even greater utility in patients

Table 1 Comparative Effect of c-myb and c-kit Targeted ODN on Primary CML Cell Colony Growth

	Anti-Myb oligo exp		Anti-Kit oligo exp	
	# Responders (decreased colonies)	% CFU-GM ↓	# Responders (decreased colonies)	% CFU-GM ↓
Chronic myelogenous leukemia	11/15	77 ± 13%	8/15	76 ± 24%

Cells were derived from patients undergoing treatment at the University of Pennsylvania. They were exposed to oligomers and cultured as described in Ref. 16.

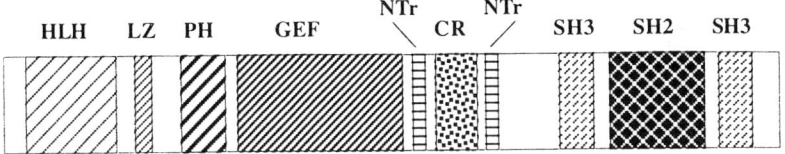

Figure 3 Predicted functional domains of proto-vav.

with hematologic malignancies, is signaling protein encoded by the vav protooncogene (69,70). The vav oncogene was discovered by Katzav et al. while screening esophageal carcinomas for transforming oncogenes (71). Its normal cellular counterpart, the *vav* protooncogene (proto-*Vav*), was subsequently cloned from a tumor cell cDNA library using a fragment of the transforming gene as a probe. Initial sequence analysis of Vav predicted that the encoded protein would be functionally complex, and this has since been verified (72–77). At its amino terminus, Vav has been shown to contain helix-loop-helix (HLH) and leucine zipper (LZ)-like motifs (Fig. 3), suggesting possible transcriptional control functions (72,78,79). Adjacent to the HLH and LZ domains is a region with multiple homologies to genes which encode proteins with the potential to function as guanine nucleotide exchange factors (GEFs) for Ras-like proteins. This suggests that Vav may function as a signaling molecule (40). Following downstream of the GEF domain are two nuclear translocation (NTr) signal motifs, further suggesting that Vav may play some role in regulating gene expression (33). Finally, it has also been shown that at its carboxy terminus, Vav contains an src homology 2 (SH2) domain flanked by two src homology 3 (SH3) domains (41).

Vav is expressed exclusively in hematopoietic cells where, as the above discussion indicates, it is assumed to play a role in signaling. The importance of this role is uncertain, in part because of conflicting functional studies which have employed different strategies for abrogating Vav gene expression in murine embryonic stem cells (80–83). Our studies with vav-targeted oligonucleotides lend some support to each of the conflicting reports cited above and imply that vav would be a therapeutically attractive target in CML (84). We have found that while vav appears to be required for erythropoiesis in both normal and malignant hematopoietic cells, *malignant* myeloid cell growth, in particular myeloid cells derived from CML patients, does appear to be dependent of Vav expression (84). The rationale for Vav as an antisense target is therefore anchored in the fact that it is differentially used in normal and malignant cells.

USE OF ANTISENSE OLIGONUCLEOTIDES IN A CLINICAL SETTING

Based on the studies reviewed above, we initiated clinical trials to evaluate the effectiveness of phosphorothioate-modified ODN antisense to the c-myb gene as marrow-purging agents for chronic phase (CP) or accelerated phase (AP) CML patients, and a Phase I intravenous infusion study for blast crisis (BC) patients, and patients with other refractory leukemias (85). ODN purging was carried out for 24 hours on CD34+ marrow cells. Patients received busulfan and cytoxan, followed by reinfusion of previously cryopreserved P-ODN-purged MNC. In the pilot marrow purging study seven CP and one AP CML patients have been treated, 7/8 engrafted. In 4/6 evaluable CP patients, metaphases were 85–100% normal 3 months after engraftment, suggesting that a significant purge had taken place in the marrow graft. Five CP patients have demonstrated marked, sustained, hematologic improvement with essential normalization of their blood counts. Follow-up ranges from 6 months to ~2 years. In an attempt to further increase purging efficiency, we incubated patient MNC for 72 hours in the P-ODN. Though PCR and LTCIC studies suggested that a very efficient purge had occurred, engraftment in five patients was poor. In the Phase I systemic infusion study, 18 refractory leukemia patients (two patients were treated at two different dose levels; 13 had AP or BC CML). Myb antisense ODN was delivered by continuous infusion at dose levels ranging between (0.3 mg/kg/day × 7 days) to (2.0 mg/kg/day × 7 days). No recurrent dose-related toxicity has been noted, though idiosyncratic toxicities, not clearly drug-related, were observed (one transient renal insufficiency; one pericarditis). One BC patient survived ~14 months with transient restoration of CP disease. These studies show that ODN may be administered safely to leukemic patients. Whether patients treated on either study derived clinical benefit is uncertain, but the results of these studies suggest to us that ODN may eventually demonstrate therapeutic utility in the treatment of human leukemias.

Some clinical experience with bcr/abl targeted antisense oligonucleotides has also been reported. De Fabritis and colleagues treated a patient with chronic myeloid leukemia in accelerated phase with autologous bone marrow transplantation. Before reinfusion, cells were purged in vitro with a 26-mer phosphorothioate antisense oligodeoxynucleotide specific for the B2A2 junction. This treatment resulted in a 24% and 41% reduction of CFU-GM and CD34+ cells, respectively. The patient was successfully engrafted with the purged marrow cells after 17 and 25 days for platelets and neutrophils, respectively. Using fluorescence in situ hybridization in interphase nuclei, some Ph-negative cells were found after the autograft. The patient was reported to be in a complete hematologic remission at 9 months posttreatment.

FUTURE PROSPECTS FOR "ANTISENSE" THERAPY

The notion of antisense-mediated gene disruption remains as attractive as any other form of gene therapy. Tantalizing preliminary data also suggest that these compounds may have some therapeutic efficacy, likely through a combination of antisense and nonsequence-dependent effects on gene function. For the field to move forward, however, a number of important technical issues will need to be solved.

The ability to deliver ODN into cells and have them reach their target in a bioavailable form also remains problematic (20). Without this ability, it is clear that even an appropriately targeted sequence is not likely to be efficient. Native phosphodiester ODNs, and the widely used phosphorothioate-modified ODNs, which contain a single sulfur substituting for oxygen at a nonbridging position at each phosphorus atom, are polyanions. Accordingly, they diffuse across cell membranes poorly and are only taken up by cells through energy-dependent mechanisms. This appears to be accomplished primarily through a combination of adsorptive endocytosis and fluid phase endocytosis which may be triggered in part by the binding of the ODN to receptor-like proteins present on the surface of a wide variety of cells (86–89). After internalization, confocal and electron microscopy studies have indicated that the bulk of the ODNs enter the endosome/lysosome compartment. These vesicular structures may become acidified and acquire other enzymes which degrade the ODNs. Biologic inactivity is the predictable result of this process. Recently described strategies for introducing ODN into cells, including various cationic lipid formulations, may address this problem (90–92).

For an ODN to hybridize with its mRNA target, it must find an accessible sequence. Sequence accessibility is at least in part a function of mRNA physical structure, which is dictated in turn by internal base composition and associated proteins in the living cell. Attempts to describe the in vivo structure of RNA, in contrast to DNA, have been fraught with difficulty (93). Accordingly, mRNA targeting is largely a hit-or-miss process, accounting for many experiments where the addition of an ODN yields no effect on expression. Hence, the ability to determine which regions of a given mRNA molecule are accessible for ODN targeting is a significant impediment to the application of this technique in many cells systems.

Recently, Milner et al. employed a novel hybridization strategy to find oligodeoxynucleotides capable of hybridizing with specific mRNAs (94). An array of 1938 oligodeoxynucleotides, which ranged in length from monomers to 17-mers, was synthesized on the surface of a glass plate and used to determine the potential of any of the oligonucleotides to form heteroduplexes with rabbit beta-globin mRNA. The oligonucleotides were complementary to the first

122 bases of mRNA comprising the 5′ UTR and bases 1–69 of the first exon. These investigators reported that very few oligonucleotides demonstrated significant heteroduplex formation with the target. Antisense activity, measured in an RNase H assay and by in vitro translation, correlated well with yield of heteroduplex on the array. The authors point out that their results help to explain the variable success that is commonly experienced in the choice of antisense oligonucleotides. It is of interest that there were no obvious features in the mRNA sequence, or predicted secondary structure which adequately explained the variation in heteroduplex formation. The authors suggest that their method may provide a simple though empirical method of selecting effective antisense oligonucleotides. The true test of the predictive value of this method, however, must rest on the ability of the selected oligonucleotides to effectively interact with their target in vivo. Since RNA folding in vivo is likely to be quite different from that encountered in vitro, this is a critical point.

To address this problem we have begun to develop a footprinting assay to determine which physical areas of an RNA are accessible to the oligonucleotide. We have proceeded under the assumption that a sequence which remains accessible to single-stranded RNases in a more physiologic environment may also remain accessible for hybridization with an oligodeoxynucleotide. Preliminary experiments performed in our laboratory in which a labeled RNA transcript is allowed to hybridize with an oligonucleotide in the presence or absence of nuclear extracts from the cells of interest along with RNase T1 suggest that footprinting of this type is feasible. Of more interest, our preliminary results suggest that this approach may be of use in designing oligonucleotides.

CONCLUSIONS

The development of reliable gene disruption strategies and their application in living cells have proven to be an extraordinarily important advance for cell and molecular biologists. Using the various available approaches, the specific functions of any given gene may now be investigated directly in the relevant cell type. Application of similar experimental tools in a clinical setting might prove to be equally valuable and could well form the basis of a monumental advance in the practice of clinical medicine. This seems particularly true at the present time since much progress has been made in understanding the molecular pathogenesis of many diseases, including cancer.

Nevertheless, in spite of some notable successes, as was discussed above, the use of oligonucleotides to modify gene expression has been found to be variable in its efficiency and therefore wanting in terms of reliability (20,95,96). It is also widely appreciated that the use of oligonucleotides for modulating gene expression has generated controversy in regard to mechanism of action, reliability, and ultimate therapeutic utility. However, since the potential power of this approach remains undisputed, and its ultimate therapeutic utility is far-reaching, these problems are clearly worth solving. It remains the hope of my laboratory, and others, that the day will soon come when these techniques will make an important contribution to the management of CML and other neoplastic disorders.

ACKNOWLEDGMENTS

Supported by grants from the NIH and the Leukemia Society of America.

REFERENCES

1. Paterson BM, Roberts BE, Kuff EL. Structural gene identification and mapping by DNA-mRNA hybrid-arrested cell-free translation. Proc Natl Acad Sci USA 1977; 74(10):4370–4374.
2. Stephenson ML, Zamecnik PC. Inhibition of Rous sarcoma viral RNA translation by a specific oligodeoxyribonucleotide. Proc Natl Acad Sci USA 1978; 75(1):285–288.
3. Mizuno T, Chou MY, Inouye M. A unique mechanism regulating gene expression: translational inhibition by a complementary RNA transcript (micRNA). Proc Natl Acad Sci USA 1984; 81(7):1966–1970.
4. Simons RW, Kleckner N. Biological regulation by antisense RNA in prokaryotes. Annu Rev Genet 1988; 22:567–600.
5. Izant JG, Weintraub H. Constitutive and conditional suppression of exogenous and endogenous genes by anti-sense RNA. Science 1985; 229(4711):345–352.
6. Izant JG, Weintraub H. Inhibition of thymidine kinase gene expression by antisense RNA: a molecular approach to genetic analysis. Cell 1984; 36(4):1007–1015.
7. Melton DW. Gene targeting in the mouse. Bioessays 1994; 16(9):633–638.
8. Helene C. Rational design of sequence-specific oncogene inhibitors based on antisense and antigene oligonucleotides. Eur J Cancer 1991; 27(11):1466–1471.
9. Sharma HW, Perez JR, Higgins-Sochaski K, Hsiao R, Narayanan R. Transcription factor decoy approach to decipher the role of NF-kappa B in oncogenesis. Anticancer Res 1996; 16(1):61–69.
10. Morishita R, Gibbons GH, Horiuchi M, et al. A gene therapy strategy using a transcription factor decoy of the E2F binding site inhibits smooth muscle proliferation in vivo. Proc Natl Acad Sci USA 1995; 92(13):5855–5859.
11. Gunther EJ, Yeasky TM, Gasparro FP, Glazer PM. Mutagenesis by 8-methoxypsoralen and 5-methylangelicin photoadducts in mouse fibroblasts: mutations at cross-linkable sites induced by offoadducts as well as cross-links. Cancer Res 1995; 55(6):1283–1288.
12. Gunther EJ, Havre PA, Gasparro FP, Glazer PM. Triplex-mediated, in vitro target-

ing of psoralen photoadducts within the genome of a transgenic mouse. Photochem Photobiol 1996; 63(2):207–212.
13. Raha M, Wang G, Seidman MM, Glazer PM. Mutagenesis by third-strand-directed psoralen adducts in repair-deficient human cells: high frequency and altered spectrum in a xeroderma pigmentosum variant. Proc Natl Acad Sci USA 1996; 93(7): 2941–2946.
14. Nellen W, Lichtenstein C. What makes an mRNA anti-sense-itive? Trends Biochem Sci 1993; 18(11):419–423.
15. Shakin SH, Liebhaber SA. Destabilization of messenger RNA/complementary DNA duplexes by the elongating 80 S ribosome. J Biol Chem 1986; 261(34): 16018–16025.
16. Ratajczak MZ, Luger SM, DeRiel K, Abrahm J, Calabretta B, Gewirtz, AM. Role of the KIT protooncogene in normal and malignant human hematopoiesis. Proc Natl Acad Sci USA 1992; 89(5):1710–1714.
17. Metcalf D. Blood. Thrombopoietin—at last [news; comment]. Nature 1994; 369(6481):519–520.
18. Methia N, Louache F, Vainchenker W, Wendling F. Oligodeoxynucleotides antisense to the proto-oncogene c-mpl specifically inhibit in vitro megakaryocytopoiesis. Blood 1993; 82(5):1395–1401.
19. Gewirtz AM, Calabretta B. A c-myb antisense oligodeoxynucleotide inhibits normal human hematopoiesis in vitro. Science 1988; 242(4883):1303–1306.
20. Gewirtz AM, Stein CA, Glazer PM. Facilitating oligonucleotide delivery: helping antisense deliver on its promise. Proc Natl Acad Sci USA 1996; 93(8):3161–3163.
21. Ratajczak MZ, Luger SM, Gewirtz AM. The c-kit proto-oncogene in normal and malignant human hematopoiesis. Int J Cell Cloning 1992; 10(4):205–214.
22. Gewirtz AM. Potential therapeutic applications of antisense oligodeoxynucleotides in the treatment of chronic myelogenous leukemia. Leuk Lymph 1993; 11(suppl 1):131–137.
23. Gewirtz AM. Treatment of chronic myelogenous leukemia (CML) with c-myb antisense oligodeoxynucleotides. Bone Marrow Transplant 1994; 14(suppl 3):S57–61.
24. Melo JV. The diversity of BCR-ABL fusion proteins and their relationship to leukemia phenotype [editorial; comment] [see comments]. Blood 1996; 88(7):2375–2384.
25. Szczylik C, Skorski T, Nicolaides NC, et al. Selective inhibition of leukemia cell proliferation by BCR-ABL antisense oligodeoxynucleotides. Science 1991; 253 (5019):562–565.
26. Skorski T, Szczylik C, Malaguarnera L, Calabretta B. Gene-targeted specific inhibition of chronic myeloid leukemia cell growth by BCR-ABL antisense oligodeoxynucleotides. Folia Histochem Cytobiol 1991; 29(3):85–89.
27. Wu AG, Joshi SS, Chan WC, et al. Effects of BCR-ABL antisense oligonucleotides (S-ODN) on human chronic myeloid leukemic cells: AS-ODN as effective purging agents. Leuk Lymph 1995; 20(1–2):67–76.
28. De Fabritiis P, Amadori S, Calabretta B, Mandelli F. Elimination of clonogenic Philadelphia-positive cells using BCR-ABL antisense oligodeoxynucleotides. Bone Marrow Transplant 1993; 12(3):261–265.
29. De Fabritiis P, Skorski T, De Propris MS, et al. Effect of bcr-abl oligodeoxynucleo-

tides on the clonogenic growth of chronic myelogenous leukaemia cells. Leukemia 1997; 11(6):811–819.
30. Chasty R, Whetton A, Lucas G. A comparison of the effect of bcr/abl breakpoint specific phosphothiorate oligodeoxynucleotides on colony formation by bcr/abl positive and negative, CD34 enriched mononuclear cell populations. Leuk Res 1996; 20(5):391–395.
31. O'Brien SG, Kirkland MA, Melo JV, et al. Antisense BCR-ABL oligomers cause non-specific inhibition of chronic myeloid leukemia cell lines. Leukemia 1994; 8(12):2156–2162.
32. Kirkland MA, O'Brien SG, McDonald, C, Davidson RJ, Cross NC, Goldman JM. BCR-ABL antisense purging in chronic myeloid leukaemia [letter; comment]. Lancet 1993; 342(8871):614.
33. Maekawa T, Kimura S, Hirakawa K, Murakami A, Zon G, Abe T. Sequence specificity on the growth suppression and induction of apoptosis of chronic myeloid leukemia cells by BCR-AML anti-sense oligodeoxynucleoside phosphorothioates. Int J Cancer 1995; 62(1):63–69.
34. Smetsers TF, van de Locht LT, Pennings AH, Wessels HM, de Witte TM, Mensink EJ. Phosphorothioate BCR-ABL antisense oligonucleotides induce cell death, but fail to reduce cellular bcr-abl protein levels. Leukemia 1995; 9(1):118–130.
35. Vaerman JL, Lammineur C, Moureau P, et al. BCR-ABL antisense oligodeoxyribonucleotides suppress the growth of leukemic and normal hematopoietic cells by a sequence-specific but nonantisense mechanism. Blood 1995; 86(10):3891–3896.
36. Mahon FX, Ripoche J, Pigeonnier V, et al. Inhibition of chronic myelogenous leukemia cells harboring a BCR-ABL B3A2 junction by antisense oligonucleotides targeted at the B2A2 junction. Exp Hematol 1995; 23(14):1606–1611.
37. Leopold LH, Shore SK, Reddy EP. Multi-unit anti-BCR-ABL ribozyme therapy in chronic myelogenous leukemia. Leuk Lymph 1996; 22(5–6):365–373.
38. Lange W, Daskalakis M, Finke J, Dolken G. Comparison of different ribozymes for efficient and specific cleavage of BCR/ABL related mRNAs. FEBS Lett 1994; 338(2):175–178.
39. Pachuk CJ, Yoon K, Moelling K, Coney LR. Selective cleavage of bcr-abl chimeric RNAs by a ribozyme targeted to non-contiguous sequences. Nucleic Acids Res 1994; 22(3):301–307.
40. Kronenwett R, Haas R, Sczakiel G. Kinetic selectivity of complementary nucleic acids: bcr-abl-directed antisense RNA and ribozymes. J Mol Biol 1996; 259(4):632–644.
41. Rittner K, Burmester C, Sczakiel G. In vitro selection of fast-hybridizing and effective antisense RNAs directed against the human immunodeficiency virus type 1. Nucleic Acids Res 1993; 21(6):1381–1387.
42. Ratajczak MZ, Kant JA, Luger SM, et al. In vivo treatment of human leukemia in a scid mouse model with c-myb antisense oligodeoxynucleotides. Proc Natl Acad Sci USA 1992; 89(24):11823–11837.
43. Skorski T, Nieborowska-Skorska M, Nicolaides NC, et al. Suppression of Philadelphia-1 leukemia cell growth in mice by BCR-ABL antisense oligodeoxynucleotide. Proc Natl Acad Sci USA 1994; 91(10):4504–4508.

44. Sawyers CL, Callahan W, Witte ON. Dominant negative MYC blocks transformation by ABL oncogenes. Cell 1992; 70(6):901–910.
45. Sawyers CL. The role of myc in transformation by BCR-ABL. Leuk Lymph 1993; 11(suppl 1):45–46.
46. Skorski T, Nieborowska-Skorska M, Campbell K, et al. Leukemia treatment in severe combined immunodeficiency mice by antisense oligodeoxynucleotides targeting cooperating oncogenes. J Exp Med 1995; 182(6):1645–1653.
47. Skorski T, Nieborowska-Skorska M, Wlodarski P, Zon G, Iozzo RV, Calabretta B. Antisense oligodeoxynucleotide combination therapy of primary chronic myelogenous leukemia blast crisis in SCID mice. Blood 1996; 88(3):1005–1012.
48. Skorski T, Nieborowska-Skorska M, Barletta C, et al. Highly efficient elimination of Philadelphia leukemic cells by exposure to bcr/abl antisense oligodeoxynucleotides combined with mafosfamide. J Clin Invest 1993; 92(1):194–202.
49. Skorski T, Nieborowska-Skorska M, Wlodarski P, et al. Treatment of Philadelphia leukemia in severe combined immunodeficient mice by combination of cyclophosphamide and bcr/abl antisense oligodeoxynucleotides [see comments]. J Natl Cancer Inst 1997; 89(2):124–133.
50. Bedi A, Zehnbauer BA, Collector MI, et al. BCR-ABL gene rearrangement and expression of primitive hematopoietic progenitors in chronic myeloid leukemia. Blood 1993; 81(11):2898–2902.
51. Bedi A, Zehnbauer BA, Barber JP, Sharkis SJ, Jones RJ. Inhibition of apoptosis by BCR-ABL in chronic myeloid leukemia. Blood 1994; 83(8):2038–2044.
52. McGahon A, Bissonnette R, Schmitt M, Cotter KM, Green DR, Cotter TG. BCR-ABL maintains resistance of chronic myelogenous leukemia cells to apoptotic cell death [published erratum appears in Blood 1994 Jun 15;83(12):3835]. Blood 1994; 83(5):1179–1187.
53. Kanei-Ishii C, Nomura T, Ogata K, et al. Structure and function of the proteins encoded by the myb gene family. Curr Top Microbiol Immunol 1996; 211:89–98.
54. Nomura N, Zu YL, Maekawa T, Tabata S, Akiyama T, Ishii S. Isolation and characterization of a novel member of the gene family encoding the cAMP response element-binding protein CRE-BP1. J Biol Chem 1993; 268(6):4259–4266.
55. Biedenkapp H, Borgmeyer U, Sippel AE, Klempnauer KH. Viral myb oncogene encodes a sequence-specific DNA-binding activity. Nature 1988; 335(6193):835–837.
56. Siu G, Wurster AL, Lipsick JS, Hedrick SM. Expression of the CD4 gene requires a Myb transcription factor. Mol Cell Biol 1992; 12(4):1592–1604.
57. Melotti P, Ku DH, Calabretta B. Regulation of the expression of the hematopoietic stem cell antigen CD34: role of c-myb. J Exp Med 1994; 179(3):1023–1028.
58. Gewirtz AM, Anfossi G, Venturelli D, Valpreda S, Sims R, Calabretta B. G1/S transition in normal human T-lymphocytes requires the nuclear protein encoded by c-myb. Science 1989; 245(4914):180–183.
59. Caracciolo D, Venturelli D, Valtieri M, Peschle C, Gewirtz AM, Calabretta B. Stage-related proliferative activity determines c-myb functional requirements during normal human hematopoiesis. J Clin Invest 1990; 85(1):55–61.
60. Mucenski ML, McLain K, Kier AB, et al. A functional c-myb gene is required for normal murine fetal hepatic hematopoiesis. Cell 1991; 65(4):677–689.

61. Anfossi G, Gewirtz AM, Calabretta B. An oligomer complementary to c-myb-encoded mRNA inhibits proliferation of human myeloid leukemia cell lines. Proc Natl Acad Sci USA 1989; 86(9):3379–3383.
62. Calabretta B, Sims RB, Valtieri M, et al. Normal and leukemic hematopoietic cells manifest differential sensitivity to inhibitory effects of c-myb antisense oligodeoxynucleotides: an in vitro study relevant to bone marrow purging. Proc Natl Acad Sci USA 1991; 88(6):2351–2355.
63. Ratajczak MZ, Hijiya N, Catani L, et al. Acute- and chronic-phase chronic myelogenous leukemia colony-forming units are highly sensitive to the growth inhibitory effects of c-myb antisense oligodeoxynucleotides. Blood 1992; 79(8):1956–1961.
64. Melotti P, Calabretta B. Induction of hematopoietic commitment and erythromyeloid differentiation in embryonal stem cells constitutively expressing c-myb. Blood 1996; 87(6):2221–2234.
65. Vandenbark GR, Chen Y, Friday E, et al. Complex regulation of human c-kit transcription by promoter repressors, activators, and specific myb elements. Cell Growth Differ 1996; 7(10):1383–1392.
66. Ratajczak MZ, Perrotti D, Melotti P, et al. Myb and Ets proteins are candidate regulators of c-kit expression in human hematopoietic cells. Blood. 1998; 91:1934–1946.
67. Yu H, Bauer B, Lipke GK, Phillips RL, Van Zant G. Apoptosis and hematopoiesis in murine fetal liver. Blood 1993; 81(2):373–384.
68. Carson WE, Haldar S, Baiocchi RA, Croce CM, Caligiuri MA. The c-kit ligand suppresses apoptosis of human natural killer cells through the upregulation of bcl-2. Proc Natl Acad Sci USA 1994; 91(16):7553–7557.
69. Bonnefoy-Berard N, Munshi A, Yron I, et al. Vav: function and regulation in hematopoietic cell signaling. Stem Cells 1996; 14(3):250–268.
70. Katzav S. vav: a molecule for all haemopoiesis? Br J Haematol 1992; 81(2):141–144.
71. Katzav S, Martin-Zanca D, Barbacid M. vav, a novel human oncogene derived from a locus ubiquitously expressed in hematopoietic cells. EMBO J 1989; 8(8):2283–2290.
72. Katzav S, Cleveland JL, Heslop HE, Pulido D. Loss of the amino-terminal helix-loop-helix domain of the vav proto-oncogene activates its transforming potential. Mol Cell Biol 1991; 11(4):1912–1920.
73. Galland F, Katzav S, Birnbaum D. The products of the mcf-2 and vav proto-oncogenes and of the yeast gene cdc-24 share sequence similarities. Oncogene 1992; 7(3):585–587.
74. Cen H, Papageorge AG, Zippel R, Lowy DR, Zhang K. Isolation of multiple mouse cDNAs with coding homology to *Saccharomyces cerevisiae* CDC25: identification of a region related to Bcr, Vav, Dbl and CDC24. EMBO J 1992; 11(11):4007–4015.
75. Alai M, Mui AL, Cutler RL, et al. Steel factor stimulates the tyrosine phosphorylation of the proto-oncogene product, p95vav, in human hemopoietic cells. J Biol Chem 1992; 267(25):18021–18025.
76. Clevenger CV, Ngo W, Sokol DL, Luger SM, Gewirtz AM. Vav is necessary for prolactin-stimulated proliferation and is translocated into the nucleus of a T-cell line. J Biol Chem 1995; 270(22):13246–13253.

77. Marengere LE, Mirtsos C, Kozieradzki I, Veillette A, Mak TW, Penninger JM. Proto-oncoprotein Vav interacts with c-Cbl in activated thymocytes and peripheral T cells. J Immunol 1997; 159(1):70–76.
78. Coppola J, Bryant S, Koda T, Conway D, Barbacid M. Mechanism of activation of the vav protooncogene. Cell Growth Differ 1991; 2(2):95–105.
79. Adams JM, Houston H, Allen J, Lints T, Harvey R. The hematopoietically expressed vav proto-oncogene shares homology with the dbl GDP-GTP exchange factor, the bcr gene and a yeast gene (CDC24) involved in cytoskeletal organization. Oncogene 1992; 7(4):611–618.
80. Wulf GM, Adra CN, Lim B. Inhibition of hematopoietic development from embryonic stem cells by antisense vav RNA. EMBO J 1993; 12(13):5065–5074.
81. Zhang R, Tsai FY, Orkin SH. Hematopoietic development of vav-/-mouse embryonic stem cells. Proc Natl Acad Sci USA 1994; 91(26):12755–12759.
82. Zmuidzinas A, Fischer KD, Lira SA, et al. The vav proto-oncogene is required early in embryogenesis but not for hematopoietic development in vitro. EMBO J 1995; 14(1):1–11.
83. Zhang R, Alt FW, Davidson L, Orkin SH, Swat W. Defective signalling through the T- and B-cell antigen receptors in lymphoid cells lacking the vav proto-oncogene. Nature 1995; 374(6521):470–473.
84. Luger SM, Ratajczak J, Ratajczak MZ, et al. A functional analysis of protooncogene Vav's role in adult human hematopoiesis. Blood 1996; 87(4):1326–1334.
85. Gewirtz AM, Luger S, Sokol D, et al. Oligodeoxynucleotide therapeutics for human myelogenous leukemia: interim results. Blood 1996; 88(suppl 1)(10):270a.
86. Loke SL, Stein CA, Zhang XH, et al. Characterization of oligonucleotide transport into living cells. Proc Natl Acad Sci USA 1989; 86(10):3474–3478.
87. Beltinger C, Saragovi HU, Smith RM, et al. Binding, uptake, and intracellular trafficking of phosphorothioate-modified oligodeoxynucleotides. J Clin Invest 1995; 95(4):1814–1823.
88. Stein CA, Mori K, Loke SL, et al. Phosphorothioate and normal oligodeoxyribonucleotides with 5'-linked acridine: characterization and preliminary kinetics of cellular uptake. Gene 1988; 72(1–2):333–341.
89. Geselowitz DA, Neckers LM. Analysis of oligonucleotide binding, internalization, and intracellular trafficking utilizing a novel radiolabeled crosslinker. Antisense Res Dev 1992; 2(1):17–25.
90. Spiller DG, Tidd DM. Nuclear delivery of antisense oligodeoxynucleotides through reversible permeabilization of human leukemia cells with streptolysin O. Antisense Res Dev 1995; 5(1):13–21.
91. Lewis JG, Lin KY, Kothavale A, et al. A serum-resistant cytofectin for cellular delivery of antisense oligodeoxynucleotides and plasmid DNA. Proc Natl Acad Sci USA 1996; 93(8):3176–3181.
92. Bergan R, Hakim F, Schwartz GN, et al. Electroporation of synthetic oligodeoxynucleotides: a novel technique for ex vivo bone marrow purging. Blood 1996; 88(2):731–741.
93. Baskerville S, Ellington AD. RNA structure. Describing the elephant. Curr Biol 1995; 5(2):120–123.

94. Milner N, Mir KU, Southern EM. Selecting effective antisense reagents on combinational oligonucleotide arrays [see comments]. Nat Biotechnol 1997; 15(6):537–541.
95. Wagner RW. The state of the art in antisense research. Nat Med 1995; 1(11): 1116–1118.
96. Stein CA, Krieg AM. Problems in interpretation of data derived from in vitro and in vivo use of antisense oligodeoxynucleotides [editorial]. Antisense Res Dev 1994; 4(2):67–69.

18
Roles of Cytokines and Adhesion Molecules in Chronic Myelogenous Leukemia

Luis Fayad and Zeev Estrov
M.D. Anderson Cancer Center, Houston, Texas

INTRODUCTION

Chronic myelogenous leukemia (CML) is a clonal hematopoietic stem cell disorder characterized by the presence of a reciprocal translocation between chromosomes 9 and 22, t(9;22) (q34;q11), termed Philadelphia chromosome (Ph) (1). This translocation results in the fusion gene *bcr/abl* that produces the *bcr/abl* protein, a constitutively activated tyrosine kinase (2). Early in the course of CML, there is an increase in the proliferation of the leukemic myeloid clone. Later, CML progresses by transition from the chronic phase to the accelerated phase; the final stage is blastic transformation, which resembles an acute myeloid or lymphoblastic leukemia (AML or ALL).

Several hematopoietic growth factors, cytokines, and adhesion molecules have been implicated in the pathogenesis, evolution, and disease progression of CML. Other cytokines—in particular, interferon-α (IFN-α)—significantly suppress the leukemic CML clone.

IFN-α has been shown to change the natural course of CML by unknown mechanisms. Research has also shown that in approximately 20% of CML patients IFN-α induces a total suppression of the leukemic Ph+ clone (3,4); in recent years, IFN-α became the drug of choice in CML. The therapeutic effects of IFN and its possible mechanisms of action are discussed in other chapters of this book.

It has been determined that several stimulatory cytokines play a role in the pathophysiology of CML (5). Because it has been found that cytokines such as interleukin-1 (IL-1) provide the leukemic cells with growth advantage (6), several means to inhibit their activity are currently being investigated in clinical trials.

Few clinical trials that test the efficacy of stimulatory cytokines when combined with antileukemic agents have been carried out (7). The effects of these molecules and their possible clinical implications are discussed in this chapter.

STIMULATORY CYTOKINES

Interleukin-1

Interleukin-1 (IL-1) is a polypeptide hormone that exhibits a wide spectrum of biological activities. The two distinct forms of IL-1 identified interleukin-1α (IL-1α) and interleukin-1β (IL-1β), together with the interleukin-1 receptor antagonist protein (IL1-RA) are members of a family of cytokines (8,9) found predominantly in monocytes; they are also produced by various normal and neoplastic cells (9,10).

IL-1α and IL-1β share 26 amino acids homology; they bind to the same receptor and they exhibit identical biological activities (10,11). In contrast, IL-1RA is a specific antagonist of IL-1 that acts by blocking the binding of IL-1 to its cell surface receptors (12–15). IL-1RA, which can be induced by IL-1β (16), may function to buffer IL-1β activity.

The translation products of both IL-1α and IL-1β are 31-kD precursor (pro) forms; both of these cytokines are cleaved by different proteases into 17.5-kD proteins. While pro-IL-1α is biologically active, only the cleaved form of IL-1β is biologically active. Pro-IL-1β is cleaved to its mature form by a cytoplasmic enzyme termed IL-1β converting enzyme (ICE) (17–20). ICE requires processing before it becomes active. It is synthesized as a 45-kD protein that undergoes autocatalytic activity. The enzyme is active when a 13-kD precursor domain and a 2-kD interverting piece are removed. The now-active ICE is a complex of freely dissociable monomers (20). Five isoforms of ICE have been described: α, β, μ, γ, and, ε (21). The ICE-α isoform possesses pro-IL-1β cleavage activity.

IL-1β is the prominent form of IL-1, and the amount of IL-1β mRNA found in activated cells is about 10- to 50-fold greater than the amount of IL-1-α mRNA (9). The mature form of IL-1β is not found intracellularly, and only little pro-IL-1β can be found outside the cell.

Two types of IL-1 receptors (IL-1R), the product of two different genes (22), have been identified. Type I IL-1R (IL-1RI) is an 80-kD molecule which is found in most of the cells; it has the ability to internalize and transduce the IL-1 signal. The type II IL-1R—IL-1RII—is a 68-kD molecule. First identified on Epstein-Barr virus (EBV)-transformed B cells and later found to be present in neutrophils, monocytes, and bone marrow cells, its function is not totally clear. IL-1RII binds both IL-1α and IL-1β but it does not transduce a signal. Because it acts as a "sink" for IL-1β, IL-1RII was described as a "decoy" receptor by Colotta and colleagues (23).

The extracellular domains of both IL-1RI and IL-1RII exist as soluble forms. Their unbound soluble forms circulate and function as buffers, binding IL-1α, IL-1β, and IL-1RA.

The interaction between IL-1 and other cytokines has been found to be important in early events of hematopoiesis (24–27). IL-1 induces the production of several cytokines and hematopoietic growth factors: granulocyte colony-stimulating factor (G-CSF); granulocyte-macrophage colony-stimulating factor (GM-CSF), macrophage colony-stimulating factor (M-CSF), stem cell factor (SCF), IL-2, IL-3, IL-6, IL-7, IL-8, and tumor necrosis factor (TNF-α). It also induces the production of other cytokines such as leukemia inhibitory factor (LIF); IFN-α, β, and δ; and macrophage inflammatory protein-1α (MIP-1α) (28–31). IL-1 upregulates the cell surface expression of many cytokines and, while it has no stimulating effect by itself, it synergizes with several growth factors in stimulating hematopoietic progenitor proliferation (9,24–26,32). IL-1 also increases the survival rate of progenitor cells in vivo and in vitro, and it has been shown to protect mice from lethal irradiation and to accelerate both granulocyte and platelet recovery after chemotherapy both in mice and in nonhuman primate models (33–36).

In patients with advanced CML, we have found that bone marrow cells produce large quantities of IL-1β. We have also discovered that this cytokine provides the cells with growth advantage (37). In marrow samples from these patients, suppression of CML colony growth was obtained with neutralizing antibodies to IL-1β, IL-1RA, and soluble IL-1 receptors (sIL-1R). Such an effect, however, was not obtained with normal marrow or with marrow cells obtained from CML patients with early stages of the disease (37).

These results were very meaningful, because a consecutive study (38) demonstrated that high IL-1β levels correlated with a poor prognosis, whereas low IL-1β and high IL-1RA levels correlated with a good prognosis. A more recent study also found that high levels of IL-1β are associated with a poor outcome, further supporting the importance of these observations (39).

Overall, these data suggest that the overproduction of IL-1β occurs in advanced stages of CML and stimulates marrow stroma and accessory cells to produce growth factors, and stimulates leukemia progenitor proliferation in a paracrine fashion.

IL-1 Inhibitors

Several naturally occurring and artificial compounds possess IL-1 inhibitory activity through a variety of mechanisms of action. As shown in Table 1, these

Table 1 IL-1 Inhibitors and Their Mechanism of Action

Reduction of IL-1 production
  Cyclo-oxygenase and lipooxygenase inhibitors
  Glucocorticoids
  n-fatty acid supplements
  Antisense IL-1 DNA
  IL-4[a]
  IL-10[a]
  TGF-β
  M20 IL-1 inhibitor
Inhibition of IL-1β processing
  IL-1β converting enzyme inhibitor
Blocking IL-1 receptors
  IL-1RA[a]
  IL-1 receptor antibodies
  Suramin
Binding and neutralizing IL-1
  sIL-1R
  IL-1 antibodies

Abbreviations: IL, interleukin; TGF, transforming growth factor.
[a]Discussed in text.

mechanisms include inhibition of IL-1 processing, blocking of IL-1 receptors, reduction of IL-1 production, and binding and neutralizing IL-1. The most important mechanisms are discussed below.

IL-1 Receptor Antagonist (IL-1RA)

IL-1RA is a 23-kD protein that was first purified from the urine of patients with monocytic leukemia and subsequently cloned (8,40–44). The gene for IL-1RA has been localized at the long arm of chromosome 2, mapping to bands 2q13–14.1 (25,45,46). The long arm of chromosome 2 also contains the genes for IL-1α and IL-1β and for both types of IL-1R.

Similar to the two IL-1 forms, α and β, the gene product of IL-1RA is pro-IL-1RA; it is cleaved to the mature form of IL-1RA. Both receptors antagonists are found as soluble IL-1RA (sIL-1RA) and intracellular IL-1RA (icIL-1RA) forms (8). Two forms of icIL-1RA have been identified, icIL-1RaI and icIL-1RaII; both are inducible in various cell types (8,47,48). The in vivo effects of IL-1RA in CML are currently under investigation in a clinical trial (Talpaz, personal communication).

Other IL-1 Inhibitors

Several other IL-1 inhibitors have been identified. In addition to IL-1RA, only interleukin-4 and interleukin-10 (discussed in the following section) are being investigated in clinical trials. Suramin was found to be active in solid tumors, but this drug was not investigated in CML. The antileukemic properties of suramin are currently under study in patients with refractory AML. (Estey, personal communication).

Interleukin-3 (IL-3)

Interleukin-3 is a pluripotent hematopoietic growth factor that stimulates multiple hematopoietic lineages. The human IL-3 gene consists of five small exons separated by one large and three small introns. A single copy of the human gene is located on the long arm of chromosome 5 q23–q31, 9 kb from the GM-CSF gene (49).

IL-3 alone (50), or in combination with SCF[51] or basic fibroblastic growth factor (bFGF) (51), can induce the proliferation of CML cells. In an IL-3-dependent murine cell line, both IL-3 and p210 *bcr/abl* activate unique and overlapping pathways of signal transduction. Transfection of a full-length 210 *bcr/abl* cDNA results in constitutively high levels of phosphorylation of >20 new proteins. Following the transfection, the cells proliferate and within 3 weeks become IL-3-independent (52). While elegant studies have been performed using this model, its relevance to the pathogenesis of CML is unclear.

A study aimed at investigating the interaction between IFN and IL-3 demonstrated that both IFN-α and -β failed to inhibit the colony formation of myeloid progenitors from chronic-phase CML patients in the presence of IL-3. In contrast, G-CSF-stimulated day 7 colony-forming unit granulocyte-macrophage (CFU-GM), and burst-forming units-erythroid (BFU-E) were inhibited by moderate doses of IFN. Suboptimal doses of IL-3 did not protect CFU-GM from the inhibitory effect of IFN (53). Further studies are required to determine whether or not IL-3 plays a unique role in CML.

Granulocyte-Macrophage Colony-Stimulating Factor (GM-CSF) and Granulocyte Colony-Stimulating Factor (G-CSF)

Murine GM-CSF, first purified from a mouse lung, conditioned medium and was found to be an N-glycosylated polypeptide of 23–29 kD (54,55). Gasson et al. (56) purified human GM-CSF from an HTLV-II T lymphoblastoid cell line. Human GM-CSF was found to have a molecular weight of 22 kD. The GM-CSF gene is located on the long arm of chromosome 5 (5q21–q32) (57,58). Alone or in combination with other cytokines, the principal biological activity of GM-CSF in the hematopoietic system is the stimulation of CFU-GM, BFU-E, and immature and megakaryocyte colony-forming cells (59,60). Expression of GM-CSF mRNA by CML blast cells is correlated with autonomous megakaryocyte-colony formation (61). This suggests that GM-CSF may act as a stimulating cytokine on CML progenitors.

G-CSF was first purified to homogeneity from the bladder carcinoma cell line 5637 (62,63). Souza and colleagues (64) isolated a full-length G-CSF DNA from a 5637 cell line cDNA library. When expressed in *E. coli*, this G-CSF DNA yielded a protein of 174 amino acids with a molecular mass of 18 kD. The G-CSF gene in humans has been located in the chromosome 17q11–q21 (65–67).

In vitro studies indicated that both GM-CSF and G-CSF stimulate leukemia progenitors and that GM-CSF stimulates ara-C metabolism in leukemia blasts of patients with AML (68). These were followed by preclinical studies using GM-CSF or G-CSF in AML and in blast crisis of CML (69–73). The hypothesis of these studies was that these cytokines may recruit these leukemia cells to the S phase of the cell cycle, thus sensitizing the neoplastic cells to the lethal effects of cell cycle-specific cytotoxic agents such as ara-C (69,71,74–77) or daunorubicine (69).

Two Phase II studies at the University of Texas M.D. Anderson Cancer Center have been performed to investigate to the use GM-CSF for priming leukemia cells in newly diagnosed AML patients (78,79). Compared with historical controls, the results of these studies were not better or worse. Numerous other studies, using growth factors in acute-leukemia patients showed diverse results: decrease in rate of infections, and greater, no change, and fewer responses to treatment (80–88). A recent randomized trial showed no increase in complete remissions obtained in patients with new AML diagnoses who were pretreated with GM-CSF prior to the chemotherapy; complete remissions decreased in patients who received GM-CSF both pre- and postinduction, or only postinduction (86). Another study, performed by the Eastern Cooperative Oncology Group (83), showed less incidence of infection and higher CR rate using, especially in older AML patients when yeast-derived GM-CSF was used. Dissimilar results of the different studies may be due to the fact the studied patients were different in their age, performance status, disease status, their cytogenetics, characteristics, schedule in cytokine administration, and use of different cytotoxic agents. Therefore, these results should be interpreted with caution. Further studies are needed to evaluate the utility of both GM-CSF and G-CSF in acute leukemia.

In an attempt to decrease the myelosuppression induced by IFN, GM-CSF was used simultaneously with IFN-α in a small group of CML patients. This approach allowed the administration of high-dose IFN and a higher-than-expected proportion of patients achieved major cytogenetic response (Talpaz, personal communication).

Interleukin-6 (IL-6)

Interleukin-6 (IL-6) is a glycoprotein with a molecular weight of 21 kD. The IL-6 gene is located on the chromosome 7p21. IL-6, a very important cytokine in aggressive lymphomas and multiple myeloma, induces hematopoietic cell differentiation with a potent effect in thrombopoiesis.

While IL-6 has been conceived as a hematopoietic growth factor, it induced a two- to 10-fold increase in the ratio of differentiated versus undifferentiated myeloid elements in 14 of 17 patients with acute leukemia (88). In M1 AML myeloblastic cells, IL-6 induces growth arrest and terminal differentiation toward monocytes; IL-6 reduced by five- to 20-fold the tyrosine phosphorylation of cellular proteins in these cells (89). The same reduction was found when M1 AML cells were transfected with the *bcr/abl* dysregulated protein-kinase; however, the level of expression of the inherent tyrosine-kinase activity of *bcr/abl* p210 was unchanged. IL-6 induced protein-tyrosine phosphate phosphatase (PTPase) activity in *bcr/abl*-transfected cells. This increase in PTPase activity did not reach the minimal protein phosphorylation activity characteristic of IL-6-treated cells. In response to IL-6, the transfected M1 clones showed normal growth and differentiation. *Bcr/abl* transfection did not alter the suppression in the levels of C-MYC and cyclin-A or -B mRNA; or c-jun mRNA induction, or dephosphorylation of retinoblastoma protein. Given this variety of findings, additional studies should be performed to investigate the role of IL-6 in CML.

Stem Cell Factor (SCF) (c-Kit Ligand, Steel Factor, Mast Cell Growth Factor)

Stem cell factor (SCF) is a multipotent hematopoietic colony-stimulating factor that binds to a specific cell surface receptor, a protein encoded by the proto-oncogen c-Kit. Whereas SCF by itself has a low capacity for inducing colony formation in hematopoietic progenitor clonogenic assays in vitro, it has strong synergistic activities with several other growth factors such as GM-CSF, G-CSF, IL-3, erythropoietin, IL-6, and IL-7.

The c-Kit proto-oncogen encodes a receptor tyrosine kinase that is considered to play an important role in hematopoiesis. The proto-oncogen c-Kit is expressed in blast cells (90) in the vast majority of AML cases, and also in some cases of CML in blastic crisis (91).

Recombinant human SCF induced a significant proliferative response in one of six CML blast crisis cell lines. Synergistic activity was found when SCF was used with GM-CSF, which suggests that SCF may act as a stimulatory cytokine of CML progenitors (92).

Based on a study which showed that very primitive normal human long-term culture-initiating cells can be maintained in a stroma completely deficient in SCF (93), Aggarwal et al. (94) investigated CML marrow cells. They found that SCF-deficient stroma provided growth advantage for nonleukemic progenitors. This suggests that a SCF-deficient culture system may be efficient for the in vitro purging of CML marrow cells or of peripheral blood cells for autologous transplantation.

Erythropoietin (EPO)

Erythropoietin (EPO) is a hormone produced by the peritubular cells in the kidney. EPO is the cytokine that exerts the primary regulation of erythropoiesis in vivo. It is widely used to treat anemia resulting from chronic renal failure, anemia associated with cancer patients, and in some patients with aplastic anemia.

In clinical studies of CML patients, EPO has been used to treat anemia in two cases (95). It has also been used to ameliorate myelosuppression without affecting adversely the response to IFN treatment (Kantarjian, personal communication), and to treat IFN-induced thrombocytopenia induced by IFN (96). It is therefore possible that EPO may have a therapeutic role in selective cases of CML.

Basic Fibroblast Growth Factor (bFGF)

Basic fibroblast growth factor (bFGF) is a hematopoietic cytokine that also plays an important role in angiogenesis and wound healing (97). bFGF, which is produced by human bone marrow stroma cells, stimulates myeloid progenitor proliferation. This effect was investigated using the adherent layer of human long-term cultures. In these studies bFGF stimulated myeloid proliferation by up to 100-fold (98,99).

In the CML blast crisis K562 cell line, bFGF had a weak stimulatory effect. However, because it synergyzed with G-CSF, GM-CSF, IL-3, and SCF, bFGF may play a role in stimulating leukemia cell proliferation (100). In addition, bFGF has been found to antagonize transforming growth factor (TGF)-β-mediated erythroid differentiation in K562 cells and downregulate the expression of glycophorin A in these cells. These data suggest that bFGF may contribute both to the proliferation and to the reduction of the differentiation of CML cells. Paradoxically, however, some investigators have reported that K562 leukemia cells have receptors only for acid fibroblastic growth factor and lack receptors for bFGF (101).

INHIBITORY CYTOKINES AND CYTOKINES WITH PLEIOTROPIC ACTIVITIES

Interleukin-2

Interleukin-2 (IL-2) is a potent cytokine with an important activity in T-cell and B-cell growth and response. The IL-2 gene exists as a single copy in human chromosome 4q26-28 (102). Four exons separated by three introns encode for a short leader sequence; this is followed by the sequence encoding the mature 133 residue protein with a molecular mass of 15 kD. The biological activity of IL-2 is mediated by interaction with cell surface receptors in T and B lymphocytes, macrophages, and natural killer (NK) cells. The receptor is a complex structure with three different chains—an α chain (IL-2Rα, p55, Tac), a β chain (IL-2Rβ, p75), and a γ chain (IL-2Rγ, p64). Discussion of the specific function of these chains is beyond the scope of this chapter.

The effects of IL-2 on CML cells has been studied in vitro. Diloo and colleagues (103) found that K562 cells express both IL-2Rα and IL-2Rβ, and the IL-2 inhibits the clonogenic growth of K562 cells in a dose-dependent manner. They have demonstrated that the IL-2-mediated inhibition of K562 proliferation is preceded by a three- to 15-fold reduction of *bcr/abl* mRNA accumulation, and a decrease in the accumulation of p210 protein levels.

Results from the work of another group also suggest that IL-2 may have a role in the suppression of CML cells. Verma and colleagues (104) found that IL-2-stimulated bone marrow cells develop a potent tumoricidal activity in vitro against K562 cells.

Studies of rats and mice suggest that IL-2 may be useful in preventing relapse in patients who undergo an allogeneic bone marrow transplantation (BMT). Pearson and colleagues (105) administered IL-2 to leukemic mice following BMT. IL-2 decreased graft-versus-host disease (GVHD) without affecting a graft-versus-leukemia (GVL) effect. Pearson proposed that this selective effect of IL-2 resulted from its effect upon CD4+ T-cells, because a dissociation between GVHD and GVL was not observed when IL-2 was administered to the recipient of CD4-depleted bone marrow (106). Similarly, Kloosterman and colleagues (107) reported an increase in the GVL effect without an increase in GVHD; this suggests that IL-2 may be useful in the setting of BMT.

The effects of IL-2 in CML have been investigated in clinical trials. IL-2 was administered in combination with IFN-α to 10 patients with Ph+ CML, all of whom had previously been treated; three had failed to respond to IFN-α prior to the study. Hematological responses were seen in 9 of the 10 patients. Elimination of the Ph clone was observed in one patient who relapsed after receiving BMT. In this patient *bcr/abl* RNA was not detected by polymerase chain reaction (108).

In an attempt to increase a GVL effect without increasing the risk of GVHD, clinical studies were performed in patients receiving allogeneic BMT. Soiffer and colleagues (109) used low-dose recombinant IL-2 (2-6 × 10^5 U/m^2/day) in 29 BMT patients with hematologic malignancies; 15 of the patients had CML. A lower incidence of relapses and superior disease-free survival was found in the study patients than in CML patients without GVHD (110). The authors noted the importance of early versus late IL-2 administration after BMT in decreasing the relapse rate by <60 days versus >60 days. They suggested that the mechanism of action of this antileukemia effect was an increase in the number of NK cells.

In patients with CML, the treatment of relapses after allogeneic BMT, stimulating the immunity of the donor cells, was first done with G-CSF (111). More recently, donor lymphocyte infusion—which induces long-lasting remissions—is becoming one of the most important therapeutic strategies, and few patients appear to be cured. The principal problem following treatment remains the mortality related to infections, veno-occlusive disease, and GVHD.

Monoclonal antibodies against IL-2 receptors, such humanized anti-Tac-IgG2a (112) and murine anti Tac (113) have been used, with responses of 40% and 9%, respectively. Studies using other anti-IL-2 receptors have also been used, with various results reported. The differences in the results in some other studies could be due to differences in patient selection, but they also could be due to the use of "humanized" versus mouse- or rat-derived antibodies (114,115).

Macrophage Inflammatory Protein-1α (MIP-1α)

Macrophage inflammatory protein-1α (MIP-1α), a member of the chemokine family of small, inducible cytokines, is a 69-amino acid peptide of 8 kD produced by stimulated macrophages. The gene of MIP-1α is located on the long arm of chromosome 17 at 11q21 (116). Several investigators have found that MIP-1α inhibits primitive hematopoietic progenitor proliferation in vitro (117–121).

We have found that MIP-1α inhibits the proliferation of AML progenitors (122). Other investigators have demonstrated that although its receptors are present on both normal and CML progenitors, this chemokine inhibits normal but not CML progenitors. The refractoriness to the suppressive effects of MIP-1α, they suggest, is due to a defect in its signaling downstream from the receptor (123). Another study, however, has shown that the daily addition of MIP-1α to adherent cultures of CML precursors produces heterogeneous responses, with duplication of CFU-GM proliferation in 26% of the cases and reduction in 44% (124).

The intriguing effects of MIP-1α in CML will require additional studies to determine its role in the disease.

Interleukin-4 (IL-4)

Interleukin-4 (IL-4) was first identified by its ability to induce the proliferation of mouse B-lymphocytes (125) and was therefore referred to as the B-cell stimulatory factor.

Human IL-4 is a glycoprotein with molecular weights of between 15 and 19 kD (113), and its gene is located on chromosome 5 at q23.3–31.2 (126). IL-4 is produced primarily by the TH_2 subset of CD4+ T cells, but it can also be produced by other subsets of cells (127,128). IL-4 has pleiotropic effects on B cells, T cells, macrophages, hematopoietic stem cells, and stroma cells.

IL-4 inhibits GM-CSF-, M-CSF-, and IL-3-induced proliferation of normal human CFU-GM colonies, and AML and CML precursors (129–134), whereas it augments the G-CSF-induced proliferation of murine and myeloid progenitors (129–131,135,136). Its effects in AML and CML in the presence of G-CSF is diverse, exerting stimulation, no effect, or inhibition (129–131). Incubation of CML bone marrow low-density cells with IL-4 results in the downregulation of the production of IL-1β and IL-6; the inhibitory effect of IL-4 in normal, CML, and AML samples can be partially reversed by IL-1β (129–131). IL-4 has also been found to upregulate the message for IL-1RA production (137).

In long-term bone marrow cultures (131,138,139) the addition of IL-4 has resulted in disruptions of their stromal architecture and the induction of significant changes in their cellular content. IL-4 decreased the number of CD34+ cells and hematopoietic progenitors in the adherent layer but increased their number in the liquid layers (140). IL-4 also changed the supernatant cytokine profile of the cultures. It upregulated the production of both M-CSF and TNF-α but decreased the levels of leukemic inhibitory factor (LIF) (141).

IL-4 inhibits IL-1β production and may therefore have a role in the therapy of IL-1-responsive neoplasms. But a therapeutic use for IL-4 in CML may be complicated by possible increments in M-CSF and TNF-α, which may produce an increase in side effects and toxicity primarily to the hematopoietic stroma.

Interleukin-8 (IL-8)

Interleukin-8 (IL-8) has also been termed monocyte chemotactic and activating factor. It is produced by many cell types upon stimulation with bacterial products or inflammation-associated cytokines. IL-8 is secreted by many cell types, including monocytes, macrophages, T-lymphocytes, endothelial cells, fibroblasts, hepatocytes, and neutrophils (142–146). Bacterial products, viruses, IL-1, and TNF-α are potent inducers of IL-8 production (144,145). IL-8 induces the expression of adhesion molecules and complement receptor type 1 (147). It also induced the release of various proteins and increases the adhesion of neutrophils to nonstimulated endothelial cells in vitro. Inhibition of IL-8 or downregulation of its production results in a reduced inflammatory response. Glucocorticoids are potent inhibitors of IL-8 (148), inhibiting both gene expression and the release of the biologically active IL-8 protein.

IL-8 is also produced by CML mononuclear cells and by fibroblasts. IFN-α may downregulate IL-8 production by fibroblasts, an effect that is similar in normal and in CML cells. IFN-α downregulated IL-8 production by CML peripheral blood cells both in vivo and in vitro, limiting the accumulation and activation of neutrophils (149). Although they may provide an explanation for some of the side effects of IFNs, the significance of these effects in CML is not clear.

Interleukin-10 (IL-10)

Interleukin-10 (IL-10) is an 18-kD polypeptide. It has been described as an immunomodulatory cytokine produced primarily by T_{H2} cells and, to a lesser extent, by B-lymphocytes as well as by macrophages, keratinocytes, and ovarian cancer cells (150). IL-10 exerts its effects through binding to a specific receptor expressed in low numbers on cells of lymphoid and myeloid origin (151). It functions primarily as an anti-inflammatory cytokine through the downregulation of interferon-γ, TNF-α, IL-1, IL-6, and GM-CSF in cells of the lymphoid lineage (152). While IL-10 is expressed in normal hematopoietic cells, its functions in normal hematopoiesis in particular in myelopoiesis are not completely understood. IL-10 inhibits spontaneous blast proliferation in AML (153). In the presence of other cytokines, IL-10 produces a wide variety of responses in different patients. IL-10 downregulates IL-1 production, but the clinical significance of this effect has yet to be explored.

Interleukin-11 (IL-11)

Interleukin-11 (IL-11) is a stromal-derived cytokine. It does not normally stimulate early progenitors by itself; rather, it exhibits synergistic activity in combination with cytokines such as IL-3, IL-4, and SCF (154). IL-11 acts at multiple stages of megakaryopoiesis, stimulates erythropoiesis, enhances immunoglobulin secretion, and promotes osteoclastogenesis; it may play a role in the maturation and activation of macrophages (155,156). IL-11 transcripts were detected in K562 cells, but the growth of K562 cells was not stimulated by IL-11.

Tumor Necrosis Factor-α (TNF-α)

Tumor necrosis factor-α (TNF-α) is a pleiotropic cytokine that has been extensively studied. It was first identified for its antitumor activity in an experimental model (157). TNF-β (lymphotoxin) is a related molecule with biological properties similar to those of TNF-α. The TNF-α gene is located on the short arm of chromosome 6, close to the major histocompatibility complex genome. Its mRNA codes for a 76-amino acid presequence followed by a 157-amino acid mature polypeptide.

TNF-α is a response modifier in inflammatory and immune reactions, affecting the proliferation, differentiation, and function of almost all cell types. It mediates cytotoxicity and plays a very important role in the pathophysiology of septic shock (158). TNF-α is produced primarily by monocytes; it has been used as a marker for monocyte function in CML. TNF-α is also produced by other hematopoietic and nonhematopoietic cells (158). Lymphotoxin, in contrast, is produced exclusively by T-lymphocytes and some T-lymphocyte-derived cell lines. Two receptors that bind both TNF-α and lymphotoxin have been identified; based on the molecular weights of their proteins, they are referred to as TNF-R55 and TNF-R75. The latter has fivefold more affinity than the former for both TNF-α and lymphotoxin.

The role of TNF-α in the hematopoietic system has been extensively investigated. While both stimulatory and inhibitory effects have been reported, depending on the nature of the cells that were analyzed (159–162), most studies emphasize its inhibitory effect.

TNF-α was studied in several hematological malignancies. TNF-α is produced by juvenile CML cells and stimulates their proliferation in an autocrine fashion (163). TNF-α may be synergetic with IL-3 and GM-CSF, thus enhancing AML progenitor proliferation (164,165), probably by upregulating their receptors (166). TNF-α also may act as an autocrine growth factor in some cases of AML (164).

In vitro studies, with cells from four CML patients, demonstrated the inhibitory effect of TNF-α in the absence of colony stimulating factors. No significant evidence of apoptosis was found, however (167). The effects of TNF-α on CML progenitors has been studied by several investigators; no direct cytotoxicity or apoptosis induced by TNF-α was found (167).

Anecdotal reports of clinical studies have suggested that TNF-α may play a role in future therapies of CML. Patients with primary or secondary resistance to IFN have received a combination therapy of IFN-α and TNF-α. A decrease in leucocyte counts was observed, but the patients failed to attain either a complete hematological remission or a cytogenetic response (168). Another clinical study using IFN-α and TNF-α in CML revealed an association between TNF-α administration, an increase in ACTH, an increase in cortisol levels, and an increase in white blood cell counts. This effect was blocked upon administration of the cortisol inhibitor metopirone (169).

Another study suggested that TNF-α may be used as a prognostic factor in CML. Elevated circulatory levels of TNF-α were predictive for resistance to treatment with IFN-α (170).

Because the elevation of TNF-α has been found to correlate with both incidence and severity GVHD, Holler and colleagues (171) treated 21 patients with hematological malignancies who had received an allogeneic BMT with monoclonal antibodies to TNF-α; 17 of the 21 patients were CML patients. A delay in the occurrence of acute GVHD was reported, with no major toxicity related to the monoclonal antibodies.

Transforming Growth Factor-β (TGF-β)

Transforming growth factor-β (TGF-β) is a pleiotropic cytokine that exerts inhibitory effects on many cell types. This cytokine, which is a member of a family of more than 20 related members, is known to arrest cells in a number of systems in mid to late G1 phase of the cell cycle.

In CML, the suppressive effect of TGF-β has been demonstrated when TGF-$β_1$ was added directly to cell cultures (172–175). The inhibitory effect of TGF-β in the presence of G-CSF was increased in chronic, accelerated, and blastic phase CML. With some patient variation, TGF-β almost completely abolished leukemia cell growth of CML in blast crisis, and of AML (173).

Using Northern blot analysis, Federico and colleagues (176) found that TGF-β mRNA was fourfold higher in K562 cells (CML blast crisis) than cells from HL-60 cells (promyelocytic leukemia). A similar pattern was found in the cells of three CML patients. The highest level of TGF-$β_1$ mRNA was found in a patient with M7 AML. The authors therefore suggested a possible correlation between the levels of TGF-β and myelofibrosis associated with hematological disorders.

ADHESION MOLECULES

A group of proteins functioning as cell adhesion and signal transduction factors have been termed adhesion molecules. These molecules have been divided into three families—the integrin family, the selectin family, and the immunoglobulin (Ig) family.

Integrins are transmembrane cell surface proteins that bind the cytoskeletal proteins and communicate with extracellular signals. This family was identified in the 1980s, and its related structures and activities have been thoroughly investigated. The integrins are involved in both cellular adhesion and signal transduction. The members of this family consist of at least 15 heterodimers of α and eight β subunits. Each β subunit associates with a number of distinct α subunits, but each α subunit only associates with one β subunit (with the exception of $α_v$). The β subfamily is the largest because it has the largest number of α subunits.

The β integrins contain a series of cellular receptors for extracellular matrix proteins, including fibronectin, collagen, laminin, and vitronectine. All share CD29 on their common β subunit (177). An important member of the β1 integrins, α4β1 (VLA-4), was identified in hematopoietic cells. It is present in lymphocytes, monocytes, eosinophils, basophils, and NK cells (178–189) but not in neutrophils (177). Another member of the β1 integrins is the fibronectin receptor α5/β1. Several investigators have demonstrated that integrin-dependent adhesion of hematopoietic cells to bone marrow stroma results in the suppression of normal progenitor proliferation (190,191). Hurley and colleagues (192) have recently shown that this inhibitory effect results from the direct engagement of the α4β1 integrin through antibody clustering.

A few studies have shown that the $β_1$ subunit plays an important role in signal transductions and oncogenesis. In lymphocytes and leukocytes the $β_1$ subunit can combine with α-actinin and vinculin, and after mitosis or antigen stimulation its level increases resulting in conformational changes in signal transduction. Receptor crosslinking of the common β1 chain of the VLA family results in rapid accumulation of transcripts for all genes induced by adherence, including the IL-1β gene; truncation of the β1 subunit abolishes integrin-mediated tyrosine phosphorylations.

When marrow cells of Ph+ CML patients are maintained in long-term bone marrow cultures, the dominant Ph+ population rapidly disappears, the Ph– normal progenitors remain detectable for periods of 2–3 months (193–195). It has been suggested that this phenomenon results from dissimilar adhesion activity of normal versus CML progenitors with the hematopoietic stroma. While normal progenitors adhere to their microenvironment and their differentiation is suppressed by stromal inhibitory molecules, CML progenitors adhere poorly and within 2–3 weeks reach terminal differentiation.

Evaluation of adhesion receptor expression demonstrated that fibronectin receptors α4, α5, and β are equally present in normal and CML marrow progenitors. Furthermore, a fraction of the CML progenitors express α2 and α6 receptors associated with laminin and collagen. Some investigators have suggested that the poor adhesion of CML progenitors to the hematopoietic stroma (196,197) may be explained by their poor adhesion to fibronectin and its domains. Although CML progenitors express normal levels of α4β1 and α5β1 integrins, they cannot adhere to fibronectin and therefore proliferate and differentiate in long-term cultures without being affected by the inhibitory properties of the stroma (198). This lack of integrin-dependent adhesion to fibronectin maybe due to either a functional or a structural abnormality in the β1 integrins (198,199).

Lundell and colleages (200) used the 8A2 antibody to activate β1 integrin. They have demonstrated an increment in the adhesion of K562 cells to fibronectin through the α5β1 integrin, which resulted in a reduction in K562 proliferation. IFN-α, the drug of choice in the therapy of CML, has been shown to increase the adhesion of CML progenitors to fibronectin (201). While it is possible that increased adhesion is the mechanism of action of IFN-α, clinical trials aimed at using the defective adhesion properties of CML progenitors are being conducted to fractionate CML bone marrow prior to autologous marrow transplantation (202,203).

SUMMARY AND CONCLUSIONS

CML is a disease characterized by the proliferation of clonal Ph+ leukemia cells. The cornerstone of the treatment of CML continues to be IFN-α and, in some younger patients, allogeneic BMT. Because age and the lack of a matching sibling donor are limiting factors for BMT, and since under the best circumstances this treatment has a related mortality rate of about 20%, IFN is the frontline treatment for most of the CML patients.

The mechanisms by which IFN-α controls CML are poorly understood. Other cytokines and adhesion molecules may play a pathophysiological role in the disease or provide new therapeutic modalities. The different activities of various cytokines in normal and in CML hematopoiesis, either in vitro or in vivo, are discussed in this chapter and are summarized in Table 2. The possible clinical applications of this cytokine armamentarium is summarized in Table 3. As shown in Table 3, IL-2 can be an important inhibitor of relapses following allogeneic BMT. Its inhibition may decrease the possibility that acute GVHD, one of the most significant causes of death in CML patients, will develop. Other cytokines such as G-CSF and GM-CSF has been used in an attempt to increase the sensitivity of the blasts to different chemotherapy regimens, with various results. Stimulatory hematopoietic growth factors, such as IL-3 and EPO, have been used to ameliorate the neutropenia and infectious complications related to chemotherapy regimens and BMT, and GM-CSF was used in combination with IFN-α to allow increments in the dose of IFN. The use of inhibitors, antagonists, and antibodies to certain cytokines such as IL-1RA for the treatment of CML and antibodies against TNF-α for the prevention of acute GVHD are currently being investigated in clinical trials.

While the data accumulating on the role of these molecules in CML are intriguing, it remains to be seen whether this knowledge will be translated and successfully used in the clinical arena.

Table 2 Role of Cytokines in Chronic Myelogenous Leukemia

Cytokine	Reference, stimulatory responses	Reference, inhibitory response	Reference, mixed responses	Reference, no activity or unclear	Comments
IL-1	9,24–26,32,38,39				Significant interaction with other cytokines
IL-2		103,104,108,109			Possible use in relapse after BMT
IL-3	50–52				Interaction with GM-CSF, SCF, and IL-4
IL-4		129–134	129–131,135,136		Primarily inhibitory, but may stimulate when used with G-CSF; may be produced by CML basophils
IL-6	88 (induces differentiation)	89			Interaction with other cytokines; may induce differentiation (in vitro)
IL-8				149	Inhibited by IFN-α
IL-10		153			Inhibitory alone; different responses when combined with other cytokines
IL-11				58	
SCF	90,92,93				Synergistic with G-CSF and GM-CSF; absence of SCF in LTC is detrimental for CML cell proliferation
EPO					Used clinically in combination with IFN-α
G-CSF	69,73			95,96	Effects similar to GM-CSF
GM-CSF	69–72				May increase incorporation of ara-C in leukemic cells; used clinically in combination with IFN-α
TNF-α	163	168			High serum levels may correlate with poor IFN-α response and advance CML
MIP-1α		122	124	123	Effect may depend upon receptor expression; IFN-α enhances expression
bFGF	100				Synergistic with G-CSF, GM-CSF, SCF, and IL-3
TGF-β		173			Inhibits proliferation of G-CSF-stimulated CML cells

Abbreviations: CML: chronic myelogenous leukemia; BMT: bone marrow transplant; IL: interleukin; SCF: stem cell factor; EPO: erythropoietin; G-CSF: granulocyte colony-stimulating factor; GM-CSF: granulocyte-macrophage colony-stimulating factor; TNF-α: tumor necrosis factor-α; MIP-α: macrophage inhibitor factor-α; bFGF: basic fibroblastic growth factor; TGF-β: transforming growth factor-β; LTC: long-term culture; IFN-α: interferon-α.

Table 3 Clinical Applications of Cytokines and Cytokine Antagonists in CML

Cytokine	Clinical use	Proposed mechanisms
Antagonists of IL-1β (e.g., IL-1RA)	In vitro decreases the proliferation of CML cells	Interrupts IL-1 autocrine and paracrine loops
IL-2	Prevents post-BMT leukemia relapse in humans and in animal models by increasing graft versus leukemia effect; used in a few patients in combination with IFN-α	T-cell-dependent immune responses; inhibition of CD4 activity; increase in NK cells
IL-2 receptor antibodies (e.g., LO-Tact-1, anti-Tac, B-B10 IgG1)	Used to prevent GVHD, with variable responses	Decreases activated T-lymphocytes; studies using humanized monoclonal antibodies obtained better results
TNF-α antibody	Delay acute GVHD after BMT	Antagonizes TNF-α an inflammatory cytokine
EPO	Decreases IFN-α-induced anemia and thrombocytopenia	Stimulates erythroid progenitors
G-CSF	Used in relapsing leukemia after BMT	Stimulates both donor and CML progenitors
GM-CSF	Decreases IFN-α-induced myelosuppression or in conjunction with chemotherapy may enhance response to ara-C	Anecdotal use for myelosuppression

Abbreviations: NK: natural killer cells; TNF: tumor necrosis factor; GVHD: graft vs. host disease; BMT: bone marrow transplant; EPO: erythropoietin.

REFERENCES

1. Rowley JD. A new consistent chromosomal abnormality in chronic myelogenous leukemia identified by quinacrine fluorescence and Giemsa staining. Nature 1973; 243:290–291.
2. Kurzrock R, Gutterman JU, Talpaz M. The molecular genetics of Philadelphia chromosome-positive leukemias. N Engl J Med 1988; 319:990–998.
3. Tura S, Baccarini M, Zuffa E, for the Italian Cooperative Study Group on Chronic Myeloid Leukemia. Interferon alfa-2a as compared with conventional chemotherapy for the treatment of chronic myeloid leukemia. N Engl J Med 1994; 330: 820–825.
4. Kantarjian HM, Smith TL, O'Brien S, et al. Prolonged survival in chronic myelog-

enous leukemia after cytogenetic response to interferon-α therapy. Ann Intern Med 1995; 122:254–261.
5. Estrov Z, Kurzrock R, Talpaz M. Cytokines and their antagonists in myeloid disorders. Semin Hematol 1995; 32:220–231.
6. Estrov Z, Kurzrock R, Talpaz M. Interleukin-1 and its inhibitors: implications for disease biology and therapy. In: Kurzrock R, ed. Cytokines: Interleukins and Their Receptors. Dordrecht: Kluwer Academic Publishers, 1995:51–82.
7. Geller RB. Use of cytokines in the treatment of acute myelocytic leukemia: a critical review. J Clin Oncol 1996; 14:1371–1382.
8. Arend WP. Interleukin-1 receptor antagonist. Adv Immunol 1993; 54:167–227.
9. Dinarello CA. Interleukin-1 and interleukin-1 antagonism. Blood 1991; 77:1627–1652.
10. Estrov Z, Kurzrock R, Talpaz M. Interruption of endoneous growth regulatory network: a novel approach to inhibition of leukemia cell proliferation. Forum Trends Clin Med 1993; 3:306–318.
11. Dower SK, Wignall JM, Schooley K, et al. Primary structure and functional expression from complementary DNA of an interleukin-1 receptor antagonist. Nature 1990; 343:341–346.
12. Arend WP, Welgus HG, Thompson RC, et al. Biological properties of recombinant human monocyte-derived interleukin-1 receptor antagonist. J Clin Invest 1990; 85:1694–1697.
13. Seckinger P, Lowenthal JW, Williamson K, et al. A urine inhibitor of interleukin-1 activity that blocks ligand binding. J Immunol 1987; 139:1546–1549.
14. Mazzei GJ, Seckinger PL, Dayer JM, Shaw AR. Purification and characterization of a 26kDa competitive inhibitor of interleukin-1. Eur J Immunol 1990; 20:683–689.
15. Eisenberg SP, Evans RJ, Arend WD, et al. Primary structure and functional expression from complementary DNA of a human interleukin-1 receptor antagonist. Nature 1990; 343:341–346.
16. Bagby GC Jr, Dinarello CA, Neerhout RC, et al. Interleukin-1 dependent paracrine granulopoiesis in chronic granulocytic leukemia of the juvenile type. J Clin Invest 1988; 82:1430–1436.
17. Black RA, Kronheim SR, Cantrell M, et al. Endogenous pyrogen production by Hodgkin's disease and human hystiocytic lymphoma cell lines in vivo. J Clin Invest 1980; 65:514–518.
18. Cerretti DP, Koslosky CJ, Mosley B, et al. Molecular cloning of the interleukin-1β converting enzyme. Science 1992; 256:97–100.
19. Kostura MJ, Tocci MJ, Limjuxo G, et al. Identification of a monocyte specific pre-interleukin-1 beta convertase activity. Proc Natl Acad Sci USA 1989; 86:5227–5231.
20. Thornberry NA, Bull HG, Calaycay JR, et al. A novel heterodimeric cysteine protease is required for interleukin-1β processing in monocytes. Nature 1992; 356:768–774.
21. Alnemri ES, Fernandez-Alnemri T, Litwack G. Cloning and expression of four novel isoforms of human interleukin-1b converting enzyme with different apoptotic activities. J Biol Chem 1995; 270:4312–4317.
22. Chizzonite R, Truitt T, Kilian PL, et al. Two high affinity interleukin-1 receptors

represent separate gene products. Proc Natl Acad Sci USA 1989; 87:8029–8033.
23. Colotta F, Dower SK, Sims JE, Mantovani A. The type II "decoy" receptor: a novel regulatory pathway for interleukin-1. Immunol Today 1994; 15:562–566.
24. Bartelmez SH, Bardley TR, Bertoncello I, et al. Interleukin-1 plus interleukin-3 plus colony-stimulating factor-1 are essential for clonal proliferation of primitive myeloid bone marrow cells. Exp Hematol 1989; 17:240–254.
25. Stanley ER, Bartocci A, Partinkin D, et al. Regulation of very primitive, multipotent, hematopoietic cells by hematopoietin-1. Cell 1986; 45:667–674.
26. Zsebo KM, Wypych J, Juschenkoff VN, et al. Effects of hematopoietin-1 and interleukin-1 activities of early hematopoietic cells of the bone marrow. Blood 1988; 71:962–968.
27. Zucali JR, Bronxmeyer HE, Dinarello CA, et al. Regulation of early human hematopoietic (BFU-E and CFU-GEMM) progenitor cells in vitro of interleukin-1 induced fibroblast medium. Blood 1987; 69:33–37.
28. Bagby GC Jr, Dinarello CA, Wallace P, et al. Interleukin-1 stimulates CM-CSF release by vascular endothelial cells. J Clin Invest 1986; 78:1316–1323.
29. Herrmann F, Oster W, Meuer SC, et al. Interleukin-1 stimulates T lymphocytes to produce granulocyte-monocyte colony-stimulating factor. J Clin Invest 1988; 81:1415–1418.
30. Rennick DG, Yang L, Gemmel L, et al. Control of hemopoiesis by a bone marrow stroma cell clone. Lipopolysaccharide and interleukin-1 inducible production of colony-stimulating factors. Blood 1987; 69:682–691.
31. Zucali JR, Dinarello CA, Oblon DJ, et al. Interleukin-1 stimulates fibroblasts to produce granulocyte-macrophage colony-stimulating activity and prostaglandin E. J Clin Invest 1986; 77:1857–1863.
32. Di Giovine FS, Duff GW. Interleukin-1 in disease. Immunol Today 1990; 11: 13–20.
33. Neta R, Oppenheim JJ, Douches SD. Interdependence of the radioprotective effects of human recombinant interleukin-1 alpha, tumor necrosis factor alpha, granulocyte colony-stimulating factor, and murine recombinant granulocyte-macrophage colony-stimulating factor. J Immunol 1988; 140:108–111.
34. Oppenheim JJ, Neta R, Tiberghien P, et al. Interleukin-1 enhances survival of lethally irradiated mice treated with allogeneic bone marrow cells. Blood 1989; 74:2257–2263.
35. Fibbe WE, van der Meer JWM, Falkenburg JHF, et al. A single low dose of human recombinant interleukin-1 accelerates the recovery of neutrophils in mice with cyclophosphamide-induced neutropenia. Exp Hematol 1989; 17:805–808.
36. Schartz GN, MacVittie TJ, Vigneulle RM, et al. Enhanced hematopoietic recovery in irradiated mice pretreated with interleukin-1 (IL-1). Immunopharmacol Immunotoxicol 1987; 9:371–389.
37. Estrov Z, Kurzrock R, Wetzler M, et al. Suppression of chronic myelogenous leukemia colony growth by IL-1 receptor antagonist and soluble IL-1 receptors: a novel application for inhibitors of IL-1 activity. Blood 1991; 78:1476–1484.
38. Wetzler M, Kurzrock R, Lowe DG, et al. Alteration in bone marrow adherent layer factor expression. A novel mechanism of chronic myelogenous leukemia progression. Blood 1990; 78:2400–2406.

39. Wetzler M, Kurzrock R, Estrov Z, et al. Altered levels of interleukin-1β and interleukin-1 receptor antagonist in chronic myelogenous leukemia. Blood 1994; 84: 3142–3147.
40. Arend WP, Gordon DF, Wood WM, et al. IL-1 beta production in cultured human mmonocytes is regulated at multiple levels. J Immunol 1989; 143:118–126.
41. Carter DB, Deibel MB Jr, Dunn CJ, et al. Purification, cloning, expression, and biological characterization of an interleukin-1 receptor antagonist protein. Nature 1990; 344:633–638.
42. Eisenberg SP, Evans RJ, Arend WP, et al. Primary structure and functional expression from complementary DNA of a human interleukin-1 receptor antagonist. Nature 1990; 343:341–346.
43. Seckinger P, Dayer JM. Interleukin-1 inhibitors. Ann Inst Pasteur/Immunol 1987; 138:486–488.
44. Shaldon S, Koch KM, Bingel M, et al. Modulation of plasma interleukin-1 and its circulating protein inhibitor (CIP) by hemodialysis and hemofiltration. Kidney Int 1987; 31:245. Abstract.
45. Lennard A, Gorman P, Carrier M, et al. Cloning and chromosome mapping of the human interleukin-1 receptor antagonist gene. Cytokine 1992; 4:83–89.
46. Peled T, Rigel M, Peritt D, et al. Effect of M-20 interleukin-1 inhibitor on normal and leukemic human myeloid progenitors. Blood 1992; 79:1172–1177.
47. Haskill S, Martin M, VanLe L, et al. cDNA cloning of a novel form of the interleukin-1 receptor antagonist associated with epithelium. Proc Natl Acad Sci USA 1991; 88:3681–3685.
48. Muzio M, Polentarutti N, Sironi M, et al. Characterization of intracellular interleukin-1 receptor antagonist II. Cytokine 1995; 7:632. Abstract.
49. LeBeau MM, Epstein N, O'Brien SJ, et al. The interleukin-3 gene is located on human chromosome 5 and is deleted in myeloid leukemias with a deletion on 5q-. Proc Natl Acad Sci USA 1987; 84:5913–5917.
50. Nomoto N, Shibata A. Capability of various cytokines to induce quiescent myeloid leukemia cells to the proliferative stage. Leuk Lymph 1992; 7:143–150.
51. Siitonen T, Zheng A, Savolainen ER, Koistinen P. The effect of mast cell growth factor on peripheral blood granulocyte-macrophage colony-forming cells in methylcellulose in myeloproliferative disorders. Eur J Haematol 1995; 55:228–234.
52. Matulonis U, Salgia R, Okuda K, et al. Interleukin-3 and p210 bcr/abl activate both unique and overlapping pathways of signal transduction in a factor-dependent myeloid cell line. Exp Hematol 1993; 21:1460–1466.
53. Despres D, Goldschmitt J, Aulitzky WE, et al. Differential effect of type I interferons on hematopoietic progenitor cells: failure of interferons to inhibit IL-3-stimulated normal and CML myeloid progenitors. Exp Hematol 1995; 23:1431–1438.
54. Burgess AW, Camakaris J, Metcalf D. Purification and properties of colony-stimulating factor from mouse lung-conditioned medium. J Biol Chem 1977; 252: 1998–2003.
55. Gough NM, Gough J, Metcalf D, et al. Molecular cloning of cDNA encoding a murine hematopoietic growth regulator, granulocyte-macrophage colony-stimulating factor. Nature 1985; 309:763–767.
56. Gasson JC, Weisbart RH, Kaufman SE, et al. Purified human granulocyte-macro-

phage colony-stimulating factor: direct action on neutrophils. Science 1984; 226: 1339–1342.
57. Huebner K, Isobe M, Corce CM, et al. The human gene encoding GM-CSF is at 5q21-q32, the chromosome region deleted in the 5q- anomaly. Science 1985; 230: 1282–1285.
58. Le Beau MM, Westbrook CA, Diaz MO, et al. Evidence of the involvement of GM-CSF and FMS in the deletion (5q) in myeloid disorders. Science 1986; 231: 984–987.
59. Ottmann OG, Abboud W, Welte K, et al. Stimulation of human hematopoietic progenitor cell proliferation and differentiation by recombinant human interleukin-3. Comparison and interactions with recombinant human granulocyte-macrophage and granulocyte colony-stimulating factors. Exp Hematol 1987; 17:191–197.
60. Lu L, Bronxmeyer HE. Induction of the release from human monocytes and PHA-stimulated T lymphocytes of hematopoietic colony stimulating and inhibiting by recombinant human B-cell growth factor-1/interleukin-4 (BSF-1/IL-4). Exp Hematol 1988; 16:505. Abstract.
61. Lajmanovich A, Berthir R, Scheitzer A, et al. Constitutive expression of GM-CSF mRNA by CML blasts cells is correlated with endogenous megacaryocytic colony formation. Leukemia 1993; 7:1211–1218.
62. Welte K, Platzer E, Lu L, et al. Purification and biochemical characterization of human pluripotent hematopoietic colony-stimulating factor. Proc Natl Acad Sci USA 1985; 82:1526–1530.
63. Platzer E, Welte K, Gabrilove JL, et al. Biological activities of a human pluripotent hematopoietic colony-stimulating factor on normal and leukemic cells. J Exp Med 1985; 162:1788–1801.
64. Souza LM, Boone TC, Gabrilove JC, et al. Recombinant human granulocyte colony-stimulating factor: effects on normal and leukemic cells. Science 1986; 232: 61–65.
65. Simmers RN, Webber LM, Shannon MF, et al. Localization of the human G-CSF gene on chromosome 17 proximal to the breakpoint of the t(15;17) in acute promyelocytic leukemia. Blood 1987; 70:330–332.
66. Le Beau MM, Lemons RS, Carrino JJ, et al. Chromosomal localization of the human G-CSF gene to 17q11 proximal to the breakpoint of the t(15;17) in acute promyelocytic leukemia. Leukemia 1987; 1:795–799.
67. Tweardy DJ, Cannizzaro LA, Palumbo AP, et al. Molecular cloning and characterization of cDNA for human granulocyte colony-stimulating factor (G-CSF) from a glioblastoma multiform cell line and localization of the G-CSF gene to chromosome band 17q21. Oncogene Res 1987; 1:209–220.
68. Gandhi V, Du M, Kantarjian HM, Plunkett W. effect of granulocyte-macrophage colony-stimulating factor on the metabolism of arabinosylcytosine triphosphate in blasts during therapy of patients with chronic myelogenous leukemia. Leukemia 1994; 8:1463–1468.
69. Tafuri A, Andreeff M. Kinetic rationale for cytokine-induced recruitment of myeloblastic leukemia followed by cycle-specific chemotherapy in vitro. Leukemia 1990; 4:826–834.

70. Aglietta M, Piacibello W, Sanavio F, et al. Kinetics of human hematopoietic cells after in vivo administration of granulocyte-macrophage colony-stimulating factor. J Clin Invest 1989; 83:551–557.
71. Cannistra SA, Groshek P, Griffin JD. Granulocyte-macrophage colony-stimulating factor enhances the cytotoxic effect of cytosine arabinoside in acute myeloblastic leukemia and in the myeloid blast crisis phase of chronic myeloid leukemia. Leukemia 1989; 3:328–334.
72. Griffin JD, Young D, Hermann F, et al. Effect of recombinant human granulocyte-macrophage colony-stimulating factor on proliferation of clonogenic cells in acute myeloblastic leukemia. Blood 1986; 67:1448–1453.
73. Jakubowski A, Andreeff M, Tafuri A, et al. In vivo and in vitro studies of rhG-CSF in acute non-lymphocytic leukemia. Blood 1989; 74(suppl 1):247a. Abstract.
74. Hiddemann W, Kiehl M, Zuhlsdorf M, et al. Granulocyte-macrophage colony-stimulating factor and interleukin-3 enhance the incorporation of cytosine arabinoside into the DNA of leukemic blasts and the cytotoxic effects on clonogenic cells from patients with acute myeloid leukemia. Semin Oncol 1992; 19(suppl 4):31–37.
75. Miyauchi J, Kelleher CA, Wang C, et al. Growth factors influence the sensitivity of leukemia stem cells to cytosine arabinoside in culture. Blood 1989; 73:1272–1278.
76. Bhalla K, Birkhofer M, Arlin A, et al. Effect of recombinant GM-CSF on the metabolism of cytosine arabinoside in normal and leukemic human bone marrow cells. Leukemia 1988; 2:810–813.
77. Van der Lely N, De Witte T, Muus P, et al. Growth factors enhance the toxicity of cytosine arabinoside towards leukemic clonogenic cells with self-renewal capacity. Exp Hematol 1990; 18:615. Abstract.
78. Estey E, Thall PF, Kantarjian H, et al. Treatment of new diagnosed acute myelogenous leukemia with granulocyte-macrophage colony-stimulating factor (GM-CSF) before and during continuous-infusion high-dose ara-C+ daunorubicin: comparison with patients treated without GM-CSF. Blood 1992; 79:2246–2255.
79. Estey E, Thall P, Andreeff M, et al. Use of granulocyte colony-stimulating factor before, during, and after fludarabine plus cytarabine induction therapy of newly diagnosed acute myelogenous leukemia or myelodysplastic syndromes: comparison with fludarabine plus cytarabine without granulocyte colony-stimulating factor. J Clin Oncol 1994; 12:671–678.
80. Ohno R, Tomonaga M, Kobayashi T, et al. Effect of granulocyte colony-stimulating factor after intensive induction therapy in relapsed or refractory acute leukemia. N Engl J Med 1990; 323:871–877.
81. Ohno R, Naoe T, Kanamaru A, et al. A double-blind controlled study of granulocyte-colony-stimulating factor started two days before induction chemotherapy in refractory acute myeloid leukemia. Blood 1994; 83:2086–2092.
82. Witz F, Harousseau JL, Cahn JY, et al. GM-CSF during and after remission induction treatment for elderly patients with acute myeloid leukemia. Blood 1994; 84(suppl 1):231a. Abstract.
83. Rowe JM, Andersen JP, Mazza JJ, et al. A randomized placebo-controlled phase

III study of granulocyte-macrophage colony-stimulating factor in adult patients (>55–70 years of age) with acute myelogenous leukemia (AML): a study of the Eastern Cooperative Oncology Group (E1490). Blood 1995; 86:457–462.
84. Stone RM, George SL, Berg DT, et al. Granulocyte-macrophage colony-stimulating factor after initial chemotherapy for elderly patients with primary acute myelogenous leukemia. N Engl J Med 1995; 332:1671–1677.
85. Dombret H, Chastang C, Fenaux P, et al. A controlled study of recombinant human granulocyte colony-stimulating factor in elderly patients after treatment for acute myelogenous leukemia. N Engl J Med 1995; 332:1678–1683.
86. Heil G, Chadid L, Hoelzer D, et al. GM-CSF in a double blind randomized placebo controlled trial in therapy of adults patients with de novo acute myeloid leukemia (AML). Leukemia 1995; 9:3–9.
87. Zittoun R, Suciu S, Mandelli F, et al. Granulocyte-macrophage colony-stimulating factor associated with induction treatment of acute myelogenous leukemia: a randomized trial by the European Organization for Research and Treatment of Cancer Leukemia Cooperative Group. J Clin Oncol 1996; 14:2150–2159.
88. Revel M. Differentiation therapy. In: Waxman S, ed. New York: Raven Press, 1991:35–61.
89. Zafriri D, Argaman M, Canaani E, Kimchi A. Induction of protein-tyrosine-phosphatase activity by interleukin-6 in M1 myeloblastic cells and analysis of possible counteractions by the BCR-ABL oncogene. Proc Natl Acad Sci USA 1993; 90:477–481.
90. Ferrari S, Grande A, Manfredini R, et al. Expression of interleukins 1, 3, 6, stem cell factor and their receptors in acute leukemia blast cells and in normal peripheral lymphocytes and monocytes. Eur J Haematol 1993; 50:141–148.
91. Siitonen T, Savolainen ER, Koistinen P, et al. Expression of the c-kit proto-oncogene in myeloproliferative disorders and myelodysplastic syndromes. Leukemia 1994; 8:631–637.
92. Pietsch T, Urte K, Steffens U, et al. Effects of human stem cell factor (c-kit ligand) on proliferation of myeloid leukemia cells: heterogeneity in response and synergy with other hematopoietic growth factors. Blood 1992; 80:1199–1206.
93. Sutherland HJ, Hogge DE, Cook DE, Eaves CJ. Alternative mechanisms with or without steel factor support primitive human hematopoiesis. Blood 1993; 81:1465–1470.
94. Agarwal R, Doren S, Hicks B, Dunbar CE. Long-term culture of chronic myelogenous leukemia marrow cells on stem cell factor-deficient stroma favors benign progenitors. Blood 1995; 85:1306–1312.
95. Oster W, Herrmann F, Mertelsmann R. Erythropoietin for the treatment of patients with anemia of malignancy. In: Mertelsmann R, Herrmann F, eds. Hematopoietic Growth Factors in Clinical Applications. New York: Marcel Dekker, 1990:141–148.
96. Kitagawa S, Saito M, Miura Y. Recombinant human erythropoietin at high doses stimulates thrombopoiesis: treatment for protracted severe myelosuppression complicating interferon-alpha and busulfan therapy for chronic myelogenous leukemia (letter). Eur J Haematol 1995; 55:285–286.

97. Klagsbrun M. The fibroblast growth factor family: structural and biological properties. Prog Growth Factor Res 1989; 1:207–235.
98. Oliver LJ, Rifkin DB, Gabrilove J, et al. Long-term culture of human bone marrow stromal cells in the presence of basic fibroblast growth factor. Growth Factors 1990; 3:231–236.
99. Wilson EL, Rifkin DB, Kelly F, et al. Basic fibroblast growth factor stimulates myelopoiesis in long-term human bone marrow cultures. Blood 1991; 77:954–960.
100. Komatsu K, Nakamura H, Masaoka T, Akedo H. Synergistic effects of basic fibroblast growth factor and hematopoietic growth factors on colony formation of K562 human leukemic cells. Leukemia 1995; 9:1565–1568.
101. Armstrong E, Vainikka A, Partanen J, et al. Expression of fibroblast growth factor receptors in human leukemia cells. Cancer Res 1992; 52:2004–2007.
102. Shows T, Eddy R, Haley L, et al. Interleukin-2 (IL-2) is assigned to human chromosome 4. Somatic Cell Mol Genet 1984; 10:315–318.
103. Dilloo D, Hanenberg H, Lion T, Burdach S. IL-2 inhibits proliferation of K562 cells and reduces accumulation of bcr/abl mRNA and oncoprotein. Leukemia 1995; 9:419–424.
104. Verma UN, Bagg A, Brown E, Mazumder A. Interleukin-2 activation of human bone marrow in long-term cultures: an effective strategy for purging and generation of anti-tumor cytotoxic effectors. Bone Marrow Transplant 1994; 13:115–123.
105. Pearson DA, Abraham VS, Sachs DH, et al. Selective inhibition of CD4 graft-versus-host activity in IL-2 treated mice. FASEB J 1992; 6:1693. Abstract.
106. Abraham VS, Sachs DH, Sykes M. Mechanism of protection from graft-versus-host disease mortality by IL-2. III. Early reduction in donor T cell subsets and expansion of a CD3+CD4–CD8– cell population. J Immunol 1992; 148:3746–3752.
107. Kloosterman TC, Martens AC, Van Bekkum DW, Hagenbeek A. The graft-vs-leukemia reaction (GvLR) and interleukin-2 (IL-2) after allogeneic bone marrow transplantation (BMT): preclinical studies. Exp Hematol 1992; 20:721. Abstract.
108. Nagler A, Ackerstein A, Barak V, Slavin S. Treatment of chronic myelogenous leukemia with recombinant human interleukin-2 and interferon-alpha 2a. J Hematother 1994; 3:75–82.
109. Soiffer R, Murray C, Ritz J. Low-dose interleukin-2 (IL-2) following bone marrow transplantation (BMT) for hematological malignancy. Proc Annu Meet Am Soc Clin Oncol 1993; 12:A982. Abstract.
110. Soiffer RJ, Murray C, Gonin R, Ritz J. Effect of low-dose interleukin-2 on disease relapse after T-cell-depleted allogeneic bone marrow transplantation. Blood 1994; 84:64–71.
111. Giralt S, Escudier S, Kantarjian H, et al. Preliminary results of treatment with filgrastin for relapse leukemia and myelodysplasia after allogeneic bone marrow transplantation. N Engl J Med 1993; 329:757–761.
112. Anasetti C, Hansen JA, Waldmann TA, et al. Treatment of acuter graft-versus-host disease with humanized anti-Tac: an antibody that binds to the interleukin-2 receptor. Blood 1994; 84:1320–1327.

113. Anasetti C, Martin PJ, Hansen JA, et al. A phase I/II study evaluating the murine anti-IL-2 receptor antibody 2A3 for treatment of acute graft-versus-host disease. Transplantation 1990; 50:49–50.
114. Herve P, Wijdenes J, Bergerat JP, et al. Treatment of corticosteroid resistant graft-versus-host disease by in vivo administration of anti-interleukin-2 receptor monoclonal antibody (B-B10). Blood 1990; 75:1017–1023.
115. Ferrant A, Latinne D, Bazin H. Prophylaxis of graft-versus-host disease in identical sibling donor bone marrow transplant by anti-IL-2 receptor monoclonal antibody LO-Tact-1. Bone Marrow Transplant 1995; 16:577–581.
116. Irving SG, Zipfel PF, Balle J, et al. Two inflammatory mediator cytokine genes are closely linked and variably amplified on chromosome 17q. Nucleic Acids Res 1990; 18:3261–3270.
117. Lord BI, Wright E, Lajtha LG. Actions of the hematopoietic stem cell proliferation inhibitor. Biochem Pharmacol 1979; 28:1843–1848.
118. Wright EG, Sheridan P, Moore MAS. An inhibitor of murine stem cell proliferation produced by normal human bone marrow. Leuk Res 1980; 4:309–314.
119. Lord BI, Wright EG. Sources of hematopoietic stem cell proliferation stimulators and inhibitors. Blood Cells 1980; 6:581–594.
120. Graham GJ, Wright EG, Hewick R, et al. Identification and characterization of an inhibitor of haemopoietic stem cell proliferation. Nature 1990; 344:442–444.
121. Graham GJ, Pragnell IB. Negative regulators of hemopoiesis—current advances. Prog Growth Factor Res 1990; 2:181–192.
122. Ferrajoli A, Talpaz M, Zipf TF, et al. Inhibition of acute myelogenous leukemia progenitor proliferation by macrophage inflammatory protein 1-α. Leukemia 1994; 8:798–805.
123. Chasty RC, Lucas GS, Owen-Lynch PJ, et al. Macrophage inflammatory protein-1 alpha receptors are present on cells enriched for CD34 expression from patients with chronic myeloid leukemia. Blood 1995; 86:4270–4277.
124. Nirsimloo N, Gordon MY. Progenitor cells in the blood and marrow of patients with chronic phase myeloid leukemia respond differently to macrophage inflammatory protein-1 alpha. Leuk Res 1995; 19:319–323.
125. Paul WE: Interleukin-4. A prototypic immunoregulatory lymphokine. Blood 1991; 77:1859–1870.
126. Le Beau MM, Lemons RS, Espinoza R III, et al. Interleukin-4 and interleukin-5 map to human chromosome 5 in a region encoding growth factors and receptors and are deleted in myeloid leukemias with del(5q). Blood 1989; 73:647–650.
127. Mossmann TR, Cherwinski H, Bond MW, et al. Two types of murine helper T cell clones. Definition according to profiles of lymphokines, activities, and secreted proteins. J Immunol 1986; 136:2438–2357.
128. Plaut M, Pierce JH, Watson CJ, et al. Mast cell lines produce lymphokines in response to cross linkage of FcεR1 or to calcium ionophores. Nature 1989; 339: 64–67.
129. Estrov Z, Markowitz AB, Kurzrock R, et al. Suppression of chronic myelogenous leukemia colony growth by interleukin-4. Leukemia 1993; 7:214–220.
130. Ferrajoli A, Talpaz M, Markowitz AB, et al. Divergent effect of interleukin-4 (IL-

4) in chronic myelogenous leukemia (CML), acute myeloblastic leukemia (AML), and normal marrow progenitor proliferation. Blood 1991; 78(suppl 1):382a. Abstract.
131. Ferrajoli A, Zipf TF, Talpaz M, et al. Growth factors controlling interleukin-4 action on hematopoietic progenitors. Ann Hematol 1993; 67:227–284.
132. Perschel C, Green I, Paul WE. Interleukin-4 induces a substance in bone marrow stromal cells that reversibly inhibits factor-dependent and factor-independent cell proliferation. Blood 1989; 73:1130–1141.
133. Sonoda Y, Okuda T, Yokota S, et al. Actions of human interleukin-4/B-cell stimulatory factor on proliferation and differentiation on enriched hematopoietic progenitor cells in culture. Blood 1990; 75:1615–1621.
134. Vellenga E, de Wold J, Beentjes JAM, et al. Divergent effects of interleukin-4 (IL-4) on the granulocyte colony-stimulating factor and IL-3 supported colony formation from normal and leukemic bone marrow cells. Blood 1990; 75:633–637.
135. Rennick DG, Yang L, Muller-Sieburg C, et al. Interleukin-4 (B-cell stimulatory factor 1) can enhance and antagonize the factor dependent growth of hematopoietic progenitor cells. Proc Natl Acad Sci USA 1987; 84:6889–6893.
136. Gasparetto C, Smith C, Gillio A, et al. Enrichment of peripheral blood stem cells with cytokine treatment in a preclinical primate model. Blood 1990; 76(suppl 1):541a. Abstract.
137. Wong HL, Costa GL, Lotze MT, et al. Interleukin (IL)-4 differentially regulates monocytes IL-1 family gene expression and synthesis in vitro and in vivo. J Exp Med 1993; 177:775–781.
138. Jansen JH, Fibbe WE, Wientjens GHM, et al. Differential stimulatory and inhibitory effects of interleukin-4 on granulocyte and monocytic colony formation in human bone marrow cultures. Blood 1990; 76(suppl 1):148a. Abstract.
139. Wetzler M, Kurzrock R, Estrov Z, et al. Interleukin-4 modulates aberrant cytokine expression in adherent layers derived from myelodysplastic and acute myelogenous leukemia patients. Blood 1992; 80(suppl 1):463a.
140. Ferrajoli A, Talpazx M, Hirsch-Ginsberg C, et al. Interleukin-4 alters human bone marrow stroma formation and modulates its interaction with hematopoietic progenitors. Blood 80(suppl 1):399a. Abstract.
141. Wetzler M, Estrov Z, Talpaz M, et al. Leukemia inhibitory factor in long-term adherent layer cultures: increased levels of bioactive protein in leukemia and modulation by IL-4, IL-1-beta, and TNF-alpha. Cancer Res 1994; 54:1837–1842.
142. Lloyd AR, Oppenheim JJ. Poly's lament: the neglected role of the polymorphonuclear neutrophils in the afferent limb of the immune response. Immunol Today 1992; 13:169–172.
143. Cassatella MA, Bazzoni F, Ceska M, et al. IL-8 production by human polymorphonuclear leukocytes. J Immunol 1992; 148:3216–3220.
144. Matsushima K, Oppenheim JJ. Interleukin 8 and MCAF: novel inflammatory cytokines inducible by IL-1 and TNF. Cytokine 1989; 1:2–13.
145. Mukaida N, Harada A, Yasumoto K, et al. Properties of pro-inflammatory cell type-specific chemotactic cytokines, interleukin-8 (IL-8) and monocyte chemotactic and activating factor (MCAF). Microbiol Immunol 1992; 36:773–789.

146. Strieter RM, Kunkel SL, Showell HJ, et al. Endothelial cell gene expression of a neutrophil chemotactic factor by TNF-α, LPS, and IL-1-1β. Science 1989; 243: 1467–1469.
147. Paccaud JP, Shifferli JA, Baggiolini M. NAP-1/IL-8 induces upregulation of CR1 receptors in human neutrophil leukocytes. Biochem Biophys Res Commun 1990; 166:187–192.
148. Tobler A, Meier R, Seitz M, et al. Glucocorticoids downregulate gene expression of GM-CSF, NAP-1/IL-8, and IL-6, but not of M-CSF in human fibroblasts. Blood 1992; 79:45–51.
149. Aman MJ, Rudolf G, Goldschmitt J, et al. Type-I interferons are potent inhibitors of interleukin-8 production in hematopoietic and bone marrow stromal cells. Blood 1993; 82:2371–2378.
150. Moore KW, O'Garra A, de Waal Malefyt R, et al. Interleukin-10. Annu Rev Immunol 1992; 11:165–190.
151. Weber-Nordt RM, Meraz MA, Schreider RB. Lipopolysaccharide-dependent induction of IL-10 receptor expression on murine fibroblasts. J Immunol 1994; 153: 3734–3744.
152. Korsmeyer SJ, Shutter JR, Veis DJ, et al. BCL2/Bax: a rheostat that regulates an anti-oxidant pathway and cell death. Semin Cancer Biol 1993; 4:327–332.
153. Bruserud O, Tore Gjertsen B, Terje Brustugun O, et al. Effects of interleukin-10 on blast cells derived from patients with acute myelogenous leukemia. Leukemia 1995; 9:1910–1920.
154. Neben S, Turner K. The biology of interleukin-11. Stem Cells 1993; 11(suppl 2): 156–162.
155. Du XX, Williams DA. Interleukin-11. A multifunctional growth factor derived from the hematopoietic microenvironment. Blood 1994; 83:2023–2030.
156. Girasole G, Passeri G, Jika RL, Manolagas SC. Interleukin-11: a new cytokine critical for osteoclast development. J Clin Invest 1994; 93:1516–1524.
157. Nauts HC. Bacteria and cancer—antagonisms and benefits. Cancer Surv 1989; 8: 713–723.
158. Old CJ. Tumor necrosis factor. Sci Am 1988; 258:69–75.
159. Caux C, Sealand S, Favre C, et al. Tumor necrosis factor-alpha strongly potentiates interleukin-3 and granulocyte-macrophage colony-stimulating factor-induced proliferation of human CD34+ hematopoietic progenitor cells. Blood 1990; 75: 2292–2298.
160. Ferrajoli A, Talpaz M, Kurzrock R, et al. Analysis of the effects of tumor necrosis factor inhibitor in human hematopoiesis. Stem Cells 1993; 11:112–119.
161. Loetscher H, Steinmetz M, Lesslauer W. Tumor necrosis factor. Receptors and inhibitors. Cancer Cells 1991; 3:221–226.
162. Murphy M, Perussia B, Trinchieri G. Effects of recombinant tumor necrosis factor, lymphotoxin, and immune interferon on proliferation and differentiation of enriched hematopoietic precursor cells. Exp Hematol 1988; 16:131–138.
163. Freedman MH, Cohen A, Grunberger T, et al. Central role of tumor necrosis factor and GM-CSF in the pathogenesis of juvenile chronic myelogenous leukemia. Br J Haematol 1992; 80:40–48.

164. Hoang T, Levy B, Onetto N, et al. Tumor necrosis factor-alpha stimulates the growth of clonogenic cells of acute myeloblastic leukemia in synergy with granulocyte/macrophage colony-stimulating factor. J Exp Med 1989; 170:15–26.
165. Salem M, Dewel R, Touw I, et al. Modulation of colony-stimulating factor-dependent growth of acute myeloid leukemia by tumor necrosis factor. Leukemia 1987; 4:37–45.
166. Elbaz O, Budel LM, Hoogerbrugge H, et al. Tumor necrosis factor regulates the expression of granulocyte-macrophage colony-stimulating factor and interleukin-3 receptors on human acute myeloid leukemia cells. Blood 1991; 77:989–995.
167. Munker R, Greither L, Darsow M, et al. Effects of tumor necrosis factor on primary human leukemia cells: ultrastructural changes. Acta Haematol 1993; 90:77–83.
168. Moritz T, Kloke O, Nagel-Hiemke M, et al. Tumor necrosis factor alpha modifies resistance to interferon alpha in vivo: first clinical data. Cancer Immunol Immunother 1992; 35:342–346.
169. Nagel-Hiemke M, Hiemke C, Kummer G, et al. Relation between leukocyte counts and cortisol secretion in CML patients undergoing combined TNF alpha/IFN alpha therapy. Ann Hematol 1992; 65:116–120.
170. Herrmann F, Helfrich SG, Lindemann A, et al. Elevated circulating levels of tumor necrosis factor predict unresponsiveness to treatment with interferon alfa-2b in chronic myelogenous leukemia. J Clin Oncol 1992; 10:631–634.
171. Holler E, Kolb HJ, Mittermüller J, et al. Modulation of acute graft-versus-host disease after allogeneic bone marrow transplantation by tumor necrosis factor α (TNFα) release in the course of pretransplant conditioning: role of conditioning regimens and prophylactic application of a monoclonal antibody neutralizing human TNFα (MAK 195F). Blood 1995; 86:890–899.
172. Holyoake TL, Freshney MG, Sproul AM, et al. Contrasting effects of rh-MIP-1 alpha and TGF-beta 1 on chronic myeloid leukemia progenitors in vitro. Stem Cells 1993; 11:122–128.
173. Murohashi I, Endho K, Nishida S, et al. Differential effects of TGF-beta 1 on normal and leukemic human hematopoietic cell proliferation. Exp Hematol 1995; 23:970–977.
174. Motyl T, Kasterka M, Grzelkowska K, et al. TGF-beta 1 inhibits polyamine biosynthesis in K562 leukemic cells. Ann Hematol 1993; 67:285–288.
175. Cashman JD, Eaves AC, Eaves CJ. Granulocyte-macrophage colony-stimulating factor modulation of the inhibitory effect of transforming growth factor-beta on normal and leukemic human hematopoietic progenitor cells. Leukemia 1992; 6:886–892.
176. Federico MH, Snitcovsky I, Maistro S, et al. Integrin receptors and TGF-beta expression in chronic myeloid leukemia cells. Braz J Med Biol Res 1994; 27:2267–2271.
177. Hemler ME. VLA proteins in the integrin family: structures, functions, and their role in leukocytes. Annu Rev Immunol 1990; 8:365–400.
178. Elices MJ, Osborn L, Takada Y, et al. VCAM-1 on activated endothelium interact

with the leukocyte integrin VLA-4 at a site distinct from VLA-4/fibronectin binding site. Cell 1990; 60:577–584.
179. Schwartz BR, Wayner EA, Carlos TM, et al. Identification of surface proteins mediating adherence of CD11/CD18-deficient lymphoblastoid cells to cultured human endothelium. J Clin Invest 1990; 85:2019–2022.
180. Shimizu Y, Shaw S. Lymphocyte adhesion mediated by VLA (beta 1) integrins. Chem Immunol 1991; 50:34–54.
181. Vennegoor CJ, van de Wiel–van Kemenade E, Huijbens RJF, et al. Role of LFA-1 and VLA-4 in the adhesion of cloned normal and LFA-1 (CD11/CD18)-deficient T cells to cultured endothelial cells: indication for a new adhesion pathway. J Immunol 1992; 148:1093–1101.
182. Vonderheide RH, Springer TA. Lymphocyte adhesion through very late antigen 4: evidence for a novel binding site in the alternative spliced domain of vascular adhesion molecule 1 and an additional α4 integrin counter-receptor on stimulated endothelium. J Exp Med 1992; 175:1433–1442.
183. van Kooyk Y, van de Wiel–van Kemenade E, Weder P, et al. Lymphocyte function-associated antigen 1 dominates very late antigen 4 in binding of activated T cells to endothelium. J Exp Med 1993; 177:185–190.
184. Carlos T, Kovach N, Schwartz B, et al. Human monocytes bind to two cytokine-induced adhesive ligands on cultured human endothelial cells; endothelial-leukocyte adhesion molecule-1 and vascular cell adhesion molecule-1. Blood 1991; 77:2266–2271.
185. Jonjic N, Jilek P, Bernasconi S, et al. Molecules involved in the adhesion and cytotoxicity of activated monocytes on endothelial cells. J Immunol 1992; 148:2080–2083.
186. Dobrina A, Menegazzi R, Carlos TM, et al. Mechanisms of eosinophil adherence to cultured vascular endothelial cells: eosinophils bind to the cytokine-induced endothelial ligand vascular cell adhesion molecule-1 via the very late activation antigen-4 integrin receptor. J Clin Invest 1991; 88:20–26.
187. Bochner BS, Luscinskas FW, Gimbrone MA Jr, et al. Adhesion of human basophils, eosinophils, and neutrophils to interleukin-1 activated human vascular endothelial cells: contribution of endothelial cell adhesion molecules. J Exp Med 1991; 173:1553–1557.
188. Schleimer RP, Sterbinsky SA, Kayser J, et al. IL-4 induces adherence of human eosinophils and basophils but no neutrophils to endothelium: association with expression of VCAM-1. J Immunol 1992; 148:1086–1092.
189. Allavena P, Paganin C, Martin-Padura I, et al. Molecules and structures involved in the adhesion of natural killer cells to vascular endothelium. J Exp Med 1991; 173:439–448.
190. Verfaillie CM. Direct contact between human primitive hematopoietic progenitors and bone marrow stroma is not required for long term in vitro hematopoiesis. Blood 1992; 79:2821–2826.
191. Hurley R, McCarthy JB, Verfaillie CM. Direct adhesion to bone marrow stroma via fibronectin receptors inhibits hematopoietic progenitor proliferation. J Clin Invest 1995; 96:511.
192. Hurley R, McCarthy JB, Verfaillie CM. Actin polymerization is required for a4b1

integrin dependent inhibition of hematopoietic progenitor proliferation. Blood 1994; 84(suppl 1):416a. Abstract.
193. Dube ID, Kalousek DK, Coulombel L, et al. Cytogenetic studies of early myeloid progenitor compartments in Ph1-positive chronic myeloid leukemia. II. Long-term culture reveals the persistence of Ph1-negative progenitors in treated as well as newly diagnosed patients. Blood 1984; 63:1172–1177.
194. Dube ID, Gupta CM, Kalousek DK, et al. Cytogenetic studies of early myeloid progenitor compartments in Ph1-positive chronic myeloid leukemia (CML). I. Persistence of Ph1-negative committed progenitors that are suppressed from differentiation in vivo. Br J Haematol 1984; 54:633–644.
195. Coulombel L, Kalousek DK, Eaves CJ, et al. Long-term marrow culture reveals chromosomally normal hematopoietic progenitor cells in patients with Philadelphia chromosome-positive chronic myelogenous leukemia. N Engl J Med 1983; 308:1493–1498.
196. Gordon MY, Dowding CR, Riley GP, et al. Altered adhesive interactions with marrow stroma of hematopoietic progenitor cells in chronic myelogenous leukemia. Nature 1987; 328:342–344.
197. Verfaillie CM, McCarthy JB, McGlave PB. Mechanisms underlying abnormal trafficking of malignant progenitors in chronic myelogenous leukemia. Decreased adhesion to stroma and fibronectin but increased adhesion to the basement membrane components laminin and collagen type IV. J Clin Invest 1992; 90:1232–1241.
198. Eaves AC, Cashman JD, Gaboury LA, et al. Unregulated proliferation of primitive chronic myeloid leukemia progenitors in the presence of normal marrow adherent cells. Proc Natl Acad Sci USA 1986; 83:5306–5310.
199. Dowding CR, Gordon MY, Goldman JM. Primitive progenitor cells in the blood of patients with chronic granulocytic leukemia. Int J Cell Cloning 1986; 4:331–340.
200. Lundell BI, McCarthy JB, Kovach NL, Verfaillie CM. Activation-dependent $\alpha 5\beta 1$-integrin-mediated adhesion to fibronectin decreases proliferation of chronic myelogenous leukemia progenitors and K562 cells. Blood 1996; 87:2450–2458.
201. Gutterman JU. Cytokine therapeutics: lessons from interferon-α. Proc Natl Acad Sci USA 1994; 91:1198–1205.
202. Sutherland HJ, Hogge DE, Lansdorp PM, et al. Quantitation, mobilization, and clinical use of long-term culture-initiating cells in blood cell autografts. J Hematotherapy 1995; 4:3–10.
203. Eaves CJ, Barnett MJ, Eaves AC. In vitro culture of bone marrow cells for autografting in CML. Leukemia 1993; 7(suppl 2):S126–S129.

19
ABL Protein Tyrosine Kinase Inhibitors
Potential Clinical Role in CML

Brian J. Druker
Oregon Health Sciences University, Portland, Oregon

INTRODUCTION

The discovery of a tyrosine kinase oncogene as the transforming protein of the Rous sarcoma virus has led to the recognition of the prominent role of tyrosine kinases in cellular growth, differentiation, and signaling. Despite the growing number of tyrosine kinases, approximately 100, and their clear association with acutely transforming retroviruses, the association between tyrosine kinases and human cancers has been limited. Chronic myelogenous leukemia (CML) was the first human disease discovered to be associated with a constitutively activated tyrosine kinase, the ABL protein tyrosine kinase, and CML remains one of the few human cancers where a tyrosine kinase appears to have a causative role.

The molecular consequences of the translocation resulting in the Philadelphia (Ph) chromosome are the juxtaposition of BCR-encoded sequences on chromosome 22 with c-ABL sequences translocated from chromosome 9 (1–3). The BCR-ABL fusion gene is transcribed and translated into a 210-kD chimeric protein in which the first exon of a c-ABL is replaced by BCR sequences (4,5). The fusion protein, p210BCR-ABL, has increased protein tyrosine kinase activity compared to c-ABL (6). A large body of scientific evidence, including animal studies described in Chapter 3 supports BCR-ABL being the cause of CML. Numerous studies have shown that the ABL protein tyrosine kinase activity is required for the transforming activities of the BCR-ABL oncoprotein (7,8). Although the BCR protein has several biochemical activities, one of the most important functions of the BCR protein in the BCR-ABL fusion protein is to activate the protein tyrosine kinase activity of ABL (9,10). Further, the tyrosine kinase activity of the BCR-ABL fusion protein correlates with the aggressiveness of the disease. Thus, the p185 version of BCR-ABL, associated with acute lymphoblastic leukemia, has nearly 10-fold greater tyrosine kinase activity than the p210 form seen in CML (7). Because the BCR-ABL protein is a novel intracellular protein with elevated tyrosine kinase activity, an inhibitor of the ABL protein tyrosine kinase could be a potentially useful therapeutic agent for CML. A further impetus to develop agents targeted against the molecular abnormality in CML has come from studies of interferon-alpha demonstrating that a cytogenetic response is independently associated with a survival advantage (11–13). Thus, an ABL protein tyrosine kinase inhibitor, if capable of decreasing the percentage of BCR-ABL-positive cells, might prolong survival of patients with CML. Specific inhibitors of the ABL protein tyrosine kinase have been synthesized, have shown promise in preclinical testing, and are likely to enter clinical trials in the near future.

REQUIREMENTS FOR SUCCESS

For therapy with an ABL protein tyrosine kinase inhibitor to be successful, either as an in vivo therapy or ex vivo as a purging agent for autologous bone marrow transplantation, several conditions must be satisfied: (1) BCR-ABL protein must be expressed; (2) BCR-ABL-negative hematopoietic progenitors must be present; (3) the inhibitor must be sufficiently selective to kill BCR-ABL-positive but not BCR-ABL-negative cells (as a corollary to this, inhibition of normal cellular ABL protein tyrosine kinase activity must not be toxic to cells); and (4) other physical properties of the inhibitor must be favorable. For example, since BCR-ABL is an intracellular protein, the inhibitor must be cell-permeable.

BCR-ABL Protein Expression

There is ample evidence for the presence of BCR-ABL protein in peripheral blood samples from CML stable-phase patients (14,15). However, the issue is whether or not there are hematopoietic progenitor cells that are positive at the DNA level for the Ph chromosome, but do not express BCR-ABL RNA or protein. There was one report of such cells in colony-forming assays of hematopoietic progenitors from CML patients (16). That is, these cells contained the Ph chromosome, but were negative for BCR-ABL RNA by polymerase chain reaction (PCR). However, a subsequent report suggests that virtually all Ph chromosome-positive cells are positive for BCR-ABL transcripts (17). Since these studies were done with only 50–100 cells, analysis of protein was not possible.

Nevertheless, the evidence suggests that BCR-ABL is expressed in Ph chromosome-positive hematopoietic progenitor cells. This is consistent with models of CML in which the constitutively activated ABL protein tyrosine kinase drives the excess myeloid proliferation characteristic of the disease.

Presence of BCR-ABL-Negative Hematopoietic Progenitor Cells

If all of the hematopoietic progenitor cells in CML patients express BCR-ABL protein, then treatment with an agent that eliminated BCR-ABL-positive cells might result in severe bone marrow aplasia. However, several approaches have demonstrated the presence of Ph chromosome-negative or BCR-ABL-negative hematopoietic progenitor cells in a significant percentage of CML patients (18,19). For years, it has been known that a proportion of patients treated with busulfan or combination chemotherapy will recover with Ph chromosome-negative hematopoiesis (20–24). This observation has been exploited in clinical trials of autologous peripheral blood stem cell transplantation. In these clinical trials, the Ph chromosome-negative hematopoietic progenitors, which predominate on recovery from intensive chemotherapy, have been collected for autologous peripheral blood stem cell transplantation (25,26).

Recent experience with interferon-alpha has demonstrated that partial or complete cytogenetic responses are possible (27,28), again supporting the notion that Ph chromosome-negative hematopoiesis is present but suppressed in CML patients. This concept has also been demonstrated in long-term bone marrow culture with the finding that in the majority of cases, marrow from CML patients will produce Ph chromosome-negative hematopoietic cells, and that under certain culture conditions the Ph chromosome negative cells may have a growth advantage (29). This finding was the basis of a clinical trial in which patients underwent autologous bone marrow transplantation using bone marrow that had been cultured for 10 days (30). Thirteen of 21 patients engrafted with 100% Ph chromosome-negative hematopoiesis, however, all evaluable patients, had detectable Ph chromosome positivity at a median of 12 months following transplantation (30). Although ample evidence supports the presence of Ph chromosome-negative hematopoiesis in CML patients, one of the major obstacles to autologous transplantation has been the infusion of a significant number of Ph chromosome-positive cells. Methods to improve selection of Ph chromosome-negative cells or to purge the Ph chromosome-positive cells might improve the success of autologous transplantation.

Inhibition of Normal Cellular ABL Protein Tyrosine Kinase

Although it may be theoretically possible to synthesize a compound that would selectively inhibit activated forms of the ABL protein tyrosine kinase, such as

BCR-ABL, it is more likely that a compound with selectivity for the ABL protein tyrosine kinase will also inhibit the function of the normal cellular ABL protein tyrosine kinase. c-ABL is ubiquitously expressed and, although its function is currently unknown, there are several lines of evidence supporting possible functions. There is no clear evidence that c-ABL is required for cellular proliferation, and results of overexpression of c-ABL have suggested that it may negatively regulate cellular proliferation (31). ABL knockout mice have decreased neonatal viability and lymphopenia (32,33), suggesting a role for ABL in lymphoid development. However, studies with antisense oligonucleotides to c-ABL have shown an inhibition of colony formation by committed hematopoietic progenitor cells (34). This finding potentially limits the therapeutic usefulness of an ABL protein tyrosine kinase inhibitor and will be addressed later.

Other Considerations

Other considerations critical to the success of an ABL protein tyrosine kinase inhibitor include the potency and specificity of the inhibitor. Since BCR-ABL is an intracellular enzyme, another equally important feature is cell permeability to enable a compound to reach its target. Tissue distribution, specifically to the bone marrow, would be required for therapeutic use in vivo but would not be required for ex vivo purging. Other physical properties of an inhibitor, including its stability, metabolism to active or inactive products, and solubility, may also affect the therapeutic success of an inhibitor, both in vivo and in vitro. Lastly, the toxicity profile of the inhibitor in vivo will determine whether a therapeutic window for such a compound exists. However, many of these potential problems, including in vivo toxicity, would not necessarily prevent successful use for ex vivo purging of hematopoietic cells for autologous transplantation.

TYROSINE KINASE INHIBITORS

History

Because of the central role of protein tyrosine kinases in cellular proliferation, considerable effort has been directed toward the development of inhibitors of this enzyme activity as potential antineoplastic agents. Compounds that possess inhibitory activity for protein tyrosine kinases were initially isolated from natural sources in the early to mid-1980s and include the flavonoid, quercetin; the isoflavonoid, genistein; the antibiotic, herbimycin A; and erbstatin (35–37). Although these compounds have shown some specific activity by reverting of cells transformed by tyrosine kinase oncogenes to a nontransformed phenotype, none of these compounds have demonstrated specificity among tyrosine kinases.

ABL Protein Tyrosine Kinase Inhibitors

Moreover, many of these and similar compounds have activities independent of or in addition to their tyrosine kinase inhibitory activity that may contribute to cellular cytotoxicity. For example, genistein can inhibit topoisomerases and induce DNA strand breakage in vivo (36).

The next group of tyrosine kinase inhibitors reported was a series of synthetic compounds. One of the first steps toward producing a useful drug was reported by Yaish et al., who synthesized compounds, referred to as tyrphostins, that display specificity for individual tyrosine kinases (38). These and similar compounds and their potential uses in cancer and other diseases that involve tyrosine kinase-induced cellular proliferation have been reviewed (39). One of the tyrphostins, AG1112, capable of specifically inhibiting the ABL protein tyrosine kinase, was reported to induce differentiation and death of a BCR-ABL-positive, erythroid blast crisis, CML cell line, K562 (40,41). Similar data for induction of K562 differentiation has been obtained with genistein, herbimycin A, and erbstatin (42–44). However, only limited data regarding the selectivity of these compounds for BCR-ABL-transformed cells are available.

As the crystal structure of several protein kinases has been determined, it is now possible to rationally design compounds based on structure of the ATP binding site or active site of the enzyme. This, in combination with the knowledge of the structure of protein tyrosine kinase inhibitors, has allowed for the synthesis of inhibitors with increased potency and specificity. One such class of compounds are 2-phenylaminopyrimidine derivatives. One compound in this class, referred to as CGP 57148, is a potent inhibitor of the ABL protein tyrosine kinase (45). The chemical structures of several tyrosine kinase inhibitors is shown in Figure 1.

CGP 57148

In Vitro Profiling of CGP 57148

The ability of CGP 57148 to inhibit a panel of protein tyrosine and serine/threonine kinases is presented in Table 1. The concentration of compound resulting in a 50% reduction of kinase activity measured in vitro or a 50% reduction in tyrosine phosphorylation of the specific tyrosine kinase (IC50) is reported. These results shown that CGP 57148 is a potent inhibitor of the ABL protein tyrosine kinases with an IC50 of 0.038 µM in vitro for substrate phosphorylation by v-ABL, 0.025 µM for BCR-ABL and c-ABL, and 0.25 µM in cell-based assays of autophosphorylation of v-ABL or BCR-ABL (Table 1). This compares to an IC50 of 0.8 µM for inhibition of in vitro phosphorylation by the tyrphostin AG1112 (41). CGP 57148 did not significantly inhibit other protein kinases tested with the exception of the platelet-derived growth factor (PDGF) receptor tyrosine kinase and does not inhibit BCR-ABL protein expression.

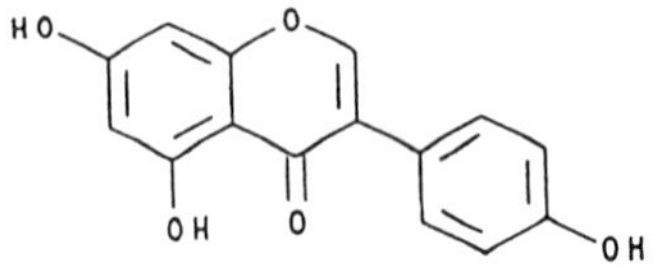

Genistein

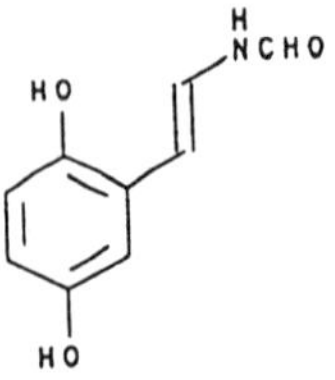

Erbstatin

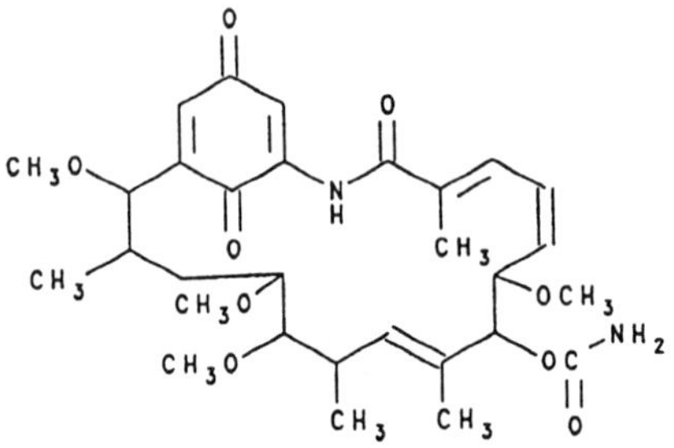

Herbimycin A

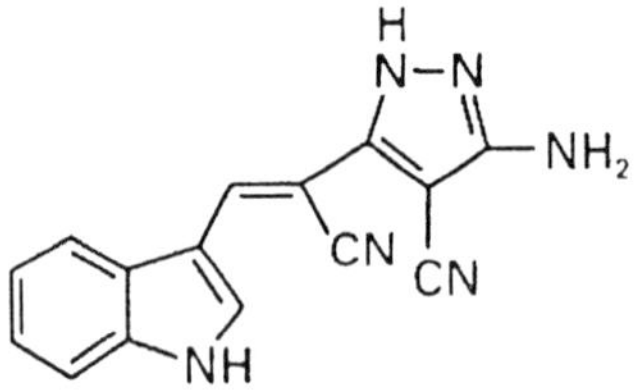

Tyrphostin AG1112

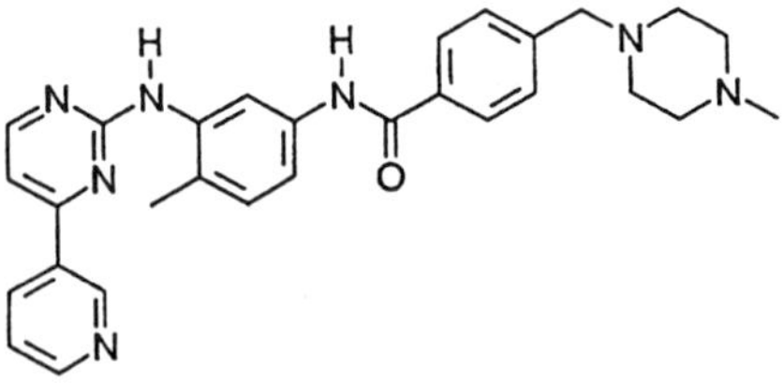

CGP 57148

Figure 1 Structure of various tyrosine kinase inhibitors.

Table 1 Profile of Inhibition of Protein Kinases by CGP 57148

Protein kinase	Substrate phosphorylation IC50 value (µM)	Cellular tyrosine phosphorylation IC50 (µM)
v-Abl	0.038	0.25
Bcr-Abl	0.025	0.25
c-Abl	0.025	
EGFR-R -ICD	>100	>100
Her-2/neu		>100
Insulin receptor		>100
IGF-1R		>100
PDGF-R		0.3
c-Src	>100	
V-Src		>100
c-Fgr	>100	
c-Lyn	>100	
v-Fms		>100
TPK-IIB	>100	
PKA	>500	
PPK	>100	
PKC α, β1, β2, γ, ε, σ, η, ζ	>100	
Casein kinases—1 and 2	>100	
cdc2/cyclin	>100	

Abbreviations: EGF-R -ICD, epidermal growth factor receptor–intracellular domain; IGF-1R, insulin-like growth factor-1 receptor; TPK, tyrosine protein kinase; PKA, protein kinase A; PPK, phosphorylase kinase; PKC, protein kinase C.
Reprinted with permission from Ref. 45.

Inhibition of Cellular Proliferation by CGP 57148

Although the in vitro profiling of CGP 57148 demonstrated a high degree of specificity, assays of cellular proliferation allow testing for inhibition of other kinases that might be required for cellular growth and proliferation. At a concentration of 1 and 10 µM CGP 57148 did not inhibit proliferation of a variety of myeloid cell lines, including 32Dcl3, MO7, and HL-60 (45). Since these concentrations are well above the IC50 for c-ABL, the results suggest that inhibition of c-ABL protein tyrosine kinase activity is not cytotoxic. Similarly, the absence of inhibition of IL-3-dependent cells such as 32Dcl3 and MO7 suggests that CGP 57148 does not inhibit tyrosine kinases, such as Jak-2, that are known to be required for IL-3-induced mitogenesis (46).

In contrast, derivatives of 32Dcl3 and MO7 that express BCR-ABL (32Dp210 and MO7p210) and are factor-independent for proliferation, undergo an apoptotic cell death within 24–48 hours of incubation with doses of 1 or 10 µM CGP 57148 in the absence of exogenous growth factor (45). Similar results have been obtained with 32Dcl3 derivative that expresses the p185 form of BCR-ABL. Addition of growth factor did not rescue the MO7p210 cells, but resulted in survival without proliferation of the 32Dp210 cells. The reason for the discrepancy between these two cell lines is not clear. CGP 57148 also induces erythroid differentiation and cell death of the human BCR-ABL-positive K562 cell line (45). The proliferation of a derivative of 32Dcl3 cells that express v-SRC was not affected by incubation with either 1 or 10 µM CGP 57148. Thus, the compound appears to be selectively toxic to cells expressing the constitutively active BCR-ABL protein tyrosine kinase.

32Dcl3 cells expressing BCR-ABL or v-SRC are capable of forming tumors in syngeneic mice. In assays of tumor formation, in which syngeneic mice were inoculated with 32Dp210 or 32Dv-SRC cells followed by treatment with CGP 57148, there was a dose-dependent inhibition of tumor growth of BCR-ABL-inoculated mice with no effects on animals inoculated with v-SRC-expressing cells (45). However, this compound has not been tested in animal models of CML, such as SCID/NOD mouse models using human CML cells or murine models using retroviral expression of BCR-ABL in hematopoietic progenitors cells.

Inhibition of Colony Formation of Hematopoietic Cells by CGP 57148

CGP 57148 has also been tested in assays of hematopoietic colony formation (45). Because of the report of antisense oligonucleotides to c-ABL-inhibiting colony formation (34), bone marrow samples from patients undergoing bone marrow transplantation for a variety of nonleukemic disorders were analyzed for colony formation in the presence of CGP 57148. At doses of 1 µM, there was no inhibition of BFU-E or CFU-GM colony formation, and only a 10–15% inhibition occurred at a dose of 10 µM. The difference between these results and those using an antisense oligonucleotide strategy to target c-ABL could reflect nonspecific toxicity of the antisense constructs or a kinase-independent function of c-ABL in supporting hematopoietic colony formation.

In contrast, when peripheral blood or bone marrow from CML patients known to be BCR-ABL-positive was incubated with CGP 57148 at a concentration of 1 µM, a 60–80% inhibition of colony formation of committed progenitor cells was seen (Fig. 2). When colonies were assayed for the presence of BCR-ABL transcripts by reverse-transcriptase polymerase chain reaction (RT-PCR), 92–96% of the colonies formed in the absence of inhibitor contained BCR-ABL. However, <20% of the colonies that formed in the presence of 1 µM CGP 57148

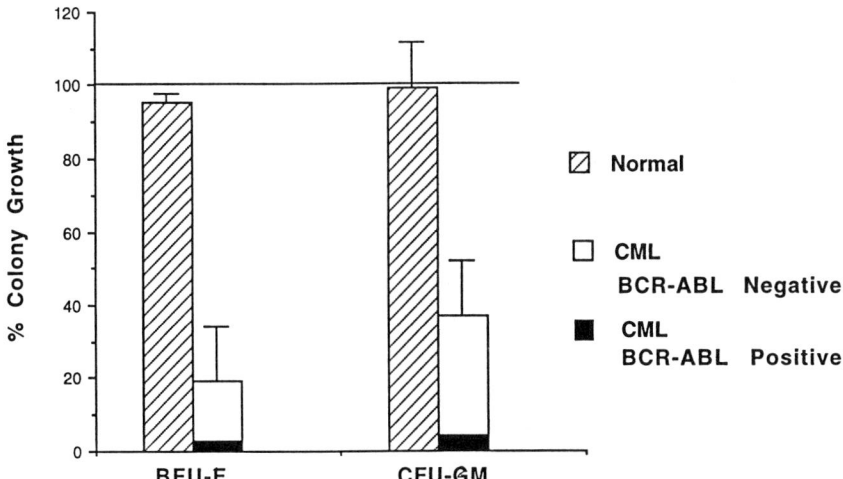

Figure 2 Colony-forming assays. Results are presented as the number of colonies formed with the line at 100% representing the average number of colonies formed without inhibitor and the columns represented the average numbers of colonies formed in the presence of inhibitor. Error bars represent standard deviations. The solid boxes represent the average number of BCR-ABL-positive colonies formed in the presence of inhibitor as assessed by RT-PCR. Reprinted with permission from Ref. 45.

contained BCR-ABL transcripts. This is represented in Figure 2 as the solid portion of the graph of CML colonies. Combining these data with the 60–80% inhibition of colony formation, there was an overall 92–98% decrease in the number of BCR-ABL-positive colonies. Interestingly, CGP 57148 did not inhibit colony formation of a Ph chromosome-negative CML patient who had no BCR-ABL transcripts detected by PCR.

Thus, CGP 57148 satisfies many of the preclinical requirements of a protein tyrosine kinase inhibitor for entry into clinical trials. It is relatively specific for the BCR-ABL tyrosine kinase, is cell-permeable, and selectively kills BCR-ABL-expressing cells at micromolar concentrations. Further, it is capable of selecting for the growth of benign hematopoietic progenitor cells from CML patients with minimal effect on normal hematopoiesis. Preliminary studies in animals have shown little if any toxicity. Regardless of whether CGP 57148 or another compound reaches clinical trials, it is clear that the era of specific therapy, using compounds designed to target molecular abnormalities such as BCR-ABL, is not far away.

WILL TYROSINE KINASE INHIBITORS WORK?

Ultimately, clinical trials will be required to test the therapeutic effects of any tyrosine kinase inhibitor. There are numerous examples of anticancer drugs with promise in preclinical testing that failed to live up to their potential. The therapeutic success of a protein tyrosine kinase inhibitor in CML will depend on the answers to a number of questions including (1) its potential for cure, (2) its effectiveness in different disease stages, and (3) its associated toxicities. However, one advantage of an ABL protein tyrosine kinase inhibitor is that if the compound fails in vivo for any of the aforementioned reasons, it might still be useful for in vitro purging of hematopoietic cells for autologous bone marrow or peripheral blood stem cell transplantation.

How Effective is a Tyrosine Kinase Inhibitor Likely to Be?

One of the critical questions regarding the use of an ABL protein tyrosine kinase inhibitor for CML is whether it will induce death of BCR-ABL-expressing cells or will simply stop the proliferation of BCR-ABL-positive cells without inducing their death. The effects in vivo will in part depend on the mechanism of action of BCR-ABL in the hematopoietic cell. Specifically, there are data supporting two proposed mechanisms. Some evidence suggests that BCR-ABL drives excess hematopoietic proliferation (47,48), while other data support BCR-ABL functioning as an antiapoptotic agent, allowing accumulation of excess numbers of myeloid cells (49–51). In the former case, an ABL protein kinase inhibitor might be expected to block the proliferation of BCR-ABL-expressing cells; in the latter case, it might allow programmed cell death to occur. The preclinical data for CGP 57148 do not resolve this issue since its effects depend on the particular cell line and the in vitro growth conditions. For example, in one cell line this compound induced cell death regardless of the presence or absence of growth factor. In contrast, in another cell line, the compound induced cell death in the absence of growth factor but only stopped cellular proliferation without inducing cell death in the presence of growth factor.

If a tyrosine kinase inhibitor proves capable of inhibiting proliferation of BCR-ABL-positive cells without inducing cell death, then long-term therapy might be required. The benefit obtained would depend on its effectiveness in suppressing the proliferation of the malignant clone and allowing the recovery of normal hematopoietic elements. Even under these circumstances, it is possible that this treatment might allow for prolonged survival. Since BCR-ABL is presumably responsible for the chromosomal instability that leads to additional cytogenetic abnormalities associated with disease progression (52), suppression of the tyrosine kinase activity of BCR-ABL might prevent or delay disease progression. Suppression of BCR-ABL cellular proliferation might be even

ABL Protein Tyrosine Kinase Inhibitors

more useful following other therapies, such as an autologous transplant, in an attempt to prevent regrowth of the BCR-ABL-positive clone. Similarly, ABL protein tyrosine kinase inhibitors may also be useful following achievement of a maximal cytogenetic response with interferon-alpha or cytoreductive chemotherapy. Thus, there is a wide range of potential uses for a tyrosine kinase inhibitor for in vivo therapy of CML. Clinical trials will be required to determine whether tyrosine kinase inhibitors will be effective as single agents, how effective they will be, or whether they will be more useful in combination with other available treatments.

Similar caveats apply to the use of an ABL protein tyrosine kinase inhibitor for in vitro purging. For example, if an ABL protein tyrosine kinase inhibitor only blocks proliferation of BCR-ABL-positive cells, it is clear that elimination of all BCR-ABL-positive cells would not be possible. As seen from the colony-forming data presented above, an approximately two-log cell kill was noted with CGP 57148. This would not be sufficient to purge marrow that was 100% Ph chromosome-positive since a significant number of Ph-positive cells would remain. However, bone marrow purging with a tyrosine kinase inhibitor might be more useful in combination with other treatments that have been reported to increase the yield of Ph chromosome-negative hematopoietic progenitors. For example, purging with a tyrosine kinase inhibitor could be performed following collection of stem cells on recovery from intensive chemotherapy. Alternatively, CD34+, HLA DR– cells have been reported to contain a significant fraction of Ph chromosome-negative hematopoietic progenitors (53) and could be selected followed by culture with a tyrosine kinase inhibitor. Since long-term bone marrow culture has been reported to select for Ph-negative hematopoieses (30), perhaps a tyrosine kinase inhibitor could also be used to enhance the results of this technique as a purging strategy. As techniques for stem cell expansion improve, addition of a tyrosine kinase inhibitor to this culture system may enhance the yield of BCR-ABL-negative cells. All of these techniques would require determining the optimal conditions for combining these treatments, such as the time of incubation in culture, the proper combination of growth factors, and the optimal source of progenitor cells.

The issue of whether there are hematopoietic progenitor cells that are positive at the DNA level for the Ph chromosome, but do not express BCR-ABL RNA or protein, is critical for the success of a tyrosine kinase inhibitor both in vivo and in vitro. Although the most recent data suggest that all cells that have the Ph chromosome also express BCR-ABL RNA (17), the question of whether this RNA is translated into protein has not been addressed. If such a hematopoietic progenitor were to exist, then eradication of cells that express the BCR-ABL protein would still leave a population of cells with the Philadelphia chromosome.

A related question is whether BCR-ABL is the cause of CML or there is another abnormality that antedates the BCR-ABL rearrangement. Several patients have been described with a clinical syndrome resembling CML who were initially Ph chromosome-negative but later had a detectable Ph chromosome (54). Clearly, there are a small percentage of patients with CML-like diseases without detectable BCR-ABL rearrangements. G6PD isoenzyme analysis has demonstrated loss of heterozygosity in a small number of analyzed cases (54), although pseudoclonality or artifactual skewing toward a single isoenzyme is a possible alternative explanation. Nevertheless, these data raise the question of whether another abnormality exists in CML cells. If so, then eradication of BCR-ABL-positive cells would not be expected to be curative. Determining the effects of a selective tyrosine kinase inhibitor may resolve some of these questions.

For What Stages of CML Will a Tyrosine Kinase Inhibitor Be Useful?

As with many antineoplastic agents, one would predict that an ABL protein tyrosine kinase inhibitor might be most effective in the earliest stages of the disease. Assuming that the BCR-ABL translocation is the critical abnormality in the stable phase of the disease, an ABL protein kinase inhibitor would be most effective in the stable phase of the disease. However, this does not necessarily preclude a benefit in more advanced disease. Current models of CML predict that in the stable phase of the disease, BCR-ABL expression results in excess myeloid proliferation either directly or by its antiapoptotic effects. With disease progression, additional molecular abnormalities cause a block of differentiation. Nevertheless, BCR-ABL may continue to drive cellular proliferation directly or indirectly. In this scenario, an ABL protein tyrosine kinase inhibitor might decrease cellular proliferation or allow programmed cell death to occur, thereby resulting in a therapeutic response, even in patients with advanced disease. Although loss of the Ph chromosome has occasionally been reported in blast crisis, this is a rare finding (54,55). It is also possible that additional mutations would eliminate the requirement for BCR-ABL function with disease progression, thus limiting the effectiveness of a tyrosine kinase inhibitor. Most likely, patients with advanced disease will be a more heterogeneous group with mixed results.

What Toxicities Might Be Anticipated?

In preliminary animal experiments few if any toxicities using CGP 57148 have been observed. Whether this favorable toxicity profile will be seen in patients awaits the results of clinical trials. There are several potential adverse effects of the use of a tyrosine kinase inhibitor in CML patients. For example, rapid eradication of BCR-ABL-positive cells by an inhibitor might result in a tumor lysis syndrome or marrow aplasia. This will depend on whether the rate of cell killing with an inhibitor exceeds the time required for the regeneration of normal bone marrow elements, but will also depend on the presence of normal marrow elements in CML patients. In the absence of normal bone marrow elements, a tyrosine kinase inhibitor could theoretically cause total marrow aplasia.

The consequences of inhibition of normal cellular ABL protein tyrosine kinase activity are also likely to be seen. As previously discussed, although the function of c-ABL is unknown, it may negatively regulate cellular proliferation and be involved in lymphoid development. Thus, it is possible that cellular immunity might be depressed. The potential long-term consequences of an agent that allows cells to escape a negative growth regulatory influence are of even greater concern.

Other side effects of tyrosine kinase inhibitors will depend on the particular proteins they inhibit. Although tyrosine kinases inhibitors continue to be synthesized with greater specificity, even a compound such as CGP 57148 also inhibits the PDGF receptor protein tyrosine kinase. PDGF has been identified as a possible mediator of pathological cellular growth in tumors such as glioblastoma and nonmalignant proliferative diseases such as atherosclerosis and fibrosis (39,56). Although this compound might also be useful in diseases that involve abnormal PDGF receptor activation, it is also possible that inhibition of the PDGF receptor could interfere with processes such as wound healing. Similarly, other compounds might inhibit other cellular tyrosine kinases, resulting in unanticipated side effects.

CONCLUSIONS

CML is one of the few cancers for which a constitutively activated protein tyrosine kinase, BCR-ABL, has been implicated as the cause of the disease. Thus, CML is an ideal disease for rational therapy, designed to target the underlying pathogenic mechanism. There has been significant progress in the development of specific ABL protein tyrosine kinase inhibitors for use in this disease, and clinical trials are on the horizon. ABL protein tyrosine kinase inhibitors have potential use either as an in vivo therapy for patients or as an in vitro purging agent for autologous bone marrow or peripheral blood stem cell transplantation. Whether these inhibitors will be successful as single agents or will be more effective in combination with currently available treatments is one of the many questions that will be answered only by clinical trials.

ACKNOWLEDGMENTS

The author is grateful to Drs. Jody Kujovich and Kathryn Kolibaba for their helpful discussions and critical review of this chapter.

REFERENCES

1. Rowley JD. A new consistent abnormality in chronic myelogenous leukaemia identified by quinacrine fluorescence and giemsa staining. Nature 1973; 243:290–293.
2. Heisterkamp N, Stephenson JR, Groffen J, et al. Localization of the c-abl oncogene adjacent to a translocation break point in chronic myelocytic leukemia. Nature 1983; 306:239–242.
3. Bartram CR, de Klein A, Hagemeijer A, et al. Translocation of c-abl correlates with the presence of a Philadelphia chromosome in chronic myelocytic leukemia. Nature 1983; 306:277–280.
4. Shtivelman E, Lifshitz B, Gale RP, Canaani E. Fused transcript of abl and bcr genes in chronic myelogenous leukaemia. Nature 1985; 315:550–554.
5. Ben-Neriah Y, Daley GQ, Mes-Masson A-M, Witte ON, Baltimore D. The chronic myelogenous leukemia-specific P210 protein is the product of the bcr/abl hybrid gene. Science 1986; 233:212–214.
6. McLaughlin J, Chianese E, Witte ON. In vitro transformation of immature hematopoietic cells by the P210 BCR/ABL oncogene product of the Philadelphia chromosome. Proc Natl Acad Sci USA 1987; 84:6558–6562.
7. Lugo TG, Pendergast AM, Muller AJ, Witte ON. Tyrosine kinase activity and transformation potency of bcr-abl oncogene products. Science 1990; 247:1079–1082.
8. Oda T, Tamura S, Matsuguchi T, Griffin JD, Druker BJ. The SH2 domain of Abl is not required for factor independent growth induced by Bcr-Abl in a murine myeloid cell line. Leukemia 1995; 9:295–301.
9. Muller AJ, Young JC, Pendergast AM, et al. BCR first exon sequences specifically activate the BCR/ABL tyrosine kinase oncogene of Philadelphia chromosome-positive human leukemias. Mol Cell Biol 1991; 11:1785–1792.
10. McWhirter JR, Wang JYJ. Activation of tyrosine kinase and microfilament-binding functions of c-abl by bcr sequences in bcr/abl fusion proteins. Mol Cell Biol 1991; 11:1553–1565.
11. Kantarjian HM, Smith TL, O'Brien S, Beran M, Pierce S, Talpaz M. Prolonged survival in chronic myelogenous leukemia after cytogenetic response to interferon-alpha therapy. Ann Intern Med 1995; 122:254–261.
12. Italian Cooperative Study Group on Chronic Myeloid Leukemia. Interferon alfa-2a as compared with conventional chemotherapy for the treatment of chronic myeloid leukemia. N Engl J Med 1994; 330:820–825.
13. Allan NC, Richards SM, Shepherd P. UK Medical Research Council randomised multicentre trial of interferon-alpha n1 for chronic myeloid leukaemia: improved survival irrespective of cytogenetic response. Lancet 1995; 345:1392–1397.
14. Guo JQ, Lian JY, Xian YM, et al. BCR-ABL protein expression in peripheral blood cells of chronic myelogenous leukemia patients undergoing therapy. Blood 1994; 83:3629–3637.
15. Guo JQ, Wang JY, Arlinghaus RB. Detection of BCR-ABL proteins in blood cells of benign phase chronic myelogenous leukemia patients. Cancer Res 1991; 51:3048–3051.

16. Keating A, Wang XH, Laraya P. Variable transcription of BCR-ABL by Ph+ cells arising from hematopoietic progenitors in chronic myeloid leukemia. Blood 1994; 83:1744–1749.
17. Diamond J, Goldman J, Melo JV. BCR-ABL, ABL-BCR, BCR, and ABL genes are all expressed in individual granulocyte-macrophage colony-forming unit colonies derived from blood of patients with chronic myeloid leukemia. Blood 1995; 85: 2171–2175.
18. Dunbar CE, Stewart FM. Separating the wheat from the chaff: selection of benign progenitor cells in chronic myeloid leukemia. Blood 1992; 79:1107–1110.
19. O'Brien SG, Goldman JM. Current approaches to hematopoietic stem-cell purging in chronic myeloid leukemia. J Clin Oncol 1995; 13:541–546.
20. Goto T, Nishikori M, Arlin Z, et al. Growth characteristics of leukemic and normal hematopoietic cells in Ph^1+ chronic myelogenous leukemia and effects of intensive treatment. Blood 1982; 59:793–808.
21. Cunningham I, Gee T, Dowling M, et al. Results of treatment of Ph^1+ chronic myelogenous leukemia with an intensive treatment regimen (L-5 protocol). Blood 1979; 53:375–395.
22. Finney R, McDonald GA, Baikie AG, Douglas AS. Chronic granulocytic leukaemia with Ph 1 negative cells in bone marrow and a ten year remission after busulphan hypoplasia. Br J Haematol 1972; 23:283–288.
23. Smalley RV, Vogel J, Huguley CMJ, Miller D. Chronic granulocytic leukemia: cytogenetic conversion of the bone marrow with cycle-specific chemotherapy. Blood 1977; 50:107–113.
24. Sharp JC, Joyner MV, Wayne AW, et al. Karyotypic conversion in Ph1-positive chronic myeloid leukaemia with combination chemotherapy. Lancet 1979; 1:1370–1372.
25. Kantarjian HM, Talpaz M, Hester J, et al. Collection of peripheral-blood diploid cells from chronic myelogenous leukemia patients early in the recovery phase from myelosuppression induced by intensive-does chemotherapy. J Clin Oncol 1995; 13: 553–559.
26. Carella AM, Podesta M, Frassoni F, et al. Collection of 'normal' blood repopulating cells during early hemopoietic recovery after intensive conventional chemotherapy in chronic myelogenous leukemia. Bone Marrow Transplant 1993; 12:267–271.
27. Talpaz M, Kantarjian H, Kurzrock R, Trujillo JM, Gutterman JU. Interferon-alpha produces sustained cytogenetic responses in chronic myelogenous leukemia. Philadelphia chromosome-positive patients. Ann Intern Med 1991; 114:532–538.
28. Ozer H, George SL, Schiffer CA, et al. Prolonged subcutaneous administration of recombinant alpha 2b interferon in patients with previously untreated Philadelphia chromosome-positive chronic-phase chronic myelogenous leukemia: effect on remission duration and survival. Cancer and Leukemia Group B study 8583. Blood 1993; 82:2975–2984.
29. Turhan AG, Humphries RK, Eaves CJ, et al. Detection of breakpoint cluster region-negative and nonclonal hematopoiesis in vitro and in vivo after transplantation of cells selected in cultures of chronic myeloid leukemia marrow. Blood 1990; 76: 2402–2410.

30. Barnett MJ, Eaves CJ, Phillips GL, et al. Autografting with cultured marrow in chronic myeloid leukemia: results of a pilot study. Blood 1994; 84:724–732.
31. Sawyers CL, McLaughlin J, Goga A, Havlik M, Witte O. The nuclear tyrosine kinase c-Abl negatively regulates cell growth. Cell 1994; 77:121–131.
32. Schwartzberg PL, Stall AM, Hardin JD, et al. Mice homozygous for the ablm1 mutation show poor viability and depletion of selected B and T cell populations. Cell 1995; 65:1165–1175.
33. Tybulewicz VL, Crawford CE, Jackson PK, Bronson RT, Mulligan RC. Neonatal lethality and lymphopenia in mice with a homozygous disruption of the c-abl protooncogene. Cell 1991; 65:1153–1163.
34. Caracciolo D, Valtieri M, Venturelli D, Peschle C, Gewirtz AM, Calabretta B. Lineage-specific requirement of c-abl function in normal hematopoiesis. Science 1989; 245:1107–1110.
35. Chang C-J, Geahlen RL. Protein-tyrosine kinase inhibition: mechanism-based discovery of antitumor agents. J Natural Prod 1992; 55:1529–1560.
36. Casnellie JE. Protein kinase inhibitors: probes for the functions of protein phosphorylation. Adv Pharmacol 1991; 22:167–205.
37. Boutin JA. Tyrosine protein kinase inhibition and cancer. Int J Biochem 1994; 26:1203–1226.
38. Yaish P, Gazit A, Gilon C, Levitzki A. Blocking of EGF-dependent cell proliferation by EGF receptor kinase inhibitors. Science 1988; 242:933–935.
39. Levitzki A, Gazit A. Tyrosine kinase inhibition: an approach to drug development. Science 1995; 267:1782–1788.
40. Kaur G, Gazit A, Levitzki A, Stowe E, Cooney DA, Sausville EA. Tyrphostin induced growth inhibition: correlation with effect on p210bcr-abl autokinase activity in K562 chronic myelogenous leukemia. Anti-Cancer Drugs 1994; 5:213–222.
41. Anafi M, Gazit A, Zehavi A, Ben-Neriah Y, Levitzki A. Tyrphostin-induced inhibition of $p210^{bcr-abl}$ tyrosine kinase activity induces K562 to differentiate. Blood 1993; 82:3524–3529.
42. Honma Y, Okabe KJ, Hozumi M, Uehara Y, Mizuno S. Induction of erythroid differentiation of K562 human leukemic cells by herbimycin A, an inhibitor of tyrosine kinase activity. Cancer Res 1989; 49:331–334.
43. Honma Y, Okabe-Kado J, Kasukabe T, Hozumi M, Umezawa K. Inhibition of abl oncogene tyrosine kinase induces erythroid differentiation of human myelogenous leukemia K562 cells. Jpn J Cancer Res 1990; 81:1132–1136.
44. Kawada M, Tawara J, Tsuji T, et al. Inhibition of Abelson oncogene function of erbstatin analogues. Drugs Under Exp Clin Res 1993; 19:235–241.
45. Druker BJ, Tamura S, Buchdunger E, et al. Effects of a selective inhibitor of the ABL tyrosine kinase on the growth of BCR-ABL positive cells. Nature Med 1996; 2:561–566.
46. Silvennoinen O, Witthuhn BA, Quelle FW, Cleveland JL, Yi T, Ihle JN. Structure of the murine Jak2 protein-tyrosine kinase and its role in interleukin 3 signal transduction. Proc Natl Acad Sci USA 1993; 90:8429–8433.
47. Daley GQ, Baltimore D. Transformation of an interleukin 3-dependent hematopoietic cell line by the chronic myelogenous leukemia-specific P210bcr/abl protein. Proc Natl Acad Sci USA 1988; 85:9312–9316.

48. Carlesso N, Griffin JD, Druker BJ. Use of a temperature-sensitive mutant to define the biological effects of the p210$^{BCR-ABL}$ tyrosine kinase on proliferation of a factor-dependent murine myeloid cell line. Oncogene 1994; 9:149–156.
49. Bedi A, Zehnbauer BA, Barber JP, Sharkis SJ, Jones RJ. Inhibition of apoptosis by BCR-ABL in chronic myeloid leukemia. Blood 1994; 83:2038–2044.
50. Kabarowski JH, Allen PB, Wiedemann LM. A temperature sensitive p210 BCR-ABL mutant defines the primary consequences of BCR-ABL tyrosine kinase expression in growth factor dependent cells. EMBO J 1994; 13:5887–5895.
51. Evans CA, Owen-Lynch PJ, Whetton AD, Dive C. Activation of the Abelson tyrosine kinase activity is associated with suppression of apoptosis in hemopoietic cells. Cancer Res 1993; 53:1735–1738.
52. Laneuville P, Sun G, Timm M, Vekemans M. Clonal evolution in a myeloid cell line transformed to interleukin-3 independent growth by retroviral transduction and expression of p210bcr/abl. Blood 1992; 80:1788–1797.
53. Verfaillie CM, Miller WJ, Boylan K, McGlave PB. Selection of benign primitive hematopoietic progenitors in chronic myelogenous leukemia on the basis of HLA-DR antigen expression. Blood 1992; 79:1003–1010.
54. Raskind WH, Ferraris AM, Najfeld V, Jacobson RJ, Moohr JW, Fialkow PJ. Further evidence of the existence of a clonal Ph-negative stage in some cases of Ph-positive chronic myelocytic leukemia. Leukemia 1993; 7:1163–1167.
55. Kurzrock R, Gutterman JU, Talpaz M. The molecular genetics of Philadelphia chromosome-positive leukemias. N Engl J Med 1988; 319:990–998.
56. Heldin CH, Westermark B. Platelet-derived growth factor: mechanism of action and possible in vivo function. Cell Regul 1990; 1:555–566.

20
Immunotherapy of Chronic Myelogenous Leukemia

David A. Scheinberg, Monica Bocchia, and Richard O'Reilly
Memorial Sloan-Kettering Cancer Center, New York, New York

INTRODUCTION

Several arms of the immune system may participate in the natural immunity or induced immunity to chronic myelogenous leukemia (CML) cells. This chapter will focus on those aspects of this immunity that are specific and that can be manipulated pharmacologically. This includes the use of passive specific therapy with lineage-specific monoclonal antibodies, targeted NK cells, and specific immune T cells, or active specific therapy with leukemia-specific vaccines.

CML is a biphasic neoplastic disorder with a prolonged indolent phase lasting an average of 4 years that features uncontrolled hematopoietic cell proliferation followed by an acute phase of blastic transformation which inevitably leads rapidly to death. There is no curative therapy for CML other than allogeneic bone marrow transplantation, an option that is available only to a small fraction of patients who have both a matched donor and are young enough to tolerate the procedure. Chemotherapy may palliate the cellular proliferation, but it does not alter the progression to acute phase. Recently, alpha-interferon has been shown to induce hematological remissions in a large fraction of patients, with normalization of the white blood cell counts and differential. A smaller fraction of patients also have variable reduction or elimination of the (9;22) translocations in their cells. However, leukemia cells are still detectable in patients by more sensitive PCR methods, and patients ultimately relapse molecularly and hematologically.

Because of the unique features of this disease, in particular the hallmark (9;22) translocation and the associated oncogenic fusion proteins (P210 or P190) which characterize the neoplastic cells, and the evidence of a residual Ph-negative population in the bone marrow, an immunotherapeutic approach that could target the Ph+ clone could be a powerful tool in the treatment of CML.

T-CELL THERAPIES

Leukemic relapse is reduced in recipients of HLA matched allogeneic grafts when compared with syngeneic grafts (1); moreover, recipients of allografts developing acute or chronic graft vs. host disease (GVHD) are at lower risk of relapse than those who do not develop this complication (2). These observations provided evidence for a graft vs. leukemia (GVL) response mediated by alloreactive T cells or other cells from the donor marrow. Recently, Kolb et al. (3) provided direct evidence supporting the contribution of effector cells derived from the donor to the antileukemic effects of a marrow graft. This initial report and subsequently others by additional groups (4,5) have found that among patients transplanted for CML, over 70% of recipients of unmodified or T-cell-depleted marrow allografts who have relapsed posttransplant can be reinduced into durable molecular remissions by treatment with infusions of high doses $(0.6-12.0 \times 108/\text{kg})$ of donor-derived peripheral blood mononuclear cells (PBMC). The observation that >90% of patients who have responded have developed GVHD infers a major contribution by alloreactive T cells to this antileukemic effect. Recently, in a trial examining the effects of escalating doses of donor PMBC on the incidence of GvH and remission in patients who have relapsed with CML more than 9 months after T-cell-depleted marrow grafts, O'Reilly and colleagues at Sloan Kettering have shown that infusions of as few as 10^7 CD3+ donor T cells/kg can induce durable remissions, with a low incidence (10–15%) and severity of GVHD (4). Therefore, the effector cell populations sufficient to eliminate leukemic cell populations may differ from those necessary to induce GVHD.

The leukemia reactive cell in adoptively transferred PBMC that induced remissions has not been identified. Both CD4-positive and CD8-positive T cells are likely to play a role in the GVL effects (6). In animal models, depletion of either population leads to abrogation of the effect, but CD4 appears more important (7). Infusions of PMBC depleted of CD8+ CD3+ T cells can also induce remissions with a low incidence of GVHD (8). Studies at MSKCC have indicated that in patients given T-cell infusions who respond to this treatment, both Ph+ leukemic cells and Ph−, presumptively normal, host T cells are eradicated; thus the effectors are probably not leukemia-specific but are more likely T cells reactive against minor alloantigens expressed on both normal and leukemic hematopoietic cells of the host (4,9). Minor alloantigen-reactive T cells have been described by Jiang et al. (10) in transplant recipients treated with donor leukocytes for CML relapse. Other effector cells exhibiting more selective activity against leukemic cells may also contribute to the remissions observed. T cells reactive against leukemia-specific antigens or alloantigens preferentially expressed on leukemic cells such as have been described by Faber et al. (11) and by Hoffman et al. (12) or reactive against leukemia-specific oncogene fusion products, as recently described by our group and others (13,14) may comprise these effectors. There may also be preferential cytotoxicity against leukemic cells by natural killer (NK) cells (15–18).

Possible targets of the GVL effect include major histocompatibility antigens, as described above, minor histocompatibility antigens, which may be lineage or maturational-specific differentiation antigens, or truly tumor-specific antigens, such as those derived from the oncogene fusion breakpoint proteins P210 or P190. These latter categories of antigens are the most appropriate targets for active or passive specific therapies.

SUMMARY OF CELLULAR EFFECTOR STRATEGIES

Both in animal models and in man, adoptive transfer of ex vivo-expanded autologous lymphokine-activated killer cells (LAK) and tumor-infiltrating T lymphocytes (TIL) has shown some promise as a therapeutic modality (19–23) in the treatment of lymphomas and solid tumors. However, in large-scale clinical trials, response rates have been modest (21,23). Hence, the capacity of a patient's own unprimed T-cell and NK-cell populations to induce durable regressions of established tumors may be limited.

In contrast, high rates of response have been achieved with infusions of donor PBMC in the treatment of CML. A reduced rate of responses in patients relapsing with AML (5) and isolated case reports of responses among patients transplanted for myeloma (24) have also demonstrated the activity of adoptive immunotherapy with normal PBMC from HLA-matched allogeneic donors. These same cells are also capable of initiating severe GVHD, a problem that may limit the ultimate utility of this approach. At Sloan Kettering, in patients treated for EBV lymphomas (25) or for CML (4), a reduction in the dose of T cells administered may limit the incidence and severity of GVHD in HLA-matched recipients. However, even doses as low as 10^5–10^6 T cells/kg may induce GVHD if administered early posttransplant. The frequency of severe GVH reactions in patients treated with donor leukocytes for relapsing CML have underscored the need for developing new strategies of adoptive cell therapy that are specifically directed toward target residual leukemic cell populations. Alternatively, methods are under development to control or eliminate T cells if they induce severe GVHD following their adoptive transfer (26).

ACTIVE SPECIFIC IMMUNOTHERAPY: VACCINES

An effective vaccine consists of an identified antigen which, either administered by itself or conjugated to a protein carrier or an adjuvant, can induce a specific cellular or humoral response. In infectious diseases, the antigen is generally an inactivated bacterium or virus or an immunogenic component thereof. The induction of "memory cells" specific for the antigen generally confers to the vaccinated host a permanent intrinsic immunity against the bacteria or the virus of interest. In this context vaccines are considered "active'" immunotherapy. One of the major obstacles for developing an effective active immunotherapy against cancer has been the lack of defined tumor-specific antigens in the cancer cells. A number of antigens defined serologically have become potential targets for vaccine therapies of cancer (27). These include glycolipids and gangliosides of melanomas and carcinomas, such as GM2, and a small set of glycoproteins, such as MUC-1 and HER2/Neu. In addition, more recently, cytolytic T cell lines have been used to identify peptide antigen targets, primarily in melanoma cells, that may serve as tumor antigens (27). Viral antigen targets may be useful as well, particularly in neoplasms associated with viral expression such as in Hodgkin's disease with EBV, T-cell leukemia/lymphoma with HTLV-1, or hepatocellular carcinoma with HBV. Recently, known tumor oncogene proteins such as mutated Ras, mutated P53, and leukemia-specific fusion proteins have been objects of intensive study as potential targets for tumor vaccines. Fusion proteins derived from fused oncogenes have been identified in about half of adult leukemias.

In CML, the t(9;22) translocation results in a chimeric bcr-abl gene that encodes either a 210-kD or 190-kD fusion protein. Two chimeric P210 bcr-abl proteins comprising products of either the b2a2 exon junction or the b3a2 exon junction can be alternatively expressed in CML cells (28). The junctional sequences of P210 and P190 represent unique tumor-specific determinants, not only because they contain a joined set of amino acid sequences that are normally not expressed on the same protein but also because, at the exact fusion point, a codon for a new amino acid is present.

Although these fusion proteins represent one of the most obvious targets for an immunological approach to the treatment of this leukemia, the major obstacle in considering them as specific tumor antigens for immunotherapy has always been their intracellular location (29). Intracellular proteins were initially thought to be inaccessible to the humoral or cellular immune system. In the recent years, a new understanding of how cells communicate with the immune system and how foreign or even self-antigens are presented in the context of the major histocompatibility complex (MHC) class I or class II molecules has allowed the reconsideration of intracellular oncogenic fusion proteins as potential targets for immunotherapy.

MHC CLASS I AND CLASS II PATHWAYS

MHC class II molecules (HLA DR, DQ, DP) are found on macrophages, B cells, dendritic cells, and other "antigen-presenting cells" (APCs). In the presence of soluble foreign antigens (i.e., bacteria or toxins) the role of these cells is to internalize the extracellular agent and, by enzymatic processing, to reduce foreign proteins into peptides 12–25 amino acids long. These peptides bind the groove of class II molecules and are transported to the cell surface. Peptide-loaded class II molecules interact specifically with the T-cell receptor (TCR) of CD4+ helper T cells to ultimately generate immune responses against the peptide antigens.

MHC class I molecules (HLA A, B, C) have a different role. These molecules are located on the surface of nucleated cells and present peptides largely derived from proteins synthesized by the cell itself. Synthesized proteins are processed in the cytoplasm to peptides 8–11 amino acids long. These peptides are transported to the endoplasmic reticulum, where they bind empty class I molecules. The peptide/class I molecule complex is next transported to the cell surface. The class I molecules interact with CD8+ cytotoxic T cells (CTLs), which are able to recognize the peptides in the class I groove through their TCR (30,31).

If the peptide in the groove belongs to a constitutional, normal self-protein, immunity is likely not to be induced after this CD8/class I interaction due to tolerance or anergy developed by T cells. If the peptide belongs to a viral protein that was synthesized by the cell as consequence of integration of the viral genome into the cell, CD8+ CTLs may recognize this peptide as a new antigen and eventually respond to and kill the cell that is presenting it. Appropriate antigen recognition and T-cell activation requires the presence of additional accessory molecules as well. In this conceptual context, a fusion protein such as bcr-abl found in a transformed neoplastic cell could also be presented in the form of a small peptide in the groove of a class I molecule. Similarly, degraded leukemia cells, in which the fusion protein is processed and presented by APCs, may serve to initiate a CD4 response. Because of the unique sequences at the fusion point, the peptides could act as tumor-specific antigens able to be recognized by CD4 or CD8+ T cells. Alternatively, lineage- and maturation-specific proteins may be used as targets of vaccination (32).

Class I and class II peptides that are presented on the surface are not randomly derived from the original proteins, but must contain specific amino acids in their sequences in one or two critical positions in order to be able to bind the appropriate HLA molecules. Thus, peptide binding is HLA-restricted. The amino acid motifs responsible for specific peptide binding to HLA class I and class II molecules have been determined for the common HLA types by the use of the analysis of acid-eluted, naturally processed peptides and by using cell lines defective in intracellular peptide loading and processing (33–35). More recently, a quantitative molecular radiobinding assay for the analysis of peptide binding to purified HLA class I molecules has been developed by Sette et al. (36).

RATIONALE FOR SPECIFIC T-CELL THERAPY IN CML

Immunization of mice with synthetic peptides corresponding to the joining region of bcr/abl elicited peptide-specific CD4+, class II MHC-restricted T cells (37). Moreover, human lymphocytes in vitro are able to recognize a 24-amino acid peptide corresponding to the pml-rar-alpha fusion region (38). In addition, human CD4+ T lymphocytes specific for a peptide of single amino acid substitution in point-mutated, oncogene ras proteins, have been cloned (39).

In order to develop an effective strategy for generating CD8 T cells specific for leukemia, several critical questions must be addressed:

1. Do oncogenic fusion proteins derived from the translocations or other protein antigens contain suitable amino acid sequences and appropriate anchor motifs for binding to class I molecules?
2. Do these peptides bind with sufficiently high affinity to the groove of HLA class I molecules?
3. Do bound peptides induce a leukemia-specific T-cell response?

Bocchia et al. analyzed the ability of a series of synthetic peptides corresponding to the junctional sequences of bcr/abl proteins to bind to purified human class I molecules (40). The rationale for this approach was twofold: First, breakpoint spanning peptides able to bind class I molecules could be potential candidate antigens for active immunotherapy against these leukemias. Second, evidence that unique tumor-specific breakpoint sequences cannot be presented in the context of HLA molecules would provide a molecular basis for immune nonresponsiveness to abnormal intracellular fusion proteins in leukemic cells.

Of 76 peptides synthesized on the basis of the known sequence of bcr/abl, we found that four peptides derived from b3a2 CML breakpoint bound with high or intermediate affinity to HLA A3,A11 and B8 using a quantitative radiobinding assay (36). The 76 possible peptide sequences spanning 8, 9, 10, or 11 amino acids of the b2a2 and b3a2 junctional regions of bcr-abl proteins were analyzed for motifs with potential to bind to the most common HLA-A class I molecules (A1, A2.1, A3.2, A11, A24) and HLA-B molecules in which anchor motifs were well known (B7, B8, and B27) (41). These HLA types are among the predominant types expressed in the United States population. Lack of binding of CML peptides to HLA-A2 has been observed previously (42). Based on their sequences alone, 21 bcr-abl peptides (10 for the b2a2 breakpoint and 11 for the b3a2 breakpoint) of 8, 9, or 10 amino acids in length were predicted to have the potential of binding one or more class I molecules. The CML peptides with appropriate motifs were synthesized and tested for binding to purified HLA molecules. Six b3a2 peptides displayed significant binding affinities for both HLA A3.2 and A11. These two class I molecules have many similarities in structure and share similar binding motifs (41). One peptide bound with high affinity (<100 nM to achieve 50% inhibition) to HLA A11 and with intermediate affinity (100–500 nM required for 50% inhibition) to HLA A3.2. In contrast, a second peptide showed high-affinity binding to HLA A3.2 (43 nM for 50% inhibition) and had intermediate affinity for HLA A11 (273 nM). A third peptide was found to bind with intermediate affinity to both A3.2 and A11 (400 nM and 125 nM for 50% inhibition, respectively). The remaining three peptides bound A3.2 or A11 much more weakly (>500 nM to <6 µM to achieve 50% inhibition). In addition, two b3a2 peptides bound to HLA B8 with intermediate (190 nM) or low affinity. None of the 10 peptides belonging to the b2a2 breakpoint showed high or intermediate relative binding affinity (<500 nM affinity) for any of the purified HLA class I molecules utilized in the binding assay. Two peptides displayed low affinity for HLA A11 or B8.

This was the first evidence that tumor-specific breakpoint peptides can bind human MHC class I molecules, and it provided a rationale for developing a CD8 therapeutic vaccine strategy. Preliminary data from other groups (14) support this premise. Recent data support the hypothesis that peptides that bind to HLA with moderate to high affinity (<500 nM) are those that are capable of T-cell stimulation after natural processing and cell surface presentation within the cleft of the appropriate HLA. The importance of these moderate- to high-affinity peptides for effective stimulation of T cells is supported by additional evidence:

1. Naturally processed peptides that are found on the surface of live cells bound to HLA molecules typically have an affinity in the range described here for the CML peptides (36).
2. Only peptides that bind to HLA with affinities in this range were able to induce a cytotoxic response in in vitro and in vivo models (33,34,38,39).
3. Peptides from the intracellular protein MAGE in melanoma identified by motifs as described above have been found to be naturally expressed in the context of appropriate HLA molecules (43) and can elicit peptide-specific HLA class I-restricted cytotoxic T-cell response.

SPECIFIC CYTOTOXICITY AND PROLIFERATION OF T CELLS

We next tested the ability of these peptides to elicit specific class I-restricted cytotoxic T lymphocytes (CTLs) in vitro HLA-matched healthy donors (13). In addition, a longer b3a2 CML breakpoint derived peptide, 25 amino acids in length (b3a2-25), was studied for its ability to induce peptide-specific, class II-mediated, T-cell proliferation. In four out of four HLA-A3 donors tested, CML-A3/A11 peptide-specific CTLs were induced that killed an allogeneic HLA-A3 matched peptide pulsed leukemia cell line. In two out of three HLA-A3 donors, the CML-A3/A11 peptide was able to induce killing of autologous and allogeneic HLA matched peptide-pulsed peripheral blood mononuclear cells (PBMC). The CML-A3 peptide induced peptide-specific CTLs in one of the four HLA A3 donors tested. PBMCs from seven donors were also tested for anti-b3a2-25 peptide proliferation in a thymidine incorporation assay. Specific proliferation was detected in three donors, all of the HLA-DR11 haplotype. This confirms the work of others (44,45), who found specific proliferation in response to CML peptides and cells.

PASSIVE SPECIFIC THERAPIES WITH MONOCLONAL ANTIBODIES

Passive therapy of leukemias with monoclonal antibodies was an early goal of this modality of treatment because the leukemia cells are readily accessible to the agents, which renders them ideal targets to the large and poorly diffusable IgG molecules, complement components, or cellular effectors. In addition, a large number of relatively leukemia-selective differentiation antigens have been described (46,47). Though no truly tumor-specific antigens are known to be expressed on the surface of leukemia cells, appropriate glycoproteins and carbohydrate antigens are known that are expressed minimally outside of the myeloid cells. These include CD13, CD33, and CD15.

Because CML is likely to involve early hematopoietic progenitors, antigens present on maturing myeloid elements may not necessarily be adequate to eliminate the clonogenic cells; in contrast, antigens found on stem cells (e.g., CD34 or HLA-Dr) may be unsuitable targets because elimination of all cells bearing these targets may result in marrow aplasia. Additional obstacles to effective therapy include heterogeneity of antigen expression on target cells, which allows antigen-negative cells to escape; the lack of penetration of the antibodies into areas distant from the hematopoietic or lymphatic system; and the immune recognition of the foreign IgG (typically of murine origin).

The use of humanized or human antibodies, small antibody fragments, or conjugation of the IgG to radioisotopes that kill in a field, may overcome some of these obstacles. In addition, the use of antibodies to selectively deliver a marrow-ablative dose of radioactivity, without extramedullary toxicity, is an appealing approach in the setting of bone marrow or stem cell rescue or transplantation. Most current work involves the use of beta emitters (^{131}I, ^{90}Y) which are capable of killing cells within a 0.5- to 5-mm field, but there is considerable interest as well in alpha emitters (^{213}Bi, ^{212}Bi, ^{211}At), which would kill cells in a 0.05-mm field (i.e., one to three cells) (48). Four radiolabeled antibodies have been used in the setting of leukemia (M195, HuM195, and P67), all directed to the myeloid antigen CD33 and antibody BC8 which binds to the leukocyte common antigen CD45 (49–51). Only the M195 agents have been reported to be used for CML, although most work with these antibodies is also focused on AML and APL.

ANTI-CD33 MEDIATED LEUKEMIA CELL KILLING

The ability of lineage- and maturation-specific, murine and genetically engineered, humanized monoclonal antibodies, M195 and HuM195 (anti-CD33), to selectively target and lyse leukemia cells has been extensively investigated. Another antibody, p67, has also been used as a carrier for radioisotopes to bone marrow (49). The expression of the CD33 antigen is restricted to myelogenous leukemias and myeloid progenitor cells, but not to other normal tissues or bone marrow stem cells (52–56). In sequential phase I trials with murine M195 (anti-CD33), we have shown that M195 injected intravenously in patients with relapsed, refractory myeloid leukemia saturates all binding sites on leukemia cells at low doses, even in patients with high tumor burden (53,57). Substantial antitumor effects were not observed in initial studies with M195 because mouse M195 does not mediate immunoeffector functions with either human effector cells or human sera (i.e., complement). However, when mouse M195 was armed with the radionuclide ^{131}I, major antitumor regressions were observed, even in patients with high burden disease ($>10^{12}$ leukemic cells), with virtually no observed toxicity outside of tumor sites in the bone marrow (57). ^{131}I-M195 has demonstrated substantial activity in three pilot trials for AML and CML before allogeneic BMT and in patients with minimal residual APL after *trans* retinoic acid therapy. This last finding suggested that if M195 were modified so as to be able to mediate immune effector functions, naked M195 might mediate destruction of residual leukemia cells in vivo. Therefore, a humanized M195 (HuM195) was developed.

HuM195 is a recombinant version of mouse M195 that was constructed by engrafting complementarity-determining regions of M195 into human IgG1 (52,58). Remarkably, HuM195 has higher avidity than mouse M195 and can mediate ADCC against leukemia targets using human peripheral blood effector cells. This new HuM195 has shown significant antileukemic activity in humans against minimal residual leukemia with unexpectedly little toxicity against normal myelopoiesis.

In a phase I clinical trial designed to evaluate the toxicity, pharmacology, and dosimetry, development of human antihuman antibody (HAHA) responses, and antileukemia effects of HuM195 in relapsed or refractory leukemia patients, rapid and specific targeting of the trace ^{131}I-labeled dose to areas of leukemia in bone marrow, spleen, and liver was observed (59). No HAHA responses were noted after administration of multiple injections of HuM195 in 13 patients tested.

Based on this targeting, specificity, toxicity profile, and lack of immunogenicity, HuM195 was evaluated for activity in humans against minimal residual leukemia, in patients with APL as a model, in whom disease could be followed with RT-PCR for the t(15;17). After attaining a clinical complete remission with retinoic acid, patients received six doses of HuM195 (3 mg/m^2/dose) by intravenous infusion twice weekly for 3 weeks. The effect of therapy on minimal residual disease was monitored by serial evaluations of bone marrow using a reverse transcription PCR (RT-PCR) for PML/RAR mRNA. Fifteen patients in first remission and seven in second remission were treated. As expected, 14 of the 15 patients had RT-PCR-detectable disease at the start of HuM195 therapy. Five converted to negative with HuM195 therapy. Patients remained in clinical and molecular complete remission from 3+ to 40+ months. These results suggest that unconjugated HuM195 has antileukemic activity in the setting of minimal residual disease. Efforts to enhance the antileukemic effects by use of IL-2 activation of NK cells as had been seen in vitro (60) are now under way in vivo in clinical trials. CML, particularly when in complete hematologic or cytogenetic remission induced by interferon, is therefore an ideal target where these effects can be explored as well.

ANTIBODY-TARGETED AND -NONTARGETED NK THERAPIES OF LEUKEMIA

Activated NK cells constitute another population of effector cells that is capable of discriminating between normal and leukemic cell populations. IL-2-activated NK cells from many normal donors lyse or actively inhibit the growth of both HLA-matched and allogeneic CML cells but have little effect on the growth of normal clonogenic progenitor cells (15,61). Similar differential activity of HLA-matched NK cells against AML blasts versus normal marrow progenitors has also been reported (62). Unfortunately, IL-2-activated NK cells from only a minority of normal marrow donors exhibit significant cytotoxicity against CML cells derived from their HLA-matched siblings (15). In some instances, this may reflect a resistance of these leukemic cells to NK cell-mediated lysis; in others, an impaired capacity of the NK cells to bind to and/or lyse these targets. In our studies, patients whose donor-derived NK cells failed to lyse their leukemic cells were at high risk of leukemic relapse in the posttransplant period (15).

Several approaches have been proposed to augment the antileukemic activity of donor NK cells emerging posttransplant. Principal among these has been the administration of cytokines such as IL-2 and IL-12 known to activate and expand NK cell populations and/or potentiate the proliferation and leukemocidal activity of NK cells (63). In vivo, our group and others have shown that IL-2-inducible NK cell precursors emerge early after either unmodified or T-cell-depleted marrow grafts (64). Furthermore, these NK cells, when stimulated with IL-2 in vitro, can exhibit striking cytotoxic activity against clonogenic leukemic cells derived from the HLA-matched host. Based on these observations, Soiffer et al. (63) are conducting trials of IL-2 administered by continuous infusion at low doses designed to augment NK cell function posttransplant. In recipients of autologous or allogeneic T-cell-depleted transplants, low doses IL-2 have been associated with limited toxicity and have induced a marked increase in both the number and cytotoxic activity of NK cells emerging early posttransplant. The ultimate effects of this approach on residual leukemic cell populations remains to be ascertained.

Another approach our group has been pursuing involves the administration of the myeloid lineage-specific monoclonal antibody HuM195 (anti CD33) to direct Fc receptor-bearing effector cells such as NK cells and macrophages to lyse leukemia targets. Alone, HuM195 demonstrated modest mAb concentration and effector cell-dependent cytotoxic activity against HL60 targets (52,60). The HuM195 showed a maximum killing of 10–30% at 5 hours of incubation with HL60 target cells. Efforts were therefore made to enhance ADCC using cytokines. Interferon, GM-CSF, and G-CSF did not promote neutrophil-mediated ADCC with HuM195. However, overnight incubation of effector cells with IL-2 showed a two- to fourfold increase of ADCC. Pronounced additive effects were demonstrated with fresh myelogenous leukemia cells and HL60 cells over that seen with HuM195 or IL-2 alone. Killing was IL-2 and HuM195 concentration-dependent; IL-2 concentrations as low as 20 U/mL were as effective as higher doses. CD16+ cells were essential for IL-2-enhanced ADCC[60]. When human neutrophils were used as effector cells, low levels of killing (6–18%) were seen using humanized M195. A clinical trial exploring IL-2 with HuM195 to treat myeloid leukemias is under way.

CONCLUSIONS

A number of potent and versatile immunotherapeutic options are in development and are showing great promise to treat CML, a disease that has already demonstrated sensitivity to these approaches. Further improvements in efficacy and reductions in toxicity of these strategies will require better understanding of the basic principles of immune recognition and response to leukemia antigens, as well as a thorough characterization of the pharmacology of these new agents.

REFERENCES

1. Gale R, Champlin R. How does bone marrow transplantation cure leukaemia? Lancet 1984; 2:28–30
2. Weiden PL, Fluornoy N, Thomas ED, et al. Antileukemic effect of graft-versus-host disease in human recipients of allogeneic marrow grafts. N Engl J Med 1979; 300:1068–1073.
3. Kolb HJ, Mittermuller J, Clemm C, et al. Donor leukocyte transfusion for treatment of recurrent chronic myelogenous leukemia in marrow transplant patients. Blood 1990; 76:2462.
4. Mackinnon S, Papadopoulos EB, Carabasi MH, et al. Adoptive immunotherapy evaluating escalating doses of donor leukocytes for relapse of chronic myeloid leukemia after bone marrow transplantation: separation of graft-versus-leukemia responses from graft-versus-host disease. Blood 1995; 86:1261.
5. Kolb HJ, Schattenberg A, Goldman, JM, et al. Graft-versus-leukemia effect of donor lymphocyte transfusions in marrow grafted patients. Blood 1995; 86:2041–2050.
6. Barrett A, Jiang YZ. Immune responses to chronic myeloid leukaemia. Bone Marrow Transplant 1992; 9:305–311.
7. Greenberg PD. Adoptive T-cell therapy of tumors: mechanisms operative in the recognition and elimination of tumor cells. Adv Immunol 1991; 49:281–355.
8. Giralt S, Hester J, Hugh Y, et al. CD8+ depleted donor lymphocyte infusion as treatment for relapsed chronic myelogenous leukemia after allogeneic bone marrow transplantation: graft vs. leukemia without graft vs. host disease. Blood 1994; 84: 538a. Abstract.
9. Marjit WAF, Kernan NA, Diaz-Barrientos T, et al. Multiple minor histocompatibility antigen-specific cytotoxic T lymphocyte clones can be generated during graft rejection after HLA-identical bone marrow transplantation. Bone Marrow Transplant 1995; 16:125–132.
10. Jiang Y-Z, Cullis JO, Kanfer EJ, Goldman JM, Barrett AJ. T-cell and NK cell mediated graft-versus-leukaemia reactivity following donor buffy coat transfusion to treat relapse after marrow transplantation for chronic myeloid leukaemia. Bone Marrow Transplant 1993; 11:133–138.
11. Faber LM, van Luxemburg-Heijs SAP, Rijnbeek M, Willemze R, Falkenberg JHF. Minor histocompatibility antigen-specific, leukemia-reactive cytotoxic T cell clones can be generated in vitro without in vivo priming using chronic myeloid leukemia cells as stimulators in the presence of α interferon. Bone Marrow Transplant 1996; 2:31–36.
12. Hoffmann T, Theobald M, Bunjes D, Weiss M, Heimpel H, Heit W. Frequency of bone marrow T cells responding to HLA-identical non-leukemic and leukemic stimulator cells. Bone Marrow Transplant 1993; 12:1–8.
13. Bocchia M, Korontsvit T, Xu Q, et al. Specific human cellular immunity to bcr-abl oncogene-derived peptides. Blood 1996; 87:3587–3592.

14. Dermime S, Molldrem J, Parker KC, et al. Human CD8+ T lymphocytes recognize the fusion region of BCR/ABL hybrid protein present in chronic myelogenous leukemia. Blood 1995; 86:620a. Abstract.
15. Hauch M, Gazzola MV, Small T, et al. Antileukemia potential of interleukin-2 activated natural killer cells after bone marrow transplantation for chronic myelogenous leukemia. Blood 1990; 75:2250–2262.
16. Mackinnon S, Hows JM, Goldman JM. Induction of in vitro graft-versus-leukemia activity following bone marrow transplantation for chronic myeloid leukemia. Blood 1990; 75:2037–2045.
17. Cesano A, O'Connor R, Nowell PC, Lange B, Clark SC, Santoli D. Establishment of karyotypically normal cytotoxic leukemic T-cell line from a T-ALL sample engrafted in SCID mice. Blood 1993; 81:2714–2722.
18. Hercend T, Takvorian T, Nowill A, et al. Characterization of natural killer cells with antileukemia activity following allogeneic bone marrow transplantation. Blood 1986; 67:722–728.
19. LaFreniere R, Rosenberg SA. Successful immunotherapy of murine experimental hepatic metastasis with lymphokine-activated killer cells and recombinant interleukin-2. Cancer Res 1985; 45:3735–3741.
20. Negrier S, Philip T, Stoter G, et al. Interleukin-2 with or without LAK cells in metastatic renal cell carcinoma: a report of a European multicentre study. Eur J Cancer Clin Oncol 1989; Suppl 3:S21–S28.
21. Rosenberg SA, Lotze MT, Yang JC, et al. Prospective randomized trial of high-dose interleukin-2 alone or in conjunction with lymphokine-activated killer cells for the treatment of patients with advanced cancer. J Natl Cancer Inst 1993; 85: 622–632.
22. Rosenberg SA, Packard BS, Aebersold PM, et al. Use of tumor-infiltrating lymphocytes and interleukin-2 in the immunotherapy of patients with metastatic melanoma. A preliminary report. N. Engl J Med 1988; 319:1676–1680.
23. Dutcher JP, Gaynor ER, Boldt DH, et al. A phase II study of high-dose continuous infusion interleukin-2 with lymphokine-activated killer cells in patients with metastatic melanoma. J Clin Oncol 1991; 9:641–648.
24. Vesole D, Tricot G, Jagannath S. Induction of graft-versus-myeloma effect following allogeneic marrow transplantation. Blood 1994; 84:331a. Abstract.
25. Papadopoulos EB, Ladanyi M, Emanuel D, et al. Infusions of donor leukocytes to treat Epstein-Barr virus-associated lymphoproliferative disorders after allogeneic bone marrow transplantation. N Engl J Med 1994; 330:1185.
26. Servida P, Rossini S, Traversari C, et al. Gene transfer into peripheral blood lymphocytes for in vivo immunomodulation of donor anti-tumor immunity in a patient affected by EBV-induced lymphoma. Blood 1993; 82:214a.
27. Lewis JJ, Houghton AN. Definition of tumor antigens suitable for vaccine construction. Cancer Biol 1995; 6:321–327.
28. Ben-Neriah Y, Daley GQ, Mes-Massan AM, Wirte ON, Baltimore D. The chronic myelogenous leukemia-specific P210 protein is the product of the bcr/abl hybrid gene. Science 1986; 233:212.
29. Dhut S, Chaplin T, Young BD. BCR-ABL and BCR proteins: biochemical characterization and localization. Leukemia 1990; 4:745.

30. Braciale TJ, Braciale VL. Antigens presentation: structural themes and functional variation. Immunol Today 1991; 12:124.
31. Restifo NP. Antigen processing and presentation (Rev.). Biol Ther Cancer Updates 1996; 2:11.
32. Molldrem J, Dermime S, Parker K, et al. Cytotoxic T cells show specificity to MHC class I-restricted peptide derived from proteinase 3, a leukemia-associated protein. Blood 1995; 86:427a. Abstract.
33. Falk K, Rotzschke O, Stevanovic S, Jung G, Rammansee HG. Allele-specific motifs revealed by sequencing of self-peptides eluted from MCH molecules. Nature 1991; 351:290.
34. Hoskin NA, Bevan MJ. Defective presentation of endogenous antigen by a cell line expressing class I molecules. Science 1990; 248:367.
35. Stuber G, Modrow S, Houglund P, et al. Assessment of major histocompatibility complex class I interaction with Epstein-Barr virus and human immunodeficiency virus peptides by elevation of membrane H-2 and HLA in peptide loading-deficient cells. Eur J Immunol 1992; 22:2697.
36. Sette A, Vitiello A, Reherman B, et al. The relationship between class I binding affinity and immunogenicity of potential cytotoxic T cell epitopes. J Immunol 1994; 153:5586–5592.
37. Chen W, Peace DJ, Rovira DK, Sheng-guo Y, Cheever MA. T-cell immunity to the joining region of p210 bcr-abl protein. Proc Natl Acad Sci USA 1992; 89:1468.
38. Gambacorti-Passenini C, Grignani F, Arlend F, Pandolfi PP, Pellicci PG, Parmiani G. Human CD4 lymphocytes specifically reorganize a peptide representing the fusion of the hybrid protein PML/RARa present in acute promyelocytic leukemia cells. Blood 1993; 81:1369–1375.
39. Jung S, Schiusener HJ. Human T lymphocytes recognize a peptide of single point-mutated, oncogenic ras proteins. J Exp Med 1996; 173:273.
40. Bocchia M, Wentworth PA, Southwood S, et al. Specific binding of leukemia oncogene fusion protein peptides to HLA class I molecules. Blood 1995; 85:2680–2684.
41. Rammensee H, Friede T, Stevanovic S. MHC ligands and peptide motifs: first listing. Immunogen 1995; 41:178.
42. Cullis JO, Barret AJ, Goldman JM, Lechler RI. Binding of BCR/ABL junctional peptides to major histocompatibility complex (MHC) class I molecules: studies in antigen-processing defective cell lines. Leukemia 1994; 8:165.
43. Celis E, Tsai V, Crimi C, et al. Induction of anti-tumor cytotoxic T lymphocytes in normal humans using primary cultures and synthetic peptide epitopes. Proc Natl Acad Sci USA 1994; 91:2105.
44. ten Bosch GJA, Toornvliet AC, Friede TH, Melief CJM, Leeksma OC. Recognition of peptides corresponding to the joining region of p210 bcr-abl by human T cells. Leukemia 1995; 9:1334.
45. ten Bosch GJA, Joosten AM, Melief CJM, Leeksma OC. Specific recognition of CML blasts by bcr-abl breakpoint peptide specific human T cells. Blood 1995; 86: 158a. Abstract.
46. Foon KA, Zighelboim J, Yale C, Gale RP. Intensive chemotherapy is the treatment of choice. Blood 1981; 58:467–470.

47. Caron PC, Scheinberg DA. Immunotherapy of acute leukemia. Curr Opin Oncol 1994; 6:14–22.
48. Jurcic JG, Scheinberg DA. Recent developments in the radioimmunotherapy of cancer. Curr Opin Immunol 1994; 6:715–721.
49. Appelbaum FR, Matthews DC, Eary JF, et al. The use of radiolabeled anti-CD33 antibody to augment marrow irradiation prior to marrow transplantation for acute myelogenous leukemia. Transplantation 1992; 54:829–833.
50. Matthews DC, Appelbaum FR, Eary JF, et al. Development of a marrow transplant regimen for acute leukemia using targeted hematopoietic irradiation delivered by ^{131}I-labeled anti-CD45 antibody combined with cyclophosphamide and total body irradiation. Blood 1995; 85:1122–1131.
51. Jurcic J, Scheinberg DA, Houghton AN. Monoclonal antibody therapy. In: Longo D, ed. Cancer Chemotherapy and Biological Response Modifiers Annual #15. 15th ed. New York: Elsevier Medical Publishers, 1994.
52. Caron PC, Co MS, Bull MK, Avdalovic NM, Queen C, Scheinberg DA. Biological and immunological features of humanized M195 (anti-CD33) monoclonal antibodies. Cancer Res 1992; 52:6761–6767.
53. Scheinberg DA, Lovett DR, Divgi CR, et al. A phase I trial of monoclonal antibody M195 in acute myelogenous leukemia: specific bone marrow targeting and internalization of radionuclide. J Clin Oncol 1991; 9:478–490.
54. Scheinberg DA, Tanimoto M, McKenzie S, Strife A, Old LJ, Clarkson BD. A diagnostic marker for acute myelogenous leukemia. Leukemia 1989; 3:440–445.
55. Griffin JD, Linch D, Sabbath K, Schlossman SF. A monoclonal antibody reactive with normal and leukemic human myeloid progenitor cells. Leuk Res 1984; 8:521–534.
56. Griffin JD, Ritz J, Nadler LM, Schlossman SF. Expression of myeloid differentiation antigens on normal and malignant myeloid cells. J Clin Invest 1981; 68:932–941.
57. Schwartz MA, Lovett DR, Redner A, et al. A dose-escalation trial of M195 labeled with iodine 131 for cytoreduction and marrow ablation in relapsed or refractory myeloid leukemias. J Clin Oncol 1993; 11:294–303.
58. Co MS, Avdalovic NM, Caron PC, et al. Chimeric and humanized antibodies with specificity for the CD33 antigen. J Immunol 1992; 148:1149–1154.
59. Caron PC, Jurcic JG, Scott AM, et al. A phase 1B trial of humanized monoclonal antibody M195 (anti-CD33) in myeloid leukemia: specific targeting without immunogenicity. Blood 1994; 7:1760–1768.
60. Caron PC, Lai LT, Scheinberg DA. Interleukin-2 enhancement of cytotoxicity by humanized monoclonal antibody M195 (anti-CD33) in myelogenous leukemia. Clin Cancer Res 1995; 1:63–70.
61. Teichmann JV, Ludwig WD, Thiel E. Cytotoxicity of interleukin 2-induced lymphokine-activated killer (LAK) cells against human leukemia and augmentation of killing by interferons and tumor necrosis factor. Leuk Res 1992; 16:287–298.
62. van den Brink MRM, Voogt PJ, Marijt WAF, van Luxemburg-Heys SAP, van Rook JJ, Brand A. Lymphokine-activated killer cells selectively kill tumor cells in

bone marrow without compromising bone marrow stem cell function in vitro. Blood 1989; 74:354–360.
63. Soiffer RJ, Mauch P, Tarbell NJ, et al. Total lymphoid irradiation to prevent graft rejection in recipients of HLA nonidentical T cell-depleted allogeneic marrow. Bone Marrow Transplant 1991; 7:23–33.
64. Keever CA, Welte K, Small T, et al. Interleukin-2-activated killer cells in patients following transplants of soybean lectin-separated and E rosette-depleted bone marrow. Blood 1987; 70:1893.

Index

ABL protein tyrosine kinase inhibitors, 395–407
  BCR-ABL negative hematopoietic progenitor cells, 397
  BCR-ABL protein expression, 396–397
  CML stage, 396–397
Accelerated phase chronic myelogenous leukemia, allogeneic stem cell transplantation, 12–13
  defined, 2, 3t
  oligonucleotide purging, 352
  symptoms, 8
aCML (see Atypical chronic myelogenous leukemia)
Active specific immunotherapy, 416
Adhesion molecules, 376–378
Age, alloSCT, 230
  bone marrow transplantation, 268–269
  interferon alpha (IFN-α), 149–150
Allogeneic bone marrow transplantation, 141
  chronic myelogenous leukemia (CML), natural history, 108–109
  chronic myelomonocytic leukemia (CMML), 62–63
  interferon alpha (IFN-α), 151
  relapse, interleukin-2 (IL-2), 371–372

Allogeneic stem cell transplantation (alloSCT), 10–14, 215–238
  accelerated phase CML, 12–13
  advanced disease, 229–230
  blastic phase CML, 12
  chronic phase CML, 13–14
  complications, 225–226
  conditioning, 221–222
  graft-*versus*-host disease (GVHD), 225–226
  graft-*versus*-leukemia (GVL), 230–232
  integrated approach, 237–238
  interferon alpha (IFN-α), 14
  limitations, 237
  matched unrelated donor transplant role, 14
  minimal residual disease (MRD), 232–235
    conventional cytogenetics, 232–233
    metaphase fluorescence in situ hybridization (FISH), 234–235
    polymerase chain reaction (PCR), 233–234
  novel regimens, 224–225
  in older patients, 13
  postallogeneic stem cell transplantation relapse, 11–12
  prognosis, 230

[Allogeneic stem cell transplantation]
  relapse management, 235–237
    donor lymphocyte transfusion, 236
    interferon alpha (IFN-α), 235
    novel approaches, 236–237
    second alloSCT, 235
  results, 10–11, 226–232
    with family members, 229
    with HLA-identical sibling donors, 226–227
    with volunteer unrelated donors, 227–229
  splenectomy and splenic irradiation, 224
  standard regimens, 222–224
    chemotherapy, 223
    chemotherapy plus irradiation, 222–223
    chemotherapy vs. chemoradiotherapy, 223–224
    splenectomy, 224
  stem cell collections, 219–221
    blood stem cell harvest, 219–221
    marrow stem cell harvest, 219
  stem cell sources, 216–219
    alternative donors, 217–219
    cord blood donors, 218–219
    HLA typing, 216
    HLA-identical sibling donors, 216–217
    related donors, 218
    volunteer unrelated donors, 218
  in transformation, 12–13
All-*trans*-retinoic acid (ATRA), chronic myelomonocytic leukemia (CMML), 61
All-*trans*-retinoic acid (ATRA)+interferon-alpha (IFN-α), Australian trials, 201–206
Alternative donors, 217–219
Amitriptyline, 21, 166
Anagrelide, 10
Anemia, chronic myelomonocytic leukemia (CMML), 48

Anthracyclines, chronic myelogenous leukemia (CML), 117–118
  chronic myelomonocytic leukemia (CMML), 59
Anti-CD33 mediated leukemia cell killing, 421–422
Antigene strategies, gene expression disruption, 342–343
Antisense oligonucleotides, clinical use, 352
  future use, 353–354
Antisense strategies, gene expression disruption, 342–343
Arabinosylcytosine, 117–118
Ara-C (*see* Cytosine-arabinoside)
Arsenical solution, 1
ATRA (*see* All-*trans* retinoic acid)
ATRA syndrome, chronic myelomonocytic leukemia (CMML), 61
Atypical chronic myelogenous leukemia (aCML), 292–293
Australian trials, interferon-alpha (IFN-α), combinations, 185–193
  high dose, 191–199
  interferon-alpha (IFN-α)+all-*trans* retinoic acid (ATRA), 201–206
  interferon-alpha (IFN-α)+hydroxyurea, 199–201
Autologous stem cell transplantation, 273–280
  chronic myelogenous leukemia (CML), 26–28, 131
  chronic phase, 274–280
    stem cell sources, 277–289
    survival, 274–277
  transformation, 273–274
Autologous stem cells, ex vivo purging, 277–278
  in vivo purging, 278–280
5-Azacytidine, chronic myelomonocytic leukemia (CMML), 65
5-aza-2′-Deoxycytidine, chronic myelomonocytic leukemia (CMML), 65

Index

Basic fibroblast growth factor (bFGF), 370
BCR (*see* Breakpoint cluster region)
BCR/ABL, oligonucleotide therapeutics, 343–346
　P190 gene, 83–94
　P210 gene, 85–94
　in vivo transfer into murine bone marrow, 88–94
BCR/ABL gene, southern blotting, 328–329
　blood vs. bone marrow, 329–332
　vs. cytogenetic monitoring, 332–333
BCR/ABL mRNA, polymerase chain reaction (PCR), 306
BCR/ABL negative hematopoietic progenitor cells, ABL protein tyrosine kinase inhibitors, 397
BCR/ABL protein expression, ABL protein tyrosine kinase inhibitors, 396–397
BCR/ABL transcripts, polymerase chain reaction (PCR), 335–336
BCR/ABL transgenic mice, 82–88
BCR/ABL translocation, fluorescence in situ hybridization (FISH), 306
　western blot analysis, 306
BCR/ABL-transformed cell line propagation, mice, 79–82
Blastic phase chronic myelogenous leukemia, 9
　allogeneic stem cell transplantation, 12
　bone marrow transplantation, 265
　defined, 2, 3t
　oligonucleotide purging, 352
　symptoms, 8
Blood stem cell harvest, 219–221
Blood vs. bone marrow studies, hypermetaphase fluorescence in situ hybridization (HMF), 323–324
B-lymphoblastic leukemia, 90–91

Bone marrow aspiration, interferon-alpha (IFN-α), 168–169
Bone marrow transplantation, 141, 259–270
　age effect, 268–269
　allogeneic, 62–63, 108–109, 151, 371–372
　interferon-alpha (IFN-α), 151
　delay effect, 265–268
　leukemia-free survival, 262–264
　phase effect, 264–265
　relapse, 261–262
　survival, 260–261
　syngeneic, 141
　unrelated donors, 269–270
Bournemouth score, chronic myelomonocytic leukemia (CMML), 52–53
Breakpoint cluster region (BCR), interferon-alpha (IFN-α), 334–335
　southern blotting, 305–306
Breakpoint cluster region (BCR) breakpoint site, chronic myelogenous leukemia (CML), interferon-alpha (IFN-α), 108
Breakpoint cluster region (BCR) monitoring, M.D. Anderson Cancer Center, 303–313
Breakpoint cluster region (BCR) rearrangement, chronic myelogenous leukemia (CML), prognosis, 307
　densitometric analysis, 306
　Ph-positive chronic myelogenous leukemia (CML), interferon-alpha (IFN-α), 307–311
　quantification, 306–311
British Medical Research Council study, busulfan vs. splenic irradiation, 115
　hydroxyurea, 18
　interferon-alpha (IFN-α), 18, 121, 125, 144–147
Bryostatin, chronic myelomonocytic leukemia (CMML), 66–67

Busulfan, 1, 9–10, 114–115, 116t, 117–118
  adverse effects, 9
  vs. chlorambucil, 115
  chronic myelomonocytic leukemia (CMML), 59
  vs. dibromomannitol, 115
  dose, 9
  German study, 17–18, 121–125, 146
  hydroxyurea vs. German CML study group, 118–119
  Italian Cooperative Study Group on CML (ICSG-CML), 17
  vs. melphalan, 115
  Ph-negative, BCR-negative CML, 295
  prognosis, 104
  vs. splenic irradiation, 115
  vs. thioguanine, 115
Busulfan/cyclophosphamide (BuCy2), allogeneic stem cell transplantation (alloSCT), 223
  cyclophosphamide/total body irradiation (CyTBI) vs. allogeneic stem cell transplantation (alloSCT), 222–223

Calcitonin gene hypermethylation, chronic myelogenous leukemia (CML), interferon-alpha (IFN-α), 108
Cancer Leukemia Group B (CALGB), interferon-alpha (IFN-α), dose, 162–163
  southern blotting, 327–337
CFU-S12, 90
CGP 57148, cellular proliferation inhibition, 401–402
  hematopoietic cell colony formation inhibition, 402–403
  structure, 400f
  in vitro profiling, 399
Children, chronic myelogenous leukemia (CML), 6–7
  chronic myelomonocytic leukemia (CMML), 47–48
  Ph-negative disorders, 7
  Ph-positive disorders, 6
Chlorambucil, busulfan vs., 115
2-Chlorodeoxyadenosine (2-CDA), chronic myelogenous leukemia (CML), 130
  chronic myelomonocytic leukemia (CMML), 64–65
CHR (see Complete hematologic remission)
Chromosome 9, 286–287
Chronic myelogenous leukemia (CML), 1–30
  accelerated phase, allogeneic stem cell transplantation, 12
  bone marrow transplantation, 265
  defined, 2, 3t
  oligonucleotide purging, 352
  symptoms, 8
  allogeneic bone marrow transplantation, 108–109, 141, 151, 371–372
  allogeneic stem cell transplantation, 10–14
    chronic phase timing, 13–14
    matched unrelated donor transplant role, 14
    older patients, 13
    postallogeneic stem cell transplantation relapse, 11–12
    results, 10–11
    transformation, 12–13
  allografts, 215–238
  anagrelide, 10
  animal models, 77–94
    future, 94
  anthracyclines, 117–118
  arabinosylcytosine, 117–118
  autologous stem cell transplantation, 26–28, 131, 273–280
    stem cell sources, 277–280
    survival, 274–277
  BCR/ABL ex vivo transfer into murine bone marrow, 88–94

Index

[Chronic myelogenous leukemia]
  blastic phase, 9
    allogeneic stem cell transplantation, 12
    bone marrow transplantation, 265
    defined, 2, 3t
    oligonucleotide purging, 352
    symptoms, 8
  bone marrow transplantation, 259–270
  busulfan, 1, 9–10, 114–115, 116t, 117–118
  chemotherapy, 9–10
  2-chlorodeoxyadenosine (2-CDA), 130
  chronic myelomonocytic leukemia (CMML) vs., 50–54
  chronic phase, alloSCT results, 226–232
    autologous stem cell transplantation, 274–280
  clinical features, 7–9
  complete hematologic remission, 3–5
  conventional therapy, changing nature, 113–133
    historic development, 114t
  cyclophosphamide, 117–118
  cytogenetic clonal evolution, 9, 13
  etiology, 2
  fluorescence in situ hybridization (FISH), 317–325
  future, 30
  herbimycin A, 130–131
  homoharringtonine, 25, 130
  hydroxyurea, 1, 9–10, 118–119
    adverse effects, 9–10
  immunotherapy, 413–424
  intensive chemotherapy, with autografting, 131
  intensive combination therapy, 117–118
  investigational modalities, 25–29
    autologous stem cell transplantation, 26–28
    growth factors, 29
    intensive chemotherapy, 26
    retinoids, 28–29

[Chronic myelogenous leukemia]
  laboratory features, 7–9
  major BCR (M-BCR), 5
  median survival, 4t, 114t
  6-mercaptopurine, 117–118
  methotrexate, 117–118
  mice, BCR/ABL transgenic, 82–88
    BCR/ABL-transofrmed cell line propagation, 79–82
    human CML cell propagation, 77–79
  natural history, 22–25
    during interferon era, 108–109
  new drugs, 130–131
  oligonucleotide therapeutics, 341–355
  pathophysiology, 5–7
  Philadelphia chromosome (Ph)-negative, 7, 285–297
  Philadelphia chromosome (Ph)-positive, 1, 6–7, 144–147, 307–312
  Philadelphia (Ph) chromosome, 5–6
  prognosis, 1, 2–5, 103–106
    biological and molecular correlates, 106–108
    during interferon era, 106
    models, 105t
    prior to interferon era, 104–105
  risk groups, 2–4
  splenic irradiation, 114
  symptoms, 7–8
  therapy, 9–25
  6-thioguanine, 117–118
  thioTEPA, 10
  transformation, autologous stem cell transplantation, 273–274
  treatment, 29–30
  tumor burden correlation with survival, 115–117
  tyrosine kinase inhibitors, 398–407
  ubenimex, 130
  vincristine, 117–118
Chronic myelomonocytic leukemia (CMML), 43–67
  allogeneic bone marrow transplantation, 62–63
  anthracyclines, 59

[Chronic myelomonocytic leukemia]
  5-azacytidine, 65
  5-aza-2′-deoxycytidine, 65
  bryostatin, 66–67
  busulfan, 59
  children, 47–48
  2-chlorodeoxyadenosine (2-CdA), 64–65
  classification, 45
  clinical features, 47–48
  vs. CML, 50–54
  colony-stimulating factors, 65–66
  cytogenetics, 47
  danazol, 66–67
  etiology, 46–47
  French-American-British Cooperative Group (FAB), 44–45
  G-CSF, 65
  GM-CSF, 65–66
  hematologic features, 48
  hexamethylene bisacetamide, 61–62
  history, 43–45
  hydroxyurea, 56–57
  incidence, 46–47
  intensive chemotherapy, 59–61
  interferon alpha (IFN-α), 64
  interferon-γ, 64
  interleukin-3, 66
  interleukin-6, 66
  interleukin-10, 66
  low-dose cytosine-arabinoside (Ara-C), 57–58
  6-mercaptopurine, 59
  molecular biology, 47
  natural history, 50–54
  nucleoside analogs, 64–65
  prognosis, 51–54
  retinoids, 61
  survival, 50
  symptoms, 47–48
  therapy, 55–67
  topotecan, 63
  vitamin D derivatives, 61
  VP-16, 55–56
Chronic neutrophilic leukemia (CNL), 293

Cigarette smoking, chronic myelomonocytic leukemia (CMML), 44–45
C-Kit ligand, 369–370
C-Kit R ligand, 349
CML (*see* Chronic myelogenous leukemia)
CML 88 trial, 176–179
  adverse effects, 178–179
  design, 176–177
  hematological toxicity, 179
  patient selection, 176–177
  results, 177–178
CML 91 trial, 179–182
CML-like syndrome, 90, 92–94
CMML (*see* Chronic myelomonocytic leukemia)
C-myb, 347–350, 352
C-myc, 346
CNL (*see* Chronic neutrophilic leukemia)
Colcemid, 320
Colony-stimulating factors, chronic myelomonocytic leukemia (CMML), 65–66
Complete hematologic remission (CHR), 3–5
Cooled charged coupled device (CCD) camera, 318
Cord blood donors, 218–219
Cutaneous vasculitis, chronic myelomonocytic leukemia (CMML), 48
Cyclophosphamide, 117–118
Cyclophosphamide/total body irradiation (CyTBI), allogeneic stem cell transplantation (alloSCT), 222–223
  vs. busulfan/cyclophosphamide (BuCy2), allogeneic stem cell transplantation (alloSCT), 222–223
Cyclosporine/methotrexate, graft-*versus*-host disease, 225–226
Cytogenetic analysis, Ph chromosome translocation, 304–305

Index

Cytogenetic relapse, 234
Cytogenetic response rate, interferon-alpha (IFN-α), 147–148, 152–153
Cytogenic abnormalities, chronic myelomonocytic leukemia (CMML), 53
Cytogenic clonal evolution, interferon-alpha (IFN-α), 108
Cytokines, 363–380
  stimulatory, 364–371
Cytosine-arabinoside (Ara-C), low-dose, chronic myelomonocytic leukemia (CMML), 57–58
Cytosine-arabinoside (Ara-C)+interferon-alpha (IFN-α), 23–24, 131, 173–183
  French trials, 176–183
    CML 88 trial, 176–179
    CML 91 trial, 179–182
  low dose, Australian trials, 186–191
  rationale, 173–176

Danazol, chronic myelomonocytic leukemia (CMML), 66–67
Decitabine, 28
Densitometric analysis, breakpoint cluster region (BCR) rearrangement, 306
Depression, interferon-alpha (IFN-α), 21, 166
Dibromomannitol, busulfan vs., 115
DNA-image cytometry, chronic myelogenous leukemia (CML), interferon-alpha (IFN-α), 108
Donor lymphocyte reinfusion, postallogeneic stem cell transplantation relapse, 12
Donor lymphocyte transfusion, alloSCT relapse, 236
Donors, 216–218, 226–229, 269–279
Dusseldorf score, chronic myelomonocytic leukemia (CMML), 53

Erbstatin, structure, 400f
Erythropoietin (EPO), 370

European Bone Marrow Transplantation Registry (EBMT), 10

FAB (see French-American-British Cooperative Group)
Fatigue, chronic myelomonocytic leukemia (CMML), 48
  interferon-alpha (IFN-α), 21, 166
^{52}Fe, 225
Fibronectin receptors, 377
Fluorescence in situ hybridization (FISH), BCR/ABL translocation, 306
  chronic myelogenous leukemia (CML), 317–325
  interferon-alpha (IFN-α), 22
  Ph (VPh) translocation interphase cells, 318–319
Fluoxetine, 21, 166
Footprinting assay, oligonucleotide, 354
Fowlers solution, 1
French study, interferon-alpha (IFN-α), 121
French trials, CML 88 trial, 176–179
  CML 91 trial, 179–182
French-American-British Cooperative Group (FAB), chronic myelomonocytic leukemia (CMML), 44–45
  diagnostic criteria, 293

G-CSF (see Granulocyte colony-stimulating factor)
Gene targets, oligonucleotide therapeutics, 343–352
Genistein, structure, 400f
German CML study group, busulfan, 17–18
  busulfan vs. splenic irradiation, 115
  hydroxyurea, 17–18
  hydroxyurea vs. busulfan, 118–119
  interferon-alpha (IFN-α), 17–18, 121–125, 131–133, 144–147
    dose, 162
    vs. Italian study, 127–129
    survival rate, 164–165

GM2, 416
GM-CSF (see Granulocyte-macrophage colony-stimulating factor)
Graft-versus-host disease (GVHD), allogeneic stem cell transplantation (alloSCT), 225–226
 clinical features, 225
 prevention, 225
 treatment, 225–226
 T-cell therapy, 415
Graft-versus-leukemia (GVL), allogeneic stem cell transplantation (alloSCT), 230–232
 T-cell therapy, 415
Granulocyte colony-stimulating factor (G-CSF), 367–369
 chronic myelomonocytic leukemia (CMML), 65
 postallogeneic stem cell transplantation relapse, 12
Granulocyte-macrophage colony-stimulating factor (GM-CSF), 367–369
 chronic myelogenous leukemia (CML), 29
 chronic myelomonocytic leukemia (CMML), 65–66
 M.D. Anderson Cancer Center, 268
Growth factors, 29
GVHD (see Graft-versus-host disease)
GVL (see Graft-versus-leukemia)

Hematological relapse, 234
Hepatomegaly, chronic myelogenous leukemia (CML), 7
 chronic myelomonocytic leukemia (CMML), 48
Herbimycin A, chronic myelogenous leukemia (CML), 130–131
 structure, 400f
HER2/Neu, 416
Hexamethylene bisacetamide, chronic myelomonocytic leukemia (CMML), 61–62
HLA typing, 216
HLA-identical sibling donors, 216–217

HMF (see Hypermetaphase fluorescence in situ hybridization)
^{166}Ho, 225
Homoharringtonine, 25, 130
HuM195, 421–422, 423
Humanized anti-Tac-IgG2a, 372
Hydroxyurea, 1, 9–10, 118–119
 adverse effects, 9–10
 British Medical Research Council study, 18
 vs. busulfan, German CML study group, 118–119
 chronic myelomonocytic leukemia (CMML), 56–57
 vs. VP-16, 56–57
 German studies, 17–18, 121–125, 146
 interferon-alpha (IFN-α), 23, 146, 163
 Italian Cooperative Study Group on CML (ICSG-CML), 17
 Ph-negative, BCR-negative CML, 295
Hydroxyurea+interferon-alpha (IFN-α), Australian trials, 199–201
Hypermetaphase fluorescence in situ hybridization (HMF), 319–323
 blood vs. bone marrow studies, 323–324
 Ph-negative, BCR positive CML, 322–323
 Ph-positive cell monitoring, interferon-alpha (IFN-α), 319–321
 post allogeneic bone marrow transplantation relapse, 321–322

IFN-α (see Interferon-alpha)
IFN-γ (see Interferon-gamma)
IgH gene, 84–85
^{131}I-labeled monoclonal antibodies, 224–225
Immodulation, postallogeneic stem cell transplantation relapse, 12
Immunotherapy, 413–424
 active specific, 416
 anti-CD33 mediated leukemia cell killing, 421–422
 cellular effector strategies, 415–416

Index

[Immunotherapy]
  MHC class I and class II pathways, 417–418
  monoclonal antibodies, 420–421
  NK therapy, 422–423
  T-cell, 414–415
  T-cell cytotoxicity and proliferation, 419–420
  T-cell rationale, 418–419
Insomnia, interferon-alpha (IFN-α), 21, 166
Integrins, 376–378
Intensive combination therapy, 117–118
Interferon-alpha (IFN-α), allogeneic bone marrow transplant, 151
  allogeneic stem cell transplantation, 14
  allogeneic stem cell transplantation relapse, 235
  Australian trials, high dose, 191–199
  bone marrow aspiration difficulties, 168–169
  breakpoint cluster region (BCR) breakpoint site, 108
  British Medical Research Council study, 18, 121, 125–127
  calcitonin gene hypermethylation, 108
  chronic myelomonocytic leukemia (CMML), 64
  combinations, 120–121
    Australian trials, 185–193
  combined modality therapy, 23–25
  vs. conventional chemotherapy, randomized studies, 144–147
  cytogenetic response rate, 147–148, 152–153
  cytogenic clonal evolution, 108
  cytoreduction, 119–120
  cytosine-arabinoside (Ara-C), 23–24
  DNA-image cytometry, 108
  dose, 119–120, 161–163
    Cancer and Leukemia Group B (CALGB), 162–163
    dose intensity, 19–20
    dose modifications, 164
    duration, 21–23

[Interferon-alpha (IFN-α)]
  endpoint definition, 164–165
  French study, 121
  German CML study group, 121–125, 132–133
    dose, 162
    vs. Italian study, 127–129
    survival rate, 164–165
  guidelines, 22t
  high-dose, cytosine-arabinoside (Ara-C) addition, 197–198
    high-risk patients, 194–195
    low-risk patients, 193–194
    patient selection, 192
    results, 194–197
    treatment, 193–197
  history, 119
  hydroxyurea, 23, 163
  hypermetaphase fluorescence in situ hybridization (HMF), 319–321
  initiation, 163–168
  interleukin-1 beta levels, 108
  Italian Cooperative Study Group on CML (ICSG-CML), 17, 121, 125–127
    vs. German CML study group, 125–127
  Italian study, survival rate, 164–165
  Japanese study, 18, 121, 125–127
    dose, 162
    survival rate, 164–165
  long-term phase II observations, 120
  M. D. Anderson trials, dose, 162
  minimal residual disease (MRD), polymerase chain reaction (PCR), 335–336
  minimal tumor burden, 20–21
  multicenter studies, 142–143
  neurotoxicity management, 166–167
  patient age, 149–150
  patient communication, 166
  patient selection, 165–166
  perspectives, 129–130
  Ph-negative, BCR-positive CML, 294

[Interferon-alpha (IFN-α)]
Ph-positive chronic myelogenous leukemia (CML), breakpoint cluster region (BCR) rearrangement, 307–311
planning, 153–159
problems, 21
prognosis, 106–108
randomized studies, 17–18, 121–129
comparative assessment, 125–129
response prediction, 152–153
response to, 142–144
single-arm studies, 15–17
southern blotting, 327–337
breakpoint cluster region (BCR), 334–335
survival, 152–153, 164–165
treatment selection, 149–150
Interferon-alpha (IFN-α)+all-*trans* retinoic acid (ATRA), Australian trials, 201–206
patient selection, 203–204
results, 204–205
treatment, 204
Interferon-alpha (IFN-α)+cytosine-arabinoside (Ara-C), 173–183
French trials, 176–183
CML 88 trial, 176–179
CML 91 trial, 179–182
rationale, 173–176
Interferon-alpha (IFN-α)+hydroxyurea, Australian trials, 199–201
Interferon-alpha (IFN-α)+low-dose cytosine-arabinoside (Ara-C), 186–191
Australian trials, 186–191
adverse effects, 189–190
complete cytogenetic response, 188
molecular response predictors, 190–191
patient selection, 187
response assessment, 188
results, 188–191
treatment, 187–188
Interferon gamma (IFN-γ), ex vivo stem cell purging, 278

Interferon-γ (IFN-γ), chronic myelomonocytic leukemia (CMML), 64
Interleukin-1-beta (IL-1β), interferon-alpha (IFN-α), 108
Interleukin-1 (IL-1), 364–365
Interleukin-2 (IL-2), 371–372
postallogeneic stem cell transplantation relapse, 12
Interleukin-3 (IL-3), 367
chronic myelomonocytic leukemia (CMML), 66
Interleukin-4 (IL-4), 367, 373
Interleukin-6 (IL-6), 369
chronic myelomonocytic leukemia (CMML), 66
Interleukin-8 (IL-8), 373–374
Interleukin-10 (IL-10), 367, 374
chronic myelomonocytic leukemia (CMML), 66
Interleukin-11 (IL-11), 374
Interleukin-1 (IL-1) inhibitors, 365–366
Interleukin-1 receptor antagonist (IL-1RA), 366
Interleukin-1 receptors (IL-1R), 364–365
International Bone Marrow Transplantation Registry, 10, 168–169, 226
Interphase fluorescence in situ hybridization, peripheral blood, 323–324
Isochromosome (17q), chronic myelomonocytic leukemia (CMML), 47
Italian Cooperative Study Group on CML (ICSG-CML), busulfan, 17, 125
hydroxyurea, 17, 125
interferon-alpha (IFN-α), 17, 121, 125, 144–147
vs. German CML study group, 127–129
survival rate, 164–165

Japanese study, interferon-alpha (IFN-α), 18, 121, 125, 144–147
dose, 162
survival rate, 164–165

Index

190-kD fusion protein, 416
210-kD fusion protein, 416
Kit receptor, 350

Linomide, postalloegeneic stem cell transplantation relapse, 12
Lymphadenopathy, chronic myelomonocytic leukemia (CMML), 48
Lymphokine-activated killer cells (LAK), 415

Macrophage inflammatory protein-1a (MIP-1a), 372–373
Mafosfamide, ex vivo stem cell purging, 278
Major BCR (M-BCR), 5
Marrow stem cell harvest, 219
Mast cell growth factor, 369–370
Matched unrelated donor (MUD) transplant, 14, 29
M.D. Anderson Cancer Center, breakpoint cluster region monitoring, 303–313
  GM-CSF, 268
  Ph-positive chronic myelogenous leukemia (CML), prognosis, 106
M.D. Anderson trials, interferon-alpha (IFN-α), dose, 162
Melphalan, busulfan vs., 115
6-mercaptopurine, busulfan vs., 115
  chronic myelogenous leukemia (CML), 117–118
  chronic myelomonocytic leukemia (CMML), 59
Metaphase fluorescence in situ hybridization (M-FISH), alloSCT, 234–235
  variant Ph (VPh) translocation, 317–318
Methotrexate, 117–118
Methotrexate/cyclosporine, graft-*versus*-host disease, 225–226
MHC class I molecules, 417–418
MHC class II molecules, 417–418

Mice, BCR/ABL transgenic, 82–88
  BCR/ABL-transformed cell line propagation, 79–82
  human CML cell propagation, 77–79
  SCID, 77–79, 345–346
Minimal residual disease (MRD), conventional cytogenetics, 232–233
  hypermetaphase fluorescence in situ hybridization, 320
  interferon-alpha (IFN-α), polymerase chain reaction (PCR), 335–336
  southern blotting vs cytogenetic monitoring, 332–333
  metaphase fluorescence in situ hybridization, 234–235
  polymerase chain reaction (PCR), 233–234
Molecular markers, interferon-alpha (IFN-α), 106–108
Molecular relapse, 234
Moloney murine leukemia virus, 92–93
Monoclonal antibodies, immunotherapy, 420–421
Monosomy 7, chronic myelomonocytic leukemia (CMML), 47
MTP190 transgene, 85–86
MUC-1, 416
Murine anti-Tac-IgG2a, 372

National Marrow Donor Program, 269
Neutrophilia, chronic myelomonocytic leukemia (CMML), 48
NK therapy, 422–423
Noonan syndrome, chronic myelomonocytic leukemia (CMML), 47
Nucleoside analogs, chronic myelomonocytic leukemia (CMML), 64–65
Nucleotides, antisense, future use, 353–354

25-OH-vitamin D, chronic myelomonocytic leukemia (CMML), 61
Oligonucleotides, 341–355
  antisense, clinical use, 352
  BCR/ABL, 343–346

[Oligonucleotides]
  footprinting assay, 354
  gene expression disruption, 342–343
  gene targets, 343–352
  purging, 352
Oral alkylating agents, 1

P190 gene, BCR/ABL, 83–94
P210 gene, BCR/ABL, 85–94
P190 protein, detection, 306
P210 protein, detection, 306
Passive specific therapy, 420–421
PCR (*see* Polymerase chain reaction)
Peripheral blood interphase, 323–324
Ph (VPh) translocation interphase cells, fluorescence in situ hybridization (FISH), 318–319
Philadelphia chromosome (Ph) translocation, cytogenetic analysis, 304–305
Philadelphia chromosome (Ph)-negative, BCR-negative chronic myelogenous leukemia, 288–290
  prognosis, 295
  therapy, 295
Philadelphia chromosome (Ph)-negative, BCR-positive chronic myelogenous leukemia, 287–288
  hypermetaphase fluorescence in situ hybridization (HMF), 322–323
  interferon-alpha (IFN-α), 294
Philadelphia chromosome (Ph)-negative chronic myelogenous leukemia, 285–297
  children, 7
  clinical characteristics, 290–292
  complex translocation, 286–287
  differential diagnosis, 292–294
  masked translocation, 286
  molecular characterization, 286–290
  prognosis, 294–296
  treatment, 294–296
  variant translocation, 286–287

Philadelphia chromosome (Ph)-positive chronic myelogenous leukemia, 1, 6–7
  children, 6
  cytogenetic studies, 320
  cytogenetic vs. molecular studies, 312
  hypermetaphase FISH (HMF), 320
  interferon-alpha (IFN-α), breakpoint cluster region (BCR) rearrangement, 307–311
  randomized studies, 144–147
  treatment selection, 149–150
  investigational modalities, 25–29
  poor prognostic factors, 4t
  prognosis, 6, 106
Philadelphia (Ph) chromosome, 5–6
  detection, 306
Polymerase chain reaction (PCR), BCR-ABL, 233
  BCR/ABL mRNA, 306
  interferon-alpha (IFN-α), 22
  minimal residual disease (MRD), interferon-alpha (IFN-α), 335–336
Polymyalgia rheumatica, chronic myelomonocytic leukemia (CMML), 48
Post allogeneic bone marrow transplantation relapse, hypermetaphase fluorescence in situ hybridization (HMF), 321–322
Purging, autologous stem cells, 277–280

Ras mutations, chronic myelomonocytic leukemia (CMML), 47
Related donors, 218
Reticulin fibrosis, 8
13-cis-Retinoic acid, chronic myelomonocytic leukemia (CMML), 61
Retinoids, chronic myelogenous leukemia (CML), 28–29
  chronic myelomonocytic leukemia (CMML), 61

SCID mice, 77–79, 345–346
Seattle protocols, bone marrow transplantation, 270

Index

Serial transplantation, in vivo stem cell purging, 280
Serous effusions, chronic myelomonocytic leukemia (CMML), 48
Sertraline, 21, 166
Smoking, chronic myelomonocytic leukemia (CMML), 44–45
Southeastern Study Group, busulfan vs. chlorambucil and 6-mercaptopurine, 115
Southern blotting, BCR/ABL gene, 328–329
  blood vs. bone marrow, 329–332
  vs. cytogenetic monitoring, 332–333
  breakpoint cluster region (BCR), 305–306
  interferon-alpha (IFN-α), 327–337
Splenectomy, 141
  allogeneic stem cell transplantation (alloSCT), 224
Splenic irradiation, 1
  busulfan vs., 115
  chronic myelogenous leukemia (CML), 114
Splenomegaly, chronic myelogenous leukemia (CML), 7
  chronic myelomonocytic leukemia (CMML), 48
Steel factor, 369–370
Stem cell collections, allogeneic stem cell transplantation (alloSCT), 219–221
Stem cell factor, 369–370
Stem cell sources, allogeneic stem cell transplantation (alloSCT), 216–219
  autologous stem cell transplantation, 277–280
Stem cell transplantation, allogeneic, 10–14, 215–238
  autologous, 26–28, 131, 273–280
Stem cells, autologous, 277–280
Suramine, 367

Survival, 4t, 114t
  autologous stem cell transplantation, chronic phase, 274–277
  bone marrow transplantation, 260–264
  chronic myelomonocytic leukemia (CMML), 50
  interferon-alpha (IFN-α), 164–165
  tumor burden correlation, 115–117
Syngeneic bone marrow transplantation, 141

Tachyphylaxis, 21
T-cells, cytotoxicity and proliferation, 419–420
  immunotherapy, 414–415
  rationale, 418–419
Thioguanine, busulfan vs., 115
6-Thioguanine, 117–118
ThioTEPA, 10
Topotecan, chronic myelomonocytic leukemia (CMML), 63
Total body irradiation/cyclophosphamide, allogeneic stem cell transplantation (alloSCT), 222–223
  vs. busulfan/cyclophosphamide (BuCy2), allogeneic stem cell transplantation (alloSCT), 222–223
Transforming growth factor-β (TGF-β), 376
Transient cytogenic relapse, 233
Triple-helix-forming oligodeoxynucleotides (TFOs), gene expression disruption, 342–343
Trisomy 8, chronic myelomonocytic leukemia (CMML), 47
Tumor debulking, 21
Tumor necrosis factor-α (TNF-α), 375–376
Tumor-infiltrating T lymphocytes (TIL), 415
Tyrhostin AG1112A, structure, 400f
Tyrosine kinase inhibitors, 398–407
  CGP 57148, 399–403
  CML stages, 406

[Tyrosine kinase inhibitors]
  effectiveness, 404–406
  history, 398–399
  structure, 400f
  toxicity, 406–407

Ubenimex, 130
Umbilical cord blood (UCB) transplantation, 218–219

Vaccines, 416
Vancouver group, autologous stem cell transplantation, 27–28
Variant Ph (VPh) translocation, metaphase-fluorescence in situ hybridization (M-FISH), 317–318
Vav, 351
VH promoter, 82
Vitamin D derivatives, chronic myelomonocytic leukemia (CMML), 61
Volunteer unrelated donors, 218
VP-16, chronic myelomonocytic leukemia (CMML), 55–56

Western blot analysis, BCR/ABL translocations, 306

About the Editors

MOSHE TALPAZ is Chairman (Ad Interim) of the Bioimmunotherapy Department, Professor of Medicine, and Internist at the University of Texas M.D. Anderson Cancer Center, Houston. He is the author, coauthor, editor, or coeditor of more than 200 research papers and books, including *Biological Response Modifiers in the Treatment of Hematopoietic Neoplasia* (Marcel Dekker, Inc.). He is a member of the Texas Medical Society, the American Medical Association, the American College of Physicians, the American Association of Cancer Research, the American Society of Clinical Oncology, the American Society of Hematology, and the International Society for Interferon Research. Dr. Talpaz received the M.D. degree (1971) from Hadassah Medical School, Hebrew University, Jerusalem, Israel. He completed his residency in internal medicine in Israel and a Fellowship in medical oncology at the University of Texas M.D. Anderson Cancer Center, where he joined the faculty in 1981.

HAGOP M. KANTARJIAN is Chairman (Ad Interim) of the Leukemia Department, Professor of Medicine, and Internist at the University of Texas M.D. Anderson Cancer Center, Houston. He is the author, coauthor, editor, or coeditor of over 185 journal articles, abstracts, and book chapters, and coeditor of *Therapy of Hematopoietic Neoplasia* and *Medical Management of Hematological Malignant Diseases* (both titles, Marcel Dekker, Inc.). He is a member of the American Association for Cancer Research, the American Society of Clinical Oncology, the American Society of Hematology, the Texas Medical Association, the American Medical Association, and the American Association for the Advancement of Science. Dr. Kantarjian received the B.S. (1975), M.D. (1979), and Internal Medicine (1981) degrees from the American University of Beirut, Lebanon, and the Medical Oncology Subspecialty degree (1983) from the University of Texas M.D. Anderson Cancer Center, Houston.

RC
643
.M434
1999